CPAP Adherence

Colin M. Shapiro • Meenakshi Gupta
Dora Zalai
Editors

CPAP Adherence

Factors and Perspectives

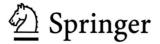 Springer

Editors
Colin M. Shapiro
University of Toronto
Toronto, ON, Canada

Meenakshi Gupta
Maple Leaf Medical Clinic
Toronto, ON, Canada

Dora Zalai
Sleep on the Bay
Toronto, ON, Canada

ISBN 978-3-030-93144-5   ISBN 978-3-030-93146-9   (eBook)
https://doi.org/10.1007/978-3-030-93146-9

Dedication to Christian Guilleminault

It is a pleasure to be asked to dedicate this book on CPAP adherence to Christian Guilleminault. "CG," as he was mostly referred to, passed away on 9 July 2019. Along with his close colleague, Dr. William C. Dement, CG founded the first sleep clinic in the world at Stanford. He also coined the term "obstructive sleep apnea" and was a driving force behind the establishment of the field of sleep medicine. CG was uniquely inventive, always looking outside of sleep medicine for new ideas. He left behind a lasting legacy of hundreds of unique scientific papers and thousands of students and trainees throughout the world, and so it was not surprising to me that Dr. Shapiro, who worked with CG as a student in the mid-1970s, wanted dedicate this book to CG. Christian was a tireless advocate of clinical research before its time, always asking the right questions with the goal of understanding all sleep pathologies, from sleep apnea across the life span to narcolepsy. His appetite for science and life in general knew no bounds! His knowledge and experience were also immense; every time a scientific presentation in sleep medicine occurred at Stanford, it was almost certain CG would have thought that he had had the idea or done something in the past related to the topic at hand. CG also had wit and suffered no fools, branding his jokingly omnipresent threat of death by "guillotine" for those who did not meet his high expectations. His persistence and dedication to sleep medicine had no match, and I'm virtually certain he would have read this book from cover to cover, wondering why he was not more cited. And yet, I'm sure he is present in many, many pages if not in name between the lines. CG made a difference in the life of many researchers and patients, and for this we are all immensely grateful.

Professor Emmanuel Mignot
Craig Reynold Professor of Sleep Medicine, Department of Psychiatry and
Behavioral Sciences, Stanford University
Director, Stanford Center for Narcolepsy
Palo Alto, CA, USA
Email: mignot@stanford.edu

In memoriam; Professor Sir Neil James Douglas
Pioneer of Sleep Medicine (1949–2020)

In 1977 I was working in the Department of Medicine at the University as an MRC Research Fellow together with Neil who had recently become a clinical lecturer. We had been classmates at Medical School in Edinburgh, often sharing the same clinical attachments. Neil had joined our year after a successful period as a pre-clinical student in St Andrews and was clearly extremely bright, capable and set fair for a glittering career. What that career was to involve became apparent when our irascible but brilliant boss, David Flenley, returned from the American Thoracic Society having just ordered a Hewlett Packard transmission oximeter. This was the first instrument to offer accurate and stable non-invasive measurement of oxygen saturation, and it opened up a new world of overnight physiological recordings. Edinburgh was fortunate as Ian Oswald was a major figure in sleep research, and Neil collaborated with his group to create our first (ad hoc) respiratory sleep laboratory in the patient waiting area of our department. Neil threw himself into this with characteristic energy and efficiency.

The results were impressive, and within 18 months, Neil was the first author of a groundbreaking Lancet paper describing the sleep stage-related pattern of oxygen desaturation in COPD patients. Over the next 10 years, Neil authored many landmark papers describing sleep disturbances in obstructive lung diseases, fitted in a visiting Fellowship to Denver where he wrote the first papers describing ventilatory control during sleep and became aware of the unrecognised and unmet needs of people with obstructive sleep apnoea. As his career in Edinburgh progressed, he developed one of the first clinical services for UK patients with sleep disorders and fought vigorously to win funding to do this, often against sceptical administrators and medical colleagues. One way in which he succeeded was through the excellence of his clinical research which showed why sleep problems were important and attracted students from across the world keen to learn from him. Unsurprisingly, this led to his appointment as Professor of Respiratory and Sleep Medicine at the University of Edinburgh. He conducted the first highly cited randomised controlled study showing that CPAP improved well-being and vitality in OSAHS patients and went on to explore all aspects of the mechanisms and impact of sleep disordered breathing, even proposing that obstructive sleep hypopnoea syndrome replace the more familiar acronym of OSA to better describe the sleep disruption associated with upper airway narrowing.

Neil knew that treatment with CPAP would only work if patients used it properly and together with the wonderful Carol Hoy (mother of a famous British Olympian) published one of the first studies showing how this could be accomplished by extending the support of CPAP users. Although Neil's career took him into other leadership roles (co-founder of the British Sleep Society, the longest serving president of the Royal College of Physicians of Edinburgh in modern times, chair of the Academy of Medical Royal Colleges), he continued to work in sleep medicine and research until he retired from clinical work. Sadly, this was not to be as long as any of us would have hoped, and his death in late summer 2020 was a huge blow. However, in a full life with so much accomplished, it will be his insights into and advocacy of the problems of sleep disordered breathing that will transform the lives of many patients and their families for years to come.

Professor Peter Calverley
Professor of Respiratory Medicine
School of Aging and Chronic Disease, University of Liverpool
Liverpool, UK
Email: pmacal@liverpool.ac.uk
February 2021

Foreword

It seems almost incredible that 40 years ago a physiological paper involving five patients with severe sleep apnea [1] launched a revolution in our understanding of the pathophysiology of this disease and established the therapeutic approach that has become common place all over the world. Indeed, continuous positive airway pressure (CPAP) has transformed the lives of countless patients, and its benefits on quality of life have definitely been remarkable.

Considering the simplicity of the idea surrounding the concept of CPAP and its implementation, one has to wonder in an era in which technological advances are amazingly fast, why a book would need to be written and be timely about CPAP so many years later. Well, to quote Bob Dylan, "the answer my friend is blowin' in the wind"! As dissemination of CPAP propagated throughout the globe, it became clear that despite all of its benefits, no one really likes to have a mask on their face the whole night and be attached to a machine like a tether, and that many factors will affect the acceptance and adherence of the nearly billion patients who need treatment for their apnea.

As sleep medicine clinicians, we have accumulated significant experience over the years in transferring the management decisions regarding patients with sleep apnea from the sleep physiology laboratory to the home setting. Furthermore, we have formulated evidence-based protocols and devised ingenious technologies that will allow for improved therapeutic implementation of CPAP. In parallel, we have explored and continue to seek alternative treatments that will relieve those patients who won't, can't, or can but only partially from the "burden" of CPAP. In the midst of all this, CPAP has changed in some ways very little: it is still based on that "pressure through the nares" [1]. And yet, it has made substantial efforts to adapt to the times we live in: lighter, quieter, softer, gentler, smaller, communicative, responsive, interfaced, ….! And yet, adherence, that magic necessity to convert a treatment to effective has not really improved by much!

HELP!!!

This new and necessary book comes at the right time and offers a comprehensive analysis and informative discussion of everything about adherence in CPAP. In a series of well-structured and logically placed sequence of chapters, this book comprehensively covers the topic of CPAP adherence, including: everything that can go wrong with CPAP adherence; everything that needs to be considered when implementing CPAP to achieve adherence; the impact that the phenotypic variance of sleep apnea imposes on adherence; who the players are in promoting adherence and their roles; the contribution of interfaces, incentives, telehealth, and economics; and a myriad of important items that anyone prescribing or treating patients who need CPAP needs to know and should know. The text is easy to read, the contributors are clearly recognized experts in their field, and each chapter provides up-to-date information and useful evidence while asking and answering pertinent questions. As such, it should become an essential guide and professional resource for many years to come.

I have already ordered my copy. Did you order yours?

David Gozal, MD, MBA, PhD (Hon)
Former President American Thoracic Society (2015–2016)
Marie M. and Harry L. Smith Endowed Chair
Chairperson, Department of Child Health
Pediatrician-in-Chief, MU Women's and Children's Hospital
University of Missouri School of Medicine
Columbia, MO, USA

Email: gozald@health.missouri.edu

Reference

1. Sullivan CE, Issa FG, Berthon-Jones M, Eves L. Reversal of obstructive sleep apnoea by continuous positive airway pressure applied through the nares. Lancet. 1981;1(8225):862–5. https://doi.org/10.1016/s0140-6736(81)92140-1. PMID: 6112294.

Preface

We cannot find a more succinct depiction of the status quo of positive airway pressure (PAP) treatment in the twenty-first century than Dickens' opening line in *A Tale of Two Cities*, "It was the best of times, it was the worst of times, it was the age of wisdom, it was the age of foolishness." [1] This is the best of times, in that there have been phenomenal developments in the usability, comfort, individualized and automated feedback of usage, as well as insurance coverage for PAP treatment in many jurisdictions. At the same time, it is the worst of times, because despite the technological advancements, the overall rate of PAP usage among those who would benefit is still low.

Recent publications question the benefit of PAP treatment on health outcomes based in part on data derived from samples with low PAP use. At the same time, there is still an insufficient recognition of sleep apnea in the medical field with only minor mention of sleep medicine in medical curricula.

A review a decade ago described the mode of CPAP adherence as 50% in clinical research studies, though one suspects that in community clinics the mode is lower [2]. The criterion for "compliance" in these studies was generally set as CPAP use of at least 4 hours, four nights per week.

In 2016, a large study found that CPAP use did not help with cardiovascular well-being [3]. However, the average nightly CPAP use was only slightly over 3 hours, and we suspect this low usage covered a very small percentage of REM sleep which comes towards the end of the night and often has the highest frequency of apneic events. It is plausible that REM sleep may be particularly significant in relation to cardiovascular well-being given the autonomic changes during this stage of sleep. The short duration of nightly CPAP use in this study raises questions about the veracity of the general conclusions.

Some of the important issues with regard to CPAP adherence include:

A. Despite accumulation of knowledge of a range of sleep disorders in the past decades, everyday sleep medicine practice often has a narrow focus on sleep apnea with an increased use of surrogate tools for apnea detection. A desire to see a large number of patients has contributed to shortened time spent in direct contact with individual patients during sleep evaluation and treatment planning. This has facilitated the emergence of fast-track "apnea medicine" as opposed to "sleep medicine" and does a disservice to our field.

   In an attempt to have the shortest face-to-face time with patients to identify and treat sleep apnea, the complexity of sleep as well as the medical, psychological, and social factors that shape patients' sleep-related quality of life, views and choices of treatment, and adherence to treatment may be overlooked. The result is that if only sleep apnea is evaluated and treated while comorbid sleep disorders and individual's life circumstances and views of their sleep are ignored, the person may choose not to start sleep apnea treatment or may arrive at erroneous conclusion that PAP treatment is not helpful. Furthermore, if the sleep study is done prior to consultation with the patient, appropriate diagnostic assessments would not be planned. As an example, if a sleep study is done as the first step for a sleepy patient without a diagnostic interview beforehand, symptoms of narcolepsy would be missed and an MSLT (multiple sleep latency test) would not be prescribed. This would diminish the likelihood of detecting narcolepsy in jurisdictions where a second study with MSLT is not possible at a later date.

B. We have a dichotomous view of PAP adherence based on an expectation of 4 hours use per night. To use an analogy, no optometrist sends a patient with myopia away with new spectacles and advises that using them for 3 to 4 hours a day will be sufficient for improved vision. When patients do not notice benefits in 3 to 4 hours of treatment use, they may give up the treatment altogether.

C. By and large, we have stuck to a single daytime treatment outcome measure – generally a scale that measures sleepiness. Sleepiness is clearly an important issue in relation to sleep apnea; however, it is not the only daytime symptom of relevance. Increasing awareness of different phenotypes of sleep apnea has led to an appreciation that some people have a more profound sense of fatigue rather than sleepiness and others have impaired alertness or problems with concentration, memory, or mood problems without sleepiness. Choosing outcome measures that capture treatment-related changes for the specific daytime symptom that the individual most cares about is more informative and meaningful both for the clinician and the patient than using the same, single measure for every person. In addition, using pre-treatment measures that assess constructs relevant to PAP adherence (PAP adherence questionnaires, claustrophobia tendency, insomnia scales, and depression scales) would allow the clinician to work closely with patients who are more likely to face challenges with PAP use.

D. PAP treatment use is shaped by the interaction of biological, social, and psychological factors. Inter-disciplinary collaboration among physicians from various disciplines, such as dentists, psychologists, in-clinic PAP coordinators, respiratory technicians, social workers, and other stakeholders in the areas of assessment, diagnosis, treatment planning, and patient support, will be essential to effectively reduce the individual and public health burden of sleep apnea. Research and social advocacy work are key to these objectives.

This book showcases perspectives, knowledge, and experience of professionals from multiple disciplines from five continents. We hope that this book will be a useful compendium of information that will be dipped into again and again with specific patients in mind.

Toronto, ON, Canada   Dora Zalai
                                                                                                     Colin M. Shapiro

References

1. Dickens C. A tale of two cities. Oxford, UK: Oxford University Press; 1998.
2. Shapiro G, Shapiro CM. Factors and influence CPAP adherence: an overview. Sleep Breath. 2010;14:323–35.
3. Doug McEvoy R, Antic NA, Heeley E, Luo Y, Ou Q, et al. CPAP for prevention of cardiovascular events in obstructive sleep apnea. N Engl J Med. 2016;375:919–31.

We thank Clodagh Ryan, Gilla Shapiro, and Andres McConnon who made a contribution to the early planning of this book.

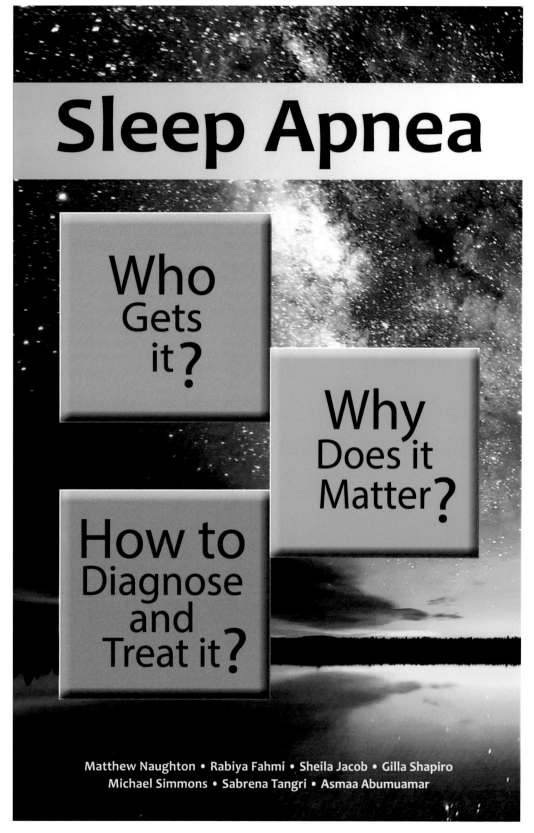

Sleep Apnea

Who Gets it?

Why Does it Matter?

How to Diagnose and Treat it?

Matthew Naughton • Rabiya Fahmi • Sheila Jacob • Gilla Shapiro
Michael Simmons • Sabrena Tangri • Asmaa Abumuamar

This educational booklet is about adult and pediatric sleep apnea and its treatment. It is richly illustrated to provide easily accessible information for patients and caregivers. For further information or copies please visit sleeponthebay.ca

Contents

Part I Approaches to Promoting PAP Adherence

1 **When to Treat with CPAP and How to Define Success** 3
Olabimpe Fashanu and Stuart F. Quan

2 **Interventions to Improve CPAP Adherence** 13
Tatyana Mollayeva

3 **Patient Adherence to CPAP: A Practical Interdisciplinary Model** 39
Colin M. Shapiro

4 **Soft Styles of Motivating Patients to Adopt CPAP** 49
Atul Khullar

5 **The Role of Education and Support in CPAP Adherence** 63
C. D. Turnbull and J. R. Stradling

6 **Role of the Behavioral Sleep Specialist Psychologist in Promoting CPAP Adherence**
71
Dora Zalai

7 **Role of the Physician in CPAP Adherence and CPAP Trials** 83
Laura H. Buckley and James R. Catterall

8 **PAP Therapy for Sleep Breathing Disorders: Good Policies and Practices** 95
Mubdiul Ali and Meir Kryger

Part II Factors Influencing PAP Adherence

9 **Socioeconomic Differences in CPAP Adherence** 103
Martha E. Billings and Susan Redline

10 **The Impact of Partner and Family Support in PAP Therapy** 109
Faith S. Luyster and Daniel J. Buysse

11 **Personality and Mental Health as Determinants of CPAP Use** 117
Royi Gilad

12 **Costs of Treatment Non-adherence in Obstructive Sleep Apnoea** 125
John O'Reilly

13 **Obstructive Sleep Apnea Phenotypes and Positive Airway Therapy Adherence** . 141
Meenakshi Gupta

Part III PAP Adherence in Medical Conditions

14 **PAP Adherence in Neurology Patients** 155
Anne Marie Morse and Sreelatha Naik

15 **Obstructive Sleep Apnea, CPAP, and Impact on Cognitive Function** 167
Miqdad Hussain Bohra and Mohammad Payman Hajiazim

16 **Sleep Apnea and Cardiovascular Disease: The Role of CPAP
and CPAP Adherence** 177
Lee A. Surkin, Asmaa M. Abumuamar, and Kathryn Hansen

17 **Cognitive Behavioral Therapy for Insomnia in Patients with Comorbid Insomnia
and Obstructive Sleep Apnea** 189
Jean-Philippe Gouin

18 **Overview of Medication Treatment for Co-Morbid Insomnia and Sleep Apnea
(COMISA)** 195
Alan D. Lowe and Megan S. Lowe

19 **CPAP Adherence in Patients with Obstructive Sleep Apnea and Depression** 203
Danielle Penney and Joseph Barbera

20 **Adherence with Treatment for Sleep Apnea in Patients with Comorbid Post-
traumatic Stress Disorder** 213
Ripu D. Jindal and Kawish Garg

21 **Relevance of CPAP in Ophthalmic Disease** 219
Tavé A. van Zyl, Bobeck S. Modjtahedi, and Louis T. van Zyl

22 **CPAP Adherence and Bariatric Surgery Patients** 227
Raed Hawa

23 **CPAP Adherence in Pregnancy** 231
Ela Kadish and Noah Gilad

Part IV   Sleep Apnea and PAP Adherence in Children and Adolescents

24 **Pathophysiology of Obstructive Sleep Apnea in Children** 239
Ian MacLusky

25 **PAP Management and Adherence for Children and Adolescents with OSAS** ... 245
Anna C. Bitners and Raanan Arens

26 **CPAP Adherence in Children with Special Health-Care Needs** 255
Anya McLaren-Barnett and Indra Narang

Part V   Alternative and Adjunct Interventions

27 **Monitoring of the Patient on CPAP and When Should Alternative Treatment
Modalities Be Considered** 279
Kin M. Yuen and Rafael Pelayo

28 **Questionnaires Evaluating Sleep Apnea and CPAP Adherence** 289
Sohaib Ahmed Shamim

29 **Compliance and Oral Appliance Use for Sleep-Related Breathing Disorders** ... 299
Michael Simmons

30 **Utilization of Wake-Promoting Drugs in Patients on CPAP Therapy** 317
Russell Rosenberg

31 **Improving CPAP Adherence Using Telehealth** 331
Ajmal Razmy

Part VI   Providers' Role and Technical Considerations

32   The CPAP Machine, Mask and Interface............................337
    Julia Lachowicz and Matthew T. Naughton

**33   How to Start Using CPAP and Benefiting From CPAP Use:
    The CPAP Vendor's Practical Information to Patients**.....................347
    Alex Novodvorets

**34   The CPAP Treatment Coordinator's Role in Helping Patients with
    CPAP Use**...355
    Elaine Huang

**35   The Respiratory Therapist and the Vendor's Perspective on
    CPAP Adherence**...363
    Barbara Capozzolo, Marcel A. Baltzan, Kateri Champagne, and Dave Johnson

Part VII   Global and Historical Perspectives

36   Global Perspective of CPAP Adherence...............................373
    Jessica Rosen, Arezu Najafi, Khosro Sadeghniiat-Haghighi, Ravi Gupta,
    Slavko M. Janković, Jianhua Shen, and Yu Jin Lee

37   The History and Future of CPAP....................................383
    Shaista Hussain

Index...387

Contributors

Asmaa M. Abumuamar, MD, MSc Department of Medicine, University of Toronto, Toronto, ON, Canada

Mubdiul Ali, MD Yale School of Medicine, Pulmonary Critical Care and Sleep Medicine, New Haven, CT, USA

Raanan Arens, MD Division of Respiratory and Sleep Medicine, Department of Pediatrics, Children's Hospital at Montefiore, Albert Einstein College of Medicine, Bronx, NY, USA

Marcel A. Baltzan, MDCM FRCPC FAASM McGill University, Faculty of Medicine, Department of Epidemiology Biostatistics and Occupational Health, Montréal, QC, Canada

Centre Intégré Universitaire des Soins et Services Sociaux du Nord de L'île de Montréal, Montréal, QC, Canada

Mount Sinai Hospital, Centre Intégré Universitaire des Soins et Services Sociaux du Centre-ouest de L'île de Montréal, Montréal, QC, Canada

Institut de Médecine du Sommeil, Montréal, QC, Canada

Joseph Barbera, MD, FRCPC Department of Psychiatry, University of Toronto, Toronto, ON, Canada

Martha E. Billings, MD, MSc Division of Pulmonary, Critical Care & Sleep Medicine, Department of Medicine, University of Washington School of Medicine, Seattle, WA, USA

Anna C. Bitners, BS Division of Respiratory and Sleep Medicine, Department of Pediatrics, Children's Hospital at Montefiore, Albert Einstein College of Medicine, Bronx, NY, USA

Miqdad Hussain Bohra, MBBS MRCPsych MSc FRCPC ESRS Department of Psychiatry, Faculty of Medicine, University of Toronto, Toronto, ON, Canada

Youthdale Child and Adolscent Sleep Center, Toronto, ON, Canada

Laura H. Buckley, BSc, MBChB, MD Department of Respiratory Medicine, University Hospitals Bristol, Bristol, UK

Daniel J. Buysse, MD University of Pittsburgh, School of Medicine, Department of Psychiatry, Pittsburgh, PA, USA

Peter Calverley, FMedSci School of Aging and Chronic Disease, University of Liverpool, Liverpool, UK

Barbara Capozzolo, MSc, RPSGT, RST, TEPM Institut de Médecine du Sommeil, Montréal, QC, Canada

James R. Catterall, BSc, MD, FRCP Department of Respiratory Medicine, University Hospitals Bristol, Bristol, UK

Kateri Champagne, MD FRCPC FAASM Institut de Médecine du Sommeil, Montréal, QC, Canada

Olabimpe Fashanu, MD, MPH Division of Sleep and Circadian Disorders, Brigham and Women's Hospital, Boston, MA, USA

Division of Sleep Medicine, Harvard Medical School, Boston, MA, USA

Kawish Garg, MD Geisinger Holy Spirit Hospital, Camp Hill, PA, USA

Noah Gilad, MD University of Toronto, Toronto, ON, Canada

Royi Gilad, MD Department of Psychiatry, University of Toronto, Toronto, ON, Canada

Youthdale Child and Adolescent Sleep Centre, Toronto, ON, Canada

Jean-Philippe Gouin, PhD Department of Psychology, Concordia University, Montreal, QC, Canada

David Gozal, MD, MBA, PhD (Hon) Department of Child Health, MU Women's and Children's Hospital, Columbia, MO, USA

University of Missouri School of Medicine, Columbia, MO, USA

Meenakshi Gupta, MD University of Saskatchewan, North Battleford, SK, Canada

Maple Leaf Medical Clinic, Toronto, ON, Canada

Ravi Gupta, MD, PhD, MAMS Department of Psychiatry and Division of Sleep Medicine, All India Institute of Medical Sciences, Rishikesh, Uttarakhand, India

Mohammad Payman Hajiazim, MD, FRCPC, ESRS Psychiatry and Sleep Medicine, Cumming School of Medicine, University of Calgary, Calgary, AB, Canada

Hotchkiss Brain Institute, University of Calgary, Calgary, AB, Canada

Kathryn Hansen, BS, CPC, CPMA, REEGT Society of Behavioral Sleep Medicine, Lexington, KY, USA

American Academy of Cardiovascular Sleep Medicine, Greenville, NC, USA

Raed Hawa, MSc MD FRCPC DABSM DABPN Faculty of Medicine, University of Toronto, Toronto, ON, Canada

University Health Network, Toronto, ON, Canada

Elaine Huang, BSc Sleep and Alertness Clinic, Toronto, ON, Canada

Shaista Hussain, BSc, MBBCh, BAO, LRCPI, LRCSI Medical Technology Solutions Laboratories, Riyadh, Saudi Arabia

Slavko M. Janković, MD, PhD Clinic of Neurology, Clinical Center of Serbia, Belgrade, Serbia

Ripu D. Jindal, MD Birmingham VA Medical Center, University of Alabama at Birmingham, Birmingham, AL, USA

Dave Johnson, BSc, RRT Institut de Médecine du Sommeil, Montréal, QC, Canada

Ela Kadish, BMesSc Hebrew University of Jerusalem, Jerusalem, Israel

Atul Khullar, MD, MSc, FRCPC, DABPN, FAASM Department of Psychiatry, University of Alberta, Edmonton, AB, Canada

Meir Kryger, MD FRCPC Yale School of Medicine, Pulmonary Critical Care and Sleep Medicine, New Haven, CT, USA

Julia Lachowicz, MBBS Alfred Hospital, Melbourne, VIC, Australia

Yu Jin Lee, MD, PhD Department of Psychiatry and Center for Sleep and Chronobiology, Seoul National University College of Medicine, Seoul, Republic of Korea

Alan D. Lowe, BSc (Phm), MD, FRCP (C) University of Toronto, Toronto, ON, Canada

Megan S. Lowe, BHSc McMaster University, Hamilton, ON, Canada

Faith S. Luyster, PhD University of Pittsburgh, School of Nursing, Pittsburgh, PA, USA

Ian MacLusky, MD Department of Pediatrics, Children's Hospital of Eastern Ontario, University of Ottawa, Ottawa, ON, Canada

Anya McLaren-Barnett, HBSc, MSc, MD Division of Pediatric Respirology, Department of Pediatrics, McMaster University, Hamilton, ON, Canada

Emmanuel Mignot, MD, PhD Department of Psychiatry and Behavioral Sciences, Stanford University, Stanford, CA, USA

Stanford Center for Narcolepsy, Palo Alto, CA, USA

Bobeck S. Modjtahedi, MD Department of Ophthalmology, Southern California Permanente Medical Group, Baldwin Park, CA, USA

Tatyana Mollayeva, MD, PhD KITE-Toronto Rehab University Health Network, Toronto, ON, Canada

Global Brain Health Institute, Institute of Neuroscience Trinity College, Dublin, Ireland

Anne Marie Morse, DO Pediatric Neurology and Pediatric Sleep Medicine, Department of Pediatrics, Janet Weis Children's Hospital, Geisinger, Danville, PA, USA

Sreelatha Naik, MD Division of Sleep Medicine, Department of Pulmonary and Critical Care, Geisinger Medical Center, Danville, PA, USA

Arezu Najafi, MD Occupational Sleep Research Center, Baharloo Hospital, Tehran University of Medical Sciences, Tehran, Iran

Indra Narang, BMEDSCI, MBBCH, MD Sleep Medicine, Division of Respiratory Medicine, Sick Children's Hospital, Toronto, ON, Canada

Matthew T. Naughton, MBBS, MD, FRACP, ATSF, FERS Alfred Hospital and Monash University, Melbourne, VIC, Australia

Alex Novodvorets, BSc, MSc CPAP Clinic, Vaughan, ON, Canada

John O'Reilly, MD Aintree University Hospital, Liverpool, UK

London Sleep Centre, London, UK

Rafael Pelayo, MD Stanford Sleep Disorders Clinic, Stanford University, Stanford, CA, USA

Danielle Penney, BSc McMaster University, Youthdale Child & Adolescent Sleep Centre, Toronto, ON, Canada

Stuart F. Quan, MD Division of Sleep and Circadian Disorders, Brigham and Women's Hospital, Boston, MA, USA

Division of Sleep Medicine, Harvard Medical School, Boston, MA, USA

Asthma and Airway Disease Research Center, University of Arizona, Tucson, AZ, USA

Edson College of Nursing and Health Innovation, Arizona State University, Tempe, AZ, USA

Ajmal Razmy, MD, FRCPC Joseph Brant Hospital, Burlington, ON, Canada

Cleveland Clinic Canada, Toronto, ON, Canada

Susan Redline, MD, MPH Division of Sleep and Circadian Disorders, Department of Medicine, Brigham and Women's Hospital, Harvard Medical School, Boston, MA, USA

Russell Rosenberg, PhD, FAASM Neurotrials Research, Atlanta, GA, USA

Jessica Rosen, MD Candidate New York Medical College, Valhalla, NY, USA

Khosro Sadeghniiat-Haghighi, MD Occupational Sleep Research Center, Baharloo Hospital, Tehran University of Medical Sciences, Tehran, Iran

Sohaib Ahmed Shamim, MBBS Dow Medical College, Karachi, Pakistan
Youthdale Child and Adolescent Sleep Centre, Toronto, ON, Canada

Colin M. Shapiro, MD University of Toronto, Toronto, ON, Canada

Jianhua Shen, MD, PhD Beijing Medipertis Sleep Medicine Center, Beijing, China

Michael Simmons, DMD, MSc, MPH Encino Center for Sleep and TMJ Disorders, Encino, CA, USA
UCLA School of Dentistry 1987–2018, Los Angeles, CA, USA

J. R. Stradling, MD Oxford National Institute of Health Research Biomedical Research Centre, University of Oxford, Oxford, UK

Lee A. Surkin, MD, FACC, FCCP, FASNC Empire Sleep Medicine, New York, NY, USA
CardioSleep Diagnostics, Greenville, NC, USA
American Academy of Cardiovascular Sleep Medicine, Greenville, NC, USA

C. D. Turnbull, DPhil Oxford National Institute of Health Research Biomedical Research Centre, University of Oxford, Oxford, UK

Louis T. van Zyl, MD, MMed Queen's University, Kingston, ON, Canada

Tavé A. van Zyl, MD Department of Ophthalmology and Visual Science, Yale School of Medicine, New Haven, CT, USA

Kin M. Yuen, MD, MS UCSF Sleep Disorders Center, Department of UCSF Pulmonary, Critical Care, Allergy and Sleep Medicine, San Francisco, CA, USA
Stanford Sleep Disorders Clinic, Stanford University, Stanford, CA, USA

Dora Zalai, MD, PhD, C. Psych Sleep on the Bay, Toronto, ON, Canada

Part I

Approaches to Promoting PAP Adherence

When to Treat with CPAP and How to Define Success

Olabimpe Fashanu and Stuart F. Quan

Abbreviations

AF	Atrial fibrillation
AHI	Apnea-hypopnea index
APAP	Auto-adjusting continuous positive airway pressure
ASV	Adaptive servo ventilation
BP	Blood pressure
BPAP	Bi-level positive airway pressure
CAD	Coronary artery disease
CHF	Congestive heart failure
CMS	Centers for Medicare and Medicaid Services
CPAP	Continuous positive airway pressure
CVD	Cardiovascular disease
ESS	Epworth Sleepiness Scale
FOSQ	Functional Outcomes of Sleep Questionnaire
LVEF	Left ventricular ejection fraction
OSA	Obstructive sleep apnea
QoL	Quality of life
SAQLI	Sleep Apnea Quality of Life Index
SF36	Medical Outcomes Study Short-Form Health Survey

O. Fashanu
Division of Sleep and Circadian Disorders, Brigham and Women's Hospital, Boston, MA, USA

Division of Sleep Medicine, Harvard Medical School, Boston, MA, USA

S. F. Quan (✉)
Division of Sleep and Circadian Disorders, Brigham and Women's Hospital, Boston, MA, USA

Division of Sleep Medicine, Harvard Medical School, Boston, MA, USA

Asthma and Airway Disease Research Center, University of Arizona, Tucson, AZ, USA

Edson College of Nursing and Health Innovation, Arizona State University, Tempe, AZ, USA
e-mail: Stuart_Quan@hms.harvard.edu

1.1 Historical Perspective and Description of Methods of Positive Airway Pressure Delivery

1.1.1 Evolution of Positive Airway Pressure

The concept of administering continuous positive airway pressure (CPAP) for treatment of lung injury began in the 1970s. However, it was not until 1980 that Colin Sullivan, an Australian physician and professor, proposed using nasal continuous positive airway pressure (CPAP) as a means to treat obstructive sleep apnea (OSA) [1]. Up until the discovery of CPAP, tracheostomy was the recommended treatment modality for severe cases of OSA [2]. The first commercially available CPAP devices in North America were manufactured in 1985. Since then, there have been improvements made to the original CPAP device, and more specialized models have been developed for alternative methods of delivery of positive airway pressure (PAP). Over the past 35 years, CPAP has become the *gold standard* and most commonly prescribed treatment for OSA worldwide.

1.1.2 Description of Various PAP Modes

Since the introduction of CPAP as a treatment for OSA, a number of refinements have been made to the method by which PAP is delivered to the patient. In general, these PAP modes were developed in response to the inability of simple CPAP to successfully treat some patients with OSA. In order to comprehend what constitutes treatment success with CPAP, it is important to understand these modes of PAP delivery as well.

1.1.2.1 Continuous and Auto-Adjusting Positive Airway Pressure (CPAP and APAP)

Continuous positive airway pressure as the name suggests delivers a relatively constant positive airway pressure during both inspiration and expiration. Auto-adjusting CPAP or

APAP functions like CPAP, but in addition, it automatically titrates the delivered pressure in response to detected upper airway narrowing or closure during episodes of apnea or hypopnea. With APAP, CPAP pressures are adjusted by using changes in airflow and vibration from sensors in the airway circuit. The algorithms are proprietary, and manufacturers' devices perform differently in simulation studies [3] suggesting that functional differences could occur in patients as well.

1.1.2.2 Bi-Level PAP (BPAP) and Auto-Adjusting BPAP

Bi-level PAP delivers higher pressures during inspiration and lower pressures during expiration. Specialized models offer a spontaneous timed (ST) mode with an option to specify a backup respiratory rate in the absence of inspiratory effort. Auto-adjusting BPAP devices automatically adjust expiratory pressures in response to detected apneas and adjust inspiratory pressures in response to hypopneas and respiratory flow limitations. BPAP is generally used for patients who either cannot tolerate or fail to be adequately treated with CPAP with mixed success [4].

1.1.2.3 Adaptive Servo Ventilation (ASV)

Adaptive servo ventilation, like BPAP, delivers higher inspiratory and lower expiratory pressures. Additionally, it varies the inspiratory pressure support on a breath-by-breath basis, within prespecified limits to achieve a target ventilatory flow. It can be set in either a fixed or variable mode with respect to delivery of expiratory pressures and backup respiratory rates. The most frequent use of ASV is for treatment of central or treatment-emergent central sleep apnea [5].

1.2 When to Treat with CPAP

The most common use of CPAP is for treatment of either symptomatic OSA or asymptomatic OSA in the setting of significant comorbid medical conditions. Additionally, CPAP is sometimes used in certain types of central sleep apnea [6].

1.2.1 Obstructive Sleep Apnea (OSA)

Obstructive sleep apnea is characterized by repetitive upper airway collapse or near collapse. The severity of OSA is defined by the apnea-hypopnea index (AHI). An AHI <5/hour is considered absent or minimal OSA. Mild OSA is defined as an AHI $\geq$5/hour and <15/hour. Moderate is defined as $\geq$15 and <30/hour and severe is $\geq$30/hour.

1.2.1.1 Treatment of Symptomatic OSA

The most common indication for the use of CPAP is to treat symptoms associated with OSA, and it remains the gold standard for therapy [7]. In the absence of complications, CPAP or APAP adequately treats the majority of patients. The following are commonly reported symptoms and their responsiveness to CPAP.

Excessive Daytime Sleepiness

Excessive daytime sleepiness is one of the cardinal symptoms of OSA and is present in up to half of patients [8]. It is generally a subjective complaint, but multiple clinical tools (see Sect. 1.3.2.1) are available for use in an attempt to achieve some uniformity in definition. The most widely used clinical questionnaire is the Epworth Sleepiness Scale (ESS). A score of >10 on ESS is consistent with excessive sleepiness. Either by self-report or by use of the ESS, CPAP has been shown to improve sleepiness after treatment in majority of sleepy patients with OSA [8].

Sleep Quality

Sleep disturbances/poor sleep quality is another common feature of the OSA with patients reporting insomnia symptoms such as difficulty falling and staying asleep and non-restorative sleep. The former may be confirmed on polysomnography. Polysomnographic electroencephalographic tracings may also suggest paradoxical insomnia, where, despite having slept during the study, the patient reports a sensation of not having slept at all likely due to the overall poor quality of sleep. Sleep quality has been shown to improve with CPAP in patients with moderate to severe OSA and comorbid insomnia, some of whom were deemed to have treatment-resistant insomnia prior to treatment of OSA. Improvements have been demonstrated using both self-reported symptoms measured via tools such as the Insomnia Severity Index and sleep quality scales (see Sect. 1.3.2.1) and objective polysomnographic findings of reduced sleep onset latency, reduced wake after sleep onset, increases in sleep efficiency, and improved sleep architecture on CPAP [9].

Snoring/Apneas

As a general rule, CPAP is not recommended for primary snoring, but when used for treatment of OSA, there is an added benefit of partial or complete resolution of snoring [10]. Apneic episodes are also observed to decrease or resolve either by apnea-sensitive patients or their bed partners with the use of CPAP. These changes have been documented objectively via reductions in the apnea-hypopnea index (AHI) either via polysomnographic monitoring or download of CPAP data [11].

Cognitive Issues

The relationship between OSA and cognition is complex, with considerable variation in reported symptoms. Common examples include difficulty concentrating, difficulty learning new material, and memory impairment (for more detail, see Sect. 1.3.2). Reports of subjective improvement in these symptoms with CPAP use are variable. Some studies have reported partial improvement in cognitive symptoms with CPAP use in severe OSA patients only [12], and others report only mild and transient improvements [13]. The consistent use of CPAP has been shown to confer some benefit in patients with mild cognitive impairment by improving cognition in some cases while slowing the rate of cognitive decline in others [14]. Thus, CPAP is sometimes initiated in patients with OSA and cognitive impairment with a primary goal to reverse or slow decline.

Mood

There is considerable overlap between symptoms of untreated OSA and depression, and many cases of OSA are misdiagnosed as depression (also see Sect. 1.3.6). Insomnia, lethargy, and psychomotor retardation can occur in either condition. CPAP has been associated with subjective improvement in mood [15], particularly those overlapping symptoms described above, and increased use of CPAP has been associated with faster rates of improvement in those same domains on the Hamilton Depression Scale [16]. Improvements in other depression scales like the Patient Health Questionnaire 9 scores have also been documented with CPAP use [17].

Overall Quality of Life (QoL)

Patients with untreated OSA often report poor quality of life mainly described as impairment in daytime function. Therefore, one of the primary indications to treat with CPAP in OSA patients is to improve their quality of life. Following treatment with CPAP, and in the absence of other comorbidities impairing daytime function, patients often report improvement in symptoms related to their quality of life. Objective data using sleep-related quality of life measurement tools such as the Calgary Sleep Apnea QoL Index (SAQLI) have shown significant improvement following the treatment of severe OSA with CPAP, but less so with mild to moderate OSA [18]. Similar improvements were demonstrated on the FOSQ-10 and the Quality of Life Enjoyment and Satisfaction questionnaires in a cohort of patients with OSA and insomnia [9]. Improvement after CPAP using general quality of life instruments has been reported but is less consistent. For example, a study in women with moderate to severe OSA documented improvement in QoL indices with CPAP use on the Quebec Sleep Questionnaire [19]. However, there was no improvement with CPAP using the Quality of Well-Being Self-Administered Questionnaire [20].

1.2.1.2 Prevent or Treat Comorbid Medical Problems

The pathophysiology of OSA strongly suggests that it is a pro-inflammatory condition. Chronic inflammation is a common underlying condition in several chronic medical diseases including cardiovascular disease. The associated chronic intermittent hypoxia and repeated arousals, which are consequences of OSA, are the underlying reason for the cascade of events which result in inflammation. Use of CPAP in OSA patients may be useful in the prevention and treatment of these conditions.

Cardiovascular Disease (CVD)

Sleep-disordered breathing has long been associated with increased cardiovascular risk in new [21] and established patients with CVD [22]. The prevalence of OSA in patients with cardiovascular disease is up to 60% [23]; see Sect. 1.3.3. OSA is associated with an increased atherosclerotic burden courtesy of systemic inflammation, which is a consequence of oxidative stress and sympathetic activation. It has been found to be an independent risk factor for atherosclerosis. Treatment of OSA has been shown to significantly improve early signs of atherosclerosis [24]. In a randomized controlled trial conducted on a cohort of patients with moderate to severe OSA, CPAP was found to improve myocardial perfusion reserve on multiple modalities of cardiovascular imaging when compared to the sham CPAP group. These findings suggest that treatment of OSA may lessen endothelial dysfunction and hence prevent the development of overt cardiovascular disease [25].

Coronary Artery Disease

Cohort studies show a clear association of incident coronary artery disease (CAD) in severe OSA [26]; also see Sect. 1.3.3. In populations with cardiovascular disease, OSA predicts subsequent major cardiovascular events [22]. Some studies indicate that the treatment of OSA with CPAP in CAD patients is associated with a decrease in the occurrence of new cardiovascular events and an increase in the time to such events [27], while some report a significant reduction in subsequent major cardiovascular events in CAD patients compared with those left untreated [28]. However, in other studies, interventions using CPAP to reduce incident or recurrent CAD have failed to provide confirmatory data. These studies have been controversial, possibly due to the heterogeneity of study populations and poor adherence to CPAP [29]. Nevertheless, the presence of CAD in those with moderate to severe OSA is an indication for treatment with CPAP even in the absence of clinical symptoms. The case for treatment in those with mild OSA is less compelling.

Atrial Fibrillation (AF) and Other Arrhythmias

Acutely, OSA causes negative intrathoracic pressure, intermittent hypoxia, and sympathetic activity which predispose to arrhythmias. Hypoxia also increases vagal tone and promotes bradycardia and heart conduction abnormalities. In the long term, OSA may cause remodelling of the heart and promote arrhythmogenicity [30]. Up to 48% of patients with OSA have been found to have arrhythmias and heart conduction abnormalities during sleep [31]. Bradycardia, heart block, non-sustained ventricular tachycardia, atrial fibrillation, and sudden cardiac death have been described in OSA. AF appears to be the most commonly described, however.

OSA is an independent risk factor for incident AF and is directly related to the severity of OSA [32]. Nocturnal palpitations can be a presenting symptom of atrial fibrillation associated with OSA. When OSA is comorbid with AF, patients have worse symptoms and higher risks of hospitalization than patients without OSA, although disease progression and outcomes are similar in both groups [33]. Furthermore, patients with untreated OSA have a higher recurrence of AF after cardioversion than patients without. Adequate treatment of OSA with CPAP has been associated with lower recurrence of AF after cardioversion or ablation [34]. However, most of the findings are from observational studies and are not always reproducible [35]. Further recent information is provided in Sect. 1.3.3.

Bradyarrhythmias including nocturnal heart block are sometimes found in OSA. One study found more than half of patients with implanted pacemakers for bradyarrhythmias had OSA defined as AHI of ≥10 events per hour of sleep [36]. Treatment of OSA with CPAP can prevent the need for a pacemaker in patients with exclusively OSA-related bradyarrhythmias which tend to occur following episodes of severe oxygen desaturation. Clear improvements in bradyarrhythmias have been demonstrated on overnight Holter monitors with CPAP [37].

Data linking OSA to the pathogenesis of cardiac arrhythmias, particularly AF, are compelling. Thus, evaluation for OSA and treatment with CPAP in the setting of new-onset or worsening arrhythmias should be performed.

Stroke

OSA is an independent risk factor for ischemic stroke through a similar pathway that predisposes to cardiovascular disease in general. Another indirect pathway is via the increased risk of AF in OSA patients which can contribute to cardioembolic strokes. However, it has been postulated that these vascular events may also occur in OSA patients through mechanisms independent of AF [38].

OSA is highly prevalent in stroke patients [39], and stroke risk increases with greater severity of OSA. Severe obstructive sleep apnea (OSA) increases the risk for incident stroke and recurrence of stroke and worsens stroke outcomes. Continuous positive airway pressure may reduce stroke risk and improve functional outcomes, particularly in treatment-compliant patients [40].

Hypertension

There is an increased prevalence of systemic hypertension in OSA, and untreated OSA contributes to resistant hypertension. The importance of OSA in the pathogenesis of hypertension was highlighted in the 7th Report of the Joint National Committee on Prevention, Detection, Evaluation, and Treatment of High Blood Pressure [41].

The severity of OSA correlates with the severity of hypertension [42]. These findings are attributed to oxidative stress and consequent endothelial dysfunction. Nocturnal non-dipping of blood pressure (BP) during sleep has been noted in OSA patients.

Use of CPAP with adequate compliance has been shown to improve blood pressure readings particularly in moderate and severe OSA patients with resistant hypertension [43]. There appears to be a strong linear dose response between duration of CPAP use and reductions in BP [44], although some studies have reported only mild BP changes [45]. Evaluation for OSA and treatment with CPAP are indicated for hypertensive patients with a history suggestive of OSA or poorly controlled hypertension.

Congestive Heart Failure (CHF)

Severe OSA has been associated with increased incidence of congestive heart failure [26]. This may be related to the degree of hypoxia associated with OSA as demonstrated by a study done on a cohort of men with OSA [46]. Use of CPAP has been shown to be helpful in CHF patients with comorbid OSA as shown by improvements in left ventricular ejection fraction (LVEF) in patients with milder degrees of systolic dysfunction (LVEF >30%) [47]. The benefits of CPAP therapy in hospitalized OSA patients with acute exacerbation of CHF have been controversial with some studies documenting reduced readmission rates for CHF [48] and others reporting no reductions in length of stay or readmission rates [49]. Nevertheless, potential benefits of treating CHF patients who have been identified as having OSA with CPAP outweigh any risks.

Type 2 Diabetes Mellitus

Obstructive sleep apnea is associated with alterations in carbohydrate metabolism, impaired glucose tolerance, and insulin resistance, and this has been found to be independent of obesity [50]. The systemic inflammatory response associated with OSA also affects appetite-regulating hormones as well as the hypothalamic-pituitary-adrenal axis. These factors suggest that OSA may be an independent risk factor for type 2 diabetes mellitus. The prevalence of OSA among individuals with type 2 diabetes mellitus is extremely high approaching 85% in one study [51]. Although the effect of treatment with CPAP in those with type 2 diabetes and OSA is conflicting, patients with type 2 diabetes mellitus should be screened for OSA and provided a trial of CPAP if OSA is present [52].

Other Medical Conditions

The presence of OSA has been implicated in the pathogenesis of several other medical conditions. For individual patients, CPAP may be indicated as adjunctive treatment.

Chronic Kidney Disease (CKD)

Obstructive sleep apnea is moderately prevalent in chronic kidney disease. It may accelerate loss of kidney function due to oxidative stress leading to endothelial dysfunction and atherosclerosis. Furthermore, OSA worsens hypertension by activating the renin-angiotensin-aldosterone axis, contributing to a decline in kidney function [53]. It has also been associated with higher risk of incident end-stage renal disease [54]. Comorbid OSA is regarded as deleterious in kidney transplant patients. Screening and management is recommended in this population [55]. In one study, CPAP has been shown to slow the progression of CKD in patients with moderate and severe OSA [56].

Non-alcoholic Fatty Liver Disease

Non-alcoholic fatty liver disease is a disorder of altered carbohydrate metabolism, which also is one of the hallmarks of OSA. This appears to be a consequence of chronic intermittent hypoxia [57]. Untreated OSA patients have been found to have increased levels of serum markers as well as cellular evidence of liver damage. However, the role of CPAP in mitigating this risk has not been confirmed.

Gastroesophageal Reflux Disease (GERD)

Gastroesophageal reflux disease has been found to be prevalent in OSA patients, and this is independent of common risk factors like obesity, age, or gender. A causal relationship has been proposed due to observation of lower esophageal relaxation in OSA. CPAP has been found to improve GERD symptoms [58].

Chronic Headaches

Morning headaches can be a presenting symptom of OSA. The underlying reason for this may be multifactorial. Potential factors include hypoxia, sleep disruption, poor sleep quality, and co-existing hypercapnia which may be observed in complicated OSA phenotypes. Patients with morning headaches should be evaluated for OSA as the use of CPAP may be beneficial in some patients [59].

Pulmonary Hypertension

Chronic intermittent hypoxia, which results from OSA, leads to pulmonary arterial vasoconstriction and pulmonary hypertension. The degree of hypoxia is more contributory to the altered dynamics in the pulmonary vasculature rather than the frequency of sleep-disordered breathing events. Nevertheless, treatment of OSA with CPAP may reduce the severity of pulmonary hypertension [60].

1.2.1.3 OSA Severity and Decision to Use CPAP

Moderate and severe OSA are established indications for treatment with CPAP to prevent well-documented acute and chronic medical complications even in the absence of clinical symptoms. However, because the impact of mild OSA on associated medical conditions is not well established, the decision to treat is largely dependent on the presence of relevant symptoms like excessive daytime sleepiness and insomnia and associated cardiovascular comorbidities or mood disorders [61].

1.2.2   Central Sleep Apnea

1.2.2.1 Closed Airway Central Sleep Apnea

Central events may occur with pharyngeal narrowing or occlusion [62]. A more compliant airway and ventilatory controller instability are predisposing factors [6]. The consequent hypoxia during these events results in compensatory hyperventilation, and the ensuing hypocapnia further drives respiratory instability and central apneas. The use of CPAP by preserving upper airway patency during central events can help reduce hypoxia and stabilize breathing [62] and be an effective treatment in those who appear to have only central sleep apnea.

1.2.2.2 Treatment-Emergent Central Sleep Apnea

The emergence of new-onset central respiratory events during sleep when a patient is started on CPAP therapy is common and has been observed in up to 6.5% of patients treated with PAP therapy. Such de novo central events (also referred to as complex sleep apnea) are thought to be transitory, and the majority will resolve within 8 weeks [63]. Persistent cases warrant a switch to an alternative mode of PAP therapy where appropriate such as ASV. Underlying risk factors for central sleep apnea should also be identified and addressed.

1.3   Defining Treatment Success

There are two general methods used to assess treatment success with PAP therapy. The first is self-report of whether there is resolution of OSA symptoms. This includes various questionnaires such as the ESS and a number of QoL tools. The second is objective determinations of CPAP adherence. Both methods should be used to ascertain treatment success.

1.3.1 Self-Report

Improvement or resolution of symptoms can only be assessed by querying the patient. At a minimum, patients should be asked about daytime sleepiness, napping, snoring, and quality of their sleep. It is especially important to inquire about episodes of inattention or frank sleepiness while driving. Documentation of the patient's bedtime, sleep latency, episodes of wake after sleep onset, and wake time may also be useful. These can then be compared to answers before starting CPAP. If available, it can be helpful to ask the same questions to a bed partner in order to corroborate the patient's answers. In some cases, patients may wish to downplay the severity of their symptoms; the bed partner's viewpoint can be a more accurate appraisal of the situation.

Complete resolution of symptoms is the best outcome. However, many patients will report improvement, but still have residual symptoms. In addition, for some patients, there unfortunately will be little or no improvement despite objective evidence of adequate or even optimum use of CPAP therapy [64]. In such cases, other explanations for lack of improvement should be sought. For example, other sleep issues may still be present such as inadequate amount of time in bed trying to sleep or disruption of sleep continuity from environmental noise. However, in a number of instances, there is persistent hypersomnia despite good CPAP adherence with no other explanation. This has been attributed to a residual effect of long-standing untreated OSA [64].

In addition to an assessment of symptoms, patients should be asked whether they use their PAP device nightly and for how long each night. If they do not use it nightly or they use it for less than their time in bed, the usage frequency and amount of time used should be ascertained. In such cases, patients often overreport their use either because they are poor at estimation or because they wish to appear compliant with therapy at the time of their clinic appointment [65]. Adverse effects from PAP use such as facial rash or sores and noticeable amounts of air leakage around the mask should be elicited.

1.3.2 Questionnaires

Various questionnaires are sometimes used to assess whether PAP treatment is beneficial. The most common instruments assess QoL or daytime sleepiness. Both of these constructs are used as quality measures by the American Academy of Sleep Medicine and are thus intended as a metric of quality of care in the practice of Sleep Medicine [66].

1.3.2.1 Quality of Life Instruments

Results from generic quality of life instruments such as the Medical Outcomes Study Short-Form Health Survey (SF36) can be inconsistent or insensitive to changes in quality of life experienced by those with OSA [67]. Although there have been few studies [68, 69], sleep-specific tools such as the Functional Outcomes of Sleep Questionnaire (FOSQ) and the Sleep Apnea Quality of Life Index (SAQLI) correlate poorly with the SF36 suggesting that they may perform better in patients with sleep apnea-related symptoms. Both are either relatively long or require in-person administration. However, short versions like the FOSQ-10 are now available and may be more useful in a clinical setting. Studies in OSA patients treated with CPAP indicate that the FOSQ and SAQLI reflect changes in QoL after treatment with CPAP [18, 70].

1.3.2.2 Assessment of Daytime Sleepiness

The most common instrument used for assessment of daytime sleepiness is the Epworth Sleepiness Scale. Originally developed by Dr. Murray Johns in 1991 [71], it has been translated and validated in multiple languages. It is a self-administered questionnaire where individuals rate their usual chances of dozing off or falling asleep in eight common situations or activities on a 4-point scale (0–3). Hence, the minimum possible score on the scale is 0 (not sleepy at all), and the maximum is 24 (extremely sleepy). Scores >10 are considered indicative of excessive sleepiness. However, it is only modestly correlated with self-reported assessments as well as with objective measures of sleepiness such as the multiple sleep latency test [72]. Unfortunately, it has been misused by insurance companies, with low scores cited as a rationale for denying approval for diagnostic testing or initiation of treatment [73]. Nevertheless, the ESS has been shown to improve after CPAP use [13].

Two other instruments, the Karolinska Sleepiness Scale and the Stanford Sleepiness Scale, are used less commonly to quantify sleepiness. The Karolinska Sleepiness Scale assesses subjective sleepiness at a particular point in time. It is a 9-point scale with a "1" indicating extreme alertness and a "9" indicating extreme sleepiness [74]. A score of 7 or higher is felt to represent significant sleepiness. The Stanford Sleepiness Scale also rates sleepiness at the time the instrument is completed. It is a 7-point scale with a "1" defined as "Feeling active, vital, alert, or wide awake" and a "7" described as "No longer fighting sleep, sleep onset soon; having dream-like thoughts" [75]. Although commonly used in research settings, normative data are not available. Inasmuch as both the Karolinska Sleepiness Scale and the Stanford Sleepiness Scale convey an assessment of sleepiness at only a single point in time, they have limited clinical utility. However, they can be administered multiple times during any time period.

1.3.3 Objective Assessment of CPAP Adherence

The limitations inherent in subjective reporting of symptoms and CPAP usage led to the evolution of objective methods of assessing sleepiness and adherence to CPAP therapy. Objective evaluation of sleepiness in the context of CPAP therapy is not usually performed because of the expense of performing studies such as the multiple sleep latency test. However, objective evaluation of CPAP adherence has become a treatment "gold standard." Early generation CPAP devices were able to provide crude determination of device usage by measuring the amount of time the device was "turned on." With the advent of advanced pressure sensors and microprocessors, new devices are now able to record the amount of time the CPAP interface or mask is worn. Initially, such data were saved on a storage card, which could be removed for data download. Currently, they are sent into the "cloud" where they can be accessed by both the patient and clinicians in near real time. Review of adherence data is now considered standard of care by sleep clinicians at the time of follow-up visits by patients with OSA; third-party reimbursement for CPAP may be contingent upon objective documentation of a minimal level of usage [76].

1.3.3.1 Interpretation of PAP Compliance Reports

Reports from CPAP devices contain data in four areas: device usage, set and delivered pressures, AHI measured from the device, and estimates of air leak. However, because CPAP devices do not have oximetry capabilities, data regarding oxygen saturation or desaturation events are not included. Device usage is generally provided as the average amount of time used over a 30-day interval. Additionally, the number and percent of days used and number and percent of nights with 4 or more hours of use are reported. For pressure data, reports specify the PAP mode (e.g., CPAP, APAP, BPAP) and the prescribed settings. For device modes which automatically adjust the therapeutic pressure such as APAP, the most important parameter provided is the 90 or 95 percentile pressure. This is the pressure at which the device spent 90 or 95% of the night at or below. For example, if an individual used the device for 10 hours and 9 hours was spent at or below 10 cm H_2O, then the 90 percentile pressure would be 10 cm H_2O. Some device manufacturers provide the 90 percentile pressure and others the 95 percentile pressure. In addition, the average peak airway pressure is provided. One of the most important metrics provided on a CPAP report is the device-measured AHI. This parameter is derived from changes in airflow measured internally by the device. It is reasonably accurate but tends to slightly overestimate severity at lower AHI values and underestimate at higher values [77]. However, differentiating between obstructive and central events may not be reliable. Finally, estimates of mask leak are provided. Some intentional leakage is inherent with the use of PAP in order to avoid CO_2 rebreathing. However, large amounts of unintentional leakage from around the mask cause facial and eye irritation and may result in poor adherence to therapy [78].

Objective evidence of treatment success is commonly defined as an AHI <5/hour and usage for at least 70% of nights for more than 4 hours per night [76]. Achievement of this goal is adversely affected by the need for high pressures and the presence of excessive amounts of unintentional leak. In a small number of cases, there will be a need to document resolution of oxygen desaturation while on PAP therapy. This will require a continuous nocturnal oximetry recording in addition to the standard PAP usage report.

1.3.3.2 What Is Treatment Success?

Successful treatment with PAP is not an all or none determination despite the large amount of pertinent information available. Improvement in symptoms whether by an individual's global impression or more formally by use of a validated instrument is an important factor. However, some persons with significant OSA are asymptomatic, and symptom improvement would not be expected. Because mild OSA is defined as an AHI ≥5/hour, a reduction in AHI below this level is considered a complete therapeutic response. However, there is controversy regarding the utility of the AHI as an index of OSA severity [79]. Thus, from a patient care perspective, can a reduction in AHI from >50/hour to 10/hour be considered a success if the patient's symptoms resolve? An AHI equal to 10/hour still is considered as mild OSA. Many clinicians would be satisfied with such a response and would be reticent to pursue additional treatment options despite the presence of residual OSA. A more complex issue is whether usage of PAP for at least 70% of nights for more than 4 hours per night defines treatment success. This amount of usage has been adopted by the Centers for Medicare and Medicaid Services (CMS) and many insurers as the minimum criteria for reimbursement for PAP therapy [76]. Unfortunately, it also has been adopted by many clinicians as the metric for treatment success. If one assumes that the amount of healthy sleep for an adult should be at least 7 hours per night [80], then over 1 month, the total amount of sleep achieved should be 210 hours. However, if a person only meets minimum CMS criteria, then the usage of PAP will only be 85 hours or 40.4% of optimum use! This calculation suggests that successful treatment should not be defined as only meeting minimum CMS criteria. Another issue is whether individuals who use PAP less than the CMS minimum will benefit from PAP. From a therapeutic perspective, it is illogical to believe that use of PAP for slightly less than 4 hours will be ineffective treatment in comparison to slightly more than 4 hours. Data examining changes in the ESS as a function of PAP usage would suggest that improvement and hence treatment success is more of a continuum rather than a threshold effect [8, 81].

1.4   Summary

Continuous positive airway pressure is indicated to treat clinical symptoms and a variety of medical conditions resulting from or occurring in association with OSA. If used for adequate amounts of time, it usually improves clinical symptoms. It also may prevent or treat some comorbid medical conditions such as hypertension and type 2 diabetes. Treatment success can be ascertained through a combination of subjective improvement in symptoms and objective documentation of adherence to therapy.

References

1. Sullivan CE, Berthon-Jones M, Issa FG, Eves L. Reversal of obstructive sleep apnoea by continuous positive airway pressure applied through the nares. Lancet. 1981;1(8225):862–5.
2. Guilleminault C, Simmons FB, Motta J, Cummiskey J, Rosekind M, Schroeder JS, et al. Obstructive sleep Apnea syndrome and tracheostomy: long-term follow-up experience. Arch Intern Med. 1981;141(8):985–8.
3. Zhu K, Roisman G, Aouf S, Escourrou SP. All APAPs are not equivalent for the treatment of sleep disordered breathing: a bench evaluation of eleven commercially available devices. J Clin Sleep Med. 2015;11(7):725–34.
4. Omobomi O, Quan SF. BPAP for CPAP failures: for the many or the few. Respirology. 2020;25(4):358–9.
5. Malfertheiner MV, Lerzer C, Kolb L, Heider K, Zeman F, Gfüllner F, et al. Whom are we treating with adaptive servo-ventilation? A clinical post hoc analysis. Clin Res Cardiol. 2017;106(9):702–10.
6. Salloum A, Rowley JA, Mateika JH, Chowdhuri S, Omran Q, Badr MS. Increased propensity for central apnea in patients with obstructive sleep apnea effect of nasal continuous positive airway pressure. Am J Respir Crit Care Med. 2010;181(2):189–93.
7. Kushida CA, Littner MR, Hirshkowitz M, Morgenthaler TI, Alessi CA, Bailey D, et al. Practice parameters for the use of continuous and bilevel positive airway pressure devices to treat adult patients with sleep-related breathing disorders. Sleep. 2006;29(3):375–80.
8. Budhiraja R, Kushida CA, Nichols DA, Walsh JK, Simon RD, Gottlieb DJ, et al. Predictors of sleepiness in obstructive sleep apnoea at baseline and after 6 months of continuous positive airway pressure therapy. Eur Respir J. 2017;50(5):1700348.
9. Krakow B, McIver ND, Ulibarri VA, Krakow J, Schrader RM. Prospective randomized controlled trial on the efficacy of continuous positive airway pressure and adaptive servo-ventilation

in the treatment of chronic complex insomnia. EClinicalMedicine. 2019;13:57–73.
10. McEvoy RD, Antic NA, Heeley E, Luo Y, Ou Q, Zhang X, et al. CPAP for prevention of cardiovascular events in obstructive sleep apnea. N Engl J Med. 2016;375(10):919–31.
11. Patil SP, Ayappa IA, Caples SM, Kimoff RJ, Patel SR, Harrod CG. Treatment of adult obstructive sleep Apnea with positive airway pressure: an American Academy of sleep medicine systematic review, {meta-analysis}, and {GRADE} assessment. J Clin Sleep Med. 2019;15(2):301–34.
12. Wang M-L, Wang C, Tuo M, Yu Y, Wang L, Yu J-T, Tan L, Chi S. Cognitive effects of treating obstructive sleep Apnea: a meta-analysis of randomized controlled trials. J Alzheimers Dis. 2020; https://doi.org/10.3233/JAD-200088. Online ahead of print.
13. Kushida CA, Nichols DA, Holmes TH, Quan SF, Walsh JK, Gottlieb DJ, et al. Effects of continuous positive airway pressure on neurocognitive function in obstructive sleep Apnea patients: the Apnea positive pressure long-term efficacy study (APPLES). Sleep. 2012;35(12):1593–602. [published correction appears in Sleep. 2016 Jul 1;39(7):1483]
14. Richards KC, Gooneratne N, Dicicco B, Hanlon A, Moelter S, Onen F, et al. CPAP adherence may slow 1-year cognitive decline in older adults with mild cognitive impairment and Apnea. J Am Geriatr Soc. 2019;67(3):558–64.
15. Yamamoto H, Akashiba T, Kosaka N, Ito D, Horie T. Long-term effects nasal continuous positive airway pressure on daytime sleepiness, mood and traffic accidents in patients with obstructive sleep apnoea. Respir Med. 2000;94(1):87–90.
16. Bucks RS, Nanthakumar S, Starkstein SS, Hillman DR, James A, McArdle N, et al. Discerning depressive symptoms in patients with obstructive sleep apnea: the effect of continuous positive airway pressure therapy on Hamilton Depression Rating Scale symptoms. Sleep. 2018;41(12) https://doi.org/10.1093/sleep/zsy178.
17. Lewis EF, Wang R, Punjabi N, Gottlieb DJ, Quan SF, Bhatt DL, et al. Impact of continuous positive airway pressure and oxygen on health status in patients with coronary heart disease, cardiovascular risk factors, and obstructive sleep apnea: a Heart Biomarker Evaluation in Apnea Treatment (HEARTBEAT) analysis. Am Heart J. 2017;189:59–67.
18. Batool-Anwar S, Goodwin JL, Kushida CA, Walsh JA, Simon RD, Nichols DA, et al. Impact of continuous positive airway pressure (CPAP) on quality of life in patients with obstructive sleep apnea (OSA). J Sleep Res. 2016;25(6):731–8.
19. Campos-Rodriguez F, Queipo-Corona C, Carmona-Berna C, Jurado-Gamez B, Cordero-Guevara J, Reyes-Nuñez N, et al. Continuous positive airway pressure improves quality of life in women with obstructive sleep apnea a randomized controlled trial. Am J Respir Crit Care Med. 2016;194(10):1286–94.
20. Batool-Anwar S, Omobomi O, Quan S. The effect of CPAP on HRQOL as measured by the quality of Well-being self-administered questionnaire (QWB-SA). Southwest J Pulm Crit Care. 2020;20(1):29–40.
21. Shahar E, Whitney CW, Redline S, Lee ET, Newman AB, Nieto FJ, et al. Sleep-disordered breathing and cardiovascular disease: cross-sectional results of the sleep heart health study. Am J Respir Crit Care Med. 2001;163(1):19–25.
22. Lee CH, Sethi R, Li R, Ho HH, Hein T, Jim MH, et al. Obstructive sleep apnea and cardiovascular events after percutaneous coronary intervention. Circulation. 2016;133(21):2008–17.
23. Mehra R. Sleep apnea and the heart. Cleve Clin J Med. 2019;86(9 Suppl 1):10–8.
24. Drager LF, Bortolotto LA, Figueiredo AC, Krieger EM, Lorenzi-Filho G. Effects of continuous positive airway pressure on early signs of atherosclerosis in obstructive sleep apnea. Am J Respir Crit Care Med. 2007;176(7):706–12.

25. Nguyen PK, Katikireddy CK, McConnell MV, Kushida C, Yang PC. Nasal continuous positive airway pressure improves myocardial perfusion reserve and endothelial-dependent vasodilation in patients with obstructive sleep apnea. J Cardiovasc Magn Reson. 2010;12(1):50.

26. Hla KM, Young T, Hagen EW, Stein JH, Finn LA, Nieto FJ, et al. Coronary heart disease incidence in sleep disordered breathing: the Wisconsin sleep cohort study. Sleep. 2015;38(5):677–84.

27. Milleron O, Pillière R, Foucher A, De Roquefeuil F, Aegerter P, Jondeau G, et al. Benefits of obstructive sleep apnoea treatment in coronary artery disease: a long-term follow-up study. Eur Heart J. 2004;25(9):728–34.

28. Capodanno D, Milazzo G, Cumbo M, Marchese A, Salemi A, Quartarone L, et al. Positive airway pressure in patients with coronary artery disease and obstructive sleep apnea syndrome. J Cardiovasc Med. 2014;15(5):402–6.

29. Furlow B. SAVE trial: no cardiovascular benefits for CPAP in OSA. Lancet Respir Med. 2016;4(11):860.

30. Geovanini GR, Lorenzi-Filho G. Cardiac rhythm disorders in obstructive sleep apnea. J Thorac Dis. 2018;10(Suppl 34):S4221–30.

31. Guilleminault C, Connolly SJ, Winkle RA. Cardiac arrhythmia and conduction disturbances during sleep in 400 patients with sleep apnea syndrome. Am J Cardiol. 1983;52(5):490–4.

32. Cadby G, McArdle N, Briffa T, Hillman DR, Simpson L, Knuiman M, et al. Severity of OSA is an independent predictor of incident atrial fibrillation hospitalization in a large sleep-clinic cohort. Chest. 2015;148(4):945–52.

33. Holmqvist F, Guan N, Zhu Z, Kowey PR, Allen LA, Fonarow GC, et al. Impact of obstructive sleep apnea and continuous positive airway pressure therapy on outcomes in patients with atrial fibrillation – results from the Outcomes Registry for Better Informed Treatment of Atrial Fibrillation (ORBIT-AF). Am Heart J. 2015;169(5):647–654.e2.

34. Fein AS, Shvilkin A, Shah D, Haffajee CI, Das S, Kumar K, et al. Treatment of obstructive sleep apnea reduces the risk of atrial fibrillation recurrence after catheter ablation. J Am Coll Cardiol. 2013;62(4):300–5.

35. Caples SM, Mansukhani MP, Friedman PA, Somers VK. The impact of continuous positive airway pressure treatment on the recurrence of atrial fibrillation post cardioversion: a randomized controlled trial. Int J Cardiol. 2019;278:133–6.

36. Garrigue S, Pépin JL, Defaye P, Murgatroyd F, Poezevara Y, Clémenty J, et al. High prevalence of sleep apnea syndrome in patients with long-term pacing: the European multicenter polysomnographic study. Circulation. 2007;115(13):1703–9.

37. Wu X, Liu Z, Chang SC, Fu C, Li W, Jiang H, et al. Screening and managing obstructive sleep apnoea in nocturnal heart block patients: an observational study. Respir Res. 2016;17:16.

38. Lipford MC, Flemming KD, Calvin AD, Mandrekar J, Brown RD, Somers VK, et al. Associations between Cardioembolic stroke and obstructive sleep Apnea. Sleep. 2015;38(11):1699–705.

39. Dong R, Dong Z, Liu H, Shi F, Du J. Prevalence, risk factors, outcomes, and treatment of obstructive sleep Apnea in patients with cerebrovascular disease: a systematic review. J Stroke Cerebrovasc Dis. 2018;27(6):1471–80.

40. Bassetti CLA, Randerath W, Vignatelli L, Ferini-Strambi L, Brill AK, Bonsignore MR, et al. EAN/ERS/ESO/ESRS statement on the impact of sleep disorders on risk and outcome of stroke. Eur J Neurol. 2020; https://doi.org/10.1111/ene.14201. Online ahead of print.

41. National High Blood Pressure Education Program. The Seventh Report of the Joint National Committee on Prevention, Detection, Evaluation, and Treatment of High Blood Pressure. Bethesda: National Heart, Lung, and Blood Institute (US); 2004. https://www.ncbi.nlm.nih.gov/books/NBK9630/.

42. Javier Nieto F, Young TB, Lind BK, Shahar E, Samet JM, Redline S, et al. Association of sleep-disordered breathing sleep apnea, and hypertension in a large community-based study. J Am Med Assoc. 2000;283(14):1829–36.

43. De Oliveira AC, Martinez D, Massierer D, Gus M, Gonçalves SC, Ghizzoni F, et al. The antihypertensive effect of positive airway pressure on resistant hypertension of patients with obstructive sleep apnea: a randomized, double-blind, clinical trial. Am J Respir Crit Care Med. 2014;190(3):345–7.

44. Barbé F, Durán-Cantolla J, Capote F, De La Peña M, Chiner E, Masa JF, et al. Long-term effect of continuous positive airway pressure in hypertensive patients with sleep apnea. Am J Respir Crit Care Med. 2010;181(7):718–26.

45. Durán-Cantolla J, Aizpuru F, Montserrat JM, Ballester E, Terán-Santos J, Aguirregomoscorta JI, et al. Continuous positive airway pressure as treatment for systemic hypertension in people with obstructive sleep apnoea: randomised controlled trial. BMJ. 2010;341:c5991.

46. Azarbarzin A, Sands SA, Taranto-Montemurro L, Vena D, Sofer T, Kim S-W, et al. The sleep apnea-specific hypoxic burden predicts incident heart failure. Chest. 2020;S0012-3692(20):30678–4.

47. Egea CJ, Aizpuru F, Pinto JA, Ayuela JM, Ballester E, Zamarrón C, et al. Cardiac function after CPAP therapy in patients with chronic heart failure and sleep apnea: a multicenter study. Sleep Med. 2008;9(6):660–6.

48. Sommerfeld A, Althouse AD, Prince J, Atwood CW, Mulukutla SR, Hickey GW. Obstructive sleep apnea is associated with increased readmission in heart failure patients. Clin Cardiol. 2017;40(10):873–8.

49. Kamel G, Munzer K, Espiritu J. Use of CPAP in patients with obstructive sleep apnea admitted to the general ward: effect on length of stay and readmission rate. Sleep Breath. 2016;20(3):1103–10.

50. Punjabi NM, Shahar E, Redline S, Gottlieb DJ, Givelber R, Resnick HE. Sleep-disordered breathing, glucose intolerance, and insulin resistance: the sleep heart health study. Am J Epidemiol. 2004;160(6):521–30.

51. Reutrakul S, Mokhlesi B. Obstructive sleep Apnea and diabetes: a state of the art review. Chest. 2017;152(5):1070–86.

52. Shaw JE, Punjabi NM, Wilding JP, Alberti KGMM, Zimmet PZ. Sleep-disordered breathing and type 2 diabetes. A report from the international diabetes federation taskforce on epidemiology and prevention. Diabetes Res Clin Pract. 2008;81(1):2–12.

53. Adeseun GA, Rosas SE. The impact of obstructive sleep apnea on chronic kidney disease. Curr Hypertens Rep. 2010;12(5):378–83.

54. Choi HS, Kim HY, Han KD, Jung JH, Kim CS, Bae EH, et al. Obstructive sleep apnea as a risk factor for incident end stage renal disease: a nationwide population-based cohort study from Korea. Clin Exp Nephrol. 2019;23(12):1391–7.

55. Parajuli S, Tiwari R, Clark DF, Mandelbrot DA, Djamali A, Casey K. Sleep disorders: serious threats among kidney transplant recipients. Transplant Rev. 2019;33(1):9–16.

56. Li X, Liu C, Zhang H, Zhang J, Zhao M, Sun D, et al. Effect of 12-month nasal continuous positive airway pressure therapy for obstructive sleep apnea on progression of chronic kidney disease. Medicine (Baltimore). 2019;98(8):e14545.

57. Aron-Wisnewsky J, Clement K, Pépin JL. Nonalcoholic fatty liver disease and obstructive sleep apnea. Metabolism. 2016;65(8):1124–35.

58. Tamanna S, Campbell D, Warren R, Ullah MI. Effect of CPAP therapy on symptoms of nocturnal gastroesophageal reflux among patients with obstructive sleep apnea. J Clin Sleep Med. 2016;12(9):1257–61.

59. Johnson KG, Ziemba AM, Garb JL. Improvement in headaches with continuous positive airway pressure for obstructive sleep apnea: a retrospective analysis. Headache. 2013;53(2):333–43.

60. Arias MA, García-Río F, Alonso-Fernández A, Martínez I, Villamor J. Pulmonary hypertension in obstructive sleep apnoea: effects of continuous positive airway pressure: a randomized, controlled cross-over study. Eur Heart J. 2006;27(9):1106–13.

61. Chowdhuri S, Quan SF, Almeida F, Ayappa I, Batool-Anwar S, Budhiraja R, et al. An official American thoracic society research statement: impact of mild obstructive sleep apnea in adults. Am J Respir Crit Care Med. 2016;193(9):e37–54.

62. Badr MS, Toiber F, Skatrud JB, Dempsey J. Pharyngeal narrowing/occlusion during central sleep apnea. J Appl Physiol. 1995;78(5):1806–15.

63. Javaheri S, Smith J, Chung E. The prevalence and natural history of complex sleep apnea. J Clin Sleep Med. 2009;5(3):205–11.

64. Santamaria J, Iranzo A, Ma Montserrat J, de Pablo J. Persistent sleepiness in CPAP treated obstructive sleep apnea patients: evaluation and treatment. Sleep Med Rev. 2007;11(3):195–207.

65. Rauscher H, Formanek D, Popp W, Zwick H. Self-reported vs measured compliance with nasal CPAP for obstructive sleep apnea. Chest. 1993;103(6):1675–80.

66. Aurora RN, Collop NA, Jacobowitz O, Thomas SM, Quan SF, Aronsky AJ. Quality measures for the care of adult patients with obstructive sleep apnea. J Clin Sleep Med. 2015;11(3):357–83.

67. Reimer MA, Flemons WW. Quality of life in sleep disorders. Sleep Med Rev. 2003;7(4):335–49.

68. Silva G, Goodwin J, Vana K, Quan S. Obstructive sleep apnea and quality of life: comparison of the SAQLI, FOSQ, and SF-36 questionnaires. Southwest J Pulm Crit Care. 2016;13(3):137–49.

69. Kasibowska-Kuźniar K, Jankowska R, Kuźniar T, Brzecka A, Piesiak P, Zwierzycki J. Comparative evaluation of two health-related quality of life questionnaires in patients with sleep apnea. Wiad Lek. 2004;57(5–6):229–32.

70. Weaver TE, Mancini C, Maislin G, Cater J, Staley B, Landis JR, et al. Continuous positive airway pressure treatment of sleepy patients with milder obstructive sleep apnea: results of the CPAP apnea trial north american program (CATNAP) randomized clinical trial. Am J Respir Crit Care Med. 2012;186(7):677–83.

71. Johns MW. A new method for measuring daytime sleepiness: the Epworth sleepiness scale. Sleep. 1991;14(6):540–5.

72. Benbadis SR, Mascha E, Perry MC, Wolgamuth BR, Smolley LA, Dinner DS. Association between the Epworth sleepiness scale and the multiple sleep latency test in a clinical population. Ann Intern Med. 1999;130(4 Pt 1):289–92.

73. Quan SF. Abuse of the Epworth sleepiness scale. J Clin Sleep Med. 2013;9(10):987.

74. Gillberg M, Kecklund G, Akerstedt T. Relations between performance and subjective ratings of sleepiness during a night awake. Sleep. 1994;17(3):236–41.

75. Hoddes E, Zarcone V, Smythe H, Phillips R, Dement WC. Quantification of sleepiness: a new approach. Psychophysiology. 1973;10(4):431–6.

76. Schwab RJ, Badr SM, Epstein LJ, Gay PC, Gozal D, Kohler M, et al. An official American Thoracic Society statement: continuous positive airway pressure adherence tracking systems the optimal monitoring strategies and outcome measures in adults. Am J Respir Crit Care Med. 2013;188(5):613–20.

77. Berry RB, Kushida CA, Kryger MH, Soto-Calderon H, Staley B, Kuna ST. Respiratory event detection by a positive airway pressure device. Sleep. 2012;35(3):361–7.

78. Valentin A, Subramanian S, Quan SF, Berry RB, Parthasarathy S. Air leak is associated with poor adherence to autopap therapy. Sleep. 2011;34(6):801–6.

79. Rapoport DM. POINT: is the apnea-hypopnea index the best way to quantify the severity of sleep-disordered breathing? Yes Chest. 2016;149(1):14–6.

80. Watson NF, Badr MS, Belenky G, Bliwise DL, Buxton OM, Buysse D, et al. Recommended amount of sleep for a healthy adult: a joint consensus statement of the American Academy of Sleep Medicine and Sleep Research Society. Sleep. 2015;38(6):843–4.

81. Weaver TE, Maislin G, Dinges DF, Bloxham T, George CFP, Greenberg H, et al. Relationship between hours of CPAP use and achieving normal levels of sleepiness and daily functioning. Sleep. 2007;30(6):711–9.

Interventions to Improve CPAP Adherence

Tatyana Mollayeva

On the neurology clinic rotation round in which you are the medical director, a senior resident with a subspecialty in sleep medicine comments that nearly half of the patients seen today have sleep apnea and were prescribed CPAP and many of these patients have difficulty tolerating this therapy and do not use it on a nightly basis. These patients are coming to the neurology clinic because of sequelae of myocardial infarction, stroke, and neuropathy, and they are only in their third decade of life. This leads to a discussion on poor CPAP adherence and its effect on cognitive and physical impairments, disability, and mortality, as well as evidence for CPAP therapy that improves these outcomes. One of the senior residents from a psychology background is convinced that multimodal cognitive behavioral therapy has to be the way to improve adherence to CPAP therapy in your patients. A medical student points out that enhancing adherence to CPAP requires not only initiatives directed at patients but also interventions enhancing the patient-provider relationship and trust and interventions focusing on continuity and coherence of care directed on optimizing sleep continuity with CPAP, which implies considerable sleep specialist and staff investment in understanding barriers to CPAP adherence in each individual patient, time, and expense to address all of the components of the patient-clinician-CPAP and environment interfaces. You remind the group that the topic of CPAP adherence, with its multiple definitions, could benefit from a well-done review of the most recent randomized clinical trials (RCTs) that address the effect of different types of interventions on CPAP adherence. The clinician-researcher on the floor, intrigued by the discussion, commits to performing such a review.

Compliance and adherence in medicine are complex terms with significant implications for patients' health and well-being, clinician's efforts, and health resources [1–3]. The *Oxford English Dictionary* defines compliance as "the acting in accordance with, or the yielding to a desire, request, condition, direction, etc.; a consenting to act in conformity with; an acceding to; practical assent" [4]. The same dictionary defines adherence as "persistence in a practice or tenet, steady observance or maintenance" [4]. Clearly, the two terms, compliance and adherence, do not hold the same meaning concerning the role of the patient and the clinician and their mutual tenacity in sticking to a proposed therapeutic regimen. Although the literature is filled with discussions on the acceptability of these terms, most recently, the term adherence is being used, which takes into account a patient's choice and is intended to be non-judgmental, unlike compliance, which reinforces patient passivity and blame [5].

The topic of patient adherence has captivated the minds of most prominent physicians and scientists for centuries [6–8]. It is believed that the recommendations of a clinician derive their value from what is by nature good for the patient and is built on the assumption that recommendations will help the patient to prevent or fight the disease. However, since ancient times, most prominent philosophers and doctors considered the needs of their patients and what they perceived as being good as part of a much broader context of patients' relations to themselves and to others, including patients' relationships with their treatment providers [9]. It is also well understood that adherence is a dynamic process that needs to be followed up by both the patient and treatment provider over a time continuum [10].

T. Mollayeva (✉)
KITE-Toronto Rehab University Health Network, Toronto, ON, Canada

Global Brain Health Institute, Institute of Neuroscience Trinity College, Dublin, Ireland
e-mail: tatyana.mollayeva@uhn.ca

Most recent estimates of patients' failure to adhere to treatment recommendations in Western medicine, in general, range from 20 to 40% for acute disease regimens, 20 to 60% for chronic disease regimens, and 50 to 80% for preventive regimens [10, 11]. Traditional facilitators to adhere to prescribed therapy are divided into patient-related factors (i.e., targeting attitudes and beliefs, perceived benefits, and lifetime habits), regimen-related factors (i.e., altering the complexity of the regimen and frequency of or duration of application), and factors related to healthcare providers, including their level of knowledge and principles of communication [11]. However, standard recommended methods for improving adherence to any therapy are still lacking. This is especially true for adherence to continuous positive airway pressure (CPAP), a noninvasive respiratory therapy technique that entails delivery to the opening of the airways, by an external interface, a positive (over atmospheric) pressure, continuously in sleep, during both expiration and inspiration [12].

Continuous positive airway pressure is the main treatment for moderate to severe obstructive sleep apnea (OSA), a chronic sleep-related breathing disorder, defined as recurrent episodes of obstructed breathing during sleep, which cause repeated arousals, sympathetic hyperactivity, and intermittent hypoxia [13]. Numerous studies controlling for confounders established that untreated OSA is a risk factor for hypertension, cardiovascular disease, strokes, car crashes, and neurocognitive dysfunction [14–17]. Other associations of OSA include impotence, depression, glucose intolerance, and reduced quality of life [18–21]. Since the approval of nasal CPAP therapy for OSA in adults in 1981 [13], numerous studies have been conducted to improve the understanding of the patient, provider, and technology's part in

adherence to this therapy, considering conservative estimations that 29 to 83% of patients are nonadherent, depending on how nonadherence is defined [22–25] (Fig. 2.1).

While there is currently no international consensus on the definition of nonadherent use of CPAP therapy, most sleep specialists agree that less than 4 hours per night can be used as a general metric [22–26], based on the results of studies that have shown that normalization of daytime sleepiness, quality of life, neurocognitive function, cardiovascular disease conditions, and diabetes improve with 4 or more hours of CPAP use per night. The Centers for Medicare and Medicaid Services require 4 hours per night for 5 out of 7 nights [27], and the American Association of Sleep Disorder defines adherence to CPAP as 4 or more hours per night and at least 9 of each of the 14 nights of ventilator use, measured by a ventilator timer recorder [28, 29]. Because the magnitude of CPAP nonadherence and the scope of nonadherence sequelae are so alarming, interests in various interventions directed toward enhancing CPAP adherence have led to the development of multiple clinical trials targeting adherence over the last decade.

Several CPAP adherence-related reviews have been published recently [22–26]. The current chapter was designed to provide an overview of the most recent (past decades) adherence-related literature within a simple hypothesized conceptual framework based on these earlier reviews on the topic (Fig. 2.2). The aim was to review and facilitate a wider application and adaptation of any new CPAP adherence interventions proved to be more efficient than standard care. Further, the author aimed to distinguish the most common types of CPAP adherence-related outcomes so that intervention effectiveness for each type of intervention can be explicitly recognized.

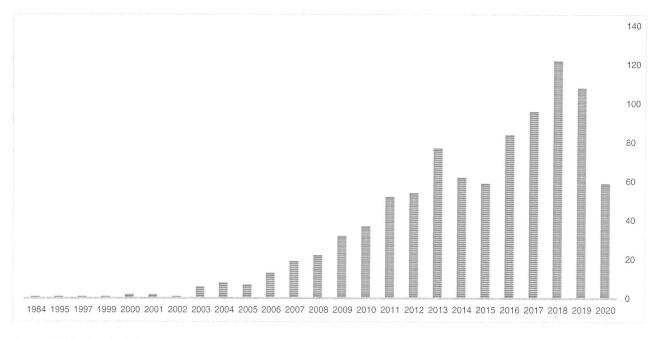

Fig. 2.1 Publications including MeSH terms Continuous Positive Airway Pressure and adherence, 1984 up to present (May 2020)

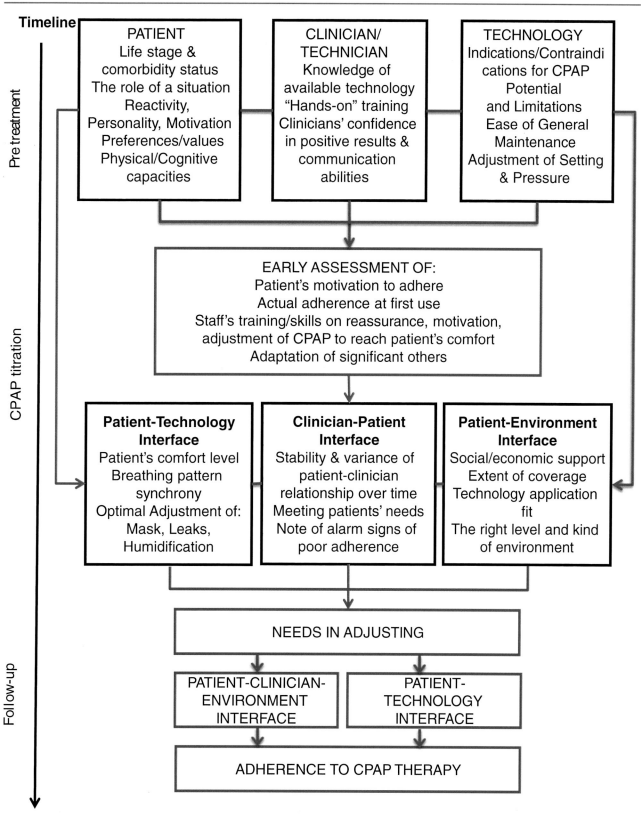

Timeline

Pre treatment

PATIENT	CLINICIAN/	TECHNOLOGY
Life stage & comorbidity status	TECHNICIAN	Indications/Contraindi cations for CPAP
The role of a situation	Knowledge of available technology	Potential
Reactivity,	"Hands-on" training	and Limitations
Personality, Motivation	Clinicians' confidence	Ease of General
Preferences/values	in positive results &	Maintenance
Physical/Cognitive	communication	Adjustment of Setting
capacities	abilities	& Pressure

EARLY ASSESSMENT OF:
Patient's motivation to adhere
Actual adherence at first use
Staff's training/skills on reassurance, motivation,
adjustment of CPAP to reach patient's comfort
Adaptation of significant others

CPAP titration

Patient-Technology Interface	**Clinician-Patient Interface**	**Patient-Environment Interface**
Patient's comfort level	Stability & variance of	Social/economic support
Breathing pattern synchrony	patient-clinician relationship over time	Extent of coverage
Optimal Adjustment of:	Meeting patients' needs	Technology application fit
Mask, Leaks,	Note of alarm signs of	The right level and kind
Humidification	poor adherence	of environment

NEEDS IN ADJUSTING

Follow-up

PATIENT-CLINICIAN-ENVIRONMENT INTERFACE	PATIENT-TECHNOLOGY INTERFACE

ADHERENCE TO CPAP THERAPY

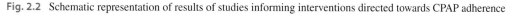

Fig. 2.2 Schematic representation of results of studies informing interventions directed towards CPAP adherence

2.1 Material and Methods

Search Procedure and Criteria for Study Inclusion
To be included in this chapter, each study had to meet the following inclusion criteria:

1. Describe at least one intervention, defined as an attempt to enhance CPAP adherence.
2. Have a control group, comparable to the intervention group in at least age and severity of sleep-disordered breathing via similar identifiers.
3. CPAP adherence was quantitatively measured via machine interrogations at both baseline and follow-up and linked to changes in any health or functional outcome.
4. The study was published in English in a peer-reviewed journal during the past decade.

Studies published before 2010 were not included in this review because they had been reviewed in the extensive bibliography and evaluation of adherence literature conducted by Sawyer et al. [23] and Rotenberg et al. [22].

A literature search of the PubMed was performed using the keywords "CPAP" intersected with "compliance" or "adherence" (restricted to focus, major keyword, or title word) and with "intervention" (in the title or abstract). Publications found through the bibliographies of identified articles and reviews were also reviewed for any relevant works.

2.1.1 Study Selection

Nine hundred and fifty-eight articles (as of May 21, 2020) using these MeSH (Medical Subject Headings) entry terms were identified. The title and abstract of the papers were scanned by two researchers to determine whether they fit the inclusion criteria. Eligible studies were selected according to the inclusion criteria by the PICOS strategy (Table 2.1).

Table 2.1 Search strategy

Population	Patients with sleep-related breathing disorders for whom CPAP was prescribed
Intervention	Any randomized parallel group studies focusing on patients' adherence to CPAP use
Comparisons	Effect of interventions versus usual care or comparisons of intervention arms
Outcome	Adherence connected to any health or functional outcome
Study design	Randomized trials with any follow-up length
Excluded	Samples with patient's age <18 years; studies in languages other than English; studies published before 2010

2.1.2 Data Extraction

Twenty-six studies met the inclusion criteria and were selected for data synthesis [30–55]. Selected studies were categorized based on the type of intervention. The information abstracted from the articles included study details (i.e., author names, publication year, and country), study characteristics (i.e., setting, design, and sample size), participant characteristics (mean age, sex, and severity of OSA), intervention type, definition of adherence and variables used to assess it, and characteristics of the intervention. The intervention was described in detail, including the focus of the intervention (educational, behavioral and affective, surgical, or technology-targeted), strategies used to deliver the intervention (such as one-to-one education, group education, or tele-monitoring), and the number of intervention strategies used in each study.

2.1.3 Data Synthesis

We used a best evidence synthesis approach to organize findings from studies of sufficient quality by tabulation and qualitative descriptions [56]. The primary outcomes considered were (1) adherence and (2) adherence-related assessments, as studied by researchers. All adherence-related assessments of outcomes relevant to patients and those relevant to healthcare were considered. Results were organized by patient population (i.e., OSA versus OSA and comorbidity; naïve versus those with poor adherence), intervention type assessed, and duration of follow-up, depicting the relative change across time within each individual study. The diversity in the content of intervention and usual care and their domains, definitions of adherence, the statistical methodologies used to quantify associations, and score assessment in the studies as well as the measures themselves ruled out application of meta-analysis in its classic form [57].

2.2 Results

Table 2.2 describes the study design, sample size and characteristics, outcome measures, and key findings of the reviewed studies, by intervention category.

2.2.1 Risk of Bias in the Included Studies

An overview of my judgments of the risk of bias for included studies (allocation, blinding, and missing data domains) is provided in Table 2.2. For most studies, information regarding the concealment of allocation could not be ascertained. For the remainder of the studies, there was insufficient infor-

Table 2.2 Selected (<10 years old) randomized clinical trials

Author (year), country, setting/population	Intervention content Control content Duration of intervention	Study design Inclusion/exclusion criteria (IC/EC)	Sample size N (T/C) Age, years Sex (%M) AHI Desaturation Withdrew Age, sex (M/F) Comparable by	Adherence definition	Outcome measures	Results	Benefits Effect size	Risk of bias assessment: sequence generation/concealment/blinding/ outcome data
Education/personalized feedback								
Chen et al. (2015), Wenzhou Medical University, Wenzhou, People's Republic of China New pts. w OSA for whom CPAP was indicated (sleep disorder clinics in Zhejiang)	Intervention arm: Nurse-led intensive support (1) hospital health education; (2) pt. self-management interventions; and (3) psychological intervention + meeting w sleep physician at 1, 3, 6, and 12 Mos Control arm: Standard support in new OSA pts. (meeting w sleep physician at 1, 3, 6, and 12 Mos) 12 Mos	Randomized, single-blinded, prospective trial IC: Legally licensed drivers with OSA EC: NR	N = 80 (40/40) Withdrew = 0 Age: 50.2 ± 10.1/50.6 ± 11.2 AHI: 55 ± 4/54 ± 4 Desaturation: NR Sex (%M): 73/70 Comparisons at BS: Age, sex, education, occupation, BMI, AHI, Q of L, mood, ESS score, symptoms – NS	$\geq$4 h/night	CPAP usage Other outcomes: Quality of life, ESS, HADS; short Form-36	Machine usage: Intervention arm longer use than control; difference statistically significant at 1, 3, 6, and 12 Mos Other outcomes: Quality of life and sleepiness improved in both arms; mood improved in intervention arm	Machine usage: Average 2.2 h/night Month 1: 6.32 ± 1.25/4.35 ± 1.71 Month 3: 6.41 ± 1.30/4.20 ± 1.20 Month 6: 6.31 ± 1.81/4.31 ± 1.25 Month 12: 6.67 ± 1.36/4.02 ± 1.23 Quality of life (SF-36) mean score mental-physical intervention group/control group: Month 1: 52–49/44–41 Month 3: 54–50/46–43 Month 6: 58–54/50–46 Month 12: 62–62/52–51 Sleepiness (arm differences NS): Month 1: 11.5 ± 1/12 ± 1 Month 3: 10.3 ± 1.4/11.2 ± 1.7 Month 6: 5.4 ± 1.4/6.4 ± 1.3 Month 12: 4.87 ± 1.5/5.36 ± 1.45 Mood: Month 1: 5.36 ± 1.54/4.59 ± 1.35 Month 3: 6.35 ± 1.25/4.05 ± 1.25 Month 6: 6.75 ± 1.48/4.21 ± 1.40 Month 12: 6.50 ± 1.6/4.00 ± 1.54	+/?/?/+ Randomization by a predetermined balanced block generated by tossing a coin Pts blinded to allocation; others: NR An intention-to-treat analysis applied
Dawson et al. (2015), University of Iowa, USA Drivers w OSA for whom CPAP was indicated	Intervention arm: Feedback regarding own naturalistic driving record (i.e., videos of three samples of pre-CPAP and three samples of post-CPAP driving shown) and CPAP compliance + general information on untreated OSA, sleep hygiene guidelines, and sleep impact on driving safety Control arm: No intervention 10 weeks	Randomized controlled trial IC: Legally licensed drivers with OSA EC: NR	N = 66 (30/36) Withdrew = NR Age: 30–60 years old AHI: NR Desaturation: NR Sex (%M): NR Comparisons: NR	$\geq$4 h/night	Mean CPAP usage Other outcomes: Driving behavior based on monitoring electronic, video, and GPS outputs	Machine usage: Intervention arm improved in weeks 1–3 from BS; effect not observed in weeks 4–10 Control arm decreased in use from BS use Other outcomes: NR	Machine usage: BS: 258 minutes/night (~4.3 h/ night) Intervention arm: Improved by 35.8 minutes/night (95% CI = 9.6, 62.0); mean 296 minutes/night Control arm: Decreased an average of 27.5 minutes/night (95% CI = 4.0, 51.0); mean 236 minutes/night Arm-specific changes higher in intervention than in control arm on weeks 1, 2, and 3 ($p < 0.001$, $p = 0.001$, and $p = 0.027$, respectively) Weeks 4 through 10, effect not significant ($p > 0.25$ in all cases)	?/?/?/?? Patients were randomized; procedure: NR Others: NR

(continued)

Table 2.2 (continued)

Author (year), country, setting/population	Intervention content / Control content / Duration of intervention	Study design / Inclusion/exclusion criteria (IC/EC)	Sample size N (T/C), Age, years, Sex (%M), AHI, Desaturation, Withdrew, Age, sex (M/F), Comparable by	Adherence definition	Outcome measures	Results	Benefits / Effect size	Risk of bias assessment: sequence generation/concealment/blinding/outcome data
Dharmakulaseelan et al. (2019), Stroke Program, Sunnybrook Health Sciences Centre, University of Toronto, Canada Pts with a history of stroke or TIA for whom CPAP was indicated	Intervention arm: Educational materials (a 5-minute animated slideshow; educational pamphlet; feedback regarding animated slideshow and pamphlet) Control arm: Usual care 6 Mos	Randomized controlled trial, blinded IC: Pts. with a history Of stroke or TIA EC: Significant physical or cognitive impairments; aphasia; inability to communicate in English; facial/bulbar weakness; life expectancy of less than 6 Mos	N = 48 (25/23) Withdrew = 0/4 Age: 71 ± 12/66 ± 19 AHI: 40.9 ± 11.1 vs 46.1 ± 25.2 Desaturation: NR Sex (%M): 56/70 Comparisons by new to CPAP to those who were not	≥28 h/week of usage	H of CPAP use/week Other outcomes: Knowledge acquisition, daytime sleepiness, functional outcomes of sleep	Machine usage: No difference in machine usage btw arms at 6-mo f/u No significant benefits were observed In knowledge acquisition, daytime sleepiness, and functional outcomes of sleep in response to intervention	Machine usage: Intervention arm: 36.4 h/week Control arm: 41.9 h/week (p = 0.506)	?/?/+/? Randomization procedure: NR Blinding: Treating physician and the outcome assessors were blinded to the treatment Others: NR
Jurado-Gamez et al. (2015), Sleep Unit of a third-level hospital/ Australia Pts w sleep apnea-hypopnea syndrome for whom CPAP was indicated	Intervention arm: Results of pts' sleep test/CPAP titration were shown (respiratory events, oxygen desaturation, impact of sleep apnea on vascular system, complications, effect on sleep quality, non-refreshing sleep, daytime sleepiness; importance of treatment adherence discussed) Control arm: No education Both arms were trained in CPAP management and in solving problems during adaptation period 6 Mos (1-, 3-, and 6-mo f/u by a nurse)	A controlled parallel arm trial IC: Pts. aged 30 to 70 years diagnosed with SAHS by PSG, with CPAP indications EC: Major psychiatric disease treated with psychotropic drugs or drug abuse	N = 330 (158/172) Withdrew = 4/5 Age: 55 ± 10.6/53 ± 9.3 AHI: 44 ± 21.2/43 ± 42.8 Desaturation (%time < 90): 10 ± 9.5/11 ± 9 Sex (% M): 70/65 Sex, treatment period, age	≥4 h/night	Average h of CPAP use/ day at 6 Mos after titration CPAP usage ≥4 h/day CPAP abandonment, % Other outcomes: Non-scheduled phone calls	H of CPAP use/night, better in intervention vs control arm # w CPAP usage ≥4 h was higher in intervention arm vs control CPAP abandonment was lower in intervention arm Others: No difference	Machine usage: Treatment arm: 5 ± 1.8 h/day Control arm: 4.3 ± 1.7; p = 0.001 CPAP usage ≥4 hour: 86% vs 76%; p = 0.031 CPAP abandonment: 13% vs 22%; p = 0.029 # of non-scheduled phone calls: 0.8 ± 0.1 vs 0.87 ± 0.1; p = 0.102	?/–/+/? Randomization: None Adequate nurse blinding/others: Unclear Others: NR

Nadeem et al. (2013), James A. Lovell Federal Health Care Center, North Chicago/USA Pts w OSA for whom CPAP was indicated	Intervention arm: Pts. were shown detailed PSG data, including graphic data from PSG prior to prescription of CPAP Control arm: Pts. were shown non-graphic paper report of PSG Pts in both arms were asked to repeat what they had learned during the session (15 minutes each) 4 weeks 1-week f/u: All pts. contacted via phone; asked to identify issues with CPAP; adherence re-emphasized	Randomized clinical trial IC: Pts. diagnosed with OSA by PSG, with CPAP indications EC: NR	*N* = 40 (20/20); 37 analyzed (18/19) Withdrew (excluded data lost/machine issues) = 4/1 Age: 57.3 ± 11.8/55.5 ± 11.6 AHI: 36.0 ± 27.8/30.5 ± 19.1 Desaturation: NR Sex (%M): 88.9/95 Sex, treatment period, age	≥4 h/night plus >70% of nights	Average h of use/night % days used CPAP adherence Health outcome: None	No difference btw arms in CPAP adherence outcomes BMI increased likelihood of improved adherence	Machine usage: Treatment arm: 3.9 ± 2.1 h/night Control arm: 4.1 ± 2.5; *p* = 0.76 # of days w CPAP usage: 20.6 ± 9.8 vs 20.8 ± 10.4; *p* = 0.59 CPAP use, % days: 58% vs 64%; *p* = 0.029 # of non-scheduled phone calls: 0.8 ± 0.1 vs 0.87 ± 0.1; *p* = 0.102 For BMI >30 kg/m², odds ratio for adherence was 13.3 (*p* < 0.007)	+/+/−/? Adequate randomization (pt picking up an envelope from a stack, which had a concealed assignment) Clinician's blinding: No Pts blinding: No – They were aware that CPAP card records adherence to therapy Others: NR
Roecklein et al. (2010), Department of Psychology, University of Pittsburgh/USA Consecutive clinic pts. w OSA intended to use CPAP/naïve CPAP users	Intervention arm: Feedback – AASM information, personal OSA severity, and risks phrased in motivational approach/ personalized feedback data before and after CPAP use: AHI, RDI, Level of blood oxygen, and daytime sleepiness Control arm: Three brochures – AASM – Entitled "obstructive sleep Apnea and snoring," "positive airway pressure therapy for sleep Apnea," and "obstructive sleep Apnea" 3 Mos (intermittent assessments at week 2)	Randomized clinical trial IC: Pts. diagnosed with OSA by PSG, with CPAP indications EC: None	*N* = 30 (14/16); 28 analyzed (13/15) Withdrew (excluded data lost/machine issues) = 4/1 Age: 46.1 ± 11.5/46.6 ± 11.3 AHI: 45.8 ± 42.38/42.69 ± 34.34 Desaturation (average O₂): 91.05 ± 4.40/91.16 ± 5.25 Sex (%M): 25/46	Not defined	Total h, average h, separate use events/day (CPAP machine reading and self-reported) Health outcome: Side effects questionnaire Calgary sleep Apnea quality of life symptoms	No difference btw arms in total h, average h, and separate use events/day at 2 weeks and 3 Mos (CPAP machine) Self-reported days using CPAP: Difference at 3 Mos Arms did not differ in rates of CPAP side effects, sleepiness, or quality of life symptoms	The likely magnitude of effect at: Week 2: Total *h* – *d* = 0.80 [95% CI = −0.01 to 1.60] Average *h*: *d* = 0.79 [95% CI = −0.02 to 1.58] Sessions: *d* = 0.77 [95%CI = −0.04 to 1.56]	+/?/−/? Adequate randomization (randomly assigned) procedure: NR Clinician's blinding: Yes (to study participation) Pt blinding: Yes (to study condition) Others: NR

(continued)

Table 2.2 (continued)

Myofunctional therapy

Author (year), country, setting/population	Intervention content Control content Duration of intervention	Study design Inclusion/exclusion criteria (IC/EC)	Sample size N (T/C) Age, years Sex (%M) AHI Desaturation Withdrew Age, sex (M/F) Comparable by	Adherence definition	Outcome measures	Results	Benefits Effect size	Risk of bias assessment: sequence generation/concealment/blinding/ outcome data
Diaféria et al. (2017), São Paulo, SP, Brazil Pts with OSA syndrome	Four arms: 1. Placebo therapy (P) (exercises without therapeutic function). 2. Myofunctional therapy (MT) (muscular endurance exercises aimed at toning oropharynx muscle arms, optimizing muscle tension mobility). 3. CPAP. 4. CPAP therapy and myofunctional therapy (CPAP + MT). 3 Mos	Randomized controlled trial IC: Newly diagnosed OSAS EC: Female gender, uncooperative, illiterate, other sleep disorders/ previous treatment for OSAS, serious or decompensated clinical or psychiatric medical illnesses	N = 100 (24/27/27/22) Withdrew = 0 Age: 48.1 ± 11.2 Sex (%M): 100 AHI: 10–30+, NS differences btw arms Desaturation: NR Age, neck circumference, BMI, ESS, snoring, snoring intensity	≥4 h/night plus at least 70% of nights	Average adherence % participants who were "adherent" at 1 week and after 3 Mos of intervention Others: ESS, snoring	Machine usage CPAP + MT Showed an increased adherence compared to CPAP ESS: All treatment arms showed decreased ESS and snoring	Machine usage: CPAP + MT: Longer use time week 1 and after month 3 compared to CPAP ($p < 0.05$) % "adherent" at 3 Mos: P: 55% MT: 63% CPAP: 30% CPAP + MT: 65%	?/?/+/? Randomly divided; procedure: NR Blinding: The evaluators were blinded Others: NR
Wang et al. (2012), School of Nursing, Central South University, China Han Chinese OSA pts	4 arms: An education (E) arm, a PMR (P) arm, an education + PMR (E + P) arm, and a control (C) arm E arm: 4-hour arm education on OSA and CPAP + a brochure CPAP therapy: a 20-min video on how to manipulate CPAP device; 24-h consultation telephone line P arm: PMR classic muscle relaxation program by Jacobson (12X40-min arm PMR practice sessions over 12 weeks, 1/week) E + P arm C arm: No intervention 12 weeks	Controlled, randomized, open-label study IC: Newly diagnosed OSA; AHI >10; education > elementary school; conscious mind; able to communicate EC: Family or personal history of mental illness; drug or alcohol abuse; severe cognitive, oncologic, or psychiatric diseases	N = 152 (38/38/38/38) Withdrew = 0 Age: 30–60+, NS differences btw arms Sex (%M): 89.5/76.3/81.6/81.6 AHI: 38.5 ± 18.7/35.7 ± 16.2/41.2 ± 21.4/43.1 ± 22.5, NS differences btw arms Desaturation: NR Age, sex, religion, living status, education, employment, education, AHI, BMI, ESS, PSQI score, HADS-D	≥4 h/night plus at least 9 of each 14 nights	Machine usage % participants who were "adherent" at 4, 8, and 12 weeks of intervention Others: ESS, PSQI, depression, anxiety	Machine usage E + P showed 31.6%, 31.5%, and 31.5% improvement in adherence over C at weeks 4, 8, and 12, respectively P showed no significant improvement over time ESS: Compared with C, E + P Improvement in ESS and PSQI score at weeks 4, 8, and 12 of intervention; E improvement at week 4 Anxiety and depression: E + P improved better than C at week 12	Machine usage: Week 4: E vs C: $\chi2 = 8.491, P = 0.004$ P vs C: $\chi2 = 6.786, P = 0.009$ E + P vs C: $\chi2 = 10.483, P = 0.001$ Week 8: E vs C: $\chi2 = 2.036, P = 0.154$ P vs C: $\chi2 = 3.7415, P = 0.053$ E + P vs C: $\chi2 = 9.212, P = 0.002$ Week 12: E vs C: $\chi2 = 1.324, P = 0.250$ P vs C: $\chi2 = 3.455, P = 0.063$ E + P vs C: $\chi2 = 8.143, P = 0.004\%$ "adherent": Week 4/week 8/week 12 C: 60.5/55.3/47.3 P: 89.5/71.1/60.5 P: 86.8/76.3/68.4 E: 92.1/86.8/78.9 No adequate statistical power	+/?/?/? Adequate randomization by block Blinding: NR Others: NR

	Intervention arm / Control arm	Design, IC, EC	Sample	Adherence definition	Outcome measures	Results	Machine usage	Quality
Family/peer support Parthasarathy et al. (2010), Academic Center, USA Recently diagnosed male pts. w OSA	Intervention arm: Pts assigned to a peer buddy system (PBS) to promote CPAP adherence (promoting self-efficacy, promoting outcome expectancies, improving risk perception, and pt. activation); 10 interactions Control arm: Usual care (CPAP initiation and education class) 90 days	Prospective, randomized, parallel arm, open-label, pilot study IC: Newly diagnosed OSA; never used CPAP; adherent to CPAP (>4 h/day of CPAP use); willing to meet with peer buddy on 2 occasions in person; able to be contacted by telephone; willing to undergo a brief training and orientation session EC: Central sleep apnea, complex sleep apnea; required oxygen on BiPAP; major medical disorders; major psychiatric illness; shift worker or frequent out-of-town traveler; unwilling to participate in orientation and training session	$N = 39$ (22/17) Withdrew = 0 Age: <65 years of age, NS differences btw arms Sex (%M): 100/100 AHI: 36.7 ± 28.6/37.5 ± 36.9, NS differences btw arms Desaturation: NR Age, BMI, race, ethnicity, education, marital status, working status, AHI, CPAP pressure, mask interface, CCI, ESS score	> 4 h/day of CPAP use	Machine usage % participants who were "adherent" on day 90 of intervention Others: Satisfaction, functional outcomes of sleep questionnaire (FOSQ), self-efficacy, and pt. activation	Machine usage Weekly CPAP adherence greater in the intervention than usual care arm No arm differences for FOSQ, vigilance, self-efficacy, or pt. activation	Machine usage: Week 1: Intervention arm: 313 ± 119 min/day (5.2 ± 2.0 h/day) Control arm: 238 ± 142 min/day or 4.0 ± 2.4 h/day; $p = 0.08$% adherent at 90 days Intervention arm: 63.6% Control arm: 40%; $p = 0.15$	?/?/?/? Randomly assigned, procedure: NR Others: NR
Remote monitoring/telemedicine Perin et al. (2019), 32 recruiting French centers, France Pts with severe OSA at high cardiovascular risk	Intervention arm: Remote multimodal telemonitoring Control arm: Usual care (CPAP initiation and education class) 6 Mos	Multicenter, open RCT IC: 18 to 75 years, with severe OSA (AHI > 30 events/h); at least one cardiovascular disease or an elevated cardiovascular risk assessed by 10-year risk of fatal cardiovascular event EC: Central sleep apnea or heart failure with a left ventricular ejection fraction <40%	$N = 306$ (157/149) Withdrew = 0 Age: 18–75 years, 61.8/60.8 NS differences btw arms Sex (%M): 74.5/73.2 AHI: 45 [35.4; 61.2]/47 [35; 60.5]; NS differences btw arms Desaturation (mean SaO₂): 92 [90; 94]/92.1 [91; 94] Age, BMI, blood pressure, history of smoking, type 2 diabetes, dyslipidemia, sedentarity, depression, ESS, fatigue, biological parameters, NS differences btw arms	≥4 h/day	Machine usage Other measures Evening SBP, change in morning and evening diastolic HBP, change in ESS score, fatigue, quality of life, physical activity, lipids, and glucose metabolism	Machine usage After 6 Mos of CPAP, significant increase in CPAP adherence and in daytime sleepiness and quality of life in favor of multimodal telemonitoring Morning systolic and diastolic HBP and evening diastolic HBP were significantly lower in both arms of CPAP treatment No difference in self-measured evening systolic BP or in steps taken per day in either arm ESS and Pichot fatigue significantly improved in both arms; range of improvement higher in intervention arm No differences btw arm in biological parameters (low-density lipoprotein, cholesterol); lowered significantly in both arms BMI did not change in either of arm	Machine usage: Significantly higher in intervention arm than in control arm: 5.28 ± 2.23 vs 4.75 ± 2.50 h, respectively	+/+/+/+ Computer-generated allocation Randomization stratified by center, home care provider, and CPAP brand Neither participants nor investigators were masked to arm assignment Data analysts blinded to arm allocation Data analyzed in intention-to-treat

(continued)

Table 2.2 (continued)

Author (year), country, setting/population	Intervention content Control content Duration of intervention	Study design Inclusion/exclusion criteria (IC/EC)	Sample size N (T/C) Age, years Sex (%M) AHI Desaturation Withdrew Age, sex (M/F) Comparable by	Adherence definition	Outcome measures	Results	Benefits Effect size	Risk of bias assessment: sequence generation/concealment/blinding/outcome data
Hoet et al. (2017), Brussels, Belgium Recently diagnosed pts. w moderate-severe OSA	Intervention arm: Telemedicine (TM) (in TM arm, a universal TM unit (T4P) was added to CPAP device) 1 month after CPAP initiation Control arm: Usual care 1 month after CPAP initiation 3 Mos (visits at 1.5 and 3 Mos)	Prospective, randomized, parallel arm, open-label, pilot study IC: 18+ years old; newly diagnosed OSA, AHI >20 EC: Previous use of CPAP; central or mixed sleep apnea; language barrier; significant comorbidity; unable to provide consent	N = 46 (23/23) Withdrew = 3/2 Age: 59 ± 13/54 ± 14, NS differences btw arms Sex (%M): 17/57 (sign diff) AHI: 50 ± 26/49 ± 24, NS differences btw arms Desaturation: NR Age, BMI, ESS, comorbidities, medication use (benzodiazepines, antidepressants), NS differences btw arms	> 4 h/night	Machine usage % participants who were "adherent" at month 3 of intervention Others: NR	Machine usage Use at 3 Mos was significantly better in TM arm In both arms, use Significantly increased between 6 weeks and 3 Mos % adherence better in TM	TM vs C 5.7 ± 1.6 vs 4.2 ± 1.9 h/night, p = 0.018 Total number of h of CPAP use 507 ± 205 h vs 387 ± 185 h; p = 0.034% adherent: 83% vs 64%	+/?/?/? Adequate randomization permuted blocks Blinding: NR Others: NR
Sparrow et al. (2010), VA Boston Healthcare System, USA Recently diagnosed pts. w OSAS	Intervention arm: Theory-driven interactive voice response system (telephone-linked communications for CPAP (TLC-CPAP)) Control arm: Placebo 12 Mos (visits at 6 and 12 Mos)	Prospective, randomized, parallel arm, open-label, pilot study IC: 18–80 years old: newly diagnosed OSA, AHI >10 EC: Previous use of CPAP; central or mixed sleep apnea; language barrier; significant comorbidity; unable to provide consent	N = 250 (124/126) Withdrew = NR Age: 55.0 years (IQR 46.0–63.0) Sex (%M): 82% AHI: 10–154 events/h, with 60% having AHI >30 Desaturation: NR Randomization stratified by sex, age, and AHI using a randomized block design to ensure balance of these factors in treatment arms	> 4 h/night	H of CPAP usage at each visit % participants who were "adherent" at months 6 and 12 of intervention Others: Functional status and depressive symptoms	Machine usage At 6 Mos, median machine use in TLC-CPAP ~1 h/night higher than in control; at 12 Mos, 2 h/night higher CPAP adherence associated with improved functional status and fewer depressive symptoms	Median usage: TLC-CPAP: 2.40 h/night and 2.98 h/night at 6 Mos and 12 Mos C: 1.48 h/night and 0.99 h/night % adherent at 12-mo TLC-CPAP intervention was associated with a 30% higher rate of CPAP use (44.7% of intervention arm using CPAP 4 h/night vs 34.5% of control arm)	+/?/+/+ Adequate randomization permuted blocks Blinding: All data were collected by research assistants blind to group assignment Analyses were performed by intention to treat
Implants Gillespie et al. (2010), four geographically dispersed tertiary sleep disorder centers, USA Recently diagnosed pts. w mild-moderate OSAS	Intervention arm: Pillar implants Control arm: Sham procedure performed in double-blind fashion 90-day f/u	A prospective, multicenter, randomized, placebo-controlled, double-blind study IC: 18+ years old; newly diagnosed OSA, AHI <15, CPAP at a level ≥ 7 Dissatisfied with CPAP EC: Soft palate unable to insert 18-mm implants, obstruction, medically unstable conditions or pregnancy, alcohol or drug abuse, and inconsistent use (1 or 2 nights/week) of sleeping meds	N = 51 (26/25) Withdrew = NR Age: 51.1 ± 9.0/52.3 ± 10.3 Sex (%M): 84/84.6 AHI: 46 ± 24/42 ± 21 Desaturation (lowest oxygen saturation, %): 82 ± 12/84 ± 4 No significant differences in pt. BS demographics between arms in sex, age, race, BMI, neck circumference, ESS, mean daily CPAP use, tongue position, tonsil size, and uvula size	≥4 h/night at least 5 nights a week	H of CPAP usage at each visit Others: Functional status and ESS scores	Machine usage No difference in average daily CPAP use between arms Improvements in ESS and functional outcomes of sleep questionnaire scores at 90 days with no differences between arms	Median usage: Pillar: 6 ± 2.5 h/night and 6 ± 2.4 h/night at BS and 90 days Sham: 5.2 ± 1.9 h/night and 5.2 ± 2.1 h/night at BS and 90 days	+/+/+/? Randomization in a double-blind fashion block randomization (by site; overall randomization ratio of 1:1) Blinding: Technician blinded to pts' treatment group Others: NR

Weight loss

Study	Intervention	Design / IC / EC	Patient characteristics	Adherence definition	Outcome measures	Results	Numeric results	Risk of bias
Hood et al. (2013), a multidisciplinary sleep center in an urban academic medical center, USA Obese men and women w mild-moderate OSA	Intervention arm: Dietary self-monitoring (SM) arm Control arm: Attention control (AC) arm 12 weeks (assessments at BS, 6 weeks (post-treatment), and 12 weeks)	A prospective randomized trial IC: OSA, currently using or initiating use of a CPAP device and having BMI between 30 and 45 kg/m EC: Another sleep disorder (e.g., narcolepsy, sleep-related seizure disorder, REM behavior disorder) or were diagnosed with anorexia nervosa, bulimia nervosa, night eating syndrome, or nocturnal sleep-related eating disorder; in pharmacological weight program	N = 40 (22/18) Withdrew = 9/7 Age: 53.7 ± 10.2/52.1 ± 13.2 Sex (%M): 45/6 AHI: NR Desaturation: NR No significant differences in pt. BS demographics between arms in sex, age, ethnicity, BMI, BS weight, education, and employment	≥4 h/night	Percent of days used >4 h Others: Weight loss	CPAP adherence at each time point by condition No difference in average daily CPAP use between arms 6-week weight loss correlated with CPAP adherence/SM participants with greater weight loss at 6 weeks had greater CPAP adherence at 6 and 12 weeks	Percent of days used >4 h: 6 weeks/12 weeks CM: 57.45 ± 37.81/61.96 ± 38.67 AC: 77.05 ± 30.79/72.13 ± 29.18 Average weight change SM: −1.44 ± 3.19 lbs. at 6 weeks (post-treatment) and − 0.52 ± 4.24 at 12 weeks (f/u); 75% lost weight at 6 weeks (range: 0.1–9.4 lbs) and 73% lost weight at 12 weeks (range: 0.1–9.8 lbs) AC: −1.38 ± 3.77 lbs. at 6 weeks (post-treatment) and − 1.22 ± 6.10 lbs. at 12 weeks	?/?/?/? Individual randomization; procedure: NR Blinding: NR Others: NR

Technology/mask interface

Study	Intervention	Design / IC / EC	Patient characteristics	Adherence definition	Outcome measures	Results	Numeric results	Risk of bias
Neuzeret and Morin (2017), ResMed Science Center, Saint Priest Cedex, France Recently diagnosed pts. w OSAHS	Intervention arm: ResMed mirage FXVR (MFX) or mask fisher and Paykel ZestVR, HC407VR, or Philips EasyLifeVR Control arm: Consistently used masks in study clinics over trial period 3 Mos of use	A prospective, multicenter, randomized, placebo-controlled, double-blind study IC: 18+ years old; newly diagnosed OSA, AHI >30, CPAP at a level ≥ 7 Dissatisfied with CPAP EC: Soft palate unable to insert 18-mm implants, obstruction, medically unstable conditions or pregnancy, alcohol or drug abuse, and inconsistent use (1 or 2 nights/week) of sleeping meds	N = 195 (85/110) Withdrew = NR Age: 53.2 ± 12.1/55.9 ± 11.9 Sex (%M): 84/84.6 AHI: 46 ± 24/42 ± 21 Desaturation (lowest oxygen saturation, %): 82 ± 12/84 ± 4 No significant differences between arms in sex, age, race, BMI, neck circumference, ESS, mean daily CPAP use, tongue position, tonsil size, and uvula size	≥4 h/night At least 5 nights a week	H of CPAP usage at each visit Others: First-line mask acceptance Pt satisfaction Contact calls and visits for mask issue Second-line mask required Duration of visit related to first-line mask only	Machine usage CPAP compliance was higher and nasal mask issue-related HCP visits were lower in MFX arm Probability of rejecting first-line nasal mask increased over time in control arm but not in MFX arm Satisfaction scores were similar in both arms No difference between arms in proportion of pts. with a first-line mask-related contact call, and call duration was similar	Median usage: CPAP compliance was higher (5.9 ± 1.8 vs 5.1 ± 1.6 h/night, p = 0.011) and nasal mask issue-related HCP visits lower (3% vs 17%, p = 0.006) in MFX arm Duration of a visit relating to a first-line nasal mask only was shorter in MFX arm, and pts. with MFX were significantly less likely to have a visit related only. Second-line mask requirement was lower in MFX arm versus control	+/?/−/+ Randomization Using a secure web platform, which displayed the assigned treatment group number Blinding: No The modified intent-to-treat population comprised all patients allocated to treatment without mouth leak during CPAP
Gulati et al. (2015), The Respiratory Support and Sleep Centre, UK Pts using CPAP <4 h/ night	Intervention arm: Bi-level PAP device Control arm: New CPAP 4 weeks long with a 2-week washout period between arms	A two-period, two-treatment crossover randomized controlled trial IC: AHI >5; CPAP prescribed for 5 weeks or more; CPAP use <4 h/ night; symptoms to suggest pressure intolerance EC: AF obstruction (FEV1/ FVC % < 60%); central sleep apnea (central events more than 50% of AHI); congestive heart failure; daytime hypercapnia (PaCO2 > 6.5 KPa); or previous bi-level PAP use	N = 28 Withdrew = NR Age: 56.7 ± 10.81 Sex (%M): 86 AHI: 35.8 ± 24.9/6.6 ± 13.4/3.7 ± 4.6 Desaturation: NR	≥4 h/night	Average number of h of PAP use, per night, by inbuilt clock counter in CPAP or bi-level PAP machine Others: ESS score, quality of life	Machine usage CPAP compliance was higher and nasal mask issue-related HCP visits were lower in MFX arm	Machine usage BS: CPAP use was of 1.49 ± 0.89 h/ night CPAP to bi-level PAP: Use 2.73 ± 1.9 h/night New CPAP brand: Use 2.23 ± 1.56/ night – All significant differences ESS BS: 13.2 (4.61) CPAP to bi-level PAP: 11.0 (4.75) New CPAP brand: 11.5 (5.34) – All significant differences Quality of life: BS: 3.7 ± 1.51 CPAP to bi-level PAP: 4.5 ± 1.46 sign New CPAP brand: 4.1 ± 1.71 NS differences	+/?/?/? Crossover randomization; procedure: NR Blinding: NR Others: NR

(continued)

Table 2.2 (continued)

Author (year), country, setting/population	Intervention content / Control content / Duration of intervention	Study design / Inclusion/exclusion criteria (IC/EC)	Sample size N (T/C) / Age, years / Sex (%M) / AHI / Desaturation / Withdrew / Age, sex (M/F) / Comparable by	Adherence definition	Outcome measures	Results	Benefits / Effect size	Risk of bias assessment: sequence generation/concealment/blinding/outcome data
Powell et al. (2012), three accredited sleep facilities, Midwestern USA. Pts w suboptimal facility-based attended CPAP titration	Intervention arm: Auto-bi-level CPAP. Control arm: CPAP. 90-day home trial period; days 7, 30, and 90	A restricted randomization procedure. IC: Adults (aged 21–75 years old); AHI ≥15; a suboptimal titration: (1) SE ≤70% and (2) ≥20 arousals/h, (3) CPAP titration aborted, or (4) low probability of CPAP compliance by judgment of physician. EC: Uncontrolled medical/psychiatric d/o; prior CPAP or bi-level use; respiratory failure/insufficiency; ENT surgery <3 Mos prior; other untreated sleep d/o; shift workers; history of alcohol/drug abuse; hypnotic use for <3 Mos; PLM arousal index ≥10	N = 48 (26/22). Withdrew: 1/1. Age: 54.1 ± 12.5/56.6 ± 9.8. Sex (%M): 81/73. AHI: 41.1 ± 22.5/39.4 ± 24.5. Desaturation: NR. No significant differences between arms in sex, age, education, neck circumference, nicotine/alcohol use, ESS, FSS, and global FOSQ. Sign difference in BMI 34.9 ± 6.5/31 ± 4.4	≥4 h/night	Average number of h of PAP use, per night, by inbuilt clock counter in CPAP or bi-level PAP machine. Others: ESS score, FSS score, global FOSQ	Proportion arm compliant. Avg use/night. % nights >4 h use. No difference in adherence between auto-bi-level and CPAP. Both arms' improvements in functional outcomes, sleepiness, and fatigue	Proportion arm compliant/avg. use/night/% nights >4 h use. Days 1–30: Bi-level CPAP: 73%/293.2 min ± 107.1/66%. CPAP: 59%/265.4 min ± 128.1/59.3%. Days 1–90: Bi-level CPAP: 62%/284.7 min ± 110.9/63.8%. CPAP: 55%/255.1 min ± 116.9/56.9%. ESS BS/day 30/day 90 Bi-level CPAP: 9.7 ± 3.9/8.2 ± 3.2/8.1 ± 3.8. CPAP: 8.2 ± 4.6/6.6 ± 4.6/6.9 ± 4.4. FSS BS/day 30/day 90 Bi-level CPAP: 4.6 ± 1.4/4.0 ± 1.2/3.7 ± 0.9. CPAP: 3.9 ± 1.0/3.7 ± 1.2/3.4 ± 1.2. Global FOSQ BS/day 30/day 90 Bi-level CPAP: 84 ± 20.9/97.5 ± 13.8/100 ± 11.3. CPAP: 91.4 ± 17.3/96.6 ± 16.6/100.1 ± 15.4	?/+/+/+ Urn randomization. Blinding: The participant, investigator, respiratory therapist, and research staff were blinded to therapy arm. Analysis based on an intent-to-treat basis
Humidification Worsnop et al. (2010), Australia	Intervention arm 1: a fisher and Paykel HC 201 CPAP pump (fisher and Paykel healthcare, Auckland, New Zealand). Control arm: HC 201 pump with the heater disabled and with no water in the chamber. Assessments at 1, 2, 4, 8, and 12 weeks	Randomized, parallel group design. IC: Aged between 30 and 80 years with a diagnosis of OSAS without regarding nose or throat complaints. EC: Development of nasal symptoms prior to trial	N = 55 (25/29). Withdrew = 0 (excluded 1, no OSA). Age: 55 ± 11/55 ± 12. Sex (%M): 84/76. AHI: 42.0 ± 23/50 ± 20. Desaturation (min): NR	NR	Adherence (h/day). Others: Nasal symptoms ESS, FOSQ, SF-36. Nasal resistance	No significant difference between arms at 1, 2, 4, 8, or 12 weeks. Intervention arm: Less blocked nose, sneezing, dry nose, stuffy nose, and a dry mouth. More satisfaction. Less pump noise versus control arm. No difference in ESS, FOSQ, and SF-36	Adherence: Intervention arm: 4.7 ± 2.4. Control arm: 4.5 ± 2.2. ESS: Intervention arm: 4.9 ± 3.6. Control arm: 5.4 ± 4.6. SF-36: Intervention arm: 76.0 ± 16.0. Control arm: 71.5 ± 19.7. Change in Rn (cmH2O/L/s) Intervention arm: 1 ± 3.8. Control arm: 2.2 ± 4.1	?/?/–/? Randomization, procedure NR; crossover design. Blinding: No. NR

Study/Population	Intervention	Sample	Threshold	Outcome measures	Results	Risk of bias
Ruhle et al., (2011), Germany. Patients with a diagnosis of OSAS without regarding nose or throat complaints	Intervention arm: Heated breathing tube humidifier (cHH). Control arm: Conventional CPAP. Assessments at 4 and 8 weeks	Prospective randomized crossover study. IC: Aged between 30 and 80 years with a diagnosis of OSAS without regarding nose or throat complaints. EC: >5 central apneas per hour of sleep, acute infection, heart failure of New York heart association classes three and four, acute pulmonary embolism, or acute coronary syndrome. $N = 44$. Withdrew = 0. Age: 51.5 ± 12.6. Sex (%M): 88.6. AHI: 43.0 ± 28.1. Desaturation (min): 81.7 ± 7.0	≥4 h/night	Average number of h of PAP use, per night, taken from devices. Others: Sleep quality (by sleep architecture). Quality of life. Side effects	At 4 weeks: Intervention versus control arm: 4.5 ± 3.0 h to 4.7 ± 3.0 h. At 8 weeks: NR. Average during the 4 weeks increased in the CPAP with cHH vs CPAP, from 4.5 ± 3.0 h to 4.7 ± 3.0 h; difference not statistically significant. Sleep quality: No significant difference between the two treatment arms. Quality of life: No significant difference between the two treatment arms. Side effects: Complaints about mouth and throat side effects lower under treatment with cHH vs without. More favorable ratings of humidity of the delivered air with ES = 0.82, followed by quality of sleep (ES = 0.67), temperature of inhaled air (ES = 0.67), dry mouth (ES = 0.64), and cold sensation in the face (ES = 0.58)	?/+/?/? Crossover randomization. Others: NR

Mixture of educational, behavioral, and affective strategies

Study/Population	Intervention	Sample	Threshold	Outcome measures	Results	Risk of bias
Aloia et al. (2013), Sleep Disorders Center of Lifespan Hospitals/ USA. Adult persons with OSA naïve to PAP therapy	Intervention arms: MET (motivational enhancement therapy): a tailored intervention providing personalized feedback using pt-centered counseling. ED (education): A didactic information about OSA and benefits of PAP. SC (standard care): a complete medical care model allowing continued interaction with physicians/ healthcare professionals, but not including counseling time. MET and ED arms each received two, 45-min, face-to-face individual counseling sessions by a trained nurse 1 week (7 ± 2 days) and 2 weeks (14 ± 2 days) after initiating PAP. 12 Mos (assessments at 3, 6, and 12 Mos)	Randomized clinical trial. IC: Moderate-severe OSA (AHI >15). EC: OSA by split-night Polysomnography, severe neurological condition or unstable psychiatric illness, a sleep disorder other than OSA (including primary central sleep apnea), congestive heart failure, and end-stage renal disease. 1:1:1 ratio (MET, ED, or SC) balancing for age, sex, education, apnea severity, and ESS score. $N = 227$ (SC74/ED80/MET73). Withdrew throughout (excluded) = SC25/ED27/MET26. Age: $52.4 \pm 11.8/47.0 \pm 11.4/51.7 \pm 10.0$ (sign diff). AHI: $48.2 \pm 26.2/46.1 \pm 23.2/45.7 \pm 23.8$. Desaturation (% < 90, diagnostic night): $27.1 \pm 28.5/25.8 \pm 28.5/24.0 \pm 26.2$. Sex (%M): 77/60/62 (borderline diff)	4 h/night	Total h, average h, separate use events/day (CPAP machine reading). Others: Decisional balance. Self-efficacy	Adherence 1/2/3/6/12mos. SC: $3.82 \pm 2.27/3.68 \pm 2.37/3.65 \pm 2.36/3.73 \pm 2.50$. ED: $4.43 \pm 2.51/4.48 \pm 2.48/4.48 \pm 2.50/4.34 \pm 2.45$. MET: $4.26 \pm 2.27/4.37 \pm 2.34/4.34 \pm 2.35/43.86 \pm 2.61$. Decisional balance BS/3/6/12mos. SC: $47.11 \pm 6.02/45.51 \pm 7.67/45.51 \pm 7.90/45.08 \pm 10.55$. ED: $46.32 \pm 5.70/46.33 \pm 7.69/46.66 \pm 9.14/45.67 \pm 8.38$. MET: $45.28 \pm 6.94/46.13 \pm 6.23/45.91 \pm 6.95/46.61 \pm 7.47$. Self-efficacy BS/3/6/12mos. SC: $20.96 \pm 2.88/20.61 \pm 4.49/21.00 \pm 5.06/19.83 \pm 6.29$. ED: $21.11 \pm 3.21/21.05 \pm 4.50/21.04 \pm 5.03/20.98 \pm 5.19$. MET: $20.63 \pm 3.26/22.48 \pm 3.08/20.96 \pm 4.23/21.25 \pm 4.84$. Adherence declined over time for all three arms. Significant interaction between level of adherence during first week of treatment and treatment arm. MET: Moderate levels of adherence during first week of PAP – More likely to adhere to treatment at f/u. ED: Persons with high levels of adherence during their first week of PAP were more likely to adhere to treatment at f/u. MET increased perception of positive aspects of PAP, but ED did not	+/–/+/– Urn randomized balancing for age, sex, education, apnea severity, and ESS. Clinician's blinding: Yes (to study participation). Pt blinding: Yes (to study condition); were informed that PAP machine would be accessed periodically to determine how the device was working. Highly nonsignificant terms were dropped from the final model to simplify the model

(continued)

Table 2.2 (continued)

Author (year), country, setting/population	Intervention content / Control content / Duration of intervention	Study design / Inclusion/exclusion criteria (IC/EC)	Sample size N (T/C) / Age, years / Sex (%M) / AHI / Desaturation / Withdrew / Age, sex (M/F) / Comparable by	Adherence definition	Outcome measures	Results	Benefits / Effect size	Risk of bias assessment: sequence generation/concealment/blinding/outcome data
Bakker et al. (2016), outpatient cardiology, diabetes, and sleep clinics/USA. Pts with moderate or severe OSA with either established cardiovascular disease (CVD) or at risk for CVD who were willing to continue with CPAP after 14 days of use	Intervention arms: CPAP + ME (motivational enhancement): Behavioral intervention devised on principles of motivational Interviewing. Control arm: CPAP only. Up to 12 months	Open-label, parallel arm, randomized controlled trial of CPAP only or CPAP + ME. IC: OSA (AHI >10; 45 to 75 years with established CVD or cardiometabolic disease, prior myocardial infarction, coronary artery revascularization procedure, ischemic stroke, or diabetes or 55 to 75 years with at least three CVD risk factors (male sex, BMI >30 kg/m², hypertension, dyslipidemia, and >10 pack-years of smoking). EC: ESS score >14 of 24, drowsy driving, commercial driving, or an uncontrolled medical condition	$N = 83$ (41/42). Withdrew = 3/2. Age: 63.8 ± 8.3/63.9 ± 7.4. AHI: 23.7 (15.9, 31.4)/21.8 (17.4, 31.0). Desaturation (% <90, diagnostic night): 3.7 (0.6, 12.3)/2.8 (0.5, 10.4). Sex (%M): 66.7/65.9	4 h/night	Average adherence across this time. The estimated difference in CPAP adherence between arms was 80. Change in CPAP adherence over time. Others: Sleep duration	Difference in adherence of 1.5 h/night (3.3 vs 4.4 h/night on average in CPAP-only and CPAP + ME arms at 6 Mos. Adherence worsened over time in both arms. Others: No significant difference in sleep duration, either over time within arms or on average between arms	Average adherence across time was 3.3 ± 2.7 and 4.4 ± 2.9 h/night in CPAP only and CPAP + ME, respectively. The estimated difference in CPAP adherence between arms was 80 minutes (95% CI, 5.0–15.2; $p = 0.04$), favoring the CPAP + ME arm; when adjusted for randomization factors, estimated difference was 99 minutes (95% CI, 33.0–164.9; $p = 0.003$). Median slope in CPAP-only and CPAP+ME arms were – 0.4 min/night (interquartile range, –22.5 to 4.9) and – 1.8 min/night (–19.5 to 1.7), respectively	+/+/+/+. Randomization was performed using a data entry system linked to an offsite server holding sequences. Randomization. In a 1:1 ratio with a block size of 4 (full night or split night with titration), site, CVD status (established or risk factors). Research assistance blinding: Yes. Statisticians: Not blinded. Others: NR
Bartlett et al. (2013), three geographically distinct clinics in Sydney, New South Wales/Australia. Pts with moderate or severe OSA and referral for a CPAP titration study	Intervention arms: Social cognitive therapy (SCT): To increase perceived self-efficacy, outcome expectations, and social support. Social interaction (SI): To ensure equal time was spent with all participants (afternoon tea (20 min) including biscuits (cookies) and decaffeinated tea and coffee +15-min CPAP educational video). Assessments at 7 nights and then 1, 3, and 6 Mos	Open-label, parallel arm, randomized controlled trial of SCT or SI. IC: OSA (AHI >10; 45 to 75 years with CVD or cardiometabolic disease, prior myocardial infarction, coronary artery revascularization procedure, ischemic stroke, or diabetes or 55 to 75 years with at least three CVD risk factors (male sex, BMI >30 kg/m², hypertension, dyslipidemia, and >10 pack-years of smoking. EC: English language barriers and any previous use of CPAP	$N = 206$ (109/97). Withdrew before 6-month visit = 10/19. Age: 46.8 ± 14.3/49.3 ± 12.3. AHI: 30.4 ± 28/39.9 ± 25.1. Desaturation: NR. Sex (%M): 70/70. No differences. In sex, education, presence of a bed partner, BMI, ESS, or any psychological factors	An average of 4 h or greater/night	Average adherence at 6 Mos. % adherent. Self-efficacy. ESS, FOSQ, DASS, FSS, PSQI, social support, outcome expectancy	No differences in CPAP adherence between arms at each of f/u- points. No difference between arms in ESS, FOSQ, DASS subscales, FSS, PSQI, social support, self-efficacy, and outcome expectancy	At 6 Mos, 54.6% were adherent in SI as compared with 47.2% in the SCT arm (difference (SCT-SI): –7.4 (22.1 to 7.2), p = 0.4). At 6 Mos, 33% in SI arm were using CPAP for ≥6 h a night, as opposed to 20.4% in SCT arm ($p = 0.06$). Higher self-efficacy (OR 2.7 per unit increase score, 95% CI 1.7–4.3, $P < 0.0001$) associated with treatment adherence at 6 Mos; neither intervention increased self-efficacy score at 6 Mos	+/+/+/+. Randomization was performed using a data entry system linked to an offsite server holding sequences. Randomization. In a 1:1 ratio with a random permuted block. Psychologist and staff administering intervention blinding: No. Other staff members' blinding: Yes. The analysis was by intention to treat

Lai et al. (2014), Sleep Disorders Centre/China Chinese pts. with newly diagnosed OSA naïve to CPAP therapy	Randomized controlled parallel arm clinical trial. Intervention arms: Brief motivational enhancement education (MEE) program standard care: 25-min video, a 20-min pt-centered interview, and a 10-min telephone f/u. Standard care (SC): Education by nurses +15-min talk to introduce basic operation of CPAP device and titration procedure + further advice (about 15 min) on the importance of CPAP therapy and care of accessories + telephone f/u at day 1 and Day3. Assessments at 1 week, 1 month, 3 Mos of f/u	IC: (1) age ≥ 18 years old with newly diagnosed OSA (apnea-hypopnea index [AHI] ≥ 5). (2) receiving in-laboratory auto-CPAP titration for the first time, and (3) no prior OSA or CPAP education classes. EC: CSA, PLMD, COPD, pregnancy, psychiatric illness on treatment, cognitive impairment, illiteracy, unstable health conditions such as end-stage renal failure on renal replacement therapy, malignancy currently on radiotherapy or chemotherapy, or dependence in daily care	N = 100 (51/49) Withdrew = 1/1 Age: 53 ± 10/51 ± 10 AHI: 30.4 ± 28/39.9 ± 25.1 Desaturation (duration of oxygen saturation < 90%, min): 21.8 (8.7, 69.8)/22.1 (5.4, 84.9) Sex (%M): 84/82 No differences In age, smoking/drinking history, education, presence of a bed partner, marital status, referral source, family members involved, CPAP level, ESS, arousal index, and other factors	At least 4 h/day	Mean daily usage, proportion of CPAP adherent, usage index, intention to use CPAP Risk perception, outcome expectations, treatment self-efficacy, improvement in daytime sleepiness	Between-arm difference estimate (95% CI), p-value Better CPAP use (higher daily CPAP usage by 2 h/d, a fourfold increase in number using CPAP for ≥70% of days with ≥4 h/d [$p < 0.001$]) and greater improvements in daytime sleepiness by 2.2 ESS units and treatment self-efficacy by 0.2 units compared with control arm	Between-arm difference estimate (95% CI), p-value Mean daily usage: 2.0 (1.3, 2.8), $p < 0.001$ Proportion of CPAP adherent: OR, 4.3 (2.0, 9.0), $p < 0.001$ Usage index, %: 31 (19, 43) Intention to use CPAP, %: 31 (20, 42), $p < 0.001$	+/+/−/? Randomization sequence was created using a computer-generated randomization program Randomization was stratified into three severity arms by AHI severity and with 1:1 allocation using a block size of 6 Blinding: No Others: NR
Lo Bue et al. (2014), Sleep Disorders Centre/Italy Pts with newly diagnosed OSA naïve to CPAP therapy	Randomized, controlled Design. Intervention arm: With support (telephone interview first week and 30th day) reinforcing interventions, consisting of motivational reinforcement and technical support in the first month of therapy. Control arm: Without support. Assessments at first, second, and third month and at second, third, and fourth quarter	IC: (1) age ≥ 18 years old with newly diagnosed OSA, consecutive. EC: Neuromuscular disease, unstable psychiatric disease or cognitive impairment, myocardial infarction, unstable angina, cardiac failure, cerebrovascular accident, lung disease with awake resting oxygen saturation of <90%	N = 40 (20/20) Withdrew = 1/2 Age: 58.55 ± 13.2/55.65 ± 8.25 AHI: 44.05 ± 16.90/44.45 ± 25.18 Desaturation (% of oxygen saturation < 90%): 20.88 ± 15.22/20.77 ± 22.03 Sex (%M): 68% No differences In age, AHI, BMI, ESS, and duration of desaturation	≥4 h/day	Mean daily usage Others: ESS	Month 1: Pts of the intervention arm showed a higher number of nights with a device use ≥4 h The difference in adherence became nonsignificant at the second and third month and at second, third, and fourth quarter ESS was lower at third, sixth, and 12th month than at BS in both arms, with no significant differences between arms	Month 1: 23.2 days in intervention arm vs 16.0 for control arm, $p = 0.022$ Treatment adherence: 77.5% in intervention arm and 55.7% in control Year 1: Mean 4.3 h/night vs 3.8 h/night and median 5.1 h/night vs 4.5 h/night – No sign difference	?/?/?/? Randomization procedure NR Blinding: NR Others: NR

(continued)

Table 2.2 (continued)

Author (year), country, setting/population	Intervention content Control content Duration of intervention	Study design Inclusion/exclusion criteria (IC/EC)	Sample size N (T/C) Age, years Sex (%M) AHI Desaturation Withdrew Comparable by	Adherence definition	Outcome measures	Results	Benefits Effect size	Risk of bias assessment: sequence generation/concealment/blinding/ outcome data
Olsen et al. (2011), Sleep Disorders Centre/ Australia Pts with newly diagnosed OSA naïve to CPAP therapy	Intervention arm: Motivational interview nurse therapy [MINT] *Motivational Enhancement Therapy Manual* developed by Miller and colleagues (Miller, Zweben, DiClemente, & Rychtarik, 1995) Sessions 1 (building motivation for change) and 2 (strengthening commitment to change) appr. 30 min (maximum 45 min) and Session 3 (booster session) approximately 20 min (maximum 30 min) Control arm: Best practice standard care (one-on-one 45-min education session conducted on the day of CPAP titration study) + questionnaire assessing CPAP-related difficulties 1 month after CPAP experience Assessments at 1-month, 2-month, 3-month, and 12-month f/us	Randomized, controlled design study IC: (1) age ≥ 18 years old with newly diagnosed OSA, consecutive EC: Neuromuscular disease, unstable psychiatric disease or cognitive impairment, myocardial infarction, unstable angina, cardiac failure, cerebrovascular accident, lung disease with awake resting oxygen saturation of <90%	$N = 106$ (53/53) Withdrew = 3/3 Age: $58.55 \pm 13.2/55.65 \pm 8.25$ AHI: $44.05 \pm 16.90/44.45 \pm 25.18$ Desaturation (% of oxygen saturation < 90%): $20.88 \pm 15.22/20.77 \pm 22.03$ Sex (%M): 69% No differences In age, AHI, BMI, and ESS MINT arm has 1.5 years more education than control arm	≥4 h/day	CPAP acceptance CPAP adherence (mean number of h of CPAP use/ night) Self-efficacy measure for sleep Apnea FOSQ Satisfaction with therapy and therapist scale–revised Behavior change Counseling index ESS	CPAP acceptance MINT versus control Rejection at 3 Mos: 6% rejection versus 28% rejection rate Rejection at 12 Mos: 4% rejection versus 26% rejection rate CPAP adherence at 3 Mos: MINT arm used CPAP significantly more h/night than control arm at all of the f/u time points up to 3-month post-treatment Initiation CPAP adherence at 12 Mos: Difference between arms marginally not significant	Adherence effect size (Cohen's d, p-value) Adherence (h/night), 1 month: 0.59, $p = 0.03$ Adherence (h/night), 2 Mos: 0.56, $p = 0.005$ Adherence (h/night), 3 Mos: 0.55, $p = 0.005$ Adherence (h/night), 12 Mos: 0.38, $p = 0.061$ Self-efficacy: MINT greater self-efficacy than control arm Risk perception: a reduction in risk perception between time 1 and 3-month f/u Perception of severity: Better functioning by 3-month f/u in MINT ESS: Difference between time 1 and time 2 nonsignificant	$-/+/?/+$ No blocking or stratification of randomization was used Randomization procedure random; no blocking or stratification of randomization Blinding: Officer, yes; patients, no; statistician, NR The adherence analyses were by intent-to-treat

Pengo et al. (2017), Sleep Disorders Centre at Guy's & St. Thomas' Hospitals/UK Consecutive pts. with newly diagnosed OSA naïve to CPAP therapy	Random allocation to one of the three arms: 1. Positively framed messages in addition to CPAP. 2. Received negatively framed messages in addition to CPAP. 3. Control: Best standard care with CPAP, but no framed messages. Assessments at 2- and 6-week f/u	Randomized, controlled design IC: Pts. with a 4% ODI ≥5/hour and typical symptoms of sleep apnea ESS >10 points or a 4% ODI > 15/hour EC: Mental or physical disability The three arms were matched for age, sex, and BMI	N = 112 (36/37/39) Withdrew = 4/6/5 Age: 46.7 ± 12.2/47.1 ± 11.7/53.5 ± 12.5 AHI: 44.05 ± 16.90/44.45 ± 25.18 Desaturation (% of oxygen saturation < 90%): 20.88 ± 15.22/20.77 ± 22.03 Sex (%M): 69/76/80 No differences in age, sex, ethnicity, ODI, BMI, pulse rise index, and nocturnal average pulse rate	≥4 h/day	Compliance, daily usage, and adherence data at 2- and 6-week f/u ESS	Week 2: Number of days of CPAP usage for >4 h was significantly higher in positively framed arms when compared with both negative framing arm and control arm Week 6: No differences between arms ESS beneficial response, no difference between arms	Week 2: % days for >4 h use – 51.6 ± 33.1/34.8 ± 33.3/35.2 ± 34.4 CPAP average daily usage: 3.7 ± 2.3/2.5 ± 2.1/2.8 ± 2.4 Week 6: % days for >4 h use – 45.7 ± 30.5/46.1 ± 32.5/50.1 ± 34.2 CPAP average daily usage: 3.5 ± 2.7/2.6 ± 2.3/3.1 ± 2.7 ESS BS 11.0 ± 6.0 vs ESS at 2 weeks 9.2 ± 5.9 points	?/?/?/?? Randomization procedure NR (note: Pts. were randomly assigned to one of the three groups) Blinding: NR Others: NR

Abbreviations: *AHI* apnea-hypopnea index, *BMI* body mass index, *BS* baseline, *CBT* cognitive-behavioral therapy, *CSA* central sleep apnea, *EDS* excessive daytime sleepiness, *ESS* Epworth sleepiness scale, *f/u* follow-up, *FSS* fatigue severity scale, *FOSQ* Functional Outcomes of Sleep Questionnaire, *h* hours, *IQR* interquartile range, *ISI* insomnia severity index, *ODI* oxygen desaturation index, *OSA* obstructive sleep apnea, *OSAS* obstructive sleep apnea syndrome, *mos* months, *NPSG* nocturnal polysomnography, *NA* not applicable, *NR* not reported, *NS* not significant, *pts.* patients, *PLMD* periodic limb movement disorder, *PSQI* Pittsburgh sleep quality index, *RDI* respiratory disturbance index, *SDB* sleep-disordered breathing

mation available to determine the extent to which studies were at risk of bias from these sources. In several studies [36, 43, 44, 47, 55], investigators attempted to blind participants to study the condition that they received. For three studies [33, 41, 44], participants would have been explicitly aware that machine usage data were assessed by study investigators; the remainder of the studies did not report how this feature of study design was addressed. In several studies [31, 32, 39, 46–49], data from all participants were collected and analyzed. Only incomplete data were available for the primary outcome in several studies [33, 34, 36, 43–45, 50, 52, 55]. For the remaining studies, it was not possible to ascertain how the intention to treat populations was composed. There was a high attrition rate in both arms (i.e., dietary self-monitoring and attention control) in one study [52], which may have affected the estimates for average machine usage.

2.2.2 Study Size and Study Characteristics

The sample size varied widely from 28 [54] to 330 patients [35]. The studies had an average sample size of 128 patients before randomization, with a male patient averaging 69% (26–100% range). None of the studies considered the effect of sex/gender on adherence to CPAP [58]. Two studies did not specify the male-to-female patient ratio [33, 37] and were not included in the calculation. Two studies included only male patients [46, 48]. All studies involved adult or elderly patients; the age ranged from 30 to >80 years; the most represented were patients within 50 to 60 years of age. Sufficient information about patients' apnea-hypopnea index (AHI) was provided in all but two studies [37, 52].

2.2.3 Study Design

Comparisons within randomized control trial studies were often complex. Nine studies [30, 34, 43–45, 47–50] reported results evaluating the effects of a single intervention in comparison to usual care, where the protocol for the usual care procedures varied from study to study. Thirteen studies [30, 36, 38, 40–42, 44, 51–55] evaluated two different interventions, and four studies reported differences between intervention and no intervention [31, 32, 35, 37]. Two studies evaluated three different interventions [34, 44], and two presented an analysis of four different interventions [39, 46].

2.2.4 Country of Study Origin and Setting

The studies were conducted in a variety of sociocultural regions of the world, with ten occurring in the United States

[33, 36–38, 40, 44, 48, 51, 52, 55], the remainder by country being Australia [32, 35, 41, 43], China [30, 39, 47], France [49, 53], the United Kingdom [34, 54], Belgium [50], Germany [31], Canada [45], Italy [42], and Brazil [46].

2.2.5 Diagnoses

The studies represented patients with a variety of sleep-related breathing disorders and disorder severities [30–55]. One study [54] evaluated different types of interventions in patients with suboptimal CPAP adherence (defined as <4 h/night) and one [55] in patients with suboptimal facility-based attended CPAP titration; the rest tested which intervention resulted in better adherence in naïve patients or recently prescribed CPAP. Three of the included studies aimed at improving CPAP adherence in patients with cardiovascular disease risk [40, 49] and history of stroke [45] as a means to prevent adverse clinical course of these disorders due to comorbid OSA. One study evaluated CPAP adherence in response to weight reduction in patients with obesity [52].

2.2.6 Intervention Strategies

Interventions were grouped into broad categories, reflecting differences in the predominant theoretical focus or target of the intervention. The primary groupings directed toward patients were (1) educational, (2) behavioral and affective, (3) a mixture on these components, (4) surgical interventions, and (5) myofunctional therapy. The primary groupings directed toward technology were (1) additions of a heated humidification, (2) use of auto-titrating or pressure relief machines, and (3) changing types of masks to prevent leakage. No interventions were identified as directed toward clinician/staff knowledge, attitudes, or skills to detect patients at risk of nonadherence and develop individualized interventions to enhance CPAP use in these patients.

2.3 Patient-Directed Interventions

2.3.1 Education

This component of interventions generally reflected pedagogical interventions, verbal or written, with a knowledge-based emphasis designed to convey information on OSA and/or health consequences associated with untreated OSA. All these interventions were personalized, applying patient-specific data during intervention sessions in person in the clinician's office or in the community.

2.3.2 Interventions Directed toward Patient Behavior and Affective State

Behaviorally focused interventions were designed to enhance adherence to CPAP by reinforcing specific behavioral patterns of continuous CPAP use. These included strategies such as motivational enhancements [30], "reinforcing interventions" [42], remote monitoring and motivation [49], telemedicine [50], interactive voice response systems, and telephone reminders [38].

Affect-focused strategies attempted to influence compliance through appeals to (1) patients' feelings and emotions showing them results of diagnostic and treatment studies [33, 35–37] or (2) social relationships and social supports, by bringing family members and social support [30, 41] or male peer coaches [48] to influence the patients' affective state toward CPAP adherence. The results of one study relating staff communication to patient outcomes [34] reported that more positive talk predicted higher patient adherence at 2 and 6 weeks of therapy as compared to negative talk and no framed messages.

2.3.3 Surgical Modification of Patients' Upper Airway and Myofunctional Therapy

The surgical modification in patients who had difficulty tolerating CPAPs [51] and myofunctional therapy [46], which increases tongue, pharynx, and soft palate muscle tone, through isometric exercises (working with muscle tension) and isotonic exercises (improving mobility) was among patient-directed strategies directed at improving patients' adherence to CPAP. These interventions were based on the premise that surgical correction of the upper airway and strengthening of the muscular rings at the level of the oropharynx will result in reducing the required level of CPAP pressure and thereby increasing adherence to CPAP therapy.

2.4 Technology-Targeted Interventions

Several clinical trials were directed toward comparisons of the efficacy of technology-directed interventions on patients' adherence to CPAP. These interventions were either testing the (1) type of machine (continuous pressure versus bi-level) [54, 55], (2) type of mask on patients' adherence to CPAP [53], or (3) application of humidifier [31, 32].

2.4.1 Auto-Titrating or Pressure Relief Machines

CPAP pressure modifications such as auto-adjusting pressure may promote comfort and, therefore, adherence. In contrast to standard CPAP, in which the applied pressure is constant throughout the sleep period and stages of sleep, APAP devices provide variable pressure matching to breathing patterns of the patient transitioning through different stages of sleep in different body positions. If obstructive events are detected, the device will increase pressure until the events are eliminated. The device will decrease the applied pressure if no events are detected over a set period. Because the minimum pressure required to keep the airway open is used, the mean pressure applied across the night should be reduced when compared to CPAP. It has been hypothesized that this reduction in mean applied pressure may improve patient comfort and therefore tolerance, resulting in improved nightly adherence with the use of APAP compared to CPAP.

2.4.2 Types of Masks

A range of interface options for delivering positive pressure therapy exists, including nasal pillows, nasal masks, oronasal masks, and custom-made interfaces. One clinical trial [53] compared the impact of different nasal masks on CPAP adherence in patients with newly diagnosed OSA. Initial mask selection that produces minimal side effects associated with inadequate mask fit (i.e., eye irritation, silicone allergies, pain or abrasion to the bridge of the nose, pressure sores, and air leaks) enhanced tolerability of therapy and therefore adherence to CPAP.

2.4.3 Humidifier

It was hypothesized that air humidification may reduce side effects associated with CPAP therapy, such as dry mouth, throat, or nose, resulting from a unidirectional airflow. Two types of humidity that were used in the clinical trials included in this review were cold passover humidity [32] and heated humidity [31]. The hypothesized mechanism of improvement in adherence was believed to be a result of an increase in patient comfort by preventing the increase in mucosal blood flux.

2.5 Duration of Follow-Up Period

Enhancing CPAP adherence may be short-lived, with many patients reverting to previously established sleep routines (i.e., drift in patient behavior), once the stimulus for a new intervention is no longer present. The average duration of follow-up time for assessing the outcomes of interventions was 5.2 months across studies. Several studies with the longest follow-up (6–12 months) reported that adherence to CPAP worsened over time in the interventions and control groups [41, 44]; however, others did not observe this phenomenon [38, 47, 49]. Several clinical trials with the longest follow-up duration (6–12 months) [38, 43, 47, 49, 50] reported statistically significant differences in CPAP adherence between intervention(s) and control group(s); two [43, 44] observed no difference.

2.6 Adherence Measures and Outcomes

Definition of adherence, measured by a ventilator timer recorder, varied from study to study included in this review, as reflected in Table 2.1. Most studies defined adherence to CPAP as 4 or more hours of use per night or on average over the study period [30, 34, 35, 37, 38, 40, 42–44, 47–50, 52, 54, 55]; others added a condition of at least 9 of each of the 14 nights of ventilator use or more than 70% of the nights [33, 39, 46, 51, 53], which is based on the American Association of Sleep Disorder standards for CPAP use.

Although many different approaches to the study of adherence were used (Table 2.2) and minimal clinically relevant changes have not been established, some conclusions about the relative effectiveness of interventions can be drawn by examining Table 2.2. Adherence-concerning measures were more strongly affected by behavioral interventions than educational ones. More specifically, it appears that motivational enhancement [30], remote monitoring and reinforcement, telemedicine, and telephone reminders [42, 43, 49, 50] were especially effective at the early stages of intervention as compared to usual care but diminished its effectiveness with time [42, 43]. An educational intervention alone [45] had a relatively weaker impact than educational efforts in combination with components targeting patients' affect state by motivation [44, 47, 48]. The way in which motivational enhancement coming from clinicians or the "peer buddy system" had an effect on the outcome was linked to the perception of positive aspects in enhancing utilization [44] and through promoting self-efficacy, outcome expectancies, improving risk perception, and patient activation [48].

Myofascial therapy [46] and education in combination with muscle relaxation [39] were more effective than usual care for up to 3 months of follow-up. Dietary self-monitoring directed toward weight loss [52], pillar implants [51], and additions of humidifiers [31, 32] were not more effective than usual care in enhancing adherence to CPAP therapy.

The adherence-related indicators broadly represent five classes of assessments: (1) health and functional outcomes (e.g., depression, anxiety, sleepiness, fatigue, functional status, etc.), (2) direct indicators (e.g., weight loss, biological markers, etc.), (3) indirect indicators (e.g., self-efficacy, symptom load, quality of life, etc.), (4) person and significant other satisfaction reports, and (5) performance (driving behavior). Several studies have also reported changes in

patients' satisfaction with therapy and therapists, behavioral change scores, knowledge acquisition, and weight loss, as a consequence of adherence-directed interventions. Studies used between one and ten different outcome measures in their assessment of the intervention effect (Table 2.1). Two studies [33, 50] did not investigate the implications of their interventions.

2.7 Intervention Benefits Toward Health and Functional Outcomes

Different thresholds of interventions based on the probabilities of health and functional benefits were considered in intervention studies directed on CPAP adherence included in this review. The majority of studies reported no differences between intervention and control arms at the last follow-up in such outcomes as daytime sleepiness [32, 34, 36, 41, 42, 45–47, 51, 55]; sleep duration [40]; sleep quality [41]; vigilance [48]; fatigue [41, 55]; quality of life [31, 36, 41, 47]; knowledge acquisition [45]; functional outcomes [45, 48, 55]; self-efficacy [41, 48 except 30]; patient activation [48]; care satisfaction [43]; number of non-scheduled phone calls [35]; side effect associated with CPAP use [31, 32, 36]; snoring elimination [46]; proportion of patients with a first-line mask-related contact call and call duration [53]; self-measured evening systolic blood pressure [49]; steps taken per day [49]; biological parameters (low-density lipoprotein, cholesterol) [49]; and body mass index [49]. Few studies have reported differences between intervention and control arms in scores of daytime sleepiness [30, 39, 49]; anxiety, depression, and sleep quality [39]; nasal mask issue-related home care personnel visits [54]; and perception of positive aspects of PAP [31, 44].

The excess cost and efforts of an intervention (including time and effort of staff working to enhance patient adherence to CPAP over time) in reference to the usual care were not reported or discussed in the studies included in this review, a significant omission, since most interventions conferred no difference between intervention and control arms in measured health and functional outcomes.

2.8 Discussion

This chapter intended to provide an overview of the effects of interventions on measurements of CPAP machine usage, drawn from most recent randomized controlled trials. Although many studies have indicated significant beneficial effects of different types of interventions on CPAP usage versus usual care at the early stages of interventions, the effects were often not sustainable with time. The clinical and practical relevance of these results was not clear considering the frequent lack of statistically significant differences between intervention and usual care arms in terms of adherence-related outcomes relevant to patients and clinicians. Finally, studies generally recruited CPAP-naïve or recently diagnosed patients with moderate to severe OSA; patients with OSA and a significant comorbidity, to whom adherence-related concerns are of critical importance in terms of health and functional consequences of poorly managed OSA, were frequently excluded from clinical trials. While recognizing that the summary results of this evidence synthesis may not be accurate given the unknown risk of bias in most of the trials, it is interesting that there is consistently a lack of evidence, in general, that intervention improves patient outcomes better than usual care. Costs associated with intervention were not discussed yet may well have occurred to be much greater than usual care. Cost-effectiveness research in patients who are believed to be at risk of poor adherence (i.e., added vulnerability at multiple levels) may help to establish how resources should best be allocated and to whom, in implementing interventions' results into a clinical decision support system [61–63].

Inspection of the content of focus of the interventions demonstrated that the more comprehensive and personalized the program and support throughout, the stronger the outcome. Combined focus interventions were generally more effective than those with a single focus, especially education. Three-focus interventions, including those with educational, behavioral, and affective components, were the strongest of the combined focus programs, although used in only a few studies [30, 34, 40, 42–44]. A more detailed inspection of individualized intervention strategies showed that written materials were weaker than interventions [36] and that home visits [35] were not any more effective in improving adherence than remote monitoring and motivational enhancement communicated through telemedicine [49, 50]. Considering the resource-intensive nature of home visits relative to telemedicine, the latter may be considered as a more attractive alternative in the light of the COVID-19 epidemic. The effects of peer buddy interventions on patient adherence showed borderline beneficial effects on the average nightly use as well as percent of adherence at 3 months after therapy initiation, in comparison to usual care [48].

There was little ability to assess the differential impact of interventions on various diagnostic groupings; most studies used chronic comorbidities in patients with OSA as their exclusion criteria. Notably, the health and direct effects of CPAP use in both intervention and control arms were evident for patients with cardiovascular disease or an elevated cardiovascular risk [40, 49] as well as for obese patients [52] and for patients with a history of stroke or transient ischemic attack [45]. Having summarized the effects of adherence-directed interventions, it is important to recognize that evaluation of effect magnitude is a relative matter, and one must

inquire about the practical meaning and usefulness of even a small increase in adherence – the clinical and practical significance of an effect size is not necessarily tied to the magnitude of effects. This notion has rarely been discussed in the discussion section of the RCT studies included in this chapter.

In reviewing the results of RCTs, one must consider whether all important potential effects of the intervention were measured. Any intervention studies may have unintended consequences. For example, attempts to increase CPAP adherence in a clinical setting in which many patients are not adherent (because of their own values and preferences, poor accessibility, unmet expectations, etc.) may result in a decline in patient-clinician trust and/or comfort. Unintended consequences may also include the effect of clinician/staff stigma toward the nonadherent patient, low motivation, and cohesiveness toward future care. Likewise, unintended consequences are related to resources (i.e., increased cost of additional intervention to treatment as usual, decreased resources allocated to other activities). Only five studies included in this review reported on the effect of the intervention on a number of nonscheduled phone calls [35], contact calls and visits for mask issue, second-line mask required, duration of visit related to first-line mask only [53], side effects interfering with CPAP use [32, 36], and care/therapist satisfaction [43, 53]; however, cost analyses were not performed to understand the monetary values associated with such outcomes.

We can draw three implications for future research from this review. First, the construct of CPAP adherence and nonadherence, as an outcome measure, should continue to be developed based on the proven effects of CPAP on multiple levels, including but not limited to morphological, biochemical, symptoms, disease, function, morbidity, and mortality [59, 60]. The significance of these different levels to each patient to whom CPAP is prescribed, a patient's attitude toward CPAP therapy, as an important determinant of adherence, has not been studied and as such remains unknown. Second, the results tend to support the view that patients' adherence does not tend to be static over time. This brings forth the question of how adherence to CPAP is defined and measured longitudinally in different patient populations and settings. Emphasis on within-individual variability, where each person serves as their own control over time, is likely to be the best technique to analyze true change in adherence in response to interventions and to answer the question of the extent to which a person's adherence to therapy is affected by disorder-related variables, which are internally (age, sex, genetic profile, etc.) or environmentally (social desirability, support, etc.) driven. The trade-off, however, is limited standardization of individual outcome measures, and irrelevance of the current theory of psychometric properties of clinical outcome measures, applicable only in single-case experimental design studies (relevant to personalized medicine theory) and limited external validity (i.e., generalizability). Finally, one of the problems associated with understanding and making progress in CPAP adherence is that it is a very complex construct, which denotes a wide variety of efforts on the part of a patient that is labor-intensive and intrusive to their established lives. Proper maintenance of the machine, mask, and tubes, and the bedroom environment, need to apply the therapy every time someone goes to sleep, learn how to deal with equipment malfunctions and need for recalibration, which are often time-consuming and costly, accepting side effects and clearly seen benefits, which are often not perceived as drastic, and deal with cultural and social desirability and image, are among the significant challenges that not every patient that requires CPAP is willing and able to overcome. Combined with the often unstructured and chaotic nature of many patients' lives, these challenges can undermine initiating and sustaining routines that promote patient adherence to CPAP (Fig. 2.3).

2.9   Future Direction

Judgments about the effect of existing interventions targeting CPAP utility are complex and subject to biases. Traditional RCT design was prone to selection bias, influencing the conclusion regarding both the effectiveness and generalizability of interventions as well as usual care. There are numerous patient characteristics, including those concerning sex and gender (i.e., the socially constructed characteristics of women and men (i.e., norms, behaviors, relations)), that were not considered but which most likely influenced the effectiveness of interventions, especially those directed at affect and behavior [63, 64]. The range of other relevant social characteristics (i.e., education, occupation, race/ethnicity, socioeconomic status, access to technical support when needed, etc.) are likely to interact with gender, skewing results of intervention effectiveness in either direction. Unfortunately, it remains unknown how gender and interacting social variables might influence the response

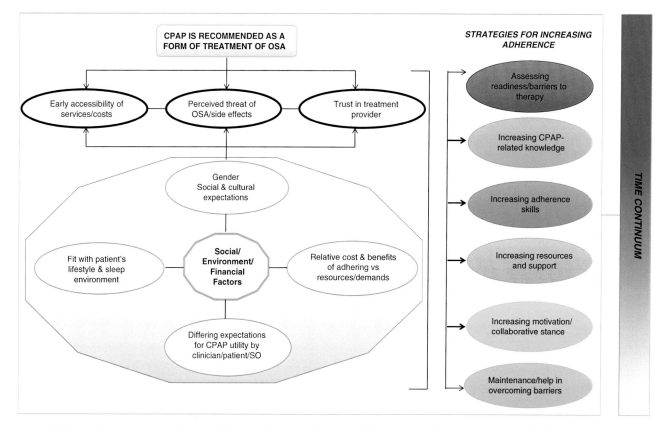

Fig. 2.3 Schematic representation of results of interventions directed toward CPAP adherence. Red colors indicate direction for future research. SO = significant others

to various types of interventions, and this is an area of investigation that solely needs research.

The relevance and impact of time is important to consider in future RCTs, where the use of simple linear changes in CPAP adherence over time is unlikely to be able to fully capture patterns of the dynamics of therapeutic change. Monitoring CPAP adherence and change in functional or health status in every patient is probably more art than science, which requires a considerable learning curve at multiple levels. It is important to recognize that adherence to CPAP is a dynamic process that varies greatly from patient to patient, and is contingent on fluctuations and adjustments within the patient-clinician, patient-technology, and patient-environment circumstances. New methods for identifying causal effects across a time continuum on CPAP utility, using social network data [65–67], is a promising future for statistical development in RCTs of complex human behaviors, as current methods have known and often unavoidable limitations. The use of network theory to analyze switching use-non-use of CPAP and vice versa across a time continuum may allow for better investigations of patients' behavior (e.g., the measure of adherence with CPAP) and the efficacy of educational, cognitive-behavioral, and other types of interventions for enhancing adherence.

The clinician-researcher summarizes the systematic review of RCTs for CPAP adherence at the quarterly team meeting. She reports that an overall number of RCTs directed toward CPAP adherence, none of which were gender-sensitive, saw a significant increase over the past decade, targeting largely naïve patients with OSA; selected subgroups of patients with comorbidity, as seen in your neurology clinic, were frequently listed among exclusion criteria. She further reports that there is little evidence that a single intervention strategy either targeting patients' knowledge, behavior, or affect or patient-technology interface exists, which has been shown to be more effective than usual care across male and female patients, conditions, and settings. After reviewing concerns about the risk of bias in RCTs that targeted patient's knowledge, behavior, and affect and those that modified patency of patients' upper airways or focused on patient-mask interface, you agree with her assessment. A discussion ensures that barriers to CPAP adherence are multiple and relate not only to the patient and their social environment but also to the patient-clinician relationships, the extent of the adherence problem, and the perceived level of untreated OSA's threatening to health and functioning. Everyone recognizes the complexity and the need for

optimizing interventions and their components directed on improving CPAP adherence in each individual patient and the population as a whole, but the specific facets that could lead to future research successes are uncertain. The clinician-researcher advocates for developing research methods of clinical trials that incorporates novel dynamical systems and network theories, which could mitigate the potential faults associated with observing group effects in the presence of clinical and behavioral heterogeneity. In the end, you conclude that although confidence is uncertain that certain type of interventions is superior to others or to usual care, all clinicians and healthcare staff in your neurology clinic should inquire and document the nightly CPAP utility in their patients across a time continuum and start developing skills in identifying and alleviating barriers to CPAP adherence.

Funding: The author was supported by Canada Research Chair Program in Neurological Disorders and Brain Health. The content is solely the author's responsibility and does not necessarily represent the official views of the Canada Research Chair Program.

References

1. Epstein LH, Masek BJ. Behavioral control of medicine compliance. J Appl Behav Anal. 1978;11(1):1–9. https://doi.org/10.1901/jaba.1978.11-1.
2. Rich A, Brandes K, Mullan B, Hagger MS. Theory of planned behavior and adherence in chronic illness: a meta-analysis. J Behav Med. 2015;38(4):673–88. https://doi.org/10.1007/s10865-015-9644-3.
3. Burke LE, Zheng Y, Wang J. Adherence. In: Principles and concepts of behavioral medicine: a global handbook. 2018.
4. Oxford English Dictionary. Oxford English dictionary online. Oxford English Dictionary 2017.
5. Gould E, Mitty E. Medication adherence is a partnership, medication compliance is not. Geriatr Nurs. 2010;31(4):290–8. https://doi.org/10.1016/j.gerinurse.2010.05.004.
6. Trostle JA. Medical compliance as an ideology. Soc Sci Med. 1988;27(12):1299–308. https://doi.org/10.1016/0277-9536(88)90194-3.
7. Wedgwood R. Plato's theory of knowledge. In: Virtue, happiness, knowledge: themes from the work of Gail fine and Terence Irwin; 2018.
8. de Bono E. Critical thinking is totally inadequate. (Can You Teach Your People to Think Smarter?)(Cover Story). Across Board CY 1996 DB Gen OneFile. 1996.
9. McCabe R, Healey PGT. Miscommunication in doctor-patient communication. Top Cogn Sci. 2018;10(2):409–24. https://doi.org/10.1111/tops.12337.

10. Dunbar-Jacob J, Mortimer-Stephens MK. Treatment adherence in chronic disease. J Clin Epidemiol. 2001;

11. O'Donohue WT, Levensky ER. Promoting treatment adherence: a practical handbook for health care providers. 2006.

12. Kakkar RK. Continuous positive airway pressure. In: Encyclopedia of sleep. 2013.

13. Sullivan CE, Issa FG, Berthon-Jones M, Eves L. Reversal of obstructive sleep apnoea by continuous positive airway pressure applied through the nares. Lancet. 1981;1(8225):862–5. https://doi.org/10.1016/s0140-6736(81)92140-1.

14. Léger D, Stepnowsky C. The economic and societal burden of excessive daytime sleepiness in patients with obstructive sleep apnea. Sleep Med Rev. 2020;51:101275. https://doi.org/10.1016/j.smrv.2020.101275.

15. Kendzerska T, Mollayeva T, Gershon AS, Leung RS, Hawker G, Tomlinson G. Untreated obstructive sleep apnea and the risk for serious long-term adverse outcomes: a systematic review. Sleep Med Rev. 2014;18(1):49–59. https://doi.org/10.1016/j.smrv.2013.01.003.

16. Djonlagic I, Guo M, Matteis P, Carusona A, Stickgold R, Malhotra A. Untreated sleep-disordered breathing: links to aging-related decline in sleep-dependent memory consolidation. PLoS One. 2014;9(1):e85918. Published 2014 Jan 29. https://doi.org/10.1371/journal.pone.0085918.

17. Morsy NE, Farrag NS, Zaki NFW, et al. Obstructive sleep apnea: personal, societal, public health, and legal implications. Rev Environ Health. 2019;34(2):153–69. https://doi.org/10.1515/reveh-2018-0068.

18. Kellesarian SV, Malignaggi VR, Feng C, Javed F. Association between obstructive sleep apnea and erectile dysfunction: a systematic review and meta-analysis. Int J Impot Res. 2018;30(3):129–40. https://doi.org/10.1038/s41443-018-0017-7.

19. Cayanan EA, Bartlett DJ, Chapman JL, Hoyos CM, Phillips CL, Grunstein RR. A review of psychosocial factors and personality in the treatment of obstructive sleep apnoea. Eur Respir Rev. 2019;28(152):190005. Published 2019 Jun 26. https://doi.org/10.1183/16000617.0005-2019.

20. Kent BD, McNicholas WT, Ryan S. Insulin resistance, glucose intolerance and diabetes mellitus in obstructive sleep apnoea. J Thorac Dis. 2015;7(8):1343–57. https://doi.org/10.3978/j.issn.2072-1439.2015.08.11.

21. Moyer CA, Sonnad SS, Garetz SL, Helman JI, Chervin RD. Quality of life in obstructive sleep apnea: a systematic review of the literature. Sleep Med. 2001;2(6):477–91. https://doi.org/10.1016/s1389-9457(01)00072-7.

22. Rotenberg BW, Murariu D, Pang KP. Trends in CPAP adherence over twenty years of data collection: a flattened curve. J Otolaryngol Head Neck Surg. 2016;45(1):43. Published 2016 Aug 19. https://doi.org/10.1186/s40463-016-0156-0.

23. Sawyer AM, Gooneratne NS, Marcus CL, Ofer D, Richards KC, Weaver TE. A systematic review of CPAP adherence across age groups: clinical and empiric insights for developing CPAP adherence interventions. Sleep Med Rev. 2011;15(6):343–56. https://doi.org/10.1016/j.smrv.2011.01.003.

24. Shapiro GK, Shapiro CM. Factors that influence CPAP adherence: an overview. Sleep Breath. 2010;14(4):323–35. https://doi.org/10.1007/s11325-010-0391-y.

25. Zampogna E, Spanevello A, Lucioni AM, et al. Adherence to continuous positive airway pressure in patients with obstructive sleep apnoea. A ten year real life study. Respir Med. 2019;150:95–100. https://doi.org/10.1016/j.rmed.2019.02.017.

26. Schwab RJ, Badr SM, Epstein LJ, et al. An official American Thoracic Society statement: continuous positive airway pressure adherence tracking systems. The optimal monitoring strategies and outcome measures in adults. Am J Respir Crit Care Med. 2013;188(5):613–20. https://doi.org/10.1164/rccm.201307-1282ST.

27. Centers of Medicare & Medicaid Services. Cms Manual System. Pub 100-03 Medicare Natl Cover Determ. 2010.

28. Patil SP, Ayappa IA, Caples SM, Kimoff RJ, Patel SR, Harrod CG. Treatment of adult obstructive sleep Apnea with positive airway pressure: an American Academy of sleep medicine systematic review, meta-analysis, and GRADE assessment. J Clin Sleep Med. 2019;15(2):301–34. Published 2019 Feb 15. https://doi.org/10.5664/jcsm.7638.

29. Kushida CA, Littner MR, Hirshkowitz M, et al. Practice parameters for the use of continuous and bilevel positive airway pressure devices to treat adult patients with sleep-related breathing disorders. Sleep. 2006;29(3):375–80. https://doi.org/10.1093/sleep/29.3.375.

30. Lai AYK, Fong DYT, Lam JCM, Weaver TE, Ip MSM. The efficacy of a brief motivational enhancement education program on CPAP adherence in OSA: a randomized controlled trial. Chest. 2014;146(3):600–10. https://doi.org/10.1378/chest.13-2228.

31. Rühle K-H, Domanski U, Schröder M, Franke KJ, Nilius G. Warmluftbefeuchtung unter CPAP mit und ohne Schlauchisolation [heated humidification during CPAP with and without tube insulation]. Pneumologie. 2010;64(5):316–9. https://doi.org/10.1055/s-0029-1244073.

32. Worsnop CJ, Miseski S, Rochford PD. Routine use of humidification with nasal continuous positive airway pressure. Intern Med J. 2010;40(9):650–6. https://doi.org/10.1111/j.1445-5994.2009.01969.x.

33. Nadeem R, Rishi MA, Srinivasan L, Copur AS, Naseem J. Effect of visualization of raw graphic polysomnography data by sleep apnea patients on adherence to CPAP therapy. Respir Care. 2013;58(4):607–13. https://doi.org/10.4187/respcare.01539.

34. Pengo MF, Czaban M, Berry MP, et al. The effect of positive and negative message framing on short term continuous positive airway pressure compliance in patients with obstructive sleep apnea. J Thorac Dis. 2018;10(Suppl 1):S160–9. https://doi.org/10.21037/jtd.2017.07.110.

35. Jurado-Gamez B, Bardwell WA, Cordova-Pacheco LJ, García-Amores M, Feu-Collado N, Buela-Casal G. A basic intervention improves CPAP adherence in sleep apnoea patients: a controlled trial. Sleep Breath. 2015;19(2):509–14. https://doi.org/10.1007/s11325-014-1038-1.

36. Roecklein KA, Schumacher JA, Gabriele JM, Fagan C, Baran AS, Richert AC. Personalized feedback to improve CPAP adherence in obstructive sleep apnea. Behav Sleep Med. 2010;8(2):105–12. https://doi.org/10.1080/15402001003622859.

37. Dawson JD, Yu L, Aksan NS, Tippin J, Rizzo M, Anderson SW. Feedback from naturalistic driving improves treatment compliance in drivers with obstructive sleep APNEA. Proc Int Driv Symp Hum Factors Driv Assess Train Veh Des. 2015;2015:30–5.

38. Sparrow D, Aloia M, Demolles DA, Gottlieb DJ. A telemedicine intervention to improve adherence to continuous positive airway pressure: a randomised controlled trial. Thorax. 2010;65(12):1061–6. https://doi.org/10.1136/thx.2009.133215.

39. Wang W, He G, Wang M, Liu L, Tang H. Effects of patient education and progressive muscle relaxation alone or combined on adherence to continuous positive airway pressure treatment in obstructive sleep apnea patients. Sleep Breath. 2012;16(4):1049–57. https://doi.org/10.1007/s11325-011-0600-3.

40. Bakker JP, Wang R, Weng J, et al. Motivational enhancement for increasing adherence to CPAP: a randomized controlled trial. Chest. 2016;150(2):337–45. https://doi.org/10.1016/j.chest.2016.03.019.

41. Bartlett D, Wong K, Richards D, et al. Increasing adherence to obstructive sleep apnea treatment with a group social cognitive therapy treatment intervention: a randomized trial. Sleep. 2013;36(11):1647–54. Published 2013 Nov 1. https://doi.org/10.5665/sleep.3118.

42. Lo Bue A, Salvaggio A, Isidoro SI, Romano S, Marrone O, Insalaco G. Usefulness of reinforcing interventions on continuous positive airway pressure compliance. BMC Pulm Med. 2014;14:78. Published 2014 May 3. https://doi.org/10.1186/1471-2466-14-78.

43. Olsen S, Smith SS, Oei TP, Douglas J. Motivational interviewing (MINT) improves continuous positive airway pressure (CPAP) acceptance and adherence: a randomized controlled trial. J Consult Clin Psychol. 2012;80(1):151–63. https://doi.org/10.1037/a0026302.

44. Aloia MS, Arnedt JT, Strand M, Millman RP, Borrelli B. Motivational enhancement to improve adherence to positive airway pressure in patients with obstructive sleep apnea: a randomized controlled trial. Sleep. 2013;36(11):1655–62. Published 2013 Nov 1. https://doi.org/10.5665/sleep.3120.

45. Dharmakulaseelan L, Kirolos N, Kamra M, et al. Educating stroke/TIA patients about obstructive sleep Apnea after stroke: a randomized feasibility study. J Stroke Cerebrovasc Dis. 2019;28(11):104317. https://doi.org/10.1016/j.jstrokecerebrovasdis.2019.104317.

46. Diaféria G, Santos-Silva R, Truksinas E, et al. Myofunctional therapy improves adherence to continuous positive airway pressure treatment. Sleep Breath. 2017;21(2):387–95. https://doi.org/10.1007/s11325-016-1429-6.

47. Chen X, Chen W, Hu W, Huang K, Huang J, Zhou Y. Nurse-led intensive interventions improve adherence to continuous positive airway pressure therapy and quality of life in obstructive sleep apnea patients. Patient Prefer Adherence. 2015;9:1707–13. Published 2015 Nov 26. https://doi.org/10.2147/PPA.S90846.

48. Parthasarathy S, Wendel C, Haynes PL, Atwood C, Kuna S. A pilot study of CPAP adherence promotion by peer buddies with sleep apnea. J Clin Sleep Med. 2013;9(6):543–50. Published 2013 Jun 15. https://doi.org/10.5664/jcsm.2744.

49. Pépin JL, Tamisier R, Hwang D, Mereddy S, Parthasarathy S. Does remote monitoring change OSA management and CPAP adherence? Respirology. 2017;22(8):1508–17. https://doi.org/10.1111/resp.13183.

50. Hoet F, Libert W, Sanida C, Van den Broecke S, Bruyneel AV, Bruyneel M. Telemonitoring in continuous positive airway pressure-treated patients improves delay to first intervention and early compliance: a randomized trial. Sleep Med. 2017;39:77–83. https://doi.org/10.1016/j.sleep.2017.08.016.

51. Gillespie MB, Wylie PE, Lee-Chiong T, Rapoport DM. Effect of palatal implants on continuous positive airway pressure and compliance. Otolaryngol Head Neck Surg. 2011;144(2):230–6. https://doi.org/10.1177/0194599810392173.

52. Hood MM, Corsica J, Cvengros J, Wyatt J. Impact of a brief dietary self-monitoring intervention on weight change and CPAP adherence in patients with obstructive sleep apnea. J Psychosom Res. 2013;74(2):170–4. https://doi.org/10.1016/j.jpsychores.2012.12.006.

53. Neuzeret PC, Morin L. Impact of different nasal masks on CPAP therapy for obstructive sleep apnea: a randomized comparative trial. Clin Respir J. 2017;11(6):990–8. https://doi.org/10.1111/crj.12452.

54. Gulati A, Oscroft N, Chadwick R, Ali M, Smith I. The impact of changing people with sleep apnea using CPAP less than 4 h per night to a bi-level device. Respir Med. 2015;109(6):778–83. https://doi.org/10.1016/j.rmed.2015.01.020.

55. Powell ED, Gay PC, Ojile JM, Litinski M, Malhotra A. A pilot study assessing adherence to auto-bilevel following a poor initial encounter with CPAP. J Clin Sleep Med. 2012;8(1):43–7. Published 2012 Feb 15. https://doi.org/10.5664/jcsm.1658.

56. Slavin RE. Best evidence synthesis: an intelligent alternative to meta-analysis. J Clin Epidemiol. 1995;48(1):9–18. https://doi.org/10.1016/0895-4356(94)00097-a.

57. Johnson BT, Huedo-Medina TB. Meta-analytic statistical inferences for continuous measure outcomes as a function of effect size metric and other assumptions. Rockville: Agency for Healthcare Research and Quality (US); 2013.

58. Tannenbaum C, Ellis RP, Eyssel F, Zou J, Schiebinger L. Sex and gender analysis improves science and engineering. Nature. 2019;575(7781):137–46. https://doi.org/10.1038/s41586-019-1657-6.

59. Pascual M, de Batlle J, Barbé F, et al. Erectile dysfunction in obstructive sleep apnea patients: a randomized trial on the effects of Continuous Positive Airway Pressure (CPAP). PLoS One. 2018;13(8):e0201930. Published 2018 Aug 8. https://doi.org/10.1371/journal.pone.0201930.

60. Gaines J, Vgontzas AN, Fernandez-Mendoza J, Bixler EO. Obstructive sleep apnea and the metabolic syndrome: the road to clinically-meaningful phenotyping, improved prognosis, and personalized treatment. Sleep Med Rev. 2018;42:211–9. https://doi.org/10.1016/j.smrv.2018.08.009.

61. Carberry JC, Amatoury J, Eckert DJ. Personalized management approach for OSA. Chest. 2018;153(3):744–55. https://doi.org/10.1016/j.chest.2017.06.011.

62. McDaid C, Griffin S, Weatherly H, et al. Continuous positive airway pressure devices for the treatment of obstructive sleep apnoea-hypopnoea syndrome: a systematic review and economic analysis. Health Technol Assess. 2009;13(4):iii–274. https://doi.org/10.3310/hta13040.

63. Beghi E, Logroscino G. General overview, conclusions, and future directions. Front Neurol Neurosci. 2016;39:154–62. https://doi.org/10.1159/000445456.

64. Clayton JA, Tannenbaum C. Reporting sex, gender, or both in clinical research? JAMA. 2016;316(18):1863–4. https://doi.org/10.1001/jama.2016.16405.

65. Kolaczyk ED, Csárdi G. Statistical analysis of network data with R, vol. 65. New York: Springer; 2014.

66. Christakis NA, Fowler JH. Social contagion theory: examining dynamic social networks and human behavior. Stat Med. 2013;32(4):556–77. https://doi.org/10.1002/sim.5408.

67. Gronchi G. The use of network theory for analyzing switching behaviors: assessing cognitive and educational-based intervention for promoting health. Front Psychol. 2018;9:1095. Published 2018 Jun 26. https://doi.org/10.3389/fpsyg.2018.01095.

Patient Adherence to CPAP: A Practical Interdisciplinary Model

Colin M. Shapiro

3.1 Introduction

When studies about CPAP first came out the arbitrary bar for use was set at 4 hours four nights a week. The advantage of this was in establishing a common language about adherence, but with the benefit of hindsight it was probably a practical decision based on the resources at the time and the limitations of the available equipment 40 years ago.

If one thinks that some of the pathophysiology of sleep apnea is consequent on the often high rates of apnea in REM sleep and one is aware that in the first 4 hours of sleep there is a relative paucity of REM sleep, to think that a large study, which recorded an average CPAP usage of 3.3 hours, might have something relevant to say about the impact of CPAP on any of the common comorbidities described in this book [e.g., hypertension, depression, arrhythmia, diabetes, etc.] seems as foolish as telling someone to wear their spectacles for part of the night when driving [if they are short-sighted] and hoping to see a decrease in motor vehicle accidents.

3.2 Style of Interaction

The models of interaction with patients have evolved over the last century from being paternalistic to collaborative. The change from the physician presuming that the patient will blindly cooperate, to a relationship of mutual participation with a patient-centered focus, has not been smooth. The recognition that the style of communication with a patient is the most salient ingredient in the soup of facilitating patient care and adherence was recognized by Sir William Osler. A recent obituary of Alwyn Lishman [1] (widely considered to be the founding father of neuropsychiatry) quoted the Mausdsley psychiatrist as saying that the fundamental skill of a psychiatrist was deceptively simple viz. "being able to talk meaningfully and helpfully with patients" This aphorism remains true. A contemporary of Lishman, Norman Geschwind (Harvard Neurologist), who is considered by many as the founding father of Behavioral Neurology, was fond of saying that one learns neurology "stroke by stroke." His point was to pay careful attention to the details of every patient's symptoms and signs, i.e., that every patient is different. This truism is equally relevant in the management of sleep apnea and CPAP treatments.

There are many factors that influence doctor–patient communication. These include personalities of both and the use of humor in the interaction [2]. Even the physical space in which the interview occurs has an influence; for example, not having garish lighting, a warm color, and art that includes scenes with water can all induce calm.

A single style for all patients is not likely to be effective. Both socioeconomic status and the age of the patient will influence what is acceptable in the interaction. The patient's personality and past experience with physicians will have a bearing on the interaction. These issues are hard to fathom and are somewhat immutable. The two keys to opening a collaborative relationship are to ensure at the outset that the patient has the opportunity to voice their concerns. This is often described as "active listening". The almost platitudinous nonverbal behaviors that facilitate adherence include smiling; facing a patient; making eye contact; and a warm voice tone, which are all well recognized [3]. Staring at a computer screen is not helpful. These authors [3] warn against fidgeting, which is indicative of impatience and comment that a comforting touch encourages and invites the patients to a partnership. However, in today's society this may be misinterpreted and an expression such as "Consider yourself metaphorically hugged" expresses the desire to comfort but at the same time shows caution toward the patient's boundaries and what has become societally acceptable.

There is a multiplicity of factors that influence CPAP adherence. These include the salience of the patient's symptoms, the contact with the referring physician or agency, the personal values of the patient vis-à-vis their health, and their

C. M. Shapiro (✉)
University of Toronto, Toronto, ON, Canada

health literacy. There will be lifestyle, economic and cultural factors, and family dynamic issues that will come into play. The persons' personality and their willingness to be open about the medical situation will have a great impact. The willingness to be open in particular has changed dramatically over the last 20 years. Previously, those requiring CPAPs were more embarrassed, but now it is widely accepted (in some but not all cultures) and the advocates among patients with positive experiences of CPAP make it easier for physicians to advocate for better adherence. The scientific literature about the consequences of sleep apnea allows one to focus on the relevant benefits of CPAP for a particular individual whether it is in the arena of sleepiness, arrhythmia, depression, etc. If the treating physician is able to cite studies that are pertinent to the patient in one's office, this can support the notion that what is being discussed is relevant to the particular patient. The history of CPAP [see final chapter in this book] is significant in this regard. Support from others, including families, especially spouse, friends, and professionals, is important and can be facilitated. Perhaps some of the most challenging factors to change are the individuals' personal values and when the values do not lead to motivation for using CPAP, one may be required to use "the big stick," which is uncomfortable, i.e., infusing safety in general (and driving safety in particular) into the discussion about adherence. This comes close to threatening and needs to be discussed with compassion.

There are over a dozen theoretical models describing the process of facilitating change in behavior and adherence to beneficial behavior. These models range from the theoretical and erudite sounding "Transtheoretical Model of Change" involving the steps of precontemplation, contemplation, preparation, action, and maintenance [4] to the more prosaic: "information motivation strategy" model, which posits that the individual must know that change is necessary; have the desire to change; and have the mechanism to achieve and maintain necessary behaviors [5].

For my money, one of the best conceptualizations of what is required to move the dial forward to improve CPAP adherence is the review by Crawford et al. [6]. These authors emphasize the biopsychosocial (BPS) model and in the title refer to the integration of psychology and medicine in achieving better adherence (see Fig. 3.1).

Engel in two papers concerning the biopsychosocial model published 20 years apart (1977 and 1997) defined the field [7, 8].

To some extent, many clinicians would instinctively use components of this conceptualization and aspects of the almost 200 references in the review cited above [6]. The authors layer the evidence relating to CPAP adherence on the well-established notion of the biopsychosocial domains and emphasize the integration of these elements. The graphic above is modeled on a figure in the review [6] and tries to emphasize the interlocking of psychological and sociological factors with clinical factors that impact on the outcome for an individual in all three domains viz. physical, psychological, and social. One may think of this as a triangle, and if one corner of the triangle is raised, the other two may drop (i.e., be neglected). Integrating all the components should be seen as a necessary condition for improving the patient/person's well-being. The implication is that all dimensions (biological, psychological, and sociological) act as a lever to facilitate improvement in the other components. Focusing on only one aspect is akin to a student getting top marks in one subject and failing in the other courses leading to a dismal report card.

For criticisms of the model, see Refs. [9, 10].

One of the last papers I accepted as an editor of the Journal of Psychosomatic Research was that by Chan et al., which included a demonstration of the way in which the BPS model pertains to end-stage renal disease [11]. This review clearly indicates how a model can confirm some expected associations but can often open an awareness of other linkages that may have not been self-evident. For example, these researchers highlight the connection between depression and specific elements of renal failure and/or dialysis, e.g., restless leg syndrome [12]. The abovementioned review [6] considers over 30 factors that may have a bearing on CPAP adherence and separate references for each item into evidence for increasing, decreasing, or not making a difference to compliance.

The NICE review on the effects of melatonin on jet lag found nine small studies (not particularly well done) in support of a benefit of melatonin in people with jet lag and one large scientifically better executed study that did *not* show benefit. This is a warning against presuming that the "louder" voice (more publications) does not make the proposal more likely to be true. This implies that a simple tally of papers "for" or "against" the impact of a particular variable of relevance to CPAP adherence cannot be simply calculated. However, it does give some insight into the perspective of different groups looking at factors that may influence adherence.

There are thirty-three topics that are considered in the review [6] and range widely from the CPAP delivery interface to the coping style of the individual. There is a wide disparity in the number of studies available to draw on to make conclusions about these postulated influences on adherence. As an example on the topic of age, there are a plethora of papers that conclude that there is no difference in adherence based on the age of the patient. There are less than a dozen papers indicating an increase in adherence with age and several papers indicating a week association. Being mindful of the caveat described above [regarding jet lag and melatonin], the following factors come out and seem to have the balance of publications increasing or decreasing adherence (see Table 3.1).

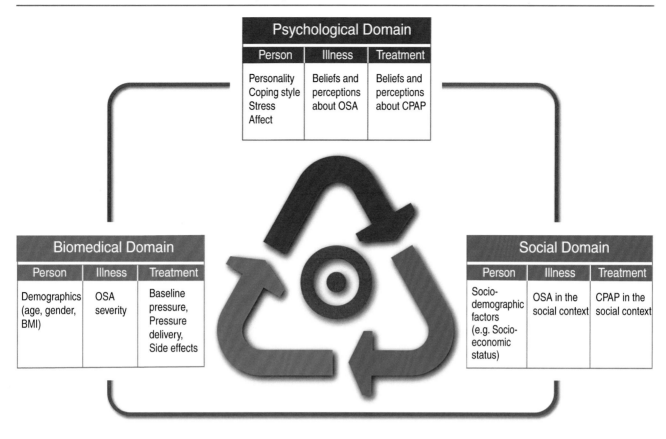

Fig. 3.1 Inter-relationship of the bio-psycho-social model vis-à-vis sleep apnea. (Based on the figure in M.R. Crawford et al. [6])

Table 3.1 Biopsychosocial factors relevant to CPAP adherence

Number of factors considered	Increasing adherence	Decreasing adherence
Biomedical sphere 15 factors considered	Treatment-specific modification in pressure, sleep quality on titration night, disease severity (weak), symptom improvement	Race ethnicity (minority) Adverse effects experienced Nasal resistance
Psychological 13 factors considered	Of the 13 categories considered, none show a clear preponderance of evidence one way or another. For example, there are 3 papers showing that negative personality factors decrease adherence and 3 studies show no difference. In general, the same applies for the other 12 factors.	
Social 6 factors considered	Higher socioeconomic class has a number of positive studies (no negative) but a slight preponderance of "no different" studies. There is no clear preponderance for any factor.	

Based on Ref. [6]

To provide the music to amplify the broad (and perhaps all embracing) concept of the biopsychosocial model (BPS), I have added the well-known mnemonic that every student of the piano learns: EGBDF (*every good boy deserves favor*). In this iteration, it would be *education,*

genetics, biodiversity, diagnostic information, and *family* support (see Fig. 3.2).

This is not to say that some/all of the items below cannot be squeezed into the rubric of the BPS model. However, this is to assist practicing clinicians to be more cognizant of crucial practical factors that are embraced by the BPS model and others that are not integral to the BPS per se.

Before elaborating on the mnemonic, there are a few general points worth noting. The recognition of comorbid conditions, and in particular, awareness of other sleep disorders, is crucial in archiving high adherence. Simply put, the patient with sleep apnea and phase delay syndrome or restless legs will be less likely to experience significant improvement from the treatment of his sleep apnea without the management of his other sleep problems.

The thoroughness of the respiratory therapist is a major but relatively under-researched factor (see Chap. 34). There are differences that CPAP companies can make in providing education (e.g., a handout booklet), and the manufacturers also have an influence particularly in the realm of the development of monitoring, which provides feedback to the patient about their usage and apnea rate.

A relatively new development of having a CPAP coordinator (see Chap. 33) in the clinic who can provide focused support and greater availability than many physicians (and

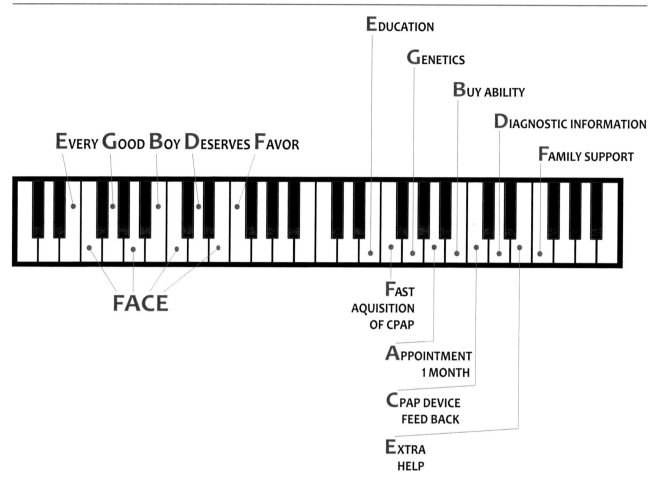

Fig. 3.2 The music of some memorable points to cover in an assessment

psychologists) can provide. They can also triage patients who need further help (e.g., referring to a psychologist).

The aphorism that it takes a village to raise a child is a truism, and there are many chapters in this book that specifically address the facets of the interconnecting components that are required to get good results with CPAP adherence. What is clear is that there is no one way to achieve the objective of high adherence. Being "patient-centric"should be the mantra. This can be with a more regimented or more egalitarian approach.

The elaboration of the mnemonic EGBDF can be amplified by the following points:

E: Education

There is no limit to the amount of education that could be provided. It is very useful to remember that the average patient seeing a family physician will retain 7 ± 2 pieces of information. This means that after giving the diagnosis, the impact of the diagnosis, a description of the treatment, and two possible side effects, some patients may be "tapped out"; i.e., they will not retain further information. The point of this is to go for the most important shots and to focus the patient

on the information that would be most relevant for that particular individual. Martin et al. [3] provide a table "What health professionals can do to help patients remember medical information" (page 55). Among the 13 recommendations, are simple suggestions such as "Speak slowly and don't rush through the information you are providing," "Pair health-behavior change information with other meaningful information," and "Put the most important information first and last." The aspects of many of these will be instinctive to some but are a useful aide memoire. For the vast majority of people acquiring CPAP internationally, they may see the treating clinician 2–4 times (e.g., assessment, post-sleep study review, and one check-up on progress) in the span of a year with or without subsequent follow-up. With this in mind, the information conveyed in the follow-up interview needs to be laser sharp in its focus. In addition, a take-away that can be digested slowly and overtime is highly desirable. After reviewing CPAP adherence [13], a small highly illustrated booklet (40 pages) "Sleep apnea, CPAP and me" [14] was developed to provide patients with digestible information. The already very good adherence in two clinics (77% and 84%, respectively, using criteria of 6 hours per night 6 nights per week) had an increase by a further 7% (in both clinics) following giving all patients illustrated educational booklet. The notion of 4 hours a night four nights a week is to build into the system an expectation of poor performance, i.e., less than a third of the sleep time in a 7-hour sleeper. Six hours six nights a week is slightly under 75% of the sleeping time and provides an emphatic expectation of being most of the time from which further gains can be made.

This $10.00 US booklet was described by many patients a pivotal, and in many cases vendors of CPAP devices distributed the booklet. My experience (in the area of "Shift Work") is that providing a hard copy of a booklet is more impactful than directing patients to a website or providing a video. An updated version, including a section on oral appliances and pediatrics, will be released to coincide with the publication of this book [15].

This chapter emphasizes a style of dialogue with the patient that is effective. Some may feel the approach is too forceful. For a more nuanced approach, see chapter (Chaps. 4 and 6). The booklet referenced above includes a graphic that emphasizes the health impact of adherence over time in those using CPAP is helpful. For patients, this is more impactful if a yardstick of the implication of CPAP use is related to a comparator with a metric that is far more readily appreciated by the patient. One such is to use a graphic which compares the patient's risk with the equivalent risk of smoking a number of cigarettes smoked per day. This is a very concrete and motivating for patients who well appreciate the consequences of smoking cessation for health reasons. The implication of stopping to breathe 32 times per hour (for example) means nothing to most people other than sounding "not good." However, if the graphic shows that this rate of breathing stops in sleep is comparable to smoking 60 cigarettes per day—this is something all patients can appreciate.

For many patients, the information about the use of CPAP is initially overwhelming. The resources for "two sessions with a therapist" are not widely available (see Chap. 6). Thus, a clear statement of the health implications in terms that the patient can relate to is very desirable. Using other members of the patients' family as "team members" and providing written material on sleep apnea are desirable.

The concept of phenotypes of sleep apnea (see Chap. 13) is no surprise. One is aware of physicians who did not want to know if their patients were sleepy as in some jurisdictions that would require the automatic referral to a government body and the invariable suspension of the patients' driving license. The license may be reinstated 3–6 months later after an on-treatment maintenance of wakefulness test (MWT) is carried out. This disruption to work and family life, especially in rural areas, is profound. One could argue that it would be better to be able to say, "you are objectively sleepy and this needs to be fixed or your license is at risk." This approach is fraught with conflicts and contradictions in the

relationship between physician and patient, but it is honest (albeit uncomfortably close to threatening). It is unquestionably galvanizing in favor of treatment. From a societal perspective, this appreciation of danger and risk of sleep apnea being untreated or undertreated is what is most required.

The knowledge about REM versus non-REM apnea rates, particularly with the increasing knowledge of specific consequences of significant REM sleep disruption by sleep apnea, allows for the possibility of using this information in a dialogue with the patient where it is pertinent, e.g., in relation to "procedural memory."

A laundry list of potential health consequences of sleep apnea may be useful for the shock value. However, to elaborate on a particular consequence, which is pertinent to the particular patient, is more impactful. In other words, if a patient has a pre-existing condition that might be impacted by sleep apnea, mentioning that that condition is likely to be improved has great relevance for the patient. It is useful to draw from the pre-sleep study consultation to be able to elaborate on particular consequences of sleep apnea whether it be cardiac, erectile function, mood, concentration, or weight management (inter alia) that are relevant to the particular patient when the patient is receiving the results of the sleep study.

G: Genetics

Sleep apnea is quintessentially a biomedical issue. However, being aware of both race and gender in the psychosocial domain is important. This is not merely the gender and race of the patient, but also the gender and race of the physician, nurse, psychologist, etc. We might wish to think that these are not relevant, but deliberately arranging for some female patients to be seen by a female respiratory therapist may make the process more comfortable and can be a "game changer" for some individuals. Describing racial factors related to the issue of sleep apnea for people with an African background or an Asian background can be helpful in indicating that one is appreciating the factors relevant to the individual patient.

B: Buy Ability

The notion of socioeconomic status may be presumed to cover this issue. However, there is an interplay between government policy and the ability to purchase a CPAP machine. For example, in Canada, some provinces will provide complete funding for people on disability and perhaps 65% funding for everyone diagnosed with sleep apnea in an accredited sleep facility. In other jurisdictions, evidence of use of CPAP is required before the money is paid out. Variability in medical modules in different nations (see Chap. 35) with different political systems will enormously impact on CPAP acquisition. The physicians' role in facilitating this process (i.e., by encouraging vendors to accept installment payments) can be enormously helpful. The simple act of communicating with the vendor in the presence of the patient adds to the perception of care and the importance of the treatment being discussed.

D: Diagnostic Information

There are wide range of methods to ascertain whether a person has sleep apnea or not and whether there are specific and relevant consequences. I would argue that more information and better quality of information facilitate a more in-depth and a more nuanced intervention. Without EEG information, many "bargaining chips" in the explanation as to why it is important that the person uses CPAP are lost. Being able, for example, to inform a patient that the amount of deep sleep they have is less than half of what most people their age have, or that they come to the surface of sleep 25 times per hour, which may be a factor in their tiredness is useful in the process of making the case for using CPAP. It is widely thought that most people suspected of having sleep apnea do not need a multiple sleep latency test (MSLT). For those who routinely do/did MSLT recordings, on the premise that sleep is to allow one to be wakeful and not sleepy (two different issues), the documentation and the awareness of the implication of objective sleepiness in relation to driving safety (and maintaining a drivers' license) are a major motivator.

F: Family Support

We do not live in a society, but societies. The difference in priorities in rural and urban environments is striking. The concurrent experience of working in a large city (Toronto—5 million) and a very small town (Parry Sound—population 6000) has highlighted the difference in attitude: to work, physicians, and family life. In a small town, most patients will come to follow-up appointments with a spouse if asked to do so. Very few patients will do so in a big city. The CPAP adherence is consistently different in the two locations (other factors being equal). The "take-away educational piece" is that it can be helpful to engage a family member, especially a spouse.

The evidence of family interaction generally shows women to be more supportive of a partner with sleep apnea than a man with a wife who has sleep apnea. However, having the husband hear the potential consequences of sleep apnea has a powerful effect.

FACE

The second mnemonic "FACE" represents:

*F*ast acquisition

There is considerable evidence that the shorter the time from the patient being told they need CPAP to actually acquire CPAP is predictive of higher adherence. Facilitating this in an ethical way is complex but can be achieved.

*A*ppointment in 1 Month after Starting CPAP

The most relevant message in this is the recognition by the patient that the physician is not simply providing a treatment, but (s)he is also concerned that the patient will benefit from it and will troubleshoot if there are difficulties. The bonus is that the patient becomes aware that they will be monitored over this month, which in itself is motivating for them to develop early patterns of usage.

*C*PAP Device Feedback

The role of the feedback that is now available from the CPAP machine is extremely powerful in facilitating adherence for many people. This is discussed later in this chapter.

*E*xtra Help

The notion that the physician is a one-person band is antiquated and, in this field, particularly inappropriate. Patients view referrals to a CPAP coordinator, psychologist and others as a sign of caring and offering specialized care, especially if they perceive that there is a good rapport between the prescriber and other members of the team.

General Issues

The inevitable question that arises is to what extent is adherence dependent on the sum of the parts of the BPS model. It would be easy to conceptualize there being person-specific factors that may play a clear role for some individuals, but not for others. If for one person the biggest factor is the disease severity, which motivates them, for a second person personality traits may be the key factor and for a third person the partner's reaction to the sleep apnea may be the most salient issue. These idiographic factors will be "drowned out" when pooling groups of people in a nomothetic analysis. Understanding what each person wants from having a sleep study is crucial. The simple question "What do I need to achieve with you for you to feel that this process of coming for a sleep evaluation was really worthwhile?" cuts to the core of what needs to be delivered for that particular person to be adherent. It is the personalized tailoring of the response to the patient's objective that one suspects is a key ingredient to providing an effective intervention. To be able to respond to one person that using a CPAP device all night every night is likely to help their depression/diabetes/hypertension personalizes the relevance of being adherent. For others, it may be the possible prophylactic benefit of guarding against potential cognitive decline, chance of having an MI, stroke or erectile dysfunction, that is motivating. For others, the prospect of a better matrimonial life may be key. The most important motivators can be established in an initial assessment before the diagnosis is made. Bringing these factors into play at the time of discussing going onto CPAP makes the process relevant.

The proverbial car salesman will try and assess if it is speed, look, power, or reliability that the customer is most concerned about and tailor the approach to the individual accordingly. The BPS plus C (culture) has the advantage of a broad interweaving perspective. In the field of psychiatry, to some extent it allowed for the melding of the biological and psychodynamic approaches. Critics may argue that the boundaries of the components are not clearly demarcated, which is true but the rejoinder could be "all the more reason to consider the intertwining influences."

One of the key issues in facilitating change in a person's actions is the relationship that has already been established. The model of the patient meeting the clinician for the first time after the sleep test does not facilitate the relationship confidence on the part of the patient. Having a focus in the interview that places the patient's needs front and center is a good opening gambit. A questions (similar to one cited above) such as "What do we need to achieve so that you will feel that this was a really useful exercise?" engenders a sense of caring for the patient. Aiming to fulfill the patient's needs while giving factual information is imperative. Providing information that supports the patient's needs but also allows for some measure of choice is likely to lead to a reasonable outcome. For example, "trying an oral appliance for your severe apnea may not be everyone's first choice. However, if that is what you want to do, I'm happy to support that, on the understanding that we check that it is being effective."

For some time, the use of CPAP was not simple nor smooth. Sorting out noise and comfort is helpful in the same way as automatic windows are a convenience to car drivers. Getting an electric car is a game changer. In a CPAP field, the advances in the equipment now provide ongoing feedback and performance measures appeal to the inherent nature of many patients (and the treating team alike). In a clinic with very high adherence, this may make a small difference (a shift from 91–94% adherence). However, if the mode of adherence is 50% (in those with heightened interest and doing research on the topic) [13], then the role of more sophisticated feedback information has the potential of being dramatic in facilitating the patient taking of "ownership" of their own usage and performance. This should in no way, however, allow clinicians to abrogate the responsibility of being involved in this process as a part of what needs to be emphasized to achieve good adherence.

Figure 3.3 elaborates on the components (steps) of the clinical contact points that can tilt the interaction between the patient and the clinic to facilitate a greater likelihood of better CPAP adherence. This graphic does not take into account many other variables that are highly relevant for example the impact of a wide range of medical including

psychiatric conditions and special circumstances such as medication being used or the change in CPAP use during the period after bariatric surgery. All of these issues are discussed in subsequent chapters in this book. What this model hopefully provides is a set of levers and strategies that help to translate the considerable cost in organizing to do a diagnostic study and the acquisition of CPAP into high usage rather than an expensive doorstop.

3.3   A Second Level of Perspective

More than most areas of medicine, the process of achieving CPAP adherence is dependent on a large number of elements in the process. The simple way to think of this is to consider the process as links in the chain. The process starts with the awareness of the referring physician/nurse and practitioner/spouse. Next is the clinical facility and the waiting time and the awareness of sleep apnea, which has had an impact on people presenting for sleep apnea assessment. The mannerisms of the clinician in the sleep clinic and the way in which the sleep study is conducted are relevant. Resources (e.g., access to psychology input) may be very variable, but until one has the full panoply of resources, the clinician is unlikely to appreciate what he or she is missing. An example of this may be the involvement of a CPAP coordinator.

More than many areas of medicine, the approach of motivational interviewing is key in the process of getting a person to make a significant change in their behavior to deal with a problem they do not fully recognize or are ambivalent about solving. The first section of this chapter may be seen as easily doable if the clinician thinks about it. This "second level" requires an acquisition of skills.

Miller and Rollnick in the book "Motivational interviewing" [16] provide an 11-point list of principles of person-centered care, which many will feel are intuitive but well worth reading as a list; see Table 3.2.

Motivational Interviews
While having a concept of the ingredients that need to be taken into account and to have the tools to facilitate that people are more likely to make a change in their behavior that leads to better health is crucial, so too is the manner in which the proposition is delivered. It is not rocket science to state the obvious that telling a person to do something "because I'm telling you it will improve your health" is not a proposition that most people would accept.

Motivational interviewing involves techniques and styles that:

A. Help the person to feel that they are part of the process.
B. Use language that resonates
C. Deal with issues that are salient for the individual

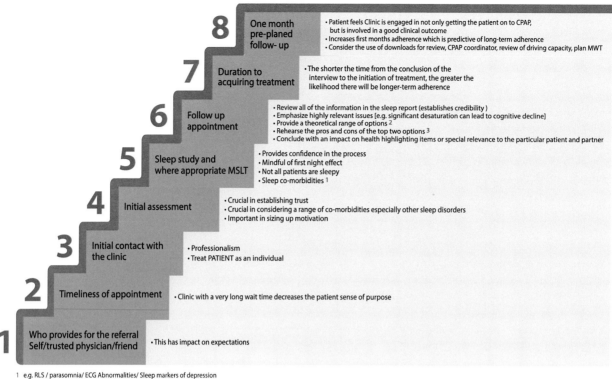

8 One month pre-planed follow-up
- Patient feels Clinic is engaged in not only getting the patient on to CPAP, but is involved in a good clinical outcome
- Increases first months adherence which is predictive of long-term adherence
- Consider the use of downloads for review, CPAP coordinator, review of driving capacity, plan MWT

7 Duration to acquiring treatment
- The shorter the time from the conclusion of the interview to the initiation of treatment, the greater the likelihood there will be longer-term adherence

6 Follow up appointment
- Review all of the information in the sleep report (establishes credibility)
- Emphasize highly relevant issues [e.g. significant desaturation can lead to cognitive decline]
- Provide a theoretical range of options 2
- Rehearse the pros and cons of the top two options 3
- Conclude with an impact on health highlighting items or special relevance to the particular patient and partner

5 Sleep study and where appropriate MSLT
- Provides confidence in the process
- Mindful of first night effect
- Not all patients are sleepy
- Sleep co-morbidities 1

4 Initial assessment
- Crucial in establishing trust
- Crucial in considering a range of co-morbidities especially other sleep disorders
- Important in sizing up motivation

3 Initial contact with the clinic
- Professionalism
- Treat PATIENT as an individual

2 Timeliness of appointment
- Clinic with a very long wait time decreases the patient sense of purpose

1 Who provides for the referral Self/trusted physician/friend
- This has impact on expectations

1 e.g. RLS / parasomnia/ ECG Abnormalities/ Sleep markers of depression
2 e.g. surgery, weight loss, drugs [not down to work], oral appliance, a postural device and Cpap. This can convey that a range of options are considered but the most appropriate is X or Y or in some cases X and Y
3 typically cost, convenience, ease of use, likelihood of effectiveness

Fig. 3.3 The steps needed to achieve high adherence

D. Allow the person to feel the change that needs to be made can be done in acceptable steps that may require different facilitators at different times in the process.

E. Do not patronize but do allow the steps to be taken to be clear and understandable.

F. Ensure that the patient has a sense of self-efficacy

G. Ensure the information shared is delivered with empathy

The key components of each of the factors are as follows:

A. A sense of trust is crucial. This is built up by the patient feeling; there is real personal interest in his/her well-being. In relatively short interactions, a key component is the perception by the patient that the clinician cares about them as a person and not merely as a CPAP client. Explicitly asking "What can I do to help you?" will open the path for this level of connection to be established. Explicitly stating what one can do is a useful starting point. This delineates the scope of practice that is available and the breadth of one's potential involvement in the pursuit of the patient's well-being. It also removes the feeling from a patient's perspective of a "chew you up and spit you out" interaction. For many patients, there is a skepticism surrounding the possibility that the motivation of the physician is increasing CPAP sales. This might taint the patient's view of physician in the sleep clinic.

B. Language is crucial, and the use of rhetoric (see the last page of this chapter) can be helpful.

Commenting to a patient that "What I lack in brains I hope to make up in perseverance" is a great line to reassure patients that this is a step-by-step relationship to facilitate their care. Some physicians might feel the statement is too self-deprecating.

C. In dealing with the issues that are relevant for the patient, there is the opportunity to be empathetic both in general and in a specific sense. For a person with a BMI (body mass index) north of 40, asking if anyone has discussed the pros and cons of bariatric surgery conveys the appreciation of the wider context. Explaining the potential links between arrhythmia/impotence/morning headaches/nocturnal enuresis in pathophysiological terms if that particular issue is relevant will allow the patient to feel that this is about them specifically. This can be as simple as telling the patient that their morning headache may be as a result of an increase in carbon dioxide and that once they are on CPAP regularly the headaches may dissipate. Similarly, indicating that they may observe an initial worsening of nocturia (for example from 4 to 6 times a night) followed by an improvement in this problem down to twice a night

Table 3.2 Strategies for increasing self-efficacy

Enactive attainments	Personal experiences of success	1. Set small steps toward behavior change so that success can be experienced early. 2. Discuss with patients their past successes so that these are salient
Vicarious experiences	Seeing the successes of similar others	1. Share with patients the success stories of others. 2. Engage patients in groups where they can view successful change. 3. Provide motivational videotapes or DVDs that combine helpful tips along with "real-life" stories of success and implementing them.
Verbal persuasion	Being told that one is capable	1. Assure the patient of his or his or her abilities; be a cheerleader. 2. Provide rationale for your beliefs about the patient's capability to be successful.
Physiological arousal		1. Help patients recognize and learn to channel the "rush of adrenaline" or "butterflies in the stomach" to motivate their successful behaviors. 2. Work with patients to manage physiological arousal that might impede their goals (consider the role of a psychologist in the team; see Chap. 6)

One key issue in facilitating adherence is improving the sense of self-efficacy. This is well summarized by the table in the book by Martin et al. [3], pp. 41. Reproduced with permission

will facilitate that the patient uses the CPAP through an initial worsening of a key symptom. Furthermore, to emphasize the role of improved cardiac function with CPAP use to bring about this change is motivating, especially for those with the problem but also as a demonstration of improving health on CPAP.

D. Pointing out that only the patients can make a behavioral change and all the clinician can do is to provide some "backup" to the steps of making the change (see Chap. 7).

Clinicians should be aware that it is important for the patient to make a strong commitment to a course of action "after weighing the pros and cons of the alternatives." It does not need to be the last word in the decision-making process. Using an example such as "many people may try either cognitive behavioral therapy or a medication to treat insomnia" but if one approach does not work after a good try one can review the choice.

E. The obvious best way to facilitate adherence to a treatment is not to patronize but to lay out all the options including relevant "straw men," e.g., "There are no known medications that fix sleep apnea," and then explain the pros and cons of each viable option and to help the patient to narrow down the choice to two options. For example, one can briefly state that "surgery is not applicable for you, that weight loss is a good idea but slow and postural device is not really an option in your case." One can then engage the patient in what may be the two best contenders for the individual (e.g., CPAP or an oral appliance). This allows a collaborative process and an enunciation of the pros and cons for each choice. It goes without saying that most people commit better to an option that they feel that they partially chose.

Some functional information (e.g., likelihood of success, cost of each option, timeline to feeling comfortable and effective resolution of symptoms) can then become part of the discussion. In this process, ensuring that the patient has the opportunity to make choices is vital to their sense of being engaged. Patients need to know that it matters less than which treatment one embarks on first, but whichever course one chooses one should give it a conscientious try and only then try the alternative.

3.4 Conclusion

I suspect that some of the above are familiar to many in the field; however, the evidence from the literature is that there is an extremely wide range of CPAP adherence in published studies and probably a much wider range of adherence among general clinicians. Using the somewhat declarative approach and appreciating the value of establishing, a relationship with the patient prior to the discussion about effectively helping them to change their behavior is key. A success rate of 85% using CPAP for 6 hours 6 nights a week is achievable, and the health outcomes are likely to be commensurately improved.

Finally, given that the form and style of speaking to a patient are always important and require skill and empathy, I have indulged myself by using a different form of rhetoric well described by Forsyth [17] in these brief (and hopefully relevant) poems (with apologies to Police, Shakespeare, and the readers).

Periodic Sentences of Our period

Every breath you choke

Every grunt is no joke

Every snort leaves the china broke

Every twitch you nearly croak

I hate watching you.

Put on your CPAP before I write another periodic sentence.

Diacope—Do Yu Cope?

Sleep or not to sleep, dream or not to dream

These are the questions to be answered by those who contemplate treatment of their apnea

To use CPAP or not to use CPAP?

Is that diacope or a rhetorical question?

And while we are about it do you want to keep

Your driving license (epiplexis)

Perhaps a maintenance of wakefulness test will suffice (procatalepsis)

Rhetorical Questions

Is sleep the restorer of the soul?

Is good deep sleep the premier brand?

Does a person with sleep apnea need to use his CPAP all night, every night?

You may question if these are "all rhetorical" questions.

References

1. David A. Obituary W Alwyn Lishman. Lancet. 2021;397:1704.
2. Francis L, Monakan K, Berger C. Laughing matter: the use of humour in medical interactions. Motiv Emot. 1999;23:155–74.
3. Martin LR, Haskard-Zolnierek KB, DiMatteo MR. Health behavior change and treatment adherence. Oxford: Oxford University Press; 2010.
4. Prochaska JO, DiClemente CC. Transtheoretical therapy: toward a more integrative model of change. Psychother Theory Res Pract. 1982;19:276–88.
5. DiMatteo RM, DiNicola DD. Achieving patient compliance. New York: Pergamon Press; 1982.
6. Crawford MR, Espie CA, Bartlett DJ, Grunstein RR. Integrating psychology and medicine in CPAP adherence-new concepts? Sleep Med Rev. 2014;18:123–39.
7. Engel GL. The need for a new medical model: a challenge for biomedicine. Science. 1977;96:129–36.
8. Engel GL. From biomedicine to biopsychosocial. Being scientific in the human domain. Psychosomatics. 1997;38:521–8.
9. Ghaemi SN. The biopsychosocial model in psychiatry: a critique. Int J Philos Relig Polit Arts. 2011;6:1–8.
10. Benning TB. Limitations of the biopsychosocial model in psychiatry. Adv Medi Educ Pract. 2015;6:347–52.
11. Chan R, Steel Z, Brooks R, Heung T, Erlich J, Chow J, Suranyi M. Psychosocial risk and protective factors for depression in the dialysis population: a systematic review and meta-regression analysis. J Psychosom Res. 2011;71:300–10.
12. Araujo SMHA, Bruin VMSD, Nepomuceno LS, Maximo ML, Daher EDF, Correia Ferrer DP. Restless legs syndrome in end-stage renal disease: clinical characteristics and associated comorbidities. Sleep Med. 2010;11:785–90.
13. Shapiro G, Shapiro CM. Factors and influence CPAP adherence: an overview. Sleep Breath. 2010;14:323–35.
14. Shapiro G, Zalai D, Trajanovic NN, Mallea J. Sleep apnea. CPAP and Me Joli Joco Publication Inc: Toronto, ON, Canada; 2011.
15. Naughton M, Fahmi R, Jacobs S, Shapiro G, Simmons M, Tangri S, Abumuamar A. Sleep Apnea – Who gets it? Why does it matter? How to diagnose and treat it? Sleep on the Bay. Toronto, ON, Canada; 2022.
16. Miller WR, Rollnick S. Application of motivational interviewing: helping people change. 3rd ed. New York, London: Guilford Press; 2013.
17. Forsyth M. The elements of eloquence: how to turn the perfect English Phase. Icon Books Ltd, London, UK; 2013.

Soft Styles of Motivating Patients to Adopt CPAP

Atul Khullar

Despite vast improvements in size, noise, and mechanical technologies over the almost 40 years since the inception of continuous positive airway pressure (CPAP), adherence to device remains middling and stagnant. Based on a total sleep time of 7 hours, a recent meta-analysis demonstrated a true adherence of 34% [1] and a recent world big data set from over 2.6 million patients indicated an average of 5.1 hours per night [2], which calculates to just over 70% of the average reported sleep time. Under this definition, the arbitrary standard Centre for Medicare and Medicaid Services (CMS) funding definition of compliance (at least four hours per day on 70% of nights) would equate to a 40% true adherence. Though this level and even more suboptimal CPAP adherence can show clinical benefits [3], it may compromise long-term outcomes [4], and good CPAP compliance is thought to be necessary to improve a wide variety of clinically relevant endpoints in several domains.

Given limited adherence and the plethora of ongoing patient-related factors that contribute, it is now postulated that though CPAP is the most efficacious treatment, it may not always be the most effective first-line treatment when considering the true levels of average adherence [5]. The concept of true AHI to compare treatments taking into account CPAP adherence has emerged as a paradigm shift given the inherent barriers and labor-intensive nature of improving compliance [6, 7]. It has been calculated that to reduce the AHI <5 score, CPAP usage should theoretically be 66–83% per night [6]. This does not even take into account device acceptance, as it has been estimated that 15–30% of people never even accept CPAP [8]. Clearly, different overall approaches to CPAP adherence and acceptance are needed, though it may be difficult to raise total compliance rates much further [9].

Much has been written about CPAP adherence, but clinically the focus has predominantly involved mechanical or "hard" approaches to optimize the airway while reducing various physical side effects. Examples include mask selection, advanced PAP interface types, nasal optimization, surgical options, and heated humidification. Some of this may be due to the marginalization of behavioral sleep medicine specialists in many jurisdictions, leading to a preponderance of breathing and surgical approaches during follow-up. Though important and helpful, "hard" approaches have shown inconsistent promise and not increased overall compliance rates significantly. They will be discussed elsewhere in the book.

This chapter will focus on reviewing underutilized non-mechanical or "soft" approaches to improve CPAP adherence and the overlapping concept of CPAP acceptance. An outline of these multifactorial approaches is in Table 4.1. These approaches will be integrated into a framework that represents the clinical management of the patient with a view to practical implementation for sleep clinicians of all disciplines.

4.1 Demographic Variables

There is a significant literature on demographic variables as they relate to CPAP adherence with marked inconsistency and weak associations. This is reviewed thoroughly elsewhere [10, 11]. Modest associations have been seen between potential nonadherence in younger age groups and people of African American heritage. Crude measures of lower socio-economic status such as lower education, unemployed status, and neighborhood demographics [12–17] also appear to be predictive of nonadherence, and this could relate to the funding availability of CPAP in a particular setting. Reimbursement did not appear directly linked to adherence in one study [18], but financial issues may be more related to actual CPAP acceptance, as low rates of uptake have been seen in studies where CPAP was not freely available [19–21]. Decreased adherence has also been seen with both habitual smoking [22, 23] and alcohol intake [24].

A. Khullar (✉)
Department of Psychiatry, University of Alberta, Edmonton, AB, Canada

© The Author(s), under exclusive license to Springer Nature Switzerland AG 2022
C. M. Shapiro et al. (eds.), *CPAP Adherence*, https://doi.org/10.1007/978-3-030-93146-9_4

Table 4.1 "Soft" approaches to CPAP acceptance/adherence

Predictive demographic variables and OSA disease factors
Nonmechanical or soft comorbidities (major mental illness, insomnia, and subjective sleep variables)
The role of the partner, spouse, or family
Adherence scales and measures
Is this the right patient and time for CPAP?
Service delivery factors
Interventions
Behavioral, supportive, and educational approaches
RHIT—Remote Health Information Technologies

Table 4.2 Suggested phenotypes of OSA [32]

Cluster 1	Female OSA
Cluster 2	Male, severe, and comorbid OSA
Cluster 3	Severe OSA syndrome
Cluster 4	Mildly symptomatic OSA
Cluster 5	Comorbid OSA

1, 4, and 5 demonstrated a higher chance of noncompliance than 3

Sex has been an inconsistent variable to predict CPAP adherence. Early studies showing higher nonadherence in men have been rightly noted to have limited nonrepresentative numbers of females due to both referral patterns and sampling in American veterans' clinics [25]. Newer, larger more inclusive studies demonstrate the female sex was more likely to correlate with a lower adherence [25, 26]. The less traditional symptom pattern in female OSA, potentially a separate phenotype, may be an influence on this. Ultimately, demographic variables show limited predictive value and are likely only proxies for true influence on CPAP use, but the ease of gathering should give them a small role in adherence and acceptance models.

4.2   OSA Disease Issues

Stronger associations between OSA disease factors and adherence have been seen, but the wide variety of subjective and objective measurements used in studies limits generalizability. A modest relation between CPAP adherence to the variables of OSA disease severity and symptomatic improvement has been noted, though it is unclear which contributes more (reviewed in Ref. [10]). Milder, yet equally symptomatic REM-related sleep-disordered breathing showed average compliance with [27], but data also exist for average adherence in minimally symptomatic populations with moderate-to-severe OSA [28]. It is likely that disease severity and symptomatic improvement have an interactive and bidirectional relationship with adherence. A limiting factor could be that many of these studies used the standard Epworth Sleepiness Scale (ESS) as a barometer of improvement and other changes in fatigue have rarely been measured in relation to adherence. Other non-airway-related symptoms such as headache [29] may also be predictive and have rarely been considered in the literature.

Obesity and BMI show mixed results in predicting adherence, but more recent studies demonstrate some association [22, 26]. It is intuitively difficult to separate weight from OSA disease severity as a predictive factor though nonobese OSA phenotypes may potentially have a higher rate of noncompliance [30].

Overall, it is clear that any model of CPAP adherence needs more inclusive multidimensional measures of OSA severity. The sleep apnea severity index (SASI), a simple composite index with four variables, showed improved predictive ability for adherence [31]. Newer research is also demonstrating distinct phenotypes of OSA (Table 4.2), which appear to impact compliance [32]. A composite approach taking into account OSA phenotypes is a promising area of further inquiry to personalize an approach to CPAP acceptance and adherence rather than discrete measures of oxygen saturation, apnea–hypopnea index, objective or subjective sleepiness.

4.3   Nonmechanical or "Soft" Comorbidities

4.3.1   Major Mental Illnesses

The bidirectional complex and overlapping relationship between OSA and depressive disorders have not been fully elucidated, but it is well known that there are high rates of major depression and depressive symptoms in OSA samples (reviewed in Ref. [33]). There have been mixed results of depression reducing adherence to CPAP (reviewed in Ref. [10]), with more recent studies demonstrating an association [16, 34]. Variability in the measurement of depressive symptoms may explain these mixed findings. Depressive symptoms also correlate with increased OSA symptoms after CPAP [35, 36], and this may indirectly lead to reduced adherence because of a perceived lack of efficacy.

Even in the absence of a direct association of depression with CPAP adherence, given the comorbid prevalence, overlap, and contribution to core symptomatology, depressive disorders must be reviewed in some fashion prior to any CPAP initiation. Depending on the severity, it may need to be treated prior to CPAP, though residual symptoms after a CPAP trial can also convince the patient that more aggressive management of depression is needed and CPAP has been shown at times itself to modestly improve depressive symptoms [37]. Potential improvement in depressive disorders and symptomatology should be considered as at least indirect means of alleviating the therapeutic burden of CPAP and enhancing treatment uptake in multiple dimensions [38].

In terms of anxiety, intuitively this would reduce CPAP adherence. Previous data sets demonstrated mixed results, but newer larger-scale data demonstrate an association with reduced CPAP adherence [16, 17, 39]. The specific anxiety of claustrophobia has also been shown to decrease CPAP adherence [40, 41].

Anxiety and depression show a great degree of overlap but are clearly different concepts with potentially different impacts on sleep. There is also a high degree of anxiety disorders with mild or limited depression; hence, screening for anxiety and depression separately can be a useful concept to help with CPAP adherence [42, 43]. Practical strategies include short patient-rated scales such as the PHQ-9 and the GAD-7 [44, 45]. Further inquiry can branch from there, or the referring provider can be notified.

Post-traumatic stress disorder (PTSD) while traditionally considered an anxiety disorder has been recently reclassified more accurately into its own chapter of trauma and trauma-related disorders [46]. In samples of veterans, the presence of PTSD correlated with significantly lower CPAP adherence [47] and insomnia, sleep disruption, and claustrophobia may be mediating factors [48]. Full diagnostic evaluation is likely not feasible outside mental health settings, but given that PTSD is a common comorbidity [47, 48], screening the potential for past trauma should be considered in certain cases and may be done clinically with the PCL-5, a simple validated scale [49], while reviewing anxiety.

Interestingly, the presence of schizophrenia was seen in one study to not affect CPAP compliance [50] indicating that there may be potential differences in the various major mental illnesses and their interaction with CPAP adherence.

4.3.2 Insomnia and Other Subjective Sleep Issues

Insomnia is commonly comorbid with OSA and may even represent a distinct phenotype of the disease [51, 52]. Insomnia has previously shown no association [14, 53, 54] with CPAP compliance, but larger studies indicate a trend toward insomnia being associated with decreased compliance [55–57], especially initial and terminal insomnia [58]. High rates of insomnia have also been seen in CPAP alternative clinics [59] indicating a potential lack of CPAP acceptance in insomnia patients. The interaction with insomnia and CPAP adherence is unclear and likely related to other comorbidities, but the presence of insomnia may represent phenotypes of OSA with lower potential CPAP adherence. Targeting insomnia with CBT-I for 4 sessions did improve adherence in a recent study [60], and for more detail about the role of CBT-I in OSA patients, see Chaps. 6 and 17. Clinically, insomnia should be noted as a potential marker for CPAP nonadherence, and re-evaluating the role and timing of CPAP in the treatment plan is then prudent.

Other subjective sleep issues such as inconsistent self-reported pretreatment bedtime [61], frequent changes in sleeping locations [62], non-supine sleep [63] as well as short sleep duration, and longer sleep latency [64] have been reported to adversely affect CPAP adherence. Again, these may be a proxy for a number of other variables such as lower socioeconomic status (SES) and insomnia, but are easy to note on a history and can be factored in.

4.3.3 Psychological Variables

There is a clear role for psychological variables in CPAP adherence as data have yielded associations that may be stronger than the traditionally assessed variables described earlier [10, 42]. A decision tree using maladaptive sleep apnea beliefs and emotional reactivity explained over 85% of nonadherent patients in one sample [65], and combination of both types of variables in a biopsychosocial (BPS) model has been conceptualized as the next dimension of predicting CPAP adherence and acceptance [10].

A number of psychological models of adherence from other health domains have been used to conceptualize CPAP adherence (see Box 4.1).

Box 4.1 A Summary of Psychological Models Studied CPAP Adherence and Acceptance

Social-cognitive theory (SCT) [66]

SCT addresses psychosocial factors and motivations influencing health behaviors and methods to promote sustained, translatable behavior change

Belief in one's ability to engage necessary behaviors to affect change (self-efficacy) is predictive for these behaviors. Knowledge and social support are important.

Transtheoretical model (TTM) [67]

Readiness to change is important. The stages are pre-contemplation, contemplation, preparation, action, and maintenance. Motivational interviewing is based on this model and has been used to enhance motivation for change in the context of CPAP use (see Chap. 6).

Social learning theory (SLT) [68]

Patient perception about level of control will determine whether they change behaviors. Value one puts on their health is the moderator as is the belief that one can overcome obstacles.

Health Belief Model (HBM) [69]

The likelihood of engaging in health behavior is based on readiness to act and the expected benefit. Readiness to act is determined by the patient's belief in susceptibility and seriousness. A cue to action acts as a trigger for change and self-efficacy continues this.

Expected perceived benefits vs barriers also play a role.

Self-Determination Theory (SDT) [70]

All behaviors lie along a continuum of relative autonomy with controlled (extrinsic) and autonomous (intrinsic) measures of motivation. Identifying where behaviors could be on the continuum can help target which interventions need to be targeted to the individual versus the system in which the individual is part of.

The data with these models related to CPAP adherence and acceptance consist of predominantly simple univariate regression, and there are clear overlapping characteristics. There are numerous interactions and moderating influences that need to be studied further, but nonetheless some trends have been seen.

Elements of SCT and TTM such as readiness, decisional balance, and self-efficacy were predictive of adherence early after a CPAP trial [71, 72], and self-efficacy alone has been seen in many studies to be predictive [73]. SCT also correlated with improved adherence in experienced CPAP users [74], and specific dimensions of SLT such as internal locus (high belief of control) over health may also be useful [75]. A small open study demonstrated the HBM predicting adherence [76] and a larger controlled study found that HBM had twice the predictive value of physiological factors [77]. Patient outcome expectancy, low perceptions of risk, and high perceived limitations due to symptoms were specific variables of the HBM that were predictive of CPAP adherence [77]. Other specific variables from psychological models that predict CPAP adherence are health value [78], elements of an active coping style [71, 73], and perceived benefits and barriers [79].

Another theme that has emerged out of this literature is the signal of different predictors of CPAP acceptance versus adherence. The SLT and TTM models were predictive after but not prior to CPAP [72]. Initial CPAP acceptance is an understudied and a key component of overall CPAP treatment. Promisingly, HBM variables above predicted adherence when measured prior to any CPAP experience [77], and a recently validated motivation to use CPAP scale [80] has been developed from SDT and could potentially be applied to both the acceptance and adherence dimensions of CPAP treatment.

Similar psychological concepts described above emerge from the user experience of CPAP. A narrative review indicates that user beliefs influence experiences, people are primed to reflect negatively to CPAP, and spouse and family influence user experience through engagement. Personality and attitude impact expectations of CPAP prior to use and reporting are very constrained by investigator-designed

assessment methods [81]. (For more details on personality and CPAP adherence, see Chap. 11.) Another recent qualitative survey also noted the concept of overall treatment ambivalence for both CPAP adherers and nonadherers [82].

There is also potential discordance between perceptions between healthcare workers (HCW) and patients on what impacts CPAP adherence. Patients perceived possibilities to learn and positive impact of education on adherence, while HCW scored higher on side effect frequency perception and its contribution to adherence [83]. This could create a basic psychological disconnect between users and their treatment providers. For example, a HCW could push mask fit, when a significant issue is lack of motivation.

Other psychological concepts that have been linked to CPAP nonadherence are type D personality type (a tendency to experience negative emotions and social inhibition) [84, 85], MMPI depression, hypochondriasis and psychopathy scales [86], and somatic–neurotic personality types [87], and neuroticism and behavioral inhibition [43]. Conversely, confidence and motivation, fun-seeking behaviors, and intellect are variables that may positively enhance CPAP adherence [88, 89]. Mindfulness has also been associated with increased adherence [90]. This is an intriguing finding since there are numerous available resources to teach mindfulness skills and has been used extensively in many other mental and physical disorders [91, 92].

4.3.4 Spousal and Partner Support

Much has been written about the dimensions that a partner or spouse brings to CPAP adherence, and it is likely a complex bidirectional relationship. Early samples were limited in scope and somewhat gender-biased to men, but a bed partner [93, 94] and being married [15] have both been seen to associate with increases in CPAP usage (see Chap. 10).

Both positive and negative spousal supports (pressure) have been seen to affect compliance positively and negatively, respectively [95, 96]. Marital conflict has predicted nonadherence but has been improved by CPAP adherence [97], and relationship satisfaction was positively associated with compliance instead of attachment style [98]. A study with a large proportion of women demonstrated spousal engagement only helped compliance in men [99], though engagement with ratings of a "high-quality marriage" was helpful in both genders in a more recent study [100]. More specifically, perceived partner autonomy support (acknowledging patient perspective, providing choices, self-initiation, and minimizing pressure) has been isolated as an independent overall factor that associates with increased CPAP adherence [101]. Thus, it is not surprising that cluster analysis noted that older retired couples, who may be likely to show many of the above factors as they remained married, were seen to have better CPAP adherence [102]. Partner sexual intimacy may also be a critical factor as good PAP adherence has been seen to relate directly and indirectly to a better intimate relationship [103], perhaps in part by helping male erectile dysfunction [104]. Conversely, the belief that less intimacy with partners could occur with CPAP was a negative predictor of adherence [105].

In summary, a dyadic perspective (i.e., how CPAP affects each partner) is likely needed with the dimensions of partners working together, perceived benefits, patient motivation for partner, and types of support, while addressing barriers of negative preconceptions, anxiety, bothersome equipment, intimacy, and image change [106, 107]. Attention to the ways couples interact as they deal with stressors and patients' response to partner involvement should also be considered. Partner involvement in the early phase of CPAP treatment was also deemed qualitatively important to adherence by patients [108].

The role of family support has not been directly studied in adult CPAP adherence, but a recent study showed improvement in self-efficacy scores and CPAP adherence with family support [109] and intuitively involving the family early on in the treatment plan would make sense, especially in some cultures that are more family-oriented.

4.3.5 Adherence Measurements

Numerous groups have tried to operationalize CPAP adherence by self-reported questionnaires integrating several key variables. However, a simple single question of whether they have encountered any problems with the device on the morning of titration also has shown prediction to adherence [93, 110]. Other pragmatic measures include the previously mentioned SASI [31], a 2-item equation of how they feel on CPAP and average usage in a 2-week trial [111], a 3-item willingness score after 4 nights of CPAP usage [112], and a 6-item CPAP questionnaire after titration [113].

More comprehensive formally validated tools include the psychological theory-based scales such as the previously mentioned Motivation to Use CPAP (MU-C) scale [80] as well as the self-efficacy measure for sleep apnea (SEMSA), a 26-item scale outlining cognitions, risk perceptions, outcome expectancies, and self-efficacy beliefs about using CPAP [114]. A more holistic scale is the Index for nonadherence to PAP (I-NAP) [115], a 19-Item scale to be given immediately after CPAP titration, that combines two components of SEMSA (self-efficacy, health literacy) BMI and demographics. Overall, the research on formal measurements that link to CPAP adherence is limited and the applicability in different clinical populations is unclear. However, designing a practical tool that helps assess the potential for nonadherence that takes into account multiple factors and

that can be delivered easily (akin to the widely adopted STOP-BANG for obstructive sleep apnea) [116] would be of great assistance.

A key limitation in developing CPAP adherence prediction models is the binary definition of adherence or nonadherence. There are likely clear clusters of CPAP adherers (Table 4.3 from Ref. [117]), which need to be better identified to obtain a clearer picture of models of nonadherence. Another latent profile analysis noted 3 groups of CPAP users, nonadherer, attempter, and adherer. Various factors predicted which subgroup a patient would be in; i.e., insomnia predicted differences between an attempters and adherers, while self-efficacy was predictive between the nonadherer and adherer groups [78]. Again this is preliminary work, but establishing clusters or phenotypes of CPAP adherence as a continuum and integrating the concept of CPAP acceptance (i.e., nonusers in Table 4.3) will be critical for adherence prediction models to progress further.

4.4 Is CPAP Right for This Patient or Is This the Right Time?

Many patients are not screened for the above concerns in standard sleep medicine clinics due to lack of awareness or training. Some of this is intermittently done at the durable medical equipment (DME) level, but given the induction to sell devices in some jurisdictions, motivation to assess softer compliance factors can be limited. Government policies can motivate this to some degree if compliance is necessary for further funding, but costs have declined so that CPAP therapy is now easily accessible to a wide cohort, and it may be that lower socioeconomic system (SES) patients that are more likely to use government support also would overlap with groups that show inherent challenges with compliance.

At a minimum, a cursory review of demographic variables and other sleep disorders (especially insomnia, depression, and anxiety) should be undertaken. Self-report questionnaires with follow-up discussion as needed can be an efficient way of reviewing this. Factoring in spousal or partner support or beliefs in some fashion is also important. Psychological variables are difficult to delineate, but basic measures such as a type D personality screen could be considered. A snapshot of patient history with risk factors should

Table 4.3 A paradigm of patterns of treatment adherence [117]

1. Good users
2. Slow improvers
3. Slow decliners
4. Variable users
5. Occasional attempters
6. Early dropouts
7. Nonusers

be taken to account as well. For example, the same severity of OSA in a healthy 30 years old and 55 years old with diabetes and hypertension would be viewed quite differently. Patients should be educated about all types of OSA treatment without distortions or pressures to purchase a CPAP machine. Other disorders may need to be addressed first, and OSA treatment can be returned to at a later point.

4.5 Delivery of Service—Diagnosis

Patient care by sleep specialist in a sleep medicine program versus primary care indicated only a trend toward improved compliance [118], but sleep specialist consultation alone has been shown to improve CPAP compliance [119].

Diagnosis by full or ambulatory study showed no difference in compliance, but both groups had better compliance than diagnosis by oximetry [120]. Early studies indicated that one night of in-laboratory titration improved compliance [121], but two nights did not [122, 123], and a split night protocol showed no difference [124] and pretreatment with CPAP showed only a trend toward greater compliance [125]. A meta-analysis of ambulatory auto-PAP vs observed titration showed no difference or increase in PAP compliance, but most of those studies had a select population where the titration was ordered by the sleep program [126, 127]. However, most retrospective databases of wider populations have not shown a difference in compliance between standard and home titration either [2].

Overall, it is unclear whether specialist consultation helps adherence and targeted studies with potential non-adherent patients are needed. It appears that for the average patient, PAP adherence may not depend on type and location of testing and titration, but again subgroups and phenotypes that could benefit from observed study and titration are likely and need to be identified. Adherence patterns are formed very quickly after beginning CPAP [93, 117, 128, 129] so any delay in appointment times to obtain specialist consultation and observed titration may offset any gains that more specialized assessment may have. Prompt intervention and support with CPAP may be more critical than type of study or specialist consultation. Clinically triaging for factors related to poor PAP compliance in addition to disease and symptom severity may help triage patients to sleep specialists more effectively. Nonetheless, specialist clinic designs need to move away from tertiary clinic models, not only finding ways to be more accessible, but also focusing resources on seeing the right patients at the right time. Care pathways for primary care physicians and utilization of alternative care providers to handle less complex OSA cases [130] and targeted use of remote technologies and virtual care may assist in this important goal.

4.6 Interventions

4.6.1 Addition of a Hypnotic to Improve Adherence

Though not truly a fully "soft" approach, this is included here as it is a nonmechanical method to possibly improve CPAP adherence. There is a paucity of data on this, which is surprising given the high comorbidity of insomnia and sleep apnea and the potential impact of insomnia on adherence. Improvement in sleep efficiency overall and one-time general sedative use on the titration night has seen to increase adherence retrospectively [131, 132], but a recent larger analysis found that there was no association [133]. Prospectively, zaleplon, a very short-acting hypnotic given on the titration night, had no association with compliance [134], but a longer-acting one, eszopiclone, was positively associated with increased CPAP adherence [135]. Many initial titrations are ambulatory now, so it is unclear how clinically useful the use of hypnotics to improve the observed titration night would be to help adherence. Intuitively, it may give a clearer titration and could be considered in patients who need or request initially observed titrations. More relevant would likely be to give a short course of hypnotic use to improve early CPAP adherence in the early critical period. One study demonstrated no change in results for 14 days of zolpidem treatment [136] and another demonstrated improvement in adherence with 14 days of eszopiclone [137]. A meta-analysis of all nonbenzodiazepine hypnotics (or z-drugs) demonstrated a net positive effect with eszopiclone having the strongest effect [138], and the longer half-life of this agent may be related to the capacity to improve adherence. Increased CPAP compliance has also been seen in PTSD patients who were on sedative medications [48].

Overall, a short course of a longer-acting hypnotic that does not affect the airway could be a potential clinical consideration to improve adherence, especially if there is significant insomnia or comorbidities that disrupt sleep. Another theory is that the arousal threshold from CPAP may increase with certain hypnotics such as eszopiclone [138] or trazodone [139], potentially increasing CPAP compliance. For more information about hypnotic medications in COMISA patients, see Chap. 18.

4.6.2 Educational, Supportive, and Behavioral Interventions for CPAP Adherence

There is a large extant literature of behavioral interventions to improve CPAP compliance. They vary significantly in control interventions, timing, design, approach, and theoretical underpinnings. Populations at risk of CPAP nonadherence were not always systematically targeted [140]. A recent full Cochrane database review on soft interventions by type for CPAP adherence is summarized in Table 4.4 [141].

In terms of delivery methods of intervention, showing the patient PSG data [142, 143], using a group approach [144] and motivational interviewing or CBT strategies [145] all appear to improve CPAP adherence. For a description of motivational interviewing and CBT, see Chap. 6. Educational videos alone appear to have inconsistent results, either trending as helpful [146], associated with increased patient follow-up with no increased adherence [147], or demonstrating no change [140].

Interventions that included home visits by healthcare professionals [148–151] appear to be effective in establishing long-term adherence but are likely impractical in most healthcare systems. Phone calls and more frequent follow-up with healthcare team on their own have had mixed positive [152, 153] and negative results [154, 155]. Other unique mechanisms with positive results have included partnering with a successful CPAP user [156], habit-forming music [157], and progressive muscle relaxation [158]. Educational literature alone had a positive effect in an early controlled study [154] and self-reported CPAP adherence in long-term users [159].

Targeted education about less commonly discussed positive outcomes of CPAP compliance that are individualized to the patient's current comorbidities may be of use in educational plans. Besides commonly known improvements in sleepiness and cardiovascular (CV) risk factors with CPAP compliance, which are usually stressed in educational programs, there are newer data for good CPAP compliance helping mild neurocognitive disorder [160, 161], gastroesophageal reflux disease (GERD) [162], and mortality from overlap syndrome (a combination of chronic obstructive pulmonary disease and OSA [163] and perhaps depression [37]).

In summary, Table 4.5 outlines the critical components of CPAP adherence interventions.

The nature of delivery of all of these components is too intensive to deliver during a routine patient encounter but does illustrate key parts of any program that can be adapted in a multimodal fashion and involve professionals from many disciplines. Although costly, an intensive multimodal

Table 4.4 Summary of evidence for psychological interventions for CPAP adherence

Type of intervention	Level of evidence certainty	Effect on adherence
Behavioral	High	Clinically significant
Supportive	Moderate	Modest
Educational/mixed	Very low	Modest

Note it is unclear if improvement in quality of life, mood/anxiety, and sleepiness improve with increased CPAP usage with these interventions

CPAP adherence program versus standard of care has demonstrated a net cost savings by increasing CPAP adherence with a commensurate reduction in CVD mortality [150]. If designed correctly with the above principles in mind, newer health information technologies and telemonitoring may further increase what can be delivered in CPAP adherence programs at reduced overall cost.

4.6.3 CPAP Adherence in Children and Adolescents

As a rule, if CPAP is selected for children and adolescents, it is likely they will have either already failed first-line treatment (adenotonsillectomy) or have other significant medical comorbidities (syndromes, malformations, obesity) that require PAP [165]. This medical complexity, along with age-related developmental and social issues, imbues a degree of complexity that likely will require some degree of soft or nonmechanical approaches to PAP adherence.

Studies of CPAP adherence in pediatric populations have shown poor-middling rates similar to adults [165, 166]. Family and demographic factors appear predictive of adherence rather than the traditional measures of severity of apnea, sleepiness, or device factors such as PAP type, mask fit, and pressure [167–169]. Key barriers were seen to be low maternal education (the most predictive), race, older patient age [169], and decreased family social support [167]. Females and developmentally delayed patients demonstrated better adherence in one study [169].

Psychosocially, noncompliance centered around the child not wanting to use it or be reminded of their OSA, the child and parent forgetting, being away from home, and the child being sick. A validated scale, the adherence barriers to continuous positive airway pressure (CPAP) questionnaire (ABCQ), has been developed to identify these barriers and is also a good summary that can be used clinically [170]. In an older adolescent-specific group, a qualitative study noted that the extent and nature of structure in the home family, style of communication, social reactions, and attitudes and perceptions of PAP benefits were all seen to affect adherence [171].

Most interventions to increase CPAP adherence in child and adolescents center around child and parent engagement, identification of specific barriers, initial acceptance, behavioral intervention, and side effects. Individual tailoring, peer support, health education, and family involvement have been seen to be helpful [171]. Other factors that have shown helpful in small studies are aligning parent-child outcomes [172] desensitization procedures to CPAP [168], brief and prolonged behavioral interventions [173], improving caregiver self-efficacy [174], and adding RT visits for low compliance

Table 4.5 Critical components of CPAP adherence interventions

Increasing knowledge

Awareness of existing attitudes (ambivalence about CPAP use, treatment expectations)

OSA, CPAP, diagnosis associated, and expected health outcomes and daily management goals

Targeting and engaging social and support factors—Including spouse, bed partner, or family

Anticipatory guidance and quickly troubleshoot problems during treatment

Assisted initial exposure to CPAP

Regular early feedback and encouragement—(automated, peers, or HCP)

Acknowledge challenges in CPAP

Problem-solving resources

Refer to a trained provider for motivational interviewing and motivational enhancement therapy, CBT for insomnia, and treatment of CPAP-related anxiety; see Chap. 6

Follow-up with sleep team in integrative fashion with above

Adapted from Refs. [81, 164]

patients [175]. Support and understanding of the challenges of PAP therapy from the team are also seen to help [167, 176].

An overall sample clinical program from a university center taking into account these factors has been outlined well [168] and good overall rates of CPAP adherence have been documented with a pediatric tertiary care program [177]. This level of care is clearly not feasible on a wide scale, but newer studies indicate that key factors can be integrated by clinicians at potentially realistic levels of manpower to improve adherence. Examples include supervised home CPAP starts with good follow-up [178] and a recent pilot study with a simple token economy table increase in young CPAP nonadherent children [179].

4.7 Approaches Using Remote Health Information Technologies (RHIT) (Telehealth, Telemonitoring, eHealth)

The use of remote health information technologies for patient self and clinician monitoring has grown in many areas of medicine as devices become more portable, powerful, and acceptable. However, remote service delivery has long been limited by antiquated face-to-face payment models and potential health information security concerns. The recent COVID-19 pandemic has caused remote strategies to grow exponentially to the point where it will likely become a primary method of service delivery if proper funding follows. Interestingly, it has been seen that the pandemic itself may increase PAP adherence of its own accord. Potential factors have been theorized as rampant media education that COVID-19 compromises the respiratory system, the high presence of comorbidities in OSA patients that clearly

increase COVID-19 risk, and more patient time and inclination to sleep with reduced activities [180].

A limitation to assessing RHIT is the lack of a standard definition. Telemedicine, telehealth, telemonitoring, eHealth (electronic health), and mobile health (mHealth) are terms used in an overlapping fashion without precision and with blurred boundaries. This is reviewed with respect to OSA elsewhere [181]. For the purposes of discussion in this chapter, we will consider them all remote health information technology (RHIT).

Sleep medicine has a robust early adopter history of adopting RHIT from performing, scoring, and interpreting sleep studies to objective remote monitoring of CPAP settings. Hence, the field is well-primed to integrate models of CPAP adherence with RHIT. With multiple designs including video [182] and Internet education [183], automated text and phone call reminders, remote troubleshooting in response to telemonitoring of CPAP data, smartphone applications, and Internet CPAP patient portals [184–186], RHIT studies to increase CPAP adherence have yielded mostly improvements versus standard of care. Two recent meta-analyses showed an overall significant short-term improvement in adherence with and quality of life with both telemonitoring care and eHealth approaches as well [187, 188].

Many of the studies analyzed were overlapping, and the effect on adherence was not maintained long term; however, many of the programs had completely ceased [187]. It is quite possible that certain phenotypes may be more suited to RHIT interventions than others [189]. Cost savings have not always been measured, but most studies demonstrated either reduction in healthcare provider time [184, 190] or an actual cost savings [191, 192], with similar patient satisfaction [183, 192]. With any RHIT-based approach, security and integrity of health data are paramount and concerns about this have been postulated as a barrier to its wide acceptance [181]. However, privacy issues were not a major concern in one large study [191] and the current pandemic has likely shifted that balance further, as less face-to-face contact, convenience, and timely access of care have become paramount [193]. Regardless, data stewardship concerns need to be outlined in any telehealth program [194].

Overall, RHIT is and will continue to be a paradigm-shifting step in all areas of medicine and major themes to ensure that CPAP adherence and overall OSA management moves forward with RHIT are as follows [195]:

1. Connect both provider and consumer technologies through electronic health records and interactive connected systems
2. Integrate care to improve risk identification with automated delivery of stepped care
3. Improve patient–provider interchange through message and predictive short surveys

4. Include team-based care in an interdisciplinary fashion with an emphasis on overall clinical outcomes.

To read more about CPAP adherence and telehealth, see Chap. 30.

4.8   Conclusion

CPAP adherence initiatives should embrace a multilevel approach taking into account the interactions between psychological, behavioral, environmental, and mechanical factors. Integrating this practically into multidisciplinary care pathways will be critical. A holistic personalized biopsychosocial (BPS) model for CPAP adherence based on key mediators has been proposed, and the specifics are outlined in Ref. [10]. The goal would be to describe certain individuals with a certain BPS profile would benefit from certain bespoke BPS interventions to improve adherence. Much of this would include the integration in a comprehensive care pathway. An analogy to the BPS management of chronic pain was made.

Though care pathways may be limited by resources, understanding the dynamic interplay of these variables and identifying major drivers of CPAP nonadherence are critical so that certain patients are not be pushed blindly toward CPAP or given extra stepped support when they most need it. A CPAP acceptance and adherence model [42] has been proposed to address some of these concerns.

Another overall heuristic could also be drawn from the evolving P4 personalized medicine approach. This consists of prediction who will develop disease, prevent disease rather than react, and personalize diagnosis/treatment and participation of patients in their own care. This model has been outlined as an approach to sleep apnea care in general [196, 197] and could be a model applied directly to CPAP adherence as per Table 4.6.

A critical part of the success of this approach CPAP adherence will be the usage of standard clinically relevant phenotypes for groups of OSA patients [198] and types of CPAP adherers rather than the traditional binary definitions. There may also be clusters of CPAP accepters. This would illustrate the point that the exact same factors may differentially affect disparate groups of OSA patients in terms of their adherence. The large data sets garnered by RHIT will be very helpful in this goal [195]. Future consumer-driven technologies and health smartphone apps may vary in accuracy but will also need to be leveraged. Medical school curricula also need to integrate this approach to RHIT, big data, clusters, and phenotypes.

The view of OSA as not just a chronic respiratory disease of airway collapsibility, but one with biopsychosocial (BPS) factors similar to depression, chronic pain, or diabetes that multiple specialities need to contribute in multiple ways will be necessary if further gains in CPAP adherence are to be materialized.

References

1. Rotenberg BW, Murariu D, Pang KP. Trends in CPAP adherence over twenty years of data collection: a flattened curve. Otolaryngol Head Neck Surg. 2016;45(1):1–9.
2. Cistulli PA, Armitstead J, Pepin J, Woehrle H, Nunez CM, Benjafield A, et al. Short-term CPAP adherence in obstructive sleep apnea: a big data analysis using real world data. Sleep Med. 2019;59:114–6.
3. Gaisl T, Rejmer P, Thiel S, Haile SR, Osswald M, Roos M, et al. Effects of suboptimal adherence of CPAP therapy on symptoms of obstructive sleep apnoea: a randomised, double-blind, controlled trial. Eur Respir J. 2020;55(3):1901526.
4. McEvoy RD, Antic NA, Heeley E, Luo Y, Ou Q, Zhang X, et al. CPAP for prevention of cardiovascular events in obstructive sleep apnea. N Engl J Med. 2016;375(10):919–31.
5. Rotenberg BW, Vicini C, Pang EB, Pang KP. Reconsidering first-line treatment for obstructive sleep apnea: a systematic review of the literature. Otolaryngol Head Neck Surg. 2016;45(1):1–9.
6. Ravesloot M, Vries ND. Reliable calculation of the efficacy of non-surgical and surgical treatment of obstructive sleep apnea revisited. Sleep. 2011;34(1):105–10.
7. Boyd SB, Walters AS. Effectiveness of treatment apnea-hypopnea index: a mathematical estimate of the true apnea-hypopnea index in the home setting. J Oral Maxillofac Surg. 2013;71(2):351–7.
8. Engleman HM, Wild MR. Improving CPAP use by patients with the sleep apnoea/hypopnoea syndrome (SAHS). Sleep Med Rev. 2003;7(1):81–99.
9. Richard W, Venker J, Herder CD, Kox D, Berg BVD, Laman M, et al. Acceptance and long-term compliance of nCPAP in obstructive sleep apnea. Eur Arch Otorhinolaryngol. 2007;264(9):1081–6.
10. Crawford MR, Espie CA, Bartlett DJ, Grunstein RR. Integrating psychology and medicine in CPAP adherence – new concepts? Sleep Med Rev. 2014;18(2):123–39.
11. Bakker JP, Weaver TE, Parthasarathy S, Aloia MS. Adherence to CPAP. Chest. 2019;155(6):1272–87.
12. Platt AB, Field SH, Asch DA, Chen Z, Patel NP, Gupta R, et al. Neighborhood of residence is associated with daily adherence to CPAP therapy. Sleep. 2009;32(6):799–806.
13. Bakker JP, O'Keeffe KM, Neill AM, Campbell AJ. Ethnic disparities in CPAP adherence in New Zealand: effects of socioeconomic status, health literacy and self-efficacy. Sleep. 2011;34(11):1595–603.
14. Billings ME, Auckley D, Benca R, Foldvary-Schaefer N, Iber C, Redline S, et al. Race and residential socioeconomics as predictors of CPAP adherence. Sleep. 2011;34(12):1653–8.
15. Gagnadoux F, Vaillant ML, Goupil F, Pigeanne T, Chollet S, Masson P, et al. Influence of marital status and employment status

Table 4.6 A personalized medicine approach to CPAP adherence

Predict—Create a reasonable set of predictive measures, perhaps validated scales

Prevent—Early intervention and possible titration interventions

Personalize—Look at ongoing partner dyad and family issues, lifestyle, phenotype

Participate—Educational programs, self-monitoring, group motivational enhancement therapy, and cognitive-behavioral therapy (CBT)

on long-term adherence with continuous positive airway pressure in sleep apnea patients. PLoS One. 2011;6(8):e22503.

16. Gulati A, Ali M, Davies M, Quinnell T, Smith I. A prospective observational study to evaluate the effect of social and personality factors on continuous positive airway pressure (CPAP) compliance in obstructive sleep apnoea syndrome. BMC Pulm Med. 2017;17(1):56.

17. Wickwire EM, Jobe SL, Oldstone LM, Scharf SM, Johnson AM, Albrecht JS. Lower socioeconomic status and co-morbid conditions are associated with reduced continuous positive airway pressure adherence among older adult Medicare beneficiaries with obstructive sleep apnea. Sleep. 2020;43(12):zsaa122.

18. Leemans J, Rodenstein D, Bousata J, Mwenge GB. Impact of purchasing the CPAP device on acceptance and long-term adherence: a Belgian model. Acta Clin Belg. 2017;73(1):34–9.

19. Riachy M, Najem S, Iskandar M, Choucair J, Ibrahim I, Juvelikian G. Factors predicting CPAP adherence in obstructive sleep apnea syndrome. Sleep Breath. 2016;21(2):295–302.

20. Lee CHK, Leow LC, Song PR, Li H, Ong TH. Acceptance and adherence to continuous positive airway pressure therapy in patients with obstructive sleep apnea (OSA) in a southeast Asian privately funded healthcare system. Sleep Sci. 2017;10(2):57–63.

21. Tan B, Tan A, Chan YH, Mok Y, Wong HS, Hsu PP. Adherence to continuous positive airway pressure therapy in Singaporean patients with obstructive sleep apnea. Am J Otolaryngol. 2018;39(5):501–6.

22. Jacobsen AR, Eriksen F, Hansen RW, Erlandsen M, Thorup L, Damgård MB, et al. Determinants for adherence to continuous positive airway pressure therapy in obstructive sleep apnea. PLoS One. 2017;12(12):e0189614.

23. Baratta F, Pastori D, Bucci T, Fabiani M, Fabiani V, Brunori M, et al. Long-term prediction of adherence to continuous positive air pressure therapy for the treatment of moderate/severe obstructive sleep apnea syndrome. Sleep Med. 2018;43:66–70.

24. Jeong JI, Kim HY, Hong SD, Ryu G, Kim SJ, Lee KE, Dhong HJ, Chung SK. Upper airway variation and frequent alcohol consumption can affect compliance with continuous positive airway pressure. Clin Exp Otorhinolaryngol. 2016;9(4):346–51.

25. Patel SR, Bakker JP, Stitt CJ, Aloia MS, Nouraie SM. Age and sex disparities in adherence to CPAP. Chest. 2021 Jan;159(1):382–9.

26. Palm A, Midgren B, Theorell-Haglöw J, Ekström M, Ljunggren M, Janson C, et al. Factors influencing adherence to continuous positive airway pressure treatment in obstructive sleep apnea and mortality associated with treatment failure – a national registry-based cohort study. Sleep Med. 2018;51:85–91.

27. Conwell W, Patel B, Doeing D, Pamidi S, Knutson KL, Ghods F, et al. Prevalence, clinical features, and CPAP adherence in REM-related sleep-disordered breathing: a cross-sectional analysis of a large clinical population. Sleep Breath. 2011;16(2):519–26.

28. Campos-Rodriguez F, Martinez-Alonso M, Sanchez-De-La-Torre M, Barbe F. Long-term adherence to continuous positive airway pressure therapy in non-sleepy sleep apnea patients. Sleep Med. 2016;17:1–6.

29. Rafael-Palou X, Turino C, Steblin A, Sánchez-De-La-Torre M, Barbé F, Vargiu E. Comparative analysis of predictive methods for early assessment of compliance with continuous positive airway pressure therapy. BMC Med Inform Decis Mak. 2018;18(1):81.

30. Gray EL, Mckenzie DK, Eckert DJ. Obstructive sleep apnea without obesity is common and difficult to treat: evidence for a distinct pathophysiological phenotype. J Clin Sleep Med. 2017;13(01):81–8.

31. Balakrishnan K, James KT, Weaver EM. Predicting CPAP use and treatment outcomes using composite indices of sleep apnea severity. J Clin Sleep Med. 2016;12(06):849–54.

32. Gagnadoux F, Le Vaillant M, Paris A, Pigeanne T, Leclair-Visonneau L, Bizieux-Thaminy A, et al. Chest. 2016;149(1):288–90.

33. Bahammam AS, Kendzerska T, Gupta R, Ramasubramanian C, Neubauer DN, Narasimhan M, et al. Comorbid depression in obstructive sleep apnea: an under-recognized association. Sleep Breath. 2015;20(2):447–56.

34. Law M, Naughton M, Ho S, Roebuck T, Dabscheck E. Depression may reduce adherence during CPAP titration trial. J Clin Sleep Med. 2014;10(02):163–9.

35. Wells RD, Freedland KE, Carney RM, Duntley SP, Stepanski EJ. Adherence, reports of benefits, and depression among patients treated with continuous positive airway pressure. Psychosom Med. 2007;69(5):449–54.

36. Gagnadoux F, Vaillant ML, Goupil F, Pigeanne T, Chollet S, Masson P, et al. Depressive symptoms before and after long-term CPAP therapy in patients with sleep apnea. Chest. 2014;145(5):1025–31.

37. Povitz M, Bolo CE, Heitman SJ, Tsai WH, Wang J, James MT. Effect of treatment of obstructive sleep apnea on depressive symptoms: systematic review and meta-analysis. PLoS Med. 2014;11(11):e1001762.

38. Cayanan EA, Bartlett DJ, Chapman JL, Hoyos CM, Phillips CL, Grunstein RR. A review of psychosocial factors and personality in the treatment of obstructive sleep apnoea. Eur Respir Rev. 2019;28(152):190005.

39. Budhiraja R, Kushida CA, Nichols DA, Walsh JK, Simon RD, Gottlieb DJ, et al. Impact of randomization, clinic visits, and medical and psychiatric comorbidities on continuous positive airway pressure adherence in obstructive sleep apnea. J Clin Sleep Med. 2016;12(03):333–41.

40. Chasens ER, Pack AI, Maislin G, Dinges DF, Weaver TE. Claustrophobia and adherence to CPAP treatment. West J Nurs Res. 2005;27(3):307–21.

41. Edmonds JC, Yang H, King TS, Sawyer DA, Rizzo A, Sawyer AM. Claustrophobic tendencies and continuous positive airway pressure therapy non-adherence in adults with obstructive sleep apnea. Heart Lung. 2015;44(2):100–6.

42. Olsen S, Smith S, Oei T. Adherence to continuous positive airway pressure therapy in obstructive sleep apnoea sufferers: a theoretical approach to treatment adherence and intervention. Clin Psychol Rev. 2008;28(8):1355–71.

43. Moran AM, Everhart DE, Davis CE, Wuensch KL, Lee DO, Demaree HA. Personality correlates of adherence with continuous positive airway pressure (CPAP). Sleep Breath. 2011;15(4):687–94.

44. Kroenke K, Spitzer RL, Williams JB. The PHQ-9: validity of a brief depression severity measure. J Gen Intern Med. 2001;16(9):606–13.

45. Spitzer RL, Kroenke K, Williams JB, Löwe B. A brief measure for assessing generalized anxiety disorder: the GAD-7. Arch Intern Med. 2006;166(10):1092–7.

46. American Psychiatric Association. Diagnostic and statistical manual of mental disorders: DSM-5. 5th ed. Arlington: American Psychiatric Association; 2013.

47. Zhang Y, Weed JG, Ren R, Tang X, Zhang W. Prevalence of obstructive sleep apnea in patients with posttraumatic stress disorder and its impact on adherence to continuous positive airway pressure therapy: a meta-analysis. Sleep Med. 2017;36:125–32.

48. Collen JF, Lettieri CJ, Hoffman M. The impact of posttraumatic stress disorder on CPAP adherence in patients with obstructive sleep apnea. J Clin Sleep Med. 2012;08(06):667–72.

49. Weathers FW, Litz BT, Keane TM, Palmieri PA, Marx BP, Schnurr PP. The PTSD checklist for DSM–5 (PCL-5). Boston: National Center for PTSD; 2013.

50. Saoud M, Saeed M, Patel S, Mador MJ. Positive airway pressure adherence in patients with obstructive sleep apnea with schizophrenia. Lung. 2019;198(1):181–5.

51. Saaresranta T, Hedner J, Bonsignore MR, Riha RL, McNicholas WT, Penzel T, et al. Clinical phenotypes and comorbidity in European sleep apnoea patients. PLoS One. 2016;11(10):e0163439.

52. Zinchuk AV, Gentry MJ, Concato J, Yaggi HK. Phenotypes in obstructive sleep apnea: a definition, examples and evolution of approaches. Sleep Med Rev. 2017;35:113–23.

53. Nguyên X-L, Chaskalovic J, Rakotonanahary D, Fleury B. Insomnia symptoms and CPAP compliance in OSAS patients: a descriptive study using data mining methods. Sleep Med. 2010;11(8):777–84.

54. Mitzkewich MP, Seda G, Jameson J, Markwald RR. Effects of insomnia and depression on CPAP adherence in a military population. Fed Pract. 2019;36(3):134–9.

55. Wickwire EM, Smith MT, Birnbaum S, Collop NA. Sleep maintenance insomnia complaints predict poor CPAP adherence: a clinical case series. Sleep Med. 2010;11(8):772–6.

56. Pieh C, Bach M, Popp R, Jara C, Crönlein T, Hajak G, et al. Insomnia symptoms influence CPAP compliance. Sleep Breath. 2012;17(1):99–104.

57. Wallace DM, Sawyer AM, Shafazand S. Comorbid insomnia symptoms predict lower 6-month adherence to CPAP in US veterans with obstructive sleep apnea. Sleep Breath. 2018;22(1):5–15.

58. Björnsdóttir E, Janson C, Sigurdsson JF, Gehrman P, Perlis M, Juliusson S, et al. Symptoms of insomnia among patients with obstructive sleep apnea before and after two years of positive airway pressure treatment. Sleep. 2013;36(12):1901–9.

59. Lam AS, Collop NA, Bliwise DL, Dedhia RC. Validated measures of insomnia, function, sleepiness, and nasal obstruction in a CPAP alternatives clinic population. J Clin Sleep Med. 2017;13(08):949–57.

60. Sweetman A, Lack L, Catcheside PG, Antic NA, Smith S, Chai-Coetzer CL, et al. Cognitive and behavioral therapy for insomnia increases the use of continuous positive airway pressure therapy in obstructive sleep apnea participants with comorbid insomnia: a randomized clinical trial. Sleep. 2019;42(12):zsz178.

61. Sawyer AM, King TS, Sawyer DA, Rizzo A. Is inconsistent pretreatment bedtime related to CPAP non-adherence? Res Nurs Health. 2014;37(6):504–11.

62. Liou HYS, Kapur VK, Consens F, Billings ME. The effect of sleeping environment and sleeping location change on positive airway pressure adherence. J Clin Sleep Med. 2018;14(10):1645–52.

63. Kim JH, Kwon MS, Song HM, Lee B-J, Jang YJ, Chung Y-S. Compliance with positive airway pressure treatment for obstructive sleep apnea. Clin Exp Otorhinolaryngol. 2009;2(2):90–6.

64. Billings ME, Rosen CL, Wang R, Auckley D, Benca R, Foldvary-Schaefer N, et al. Is the relationship between race and continuous positive airway pressure adherence mediated by sleep duration? Sleep. 2013;36(2):221–7.

65. Poulet C, Veale D, Arnol N, Lévy P, Pepin J, Tyrrell J. Psychological variables as predictors of adherence to treatment by continuous positive airway pressure. Sleep Med. 2009;10(9):993–9.

66. Bandura A. Health promotion from the perspective of social cognitive theory. Psychol Health. 2008;13:623–49.

67. Prochaska JO, Johnson S, Lee P. The transtheoretical model of behavior change. In: Shumaker SA, Schron EB, Ockene JK, McBee WL, editors. The handbook of health behavior change. New York: Springer Publishing Company; 1998. p. 59–84.

68. Wallston KA. Hocus-pocus, the focus isn't strictly on locus: Rotter's social learning theory modified for health. Cogn Ther Res. 1992;16(2):183–99.

69. Champion V, Skinner CS. The health belief model. In: Glanz K, Rimer B, Viswanath K, editors. Health behavior and health education. 4th ed. San Francisco: Jossey-Bass; 2008. p. 45–65.

70. Ryan RM, Deci EL. Self-determination theory and the facilitation of intrinsic motivation, social development, and well-being. Am Psychol. 2000;55(1):68–78.

71. Stepnowsky CJ, Bardwell WA, Moore PJ, Ancoli-Israel S, Dimsdale JE. Psychologic correlates of compliance with continuous positive airway pressure. Sleep. 2002;25(7):758–62.

72. Aloia MS, Arnedt JT, Stepnowsky C, Hecht J, Borrelli B. Predicting treatment adherence in obstructive sleep apnea using principles of behavior change. J Clin Sleep Med. 2005;01(04):346–53.

73. Saconi B, Yang H, Watach AJ, Sawyer AM. Coping processes, self-efficacy, and CPAP use in adults with obstructive sleep apnea. Behav Sleep Med. 2018;18(1):68–80.

74. Stepnowsky CJ, Marler MR, Palau J, Brooks JA. Social-cognitive correlates of CPAP adherence in experienced users. Sleep Med. 2006;7(4):350–6.

75. Wild M. Can psychological factors help us to determine adherence to CPAP? A prospective study. Eur Resp J. 2004;24(3):461–5.

76. Tyrrell J, Poulet C, Pépin J-L, Veale D. A preliminary study of psychological factors affecting patients' acceptance of CPAP therapy for sleep apnoea syndrome. Sleep Med. 2006;7(4):375–9.

77. Olsen S, Smith S, Oei T, Douglas J. Health belief model predicts adherence to CPAP before experience with CPAP. Eur Resp J. 2008;32(3):710–7.

78. Wohlgemuth WK, Chirinos DA, Domingo S, Wallace DM. Attempters, adherers, and non-adherers: latent profile analysis of CPAP use with correlates. Sleep Med. 2015;16(3):336–42.

79. Sage CE, Southcott A, Brown SL. The health belief model and compliance with CPAP treatment for obstructive sleep apnoea. Behav Change. 2001;18(3):177–85.

80. Broström A, Ulander M, Nilsen P, Lin C-Y, Pakpour AH. Development and psychometric evaluation of the Motivation to Use CPAP Scale (MUC-S) using factorial structure and Rasch analysis among patients with obstructive sleep apnea before CPAP treatment is initiated. Sleep Breath. 2020. https://doi.org/10.1007/s11325-020-02143-9.

81. Ward K, Hoare KJ, Gott M. What is known about the experiences of using CPAP for OSA from the users' perspective? A systematic integrative literature review. Sleep Med Rev. 2014;18(4):357–66.

82. Zarhin D, Oksenberg A. Ambivalent adherence and nonadherence to continuous positive airway pressure devices: a qualitative study. J Clin Sleep Med. 2017;13(12):1375–84.

83. Broström A, Strömberg A, Ulander M, Fridlund B, Mårtensson J, Svanborg E. Perceived informational needs, side-effects and their consequences on adherence—a comparison between CPAP treated patients with OSAS and healthcare personnel. Patient Educ Couns. 2009;74(2):228–35.

84. Broström A, Strömberg A, Mårtensson J, Ulander M, Harder L, Svanborg E. Association of Type D personality to perceived side effects and adherence in CPAP-treated patients with OSAS. J Sleep Res. 2007;16(4):439–47.

85. Maschauer EL, Fairley DM, Riha RL. Does personality play a role in continuous positive airway pressure compliance? Breathe. 2017;13(1):32–43.

86. Edinger JD, Carwile S, Miller P, Hope V, Mayti C. Psychological status, syndromatic measures, and compliance with nasal CPAP therapy for sleep apnea. Percept Mot Skills. 1994;78(3 Pt 2):1116–8.

87. Ekici A, Ekici M, Oğuztürk O, Karaboğa I, Cimen D, Senturk E. Personality profiles in patients with obstructive sleep apnea. Sleep Breath. 2013;17(1):305–10.

88. Mehrtash M, Bakker JP, Ayas N. Predictors of continuous positive airway pressure adherence in patients with obstructive sleep apnea. Lung. 2019;197(2):115–21.

89. Copur AS, Erik Everhart D, Zhang C, Chen Z, Shekhani H, Mathevosian S, Loveless J, Watson E, Kadri I, Wallace L, Simon E, Fulambarker AM. Effect of personality traits on adherence

with positive airway pressure therapy in obstructive sleep apnea patients. Sleep Breath. 2018;22(2):369–76.

90. Li Y, Huang X, Su J, Wang Y. Mindfulness may be a novel factor associated with CPAP adherence in OSAHS patients. Sleep Breath. 2019;24(1):183–90.

91. Carlson LE. Mindfulness-based interventions for physical conditions: a narrative review evaluating levels of evidence. ISRN Psychiatry. 2012;2012:1–21.

92. Khoury B, Lecomte T, Fortin G, Masse M, Therien P, Bouchard V, Chapleau MA, Paquin K, Hofmann SG. Mindfulness-based therapy: a comprehensive meta-analysis. Clin Psychol Rev. 2013;33(6):763–71.

93. Lewis KE, Seale L, Bartle IE, Watkins AJ, Ebden P. Early predictors of CPAP use for the treatment of obstructive sleep apnea. Sleep. 2004;27(1):134–8.

94. Cartwright R. Sleeping together: a pilot study of the effects of shared sleeping on adherence to CPAP treatment in obstructive sleep apnea. J Clin Sleep Med. 2008;04(02):123–7.

95. Baron KG, Smith TW, Berg CA, Czajkowski LA, Gunn H, Jones CR. Spousal involvement in CPAP adherence among patients with obstructive sleep apnea. Sleep Breath. 2010;15(3):525–34.

96. Baron KG, Gunn HE, Czajkowski LA, Smith TW, Jones CR. Spousal involvement in CPAP: does pressure help? J Clin Sleep Med. 2012;08(02):147–53.

97. Baron KG, Smith TW, Czajkowski LA, Gunn HE, Jones CR. Relationship quality and CPAP adherence in patients with obstructive sleep apnea. Behav Sleep Med. 2009;7(1):22–36.

98. Adams GC, Skomro R, Wrath AJ, Le T, Mcwilliams LA, Fenton ME. The relationship between attachment, treatment compliance and treatment outcomes in patients with obstructive sleep apnea. J Psychosom Res. 2020;137:110196.

99. Batool-Anwar S, Baldwin C, Fass S, Quan S. Role of spousal involvement in continuous positive airway pressure (CPAP) adherence in patients with obstructive sleep apnea (OSA). Southwest J Pulm Crit Care. 2017;14(5):213–27.

100. Gentina T, Bailly S, Jounieaux F, Codron F, Lamblin C, Verkindre C, et al. Marital quality, partners engagement and continuous positive airway pressure adherence in obstructive sleep apnea. Sleep Med. 2019 Mar;55:56–61.

101. Baron CE, Smith TW, Baucom BR, Uchino BN, Williams PG, Sundar KM, et al. Relationship partner social behavior and continuous positive airway pressure adherence: the role of autonomy support. Health Psychol. 2020;39(4):325–34.

102. Mendelson M, Gentina T, Gentina E, Tamisier R, Pépin J-L, Bailly S. Multidimensional evaluation of continuous positive airway pressure (CPAP) treatment for sleep apnea in different clusters of couples. J Clin Med. 2020;9(6):1658.

103. Lai AYK, Ip MSM, Lam JCM, Weaver TE, Fong DYT. A pathway underlying the impact of CPAP adherence on intimate relationship with bed partner in men with obstructive sleep apnea. Sleep Breath. 2015;20(2):543–51.

104. Khafagy AH. Treatment of obstructive sleep apnoea as a therapeutic modality for associated erectile dysfunction. Int J Clin Pract. 2012;66(12):1204–8.

105. Ye L, Pack AI, Maislin G, Dinges D, Hurley S, Mccloskey S, et al. Predictors of continuous positive airway pressure use during the first week of treatment. J Sleep Res. 2011;21(4):419–26.

106. Ye L, Malhotra A, Kayser K, Willis DG, Horowitz JA, Aloia MS, et al. Spousal involvement and CPAP adherence: a dyadic perspective. Sleep Med Rev. 2015;19:67–74.

107. Ye L, Antonelli MT, Willis DG, Kayser K, Malhotra A, Patel SR. Couples' experiences with continuous positive airway pressure treatment: a dyadic perspective. Sleep Health. 2017;3(5):362–7.

108. Luyster FS, Dunbar-Jacob J, Aloia MS, Martire LM, Buysse DJ, Strollo PJ. Patient and partner experiences with obstructive sleep apnea and CPAP treatment: a qualitative analysis. Behav Sleep Med. 2014;14(1):67–84.

109. Xu Q, Xie H, Lin Y, Yao Y, Ye Z, Chen J, et al. Family support is beneficial to the management and prognosis of patients with obstructive sleep apnoea. Ann Palliat Med. 2020;9(4):1375–81.

110. Guralnick AS, Pant M, Minhaj M, Sweitzer BJ, Mokhlesi B. CPAP adherence in patients with newly diagnosed obstructive sleep apnea prior to elective surgery. J Clin Sleep Med. 2012;08(05):501–6.

111. Ghosh D, Allgar V, Elliott MW. Identifying poor compliance with CPAP in obstructive sleep apnoea: a simple prediction equation using data after a two week trial. Respir Med. 2013;107(6):936–42.

112. Kreivi H-R, Maasilta P, Bachour A. Willingness score obtained after a short CPAP trial predicts CPAP use at 1 year. Sleep Breath. 2013;18(1):207–13.

113. Balachandran JS, Yu X, Wroblewski K, Mokhlesi B. A brief survey of patients' first impression after CPAP titration predicts future CPAP adherence: a pilot study. J Clin Sleep Med. 2013;09(03):199–205.

114. Weaver TE, Maislin G, Dinges DF, Younger J, Cantor C, McCloskey S, Pack AI. Self-efficacy in sleep apnea: instrument development and patient perceptions of obstructive sleep apnea risk, treatment benefit, and volition to use continuous positive airway pressure. Sleep. 2003;26(6):727–32.

115. Sawyer AM, King TS, Hanlon A, Richards KC, Sweer L, Rizzo A, et al. Risk assessment for CPAP nonadherence in adults with newly diagnosed obstructive sleep apnea: preliminary testing of the Index for Nonadherence to PAP (I-NAP). Sleep Breath. 2014;18(4):875–83.

116. Chung F, Yegneswaran B, Liao P, Chung SA, Vairavanathan S, Islam S, Khajehdehi A, Shapiro CM. STOP questionnaire: a tool to screen patients for obstructive sleep apnea. Anesthesiology. 2008;108(5):812–21.

117. Aloia MS, Goodwin MS, Velicer WF, Arnedt JT, Zimmerman M, Skrekas J, et al. Time series analysis of treatment adherence patterns in individuals with obstructive sleep apnea. Ann Behav Med. 2008;36(1):44–53.

118. Nadal N, Batlle JD, Barbé F, Marsal JR, Sánchez-De-La-Torre A, Tarraubella N, et al. Predictors of CPAP compliance in different clinical settings: primary care versus sleep unit. Sleep Breath. 2018;22(1):157–63.

119. Pamidi S, Knutson KL, Ghods F, Mokhlesi B. The impact of sleep consultation prior to a diagnostic polysomnogram on continuous positive airway pressure adherence. Chest. 2012;141(1):51–7.

120. Chai-Coetzer CL, Antic NA, Hamilton GS, Mcardle N, Wong K, Yee BJ, et al. Physician decision making and clinical outcomes with laboratory polysomnography or limited-channel sleep studies for obstructive sleep apnea. Ann Intern Med. 2017;166(5):332.

121. Means MK, Edinger JD, Husain AM. CPAP compliance in sleep apnea patients with and without laboratory CPAP titration. Sleep Breath. 2004;8(1):7–14.

122. Kaplan JL, Chung SA, Fargher T, Shapiro CM. The effect of one versus two nights of in-laboratory continuous positive airway pressure titration on continuous positive airway pressure compliance. Behav Sleep Med. 2007;5(2):117–29.

123. Shapiro GK, Shapiro CM. Factors that influence CPAP adherence: an overview. Sleep Breath. 2010;14(4):323–35.

124. Collen J, Holley A, Lettieri C, Shah A, Roop S. The impact of split-night versus traditional sleep studies on CPAP compliance. Sleep Breath. 2009;14(2):93–9.

125. Suzuki M, Saigusa H, Furukawa T. Comparison of sleep parameters at titration and subsequent compliance between CPAP-pretreated and non-CPAP-pretreated patients with obstructive sleep apnea. Sleep Med. 2007;8(7–8):773–8.

126. Ip S, D'Ambrosio C, Patel K, Obadan N, Kitsios GD, Chung M, et al. Auto-titrating versus fixed continuous positive airway pres-

sure for the treatment of obstructive sleep apnea: a systematic review with meta-analyses. Syst Rev. 2012;1:20.

127. Rosen CL, Auckley D, Benca R, Foldvary-Schaefer N, Iber C, Kapur V, et al. A multisite randomized trial of portable sleep studies and positive airway pressure autotitration versus laboratory-based polysomnography for the diagnosis and treatment of obstructive sleep apnea: the HomePAP study. Sleep. 2012;35(6):757–67.

128. Drake CL, Day R, Hudgel D, Stefadu Y, Parks M, Syron ML, et al. Sleep during titration predicts continuous positive airway pressure compliance. Sleep. 2003;26(3):308–11.

129. Budhiraja R, Parthasarathy S, Drake CL, Roth T, Sharief I, Budhiraja P, et al. Early CPAP use identifies subsequent adherence to CPAP therapy. Sleep. 2007;30(3):320–4.

130. Billings ME, Pendharkar SR. Alternative care pathways for obstructive sleep apnea and the impact on positive airway pressure adherence: unraveling the puzzle of adherence. Sleep Med Clin. 2021;16(1):61–74.

131. Somiah M, Taxin Z, Keating J, Mooney AM, Norman RG, Rapoport DM, et al. Sleep quality, short-term and long-term CPAP adherence. J Clin Sleep Med. 2012;08(05):489–500.

132. Collen J, Lettieri C, Kelly W, Roop S. Clinical and polysomnographic predictors of short-term continuous positive airway pressure compliance. Chest. 2009;135(3):704–9.

133. Holley AB, Londeree WA, Sheikh KL, Andrada TF, Powell TA, Khramtsov A, et al. Zolpidem and eszopiclone pre-medication for PSG: effects on staging, titration, and adherence. Mil Med. 2018;183(7–8):e251–6.

134. Park JG, Olson EJ, Morgenthaler TI. Impact of zaleplon on continuous positive airway pressure therapy compliance. J Clin Sleep Med. 2013;09(05):439–44.

135. Lettieri CJ, Collen JF, Eliasson AH, Quast TM. Sedative use during continuous positive airway pressure titration improves subsequent compliance. Chest. 2009;136(5):1263–8.

136. Bradshaw DA, Ruff GA, Murphy DP. An oral hypnotic medication does not improve continuous positive airway pressure compliance in men with obstructive sleep apnea. Chest. 2006;130(5):1369–76.

137. Lettieri CJ. Effects of a short course of eszopiclone on continuous positive airway pressure adherence. Ann Intern Med. 2009;151(10):696.

138. Wang D, Tang Y, Chen Y, Zhang S, Ma D, Luo Y, Li S, Su X, Wang X, Liu C, Zhang N. The effect of non-benzodiazepine sedative hypnotics on CPAP adherence in patients with OSA: a systematic review and meta-analysis. Sleep. 2021;44:zsab077.

139. Heinzer RC, White DP, Jordan AS, Lo YL, Dover L, Stevenson K, et al. Trazodone increases arousal threshold in obstructive sleep apnoea. Eur Respir J. 2008;31(6):1308–12.

140. Guralnick AS, Balachandran JS, Szutenbach S, Adley K, Emami L, Mohammadi M, et al. Educational video to improve CPAP use in patients with obstructive sleep apnoea at risk for poor adherence: a randomised controlled trial. Thorax. 2017;72(12):1132–9.

141. Askland K, Wright L, Wozniak DR, Emmanuel T, Caston J, Smith I. Educational, supportive and behavioural interventions to improve usage of continuous positive airway pressure machines in adults with obstructive sleep apnoea. Cochrane Database Syst Rev. 2020;4(4):CD007736.

142. Falcone VA, Damiani MF, Quaranta VN, Capozzolo A, Resta O. Polysomnograph chart view by patients: a new educational strategy to improve CPAP adherence in sleep apnea therapy. Respir Care. 2013;59(2):193–8.

143. Jurado-Gamez B, Bardwell WA, Cordova-Pacheco LJ, García-Amores M, Feu-Collado N, Buela-Casal G. A basic intervention improves CPAP adherence in sleep apnoea patients: a controlled trial. Sleep Breath. 2014;19(2):509–14.

144. Delanote I, Borzée P, Belge C, Buyse B, Testelmans D. Adherence to CPAP therapy: comparing the effect of three educational approaches in patients with obstructive sleep apnoea. Clin Respir J. 2016;12(1):91–6.

145. Bakker JP, Wang R, Weng J, Aloia MS, Toth C, Morrical MG, et al. Motivational enhancement for increasing adherence to CPAP. Chest. 2016;150(2):337–45.

146. Basoglu OK, Midilli M, Midilli R, Bilgen C. Adherence to continuous positive airway pressure therapy in obstructive sleep apnea syndrome: effect of visual education. Sleep Breath. 2011;16(4):1193–200.

147. Wiese HJ, Boethel C, Phillips B, Wilson JF, Peters J, Viggiano T. CPAP compliance: video education may help! Sleep Med. 2005;6(2):171–4.

148. Damjanovic D, Fluck A, Bremer H, Muller-Quernheim J, Idzko M, Sorichter S. Compliance in sleep apnoea therapy: influence of home care support and pressure mode. Eur Respir J. 2009;33(4):804–11.

149. Deng T, Wang Y, Sun M, Chen B. Stage-matched intervention for adherence to CPAP in patients with obstructive sleep apnea: a randomized controlled trial. Sleep Breath. 2012;17(2):791–801.

150. Bouloukaki I, Giannadaki K, Mermigkis C, Tzanakis N, Mauroudi E, Moniaki V, et al. Intensive versus standard follow-up to improve continuous positive airway pressure compliance. Eur Respir J. 2014;44(5):1262–74.

151. Chen Y-F, Hang L-W, Huang C-S, Liang S-J, Chung W-S. Polysomnographic predictors of persistent continuous positive airway pressure adherence in patients with moderate and severe obstructive sleep apnea. Kaohsiung J Med Sci. 2015;31(2):83–9.

152. Lewis KE, Bartle IE, Watkins AJ, Seale L, Ebden P. Simple interventions improve re-attendance when treating the sleep apnoea syndrome. Sleep Med. 2006;7(3):241–7.

153. Sedkaoui K, Leseux L, Pontier S, Rossin N, Leophonte P, Fraysse J-L, et al. Efficiency of a phone coaching program on adherence to continuous positive airway pressure in sleep apnea hypopnea syndrome: a randomized trial. BMC Pulm Med. 2015;15(1):102.

154. Chervin RD, Theut S, Bassetti C, Aldrich MS. Compliance with nasal CPAP can be improved by simple interventions. Sleep. 1997;20(4):284–9.

155. Hui DS, Chan JK, Choy DK, Ko FW, Li TS, Leung RC, Lai CK. Effects of augmented continuous positive airway pressure education and support on compliance and outcome in a Chinese population. Chest. 2000;117(5):1410–6.

156. Parthasarathy S, Wendel C, Haynes PL, Atwood C, Kuna S. A pilot study of CPAP adherence promotion by peer buddies with sleep apnea. J Clin Sleep Med. 2013;09(06):543–50.

157. Smith CE, Dauz E, Clements F, Werkowitch M, Whitman R. Patient education combined in a music and habit-forming intervention for adherence to continuous positive airway (CPAP) prescribed for sleep apnea. Patient Educ Couns. 2009;74(2):184–90.

158. Wang W, He G, Wang M, Liu L, Tang H. Effects of patient education and progressive muscle relaxation alone or combined on adherence to continuous positive airway pressure treatment in obstructive sleep apnea patients. Sleep Breath. 2011;16(4):1049–57.

159. Fuchs FS, Pittarelli A, Hahn EG, Ficker JH. Adherence to continuous positive airway pressure therapy for obstructive sleep apnea: impact of patient education after a longer treatment period. Respiration. 2010;80(1):32–7.

160. Lin S-W, Chou Y-T, Kao K-C, Chuang L-P, Yang C-M, Hu H-C, et al. Immediate and long-term neurocognitive outcome in patients with obstructive sleep apnea syndrome after continuous positive airway pressure treatment. Indian J Otolaryngol Head Neck Surg. 2014;67(S1):79–85.

161. Wang Y, Cheng C, Moelter S, Fuentecilla JL, Kincheloe K, Lozano AJ, et al. One year of continuous positive airway pressure adherence improves cognition in older adults with mild apnea and mild cognitive impairment. Nurs Res. 2020;69(2):157–64.

162. Tamanna S, Campbell D, Warren R, Ullah MI. Effect of CPAP therapy on symptoms of nocturnal gastroesophageal reflux among patients with obstructive sleep apnea. J Clin Sleep Med. 2016;12(9):1257–61.

163. Stanchina ML, Welicky LM, Donat W, Lee D, Corrao W, Malhotra A. Impact of CPAP use and age on mortality in patients with combined COPD and obstructive sleep apnea: the overlap syndrome. J Clin Sleep Med. 2013;9(8):767–72.

164. Sawyer AM, Gooneratne NS, Marcus CL, Ofer D, Richards KC, Weaver TE. A systematic review of CPAP adherence across age groups: clinical and empiric insights for developing CPAP adherence interventions. Sleep Med Rev. 2011;15(6):343–56.

165. Machaalani R, Evans CA, Waters KA. Objective adherence to positive airway pressure therapy in an Australian paediatric cohort. Sleep Breath. 2016;20(4):1327–36.

166. Marcus CL. Adherence to and effectiveness of positive airway pressure therapy in children with obstructive sleep apnea. Pediatrics. 2006;117(3):e442–51.

167. Difeo N, Meltzer LJ, Beck SE, Karamessinis LR, Cornaglia MA, Traylor J, et al. Predictors of positive airway pressure therapy adherence in children: a prospective study. J Clin Sleep Med. 2012;08(03):279–86.

168. King MS, Xanthopoulos MS, Marcus CL. Improving positive airway pressure adherence in children. Sleep Med Clin. 2014;9(2):219–34.

169. Hawkins SM, Jensen EL, Simon SL, Friedman NR. Correlates of Pediatric CPAP adherence. J Clin Sleep Med. 2016;12(06):879–84.

170. Simon SL, Duncan CL, Janicke DM, Wagner MH. Barriers to treatment of paediatric obstructive sleep apnoea: development of the adherence barriers to continuous positive airway pressure (CPAP) questionnaire. Sleep Med. 2012;13(2):172–7.

171. Prashad PS, Marcus CL, Maggs J, Stettler N, Cornaglia MA, Costa P, et al. Investigating reasons for CPAP adherence in adolescents: a qualitative approach. J Clin Sleep Med. 2013;09(12):1303–13.

172. Kirk VG, O'Donnell AR. Continuous positive airway pressure for children: a discussion on how to maximize compliance. Sleep Med Rev. 2006;10(2):119–27.

173. Koontz KL, Slifer KJ, Cataldo MD, Marcus CL. Improving pediatric compliance with positive airway pressure therapy: the impact of behavioral intervention. Sleep. 2003;26(8):1010–5.

174. Xanthopoulos MS, Kim JY, Blechner M, Chang MY, Menello MK, Brown C, et al. Self-efficacy and short-term adherence to continuous positive airway pressure treatment in children. Sleep. 2017;40(7).

175. Jambhekar SK, Com G, Tang X, Pruss KK, Jackson R, Bower C, et al. Role of a respiratory therapist in improving adherence to positive airway pressure treatment in a pediatric sleep apnea clinic. Respir Care. 2013;58(12):2038–44.

176. Katz SL, Kirk VG, Maclean JE, Bendiak GN, Harrison M-A, Barrowman N, et al. Factors related to positive airway pressure therapy adherence in children with obesity and sleep-disordered breathing. J Clin Sleep Med. 2020;16(5):733–41.

177. O'Donnell AR, Bjornson CL, Bohn SG, Kirk VG. Compliance rates in children using noninvasive continuous positive airway pressure. Sleep. 2006;29(5):651–8.

178. Perriol M-P, Jullian-Desayes I, Joyeux-Faure M, Bailly S, Andrieux A, Ellaffi M, et al. Long-term adherence to ambulatory initiated continuous positive airway pressure in non-syndromic OSA children. Sleep Breath. 2019;23(2):575–8.

179. Mendoza-Ruiz A, Dylgjeri S, Bour F, Damagnez F, Leroux K, Khirani S. Evaluation of the efficacy of a dedicated table to improve CPAP adherence in children: a pilot study. Sleep Med. 2019;53:60–4.

180. Attias D, Pepin JL, Pathak A. Impact of COVID-19 lockdown on adherence to continuous positive airway pressure by obstructive sleep apnoea patients. Eur Respir J. 2020;56(1):2001607.

181. Schutte-Rodin S. Telehealth, telemedicine, and obstructive sleep apnea. Sleep Med Clin. 2020;15(3):359–75.

182. Sparrow D, Aloia M, Demolles DA, Gottlieb DJ. A telemedicine intervention to improve adherence to continuous positive airway pressure: a randomised controlled trial. Thorax. 2010;65(12):1061–6.

183. Taylor Y, Eliasson A, Andrada T, Kristo D, Howard R. The role of telemedicine in CPAP compliance for patients with obstructive sleep apnea syndrome. Sleep Breath. 2006;10(3):132–8.

184. Munafo D, Hevener W, Crocker M, Willes L, Sridasome S, Muhsin MA. A telehealth program for CPAP adherence reduces labor and yields similar adherence and efficacy when compared to standard of care. Sleep Breath. 2016;20(2):777–85.

185. Isetta V, Torres M, González K, Ruiz C, Dalmases M, Embid C, et al. A New mHealth application to support treatment of sleep apnoea patients. J Telemed Telecare. 2016;23(1):14–8.

186. Malhotra A, Crocker ME, Willes L, Kelly C, Lynch S, Benjafield AV. Patient engagement using new technology to improve adherence to positive airway pressure therapy. Chest. 2018;153(4):843–50.

187. Chen C, Wang J, Pang L, Wang Y, Ma G, Liao W. Telemonitor care helps CPAP compliance in patients with obstructive sleep apnea: a systemic review and meta-analysis of randomized controlled trials. Ther Adv Chronic Dis. 2020;11:204062232090162.

188. Aardoom JJ, Loheide-Niesmann L, Ossebaard HC, Riper H. Effectiveness of electronic health interventions in improving treatment adherence for adults with obstructive sleep apnea: meta-analytic review. J Med Internet Res. 2020;22(2):e16972.

189. Farré R, Navajas D, Gozal D, Montserrat JM. Telematic multiphysician decision-making for improving CPAP prescription in sleep apnoea. Arch Bronconeumol. 2019;55(11):604–6.

190. Anttalainen U, Melkko S, Hakko S, Laitinen T, Saaresranta T. Telemonitoring of CPAP therapy may save nursing time. Sleep Breath. 2016;20(4):1209–15.

191. Turino C, Batlle JD, Woehrle H, Mayoral A, Castro-Grattoni AL, Gómez S, et al. Management of continuous positive airway pressure treatment compliance using telemonitoring in obstructive sleep apnoea. Eur Respir J. 2017;49(2):1601128.

192. Isetta V, Negrín MA, Monasterio C, Masa JF, Feu N, Álvarez A, et al. A Bayesian cost-effectiveness analysis of a telemedicine-based strategy for the management of sleep apnoea: a multicentre randomised controlled trial. Thorax. 2015;70(11):1054–61.

193. Bros JS, Poulet C, Arnol N, Deschaux C, Gandit M, Charavel M. Acceptance of telemonitoring among patients with obstructive sleep apnea syndrome: how is the perceived interest by and for patients? Telemed e-Health. 2018;24(5):351–9.

194. Swieca J, Hamilton GS, Meaklim H. The management, privacy and medico-legal issues of electronic CPAP data in Australia and New Zealand. Sleep Med. 2017;36(Suppl 1):S48–55.

195. Pépin JL, Tamisier R, Hwang D, Mereddy S, Parthasarathy S. Does remote monitoring change OSA management and CPAP adherence? Respirology. 2017;22(8):1508–17.

196. Lim DC, Sutherland K, Cistulli PA, Pack AI. P4 medicine approach to obstructive sleep apnoea. Respirology. 2017;22(5):849–60.

197. Pack AI. Application of personalized, predictive, preventative, and participatory (P4) medicine to obstructive sleep apnea. A roadmap for improving care? Ann Am Thorac Soc. 2016;13(9):1456–67.

198. Cistulli PA, Sutherland K. Phenotyping obstructive sleep apnoea-bringing precision to oral appliance therapy. J Oral Rehabil. 2019;46(12):1185–91.

The Role of Education and Support in CPAP Adherence

5

C. D. Turnbull and J. R. Stradling

Abbreviations

AHI	Apnoea hypopnoea index
APAP	Auto-adjusting positive airway pressure device
ATS	American Thoracic Society
CBT	Cognitive behavioural therapy
CBT-I	Cognitive behavioural therapy for insomnia
COVID-19	Coronavirus disease 2019
CPAP	Continuous positive airway pressure
ESS	Epworth sleepiness score
EU	European Union
FOSQ	Functional outcomes of sleep questionnaire
MET	Motivational enhancement therapy
MSLT	Multiple sleep latencies test
NICE	National Institute of Clinical Effectiveness
ODI	Oxygen desaturation index
OSA	Obstructive sleep apnoea
PC	Personal computer
QALY	Quality adjusted life year
UK	United Kingdom
US	United States of America

Key Points

- Adequate CPAP adherence is important to derive maximum benefit from therapy
- Thresholds defining adequate adherence are arbitrary, and treatment should focus instead on increasing hours of usage to produce the optimum symptom relief acceptable to the patient

- Specific interventions of education, eHealth, behavioural and motivational therapies and telemonitoring can all improve CPAP adherence
- The COVID-19 pandemic, requiring social distancing for aerosol-generating procedures, has limited the application of some of these face-to-face interventions

5.1 Why Is CPAP Adherence Important?

Continuous positive airway pressure (CPAP) treatment is effective in improving patient symptoms, quality of life, driving performance, blood pressure and possibly other cardiometabolic outcomes. It seems obvious that CPAP must be used to derive any benefit from it, rather than sit in a cupboard gathering dust. However, the amount of use needed to achieve a benefit from CPAP is not clear, and probably varies depending on the patient, and the desired outcome.

CPAP adherence is commonly measured with two metrics: the hours of usage per night, and the percentage of nights above an arbitrary threshold; rarely is the real desired outcome, relief of symptoms, the main outcome to which attention is paid. A threshold of adequate usage is often arbitrarily reported to be 4 h/night. Figure 5.1 displays the proportion of patients in whom the subjective sleepiness (Epworth Sleepiness Score or ESS), sleep related quality of life (Functional Outcomes of Sleep Questionnaire or FOSQ) and objective sleepiness (Multiple Sleep Latency Tests or MSLT) returned to 'normal' levels in each category of CPAP [1]. Despite the continuous nature of these relationships, this graph has been interpreted as suggesting that thresholds of 4, 6 and 7.5 h/night CPAP usage were the levels above which minimal further benefit was likely from increasing CPAP adherence for the ESS, the MSLT and the FOSQ, respectively. However, many patients in this study noticed significant improvement below these arbitrary thresholds, Table 3 in [1]. For example, the ESS returned to 'normal' values in 18/33 (55%) of patients with CPAP usage of less than 4 h/night.

C. D. Turnbull (✉) · J. R. Stradling
Oxford National Institute of Health Research Biomedical Research Centre, University of Oxford, Oxford, UK
e-mail: Christopher.Turnbull@ouh.nhs.uk

C. M. Shapiro et al. (eds.), *CPAP Adherence*, https://doi.org/10.1007/978-3-030-93146-9_5

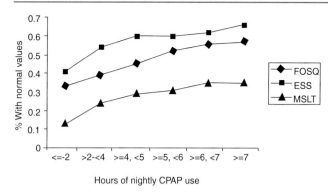

Fig. 5.1 Graph showing the proportion of patients with values that had normalised for the FOSQ, ESS and MSLT by categorical hours of night CPAP use. There is a dose response to CPAP therapy with increasing proportions of patients with normalised values with increasing usage of CPAP. ESS Epworth Sleepiness Score, FOSQ Functional Outcomes of Sleep Questionnaire, MSLT Multiple Sleep Latency Tests. (Reproduced with permission from Weaver et al. [1])

In a novel experiment, stopping CPAP for 2 weeks in patients who had previous 'suboptimal' CPAP use of only 3–4 h/night, led to significantly increased daytime sleepiness [2]. This demonstrates that some individuals derive benefit from CPAP with usage below an arbitrary 4 h/night threshold. It is important to remember that low adherence does not equal no benefit, and thus should not be used as a reason to stop a patient's therapy.

The level of CPAP adherence also has financial and driving implications. Reimbursement for CPAP in some countries is dependent on meeting adherence criteria, with the US requirements perhaps the best known: ongoing CPAP coverage requires CPAP usage for >4 h/night, for >70% of nights, in a consecutive 30-day period between the 31st and 91st days of treatment. In France, an equally arbitrary average 3 h/night usage is required for ongoing coverage. Driver licensing also requires adherence with therapy. By the end of 2015, an updated European Union (EU) directive on driving was adopted (2014/85/EU). This requires that patients with moderate to severe OSA demonstrate adherence with therapy and have ongoing 3-yearly or annual review for group 1 and group 2 license holders, respectively. The exact threshold for adherence was not set, although suggested to be >4 h/night in the UK interpretation.

Whilst health professionals should focus on the benefit a patient derives from CPAP, long-term adherence with CPAP therapy is required to make CPAP cost-effective. Figure 5.2 shows a health economic model of the cost-effectiveness of CPAP [3]. If a patient uses CPAP for less than 1 year it costs over £20,000 per quality-adjusted life year (QALY), which is above the UK National Institute for Clinical Effectiveness (NICE) threshold for cost-effectiveness. Therefore, the majority of patients need to use CPAP for over 1 year for it to be deemed cost-effective.

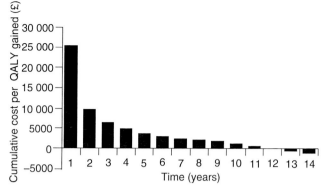

Fig. 5.2 Cumulative cost per quality adjusted life year (QALY) of continuous positive airway pressure (CPAP). (Reproduced from Guest et al. [3])

Whilst precise thresholds for usage are arbitrary, adequate CPAP adherence — *which will vary between patients* — is clearly important in terms of symptoms and may be important in terms of finances and driver licensing.

5.2 Baseline Factors Affecting Adherence

A great deal of research has focussed on trying to find factors that predict CPAP adherence [4]. Whilst no pre-treatment predictors are precise enough to guide the binary decision on whether to trial CPAP or not, a number of factors are relevant when considering how much help a patient may need when starting CPAP. Factors influencing CPAP adherence are displayed in Table 5.1.

Whilst the severity of OSA has not universally been shown to be predictive of CPAP adherence, there is a significant long-term relationship (Fig. 5.3). It is important to remember that many patients with milder OSA do adhere with therapy, and that CPAP has been shown to be effective for some, in even the mildest OSA [5]. The severity of sleepiness, as measured by the ESS, is somewhat predictive of long-term CPAP adherence [6].

The reason for referral is important to consider, as patients who initiate their referral are more likely to use CPAP [4]. Patients with minimally symptomatic OSA are less likely to use CPAP [7], and may have been referred as part of screening for OSA. Demographic factors such as age, gender, race and language have been reported to predict CPAP adherence [4]. Whilst these may not be modifiable, specific strategies to improve access, such as translating material, may be necessary, depending on the local population.

Psychological factors are important, such as co-morbid depression and personality type (See Chaps. 11 and 19). Symptoms of depression commonly co-exist with OSAS [8]. While CPAP may improve symptoms of depression, patients with a diagnosis of depression may require additional, spe-

Table 5.1 Factors with reported predictive value for CPAP adherence

OSA and symptom severity
  AHI
  ODI
  ESS
Reason for referral
  Self-initiated
  Screening
Demographic/patient factors
  Age
  Gender
  Race
  Language
  Socioeconomic status
  Smoking status
Psychosocial factors
  Personality type
  Depression
  Marital status
  Partner involvement
  Social support
  Self-efficacy
  Motivation
  Treatment outcome expectations
  Comorbid insomnia

cific treatment for their depression to enable CPAP usage. Social support networks are also important to CPAP adherence. Having a supportive partner or positive support network is helpful, whilst living alone tends to make patients less likely to use CPAP [4, 9] (See Chap. 10). Practically, this means engaging supportive partners where possible. Patients support groups and patient-run organisations can also be helpful [4, 9].

Socioeconomic status also influences CPAP adherence, and this probably relates to a patient's ability to self-finance aspects related to their healthcare. For example, those in the USA who do not meet USA Medicare CPAP adherence reimbursement criteria may then have to self-fund equipment. Other financial disincentives to treatment include the ability to attend appointments, including leave from work and travel expenses. Considering ways of minimising these barriers to healthcare can aid in the support of patients.

5.3 The Role of Education During CPAP Set-up

Education prior to setting-up CPAP is crucial and increases CPAP adherence [10]. Pre-treatment education shapes the patient's opinion of OSA and CPAP therapy. Patients will arrive at appointments with pre-conceived ideas about their condition and about CPAP therapy. Education should include information relating to the pathophysiology of OSA, the symptoms of OSA, the associated comorbidities, a descrip-

tion of CPAP, the impact of CPAP on symptoms and other outcomes, the common issues with CPAP and some basic troubleshooting.

Historically, educational material was provided on a one-to-one basis and CPAP set-up was performed with an in-lab titration. However, this is expensive, and many healthcare systems have moved away from in-lab CPAP titrations, favouring the use of auto-adjusting devices or algorithms to determine CPAP pressures. With the move away from in-lab CPAP set-up, the educational component has moved from one-to-one to group sessions. Group sessions delivered by a skilled and trained sleep practitioner are as effective as one-to-one education sessions [11]. However, it is important to consider certain situations where this might not be practical, such as in individuals with language barriers, hearing difficulties or learning disabilities.

Educational packages can also be delivered by video or web-based packages and are included as part of eHealth. eHealth represents a complex intervention variably including education, motivational interviews, telemonitoring (which will be discussed in a later section), and even financial incentives for using patient telemonitoring. eHealth has been shown to increase average CPAP usage by approximately 0.5 h/night [10]. There is of course a dilemma when gauging how enthusiastic to be when introducing CPAP, on the one hand, unless the practitioner is enthusiastic, it is unlikely the patient will be enthusiastic; on the other hand, if CPAP is being tried when it is unclear if a patient's symptoms are due to OSA or not (a diagnostic trial), then it is fair to suggest to the patient that CPAP may or may not work for them. Whilst education has an important role in ensuring optimal CPAP adherence, other methods of support are probably required in all but the most motivated patients [12].

5.4 Specific Behavioural Interventions

Behavioural interventions are sometimes incorporated into education and support pathways for CPAP set-up. Motivational enhancement therapy (MET) and cognitive behavioural therapy (CBT) are the two most researched behavioural interventions and have been shown to improve CPAP usage by about 1.5 h/night [9], although not necessarily with a commensurate further decrease in symptoms. Cognitive behavioural interventions challenge non-adaptive beliefs and decrease the frequency of non-adaptive behaviours and concurrently enhance motivation for behavioural change. These interventions require specific staff training or referral to a psychologist. Motivational interventions are most helpful for patients who are ambivalent about CPAP use, while education and social interaction probably provide similar benefits to cognitive therapy in unselected patients

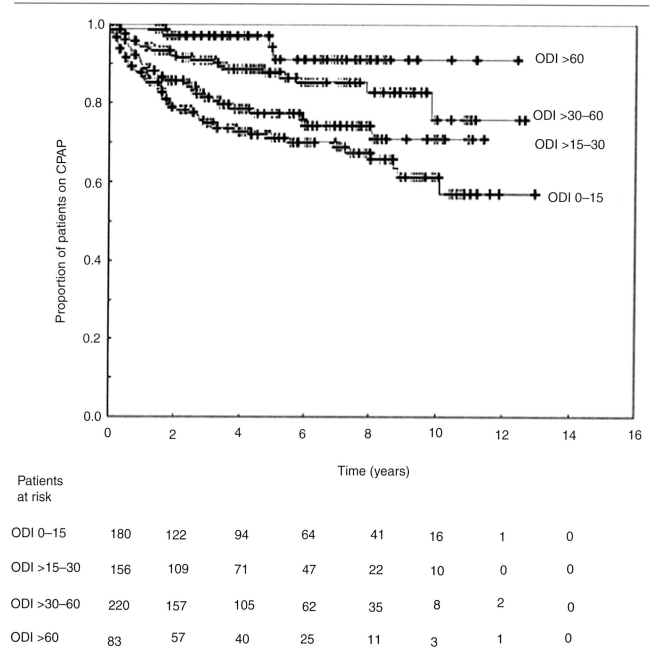

Fig. 5.3 Kaplan-Meir plot showing the proportion of patients using CPAP therapy over time. Whilst a high proportion of patients with severe OSA continued CPAP long-term, approximately 70% of patients with mild OSA were still using CPAP after 5 years of follow, and >50% at 10 years. (Reproduced with permission from Kohler et al. Thorax. 2010; 65: 829–32)

[13]. In patients with co-existent insomnia, specific CBT for insomnia (CBT-I) may be a necessary adjunct to CPAP (also see Chaps. 6 and 17).

5.5 The CPAP Interface and Adherence

Expertise and a range of equipment are required to optimise the CPAP interface during CPAP set-up. The first interface choice is between auto-adjusting positive airway pressure

device (APAP) and CPAP. Whilst APAP devices tend to deliver lower pressures throughout the night, overall adherence is similar for APAP and CPAP devices [14], except possibly in patients requiring the highest pressures. Whilst APAP devices tend to cost more than CPAP devices, the difference in price is less marked than historically. The starting choice between APAP and CPAP is usually determined by individual CPAP pathway differences and cost. Struggling patients may be switched from CPAP to APAP, or vice versa, to try to aid comfort and adherence.

A range of different mask types are now available including full face masks, oronasal masks, nasal masks and nasal pillows. There is little randomised evidence to support routine choice of one type of mask over another, and practically the choice of mask is normally determined by patient factors. Skilled, trained, enthusiastic and experienced sleep nurses/technicians/physiologists are crucial in selecting the correct mask. This also requires the availability of a variety of different sizes and mask shapes to enable a good mask fit. Full face masks may not be ideal for patients with claustrophobia, whilst those with nasal congestion or who tend breath through their mouth may struggle with nasal-only masks. Chin straps can be used as an adjunct to a nasal mask in patients who breathe through their mouth but are not popular.

When trialling different masks, it is best to have the CPAP device delivering pressures likely to occur during treatment, to gauge both comfort and likely leaks; this means that exhaled air is blown into the immediate environment, which is a potential problem when COVID-19 is prevalent. It is unclear whether removing the opportunity to trial CPAP, with the therapist actually present, will reduce the subsequent adherence and a multicentre study in the UK aims to assess this question. The alternative of full personal protection for the therapist, and adequate air changes between patients, will be very expensive and time-consuming. Humidification and heated tubing can be added to the CPAP interface, but this is usually reserved for those with specific technical issues, rather than routine usage, as they introduce additional maintenance issues for the patient.

5.6   The Pattern of CPAP Usage Is Established Early

Whilst baseline factors are not particularly helpful in determining long-term adherence, early CPAP usage does predict longer-term use (Fig. 5.4) [15]. In fact, CPAP usage is probably determined within the first 1–2 weeks. However, it is worth bearing in mind that there are still individuals who will increase their CPAP use following the first few weeks and this is probably as a result of support and 'getting used to it'. However, it is less clear if this early predictability is simply due to whether or not a patient finds it easy to get on with immediately, and whether early intervention is influential to long-term adherence.

5.7   Early Follow-up

Given that the pattern of CPAP usage is determined early, support at this time is presumably helpful. There are several aspects to follow-up, including an assessment of the acceptability and tolerability of CPAP, review of symptoms, a

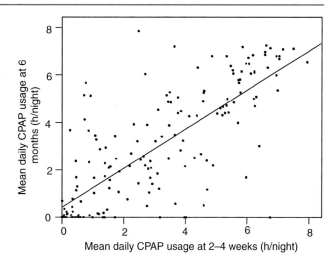

Fig. 5.4 Graph showing that correlation between the early mean daily CPAP use between weeks 2–4 and the longer-term mean daily CPAP use at 6 months in the MOSAIC trial. The pattern of usage is established early, presumably making this a crucial time to focus on education and support. However, low early low CPAP usage can be improved in some individuals represented by the points in the top left quadrant (with the converse also sometimes being true). (Adapted with permission from Turnbull et al. [15])

check of adherence and review of driver licensing. An expert panel consensus suggested that the key aspects of CPAP follow-up are: acceptability of treatment (side effects and preparedness to continue), technical aspects (mask fit, humidification, replacing parts), objective assessment of sleepiness/symptoms/quality of life, measurement of adherence, assessing sleep quality, driving/licensing issues, lifestyle issues and sleep hygiene [16].

Historically services have tried to follow-up patients within the first 2–4 weeks of starting CPAP therapy. However, as CPAP services have expanded, they have been placed under ever increasing pressure and this target has become harder and harder to achieve. Under this increasing pressure, services need to find new ways of targeting resources to ensure that standards are maintained.

5.8   The Role of Telemonitoring

Telemonitoring is the remote monitoring of CPAP adherence using wireless technology, and the ability to modify some of a machine's settings remotely as well. Telemonitoring is now available with most CPAP machines via cloud-based software. Telemonitoring usually requires an institution to pay for the service from the CPAP companies and requires patient consent to the electronic transfer of their data. During the first 3 months of CPAP set-up, use of telemonitoring increases usage with CPAP by approximately 1 h/night [17]. Whilst this increase has not been shown to translate to greater improvements in sleepiness or quality of life, studies in this area have mainly looked at CPAP usage as the main outcome and probably lack power to find small improvements in sleepiness or other symptoms.

There are several other benefits of telemonitoring, such as reducing the number of face-to-face visits to hospital. This became particularly important during the COVID-19 pandemic, but has also been helpful due to difficulties with travel and car parking when attending hospital appointments. Patients overall satisfaction with telemonitoring is mixed, with one study suggesting similar satisfaction levels to usual care and another reporting worse satisfaction [17]. A minority of patients also have concerns about privacy with electronic transfer of data. Overall, the benefits of telemonitoring probably outweigh the harms and its use was already gaining popularity even before the COVID-19 pandemic. The pandemic has merely hastened adoption, which is unlikely to reverse once over.

Some consideration does need to be given to how an individual service will utilise telemonitoring as the workload required to regularly review monitoring for all patients on CPAP will be impossible. Patient consent to data transfer, and 'contracts' whereby they agree to take responsibility for their usage of CPAP are important, as there have been concerns that sleep units might become responsible for not spotting that a patient had stopped using their machine with a resultant road traffic collision for example.

Telemonitoring is often used to monitor CPAP usage in the first days, weeks and months. It can be helpful in immediately flagging up patients who have specific issues such as low usage, high mask leak and residual events. At present there are no clear guidelines on the thresholds for these data that would lead to pro-active intervention, it being likely that this will remain different for different patients. An example of telemonitoring software output is shown in Fig. 5.5. Patients with issues can be prioritised for early face-to-face follow-up, which can help to manage increasingly high workloads. Following the first few months of successful CPAP initiation, clinical teams may decide to switch off continuing telemonitoring. Depending on the contract with the CPAP Company, telemonitoring can then be re-activated when a patient's follow-up is due or new problems arise. A final utility available through telemonitoring is the use of patient smartphone apps and PC software. Patients can use these to get feedback on their CPAP usage, possible problems such as mask leaks and highlighting sources of support for specific issues [18].

5.9   Support and Troubleshooting

The frequency of long-term follow-up for patients using CPAP is uncertain. An ATS expert panel advises follow-up at 1 week, 4–6 weeks, 12 weeks, 6 months and then annually [19]. The EU directive on driving mandates reviews of patients at least every 3 years for those with group 1 (cars) and annually for those with group 2

Fig. 5.5 Day-to-day view of two patient's CPAP adherence. The top patient has excellent hours of usage displayed with green bars (over 4 h/night) and only one red bar (less than 4 h/night). The bottom patient is doing less well with frequent low usage, although they are clearly trying to use CPAP every night. This enables rapid identification of the second patient as needing help and support to improve their CPAP adherence

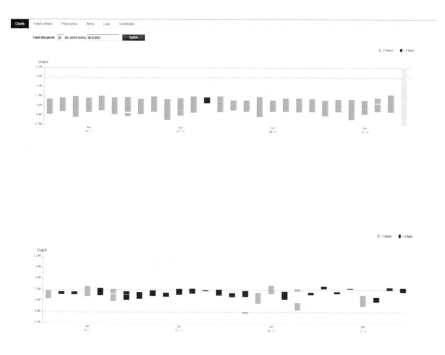

licenses (heavy goods and public service vehicles). In the UK, many services are no longer able to offer routine annual follow-up for all patients and instead offer as-required appointments. The advantage of as-required appointments is that patients utilise health care when they need it to resolve issues. However, as-required appointments place an onus on patients, and not all patients will be motivated to engage with this. CPAP filters usually need replacing every 4–6 months; CPAP masks, headgear and tubing need replacement approximately every 18 months and CPAP machines need replacement after approximately every 5–7 years depending on usage. Lack of timely replacement of parts can cause problems with mask leak or loss of pressure.

Follow-up appointments for support and troubleshooting provide another opportunity to check that patients are cleaning and maintaining their equipment. Mask cushioning should be cleaned in warm water with a mild detergent (not hand soap), then rinsed with water and left to drip-dry on a towel. This is important as the build-up of grease can affect mask seal and lead to leakage. The mask, mask cushioning, headgear and CPAP tubing should ideally be washed similarly, approximately once a week.

Troubleshooting at follow-up is an important part of CPAP support and can help to address issues with the CPAP interface and side effects (Table 5.2).

5.10   Summary

Adherence is important to derive benefits from CPAP, but exact thresholds for adherence are arbitrary. Support and education should focus on helping patients to improve their CPAP adherence to engender adequate symptom resolution, rather than achieving arbitrary thresholds of usage. Education and support can be delivered in group settings and assisted by eHealth. Specific motivational, behavioural therapies and telemonitoring are useful methods to improve CPAP adherence. In an era of pandemic virus infections such as COVID-19, maintenance of best practice will prove difficult, but ways to achieve best possible adherence must be found, despite the limitations this imposes.

Acknowledgement Dr Turnbull was supported by a National Institute of Health Research Clinical Lectureship. The authors would like to acknowledge the support of the Oxford National Institute of Health Research Biomedical Research Centre. The authors were supported by the National Institute for Health Research (NIHR) Oxford

Table 5.2 Specific CPAP issues and troubleshooting

Interface issues	Suggested solutions
Mask leak	Check mask and headgear integrity and fit and consider replacement/refitting
Rainout (water condensing in CPAP tubing which can then leak into the CPAP mask)	Consider heated tubing
Loss of pressure	Check machine, mask and headgear and consider replacing
Patient symptoms	Suggested solutions
Discomfort	Check mask and headgear integrity and fit and consider replacement/refitting
Skin issues particularly at the nasal bridge	Check mask fit and consider replacement with nasal pillows or specialised masks not involving the nasal bridge
Claustrophobia	Consider mask replacement to a nasal or specialised mask not involving the nasal bridge
Dry, stuffy nose or nosebleeds	Consider oronasal mask/full face mask, consider humidification and consider the need for treatment of rhinitis with nasal decongestants or steroids: Consider referral to ear nose and throat (ENT) specialist if no response
Dry mouth	Consider oronasal mask/full face mask, consider chin strap and consider humidification
Aural fullness	May be due to the pressure: Consider a reduction in pressure and referral to ENT
Aerophagia	May be due to the pressure: Consider a reduction in pressure and referral to ENT
Specific scenarios	Suggested solutions
Air travel/foreign travel	Advise the need for plug adapter and suggest providing patients with a letter for air travel stating the need for CPAP as carry on: Patients who frequently fly long haul may wish to consider purchasing a device with inbuilt battery
CPAP without an electricity source	Advise patients to consider hiring a rechargeable battery

Biomedical Research Centre (BRC). The views expressed are those of the authors and not necessarily of the NHS, the NIHR, or the Department of Health.

References

1. Weaver TE, Maislin G, Dinges DF, Bloxham T, George CF, Greenberg H, et al. Relationship between hours of CPAP use and achieving normal levels of sleepiness and daily functioning. Sleep. 2007;30(6):711–9.
2. Gaisl T, Rejmer P, Thiel S, Haile SR, Osswald M, Roos M, et al. Effects of suboptimal adherence of CPAP therapy on symptoms of

obstructive sleep apnoea: a randomised, double-blind, controlled trial. Eur Respir J. 2020;55(3):1901526.

3. Guest JF, Helter MT, Morga A, Stradling JR. Cost-effectiveness of using continuous positive airway pressure in the treatment of severe obstructive sleep apnoea/hypopnoea syndrome in the UK. Thorax. 2008;63(10):860–5.

4. Mehrtash M, Bakker JP, Ayas N. Predictors of continuous positive airway pressure adherence in patients with obstructive sleep apnea. Lung. 2019;197(2):115–21.

5. Wimms AJ, Kelly JL, Turnbull CD, McMillan A, Craig SE, O'Reilly JF, et al. Continuous positive airway pressure versus standard care for the treatment of people with mild obstructive sleep apnoea (MERGE): a multicentre, randomised controlled trial. Lancet Respir Med. 2019;8(4):349–58.

6. McArdle N, Devereux G, Heidarnejad H, Engleman HM, Mackay TW, Douglas NJ. Long-term use of CPAP therapy for sleep apnea/hypopnea syndrome. Am J Respir Crit Care Med. 1999;159(4 Pt 1):1108–14.

7. Gagnadoux F, Le Vaillant M, Paris A, Pigeanne T, Leclair-Visonneau L, Bizieux-Thaminy A, et al. Relationship between OSA clinical phenotypes and CPAP treatment outcomes. Chest. 2016;149(1):288–90.

8. Hobzova M, Prasko J, Vanek J, Ociskova M, Genzor S, Holubova M, et al. Depression and obstructive sleep apnea. Neuro Endocrinol Lett. 2017;38(5):343–52.

9. Weaver TE. Novel aspects of CPAP treatment and interventions to improve CPAP adherence. J Clin Med. 2019;8(12):2220.

10. Aardoom JJ, Loheide-Niesmann L, Ossebaard HC, Riper H. Effectiveness of eHealth interventions in improving treatment adherence for adults with obstructive sleep apnea: meta-analytic review. J Med Internet Res. 2020;22(2):e16972.

11. Stradling JR, Hardinge M, Smith DM. A novel, simplified approach to starting nasal CPAP therapy in OSA. Respir Med. 2004;98(2):155–8.

12. Bakker JP, Weaver TE, Parthasarathy S, Aloia MS. Adherence to CPAP: what should we be aiming for, and how can we get there? Chest. 2019;155(6):1272–87.

13. Bartlett D, Wong K, Richards D, Moy E, Espie CA, Cistulli PA, et al. Increasing adherence to obstructive sleep apnea treatment with a group social cognitive therapy treatment intervention: a randomized trial. Sleep. 2013;36(11):1647–54.

14. Nolan GM, Doherty LS, Mc Nicholas WT. Auto-adjusting versus fixed positive pressure therapy in mild to moderate obstructive sleep apnoea. Sleep. 2007;30(2):189–94.

15. Turnbull CD, Bratton DJ, Craig SE, Kohler M, Stradling JR. In patients with minimally symptomatic OSA can baseline characteristics and early patterns of CPAP usage predict those who are likely to be longer-term users of CPAP. J Thorac Dis. 2016;8(2):276–81.

16. Murphie P, Little S, Paton R, McKinstry B, Pinnock H. Defining the core components of a clinical review of people using continuous positive airway pressure therapy to treat obstructive sleep apnea: an international e-delphi study. J Clin Sleep Med. 2018;14(10):1679–87.

17. Patil SP, Ayappa IA, Caples SM, Kimoff RJ, Patel SR, Harrod CG. Treatment of adult obstructive sleep apnea with positive airway pressure: an American academy of sleep medicine systematic review, meta-analysis, and GRADE assessment. J Clin Sleep Med. 2019;15(2):301–34.

18. Hwang D, Chang JW, Benjafield AV, Crocker ME, Kelly C, Becker KA, et al. Effect of telemedicine education and telemonitoring on continuous positive airway pressure adherence. The tele-OSA randomized trial. Am J Respir Crit Care Med. 2018;197(1):117–26.

19. Schwab RJ, Badr SM, Epstein LJ, Gay PC, Gozal D, Kohler M, et al. An official American Thoracic Society statement: continuous positive airway pressure adherence tracking systems. The optimal monitoring strategies and outcome measures in adults. Am J Respir Crit Care Med. 2013;188(5):613–20.

Role of the Behavioral Sleep Specialist Psychologist in Promoting CPAP Adherence

Dora Zalai

Research and clinical practice have clearly shown that a pure biomedical view, focusing exclusively on patient demographics and disease parameters have not been sufficient to conceptualize and facilitate adherence to continuous positive airway pressure (CPAP) treatment. By and large, BMI, obstructive sleep apnea (OSA) severity, CPAP pressure, machine type, humidification or mask interface alone have been found to be poor predictors of CPAP use [1]. Notably, demographic and several illness-specific factors (e.g., OSA severity, anatomical factors that contribute to OSA, arousal threshold, nasal pressure) cannot be directly changed in a routine clinical encounter and therefore are not strategic targets when the aim is to help patients using a positive airway pressure (PAP) machine. Given their low predictive power in treatment adherence, it is not surprising that interventions focusing solely on these health/illness and treatment factors have shown limited success in substantially improving PAP adherence in the long term [2–8]. In contrast, psychological factors, including motivation, self-efficacy, coping style, as well as beliefs about sleep apnea and treatment outcomes are significant predictors of CPAP adherence [9–15]. Crucially, these psychological factors are malleable and targeting them with a combination of evidence-based methods appears to have the largest potential to effectively promote PAP adherence [16–22], also see Chap. 2 in this book.

In order to better understand CPAP adherence, we need to move beyond a purely biomedical approach and explore the dynamic interaction among biomedical, psychological, and social factors for each individual patient [23]. Working in partnership with the person with sleep apnea using a biopsychosocial model as a framework to explore factors that are relevant to the person's CPAP use, opens the possibility to plan interventions that are feasible/optimal for the individual.

Psychologists with special knowledge in behavioral sleep medicine work with clients using the framework of an integrated biopsychosocial model. They understand the biomedical factors relevant to sleep apnea and CPAP and also have experience in providing interventions that have been shown to effectively support adherence with PAP treatment, including motivational enhancement, cognitive behavioral therapy focusing on CPAP use, cognitive behavioral therapy for insomnia for those with comorbid insomnia, and evidence-based psychological interventions for patients who have mental health conditions that impede CPAP use.

Psychologists follow a collaborative case formulation-based approach when they work with clients. The psychologist and the client form a shared understanding of the factors that are relevant for the individual client with regard to their sleep, sleep apnea and its treatment. If the client wants to move toward (increased) PAP device use, the psychologist works with the client to help them achieve their goal using evidence-based methods that facilitate the desired change. At the same time, the psychologist versed in behavioral sleep medicine collaborates with other members of the health care team, including sleep specialist physician, general practitioner, CPAP coordinator, respiratory therapist. Typically, the psychologist meets with the client regularly, which helps patients to stay on track in moving toward their goals and at the same time ensures that clients do not "fall between the cracks" when regular medical follow-up is not possible.

Ideally, the behavioral sleep specialist is included in multidisciplinary teams that provide care for patients with sleep apnea as they bring to the treatment team a set of skills and knowledge that complement the expertise of physicians, respiratory therapists, and other professionals. Given that long-term adherence is influenced by early postdiagnosis CPAP use, ideally, the psychologist is invited on board soon after the diagnosis is made in situations when CPAP adherence proves to be challenging for the patient after all technical issues have been addressed. The following are typical examples where the psychologist uses evidence-based methods to help clients with CPAP treatment. Each section starts with short case summary followed by a description of research evidence.

D. Zalai (✉)
Sleep on the Bay, Toronto, ON, Canada
e-mail: drzalai@sleep-psychology.ca

© The Author(s), under exclusive license to Springer Nature Switzerland AG 2022
C. M. Shapiro et al. (eds.), *CPAP Adherence*, https://doi.org/10.1007/978-3-030-93146-9_6

6.1 When the Patient Is Ambivalent About CPAP Use: The Importance of Client-Clinician Communication

Box 1: Case Example (Mark)

Mark was referred to the sleep laboratory because he complained about nonrefreshing sleep and tiredness to the family physician during his annual medical visit. The family physician noted on the referral form that Mark snores and he has high blood pressure. The overnight PSG showed severe OSA (AHI in total sleep time = 39; AHI in supine position = 61, AHI in REM sleep = 46) and the MSLT on the next day demonstrated excessive daytime sleepiness. During the medical visit following the sleep study, the sleep specialist physician explained to Mark his sleep study results, told him what sleep apnea is and what are the medical consequences of sleep apnea (including high blood pressure), and listed the treatment options. He strongly recommended CPAP, introduced Mark to the CPAP provider at the sleep clinic, and arranged that Mark would see the sleep physician a month after his CPAP titration.

At the follow-up visit, the physician reviewed with Mark the CPAP titration study results and asked Mark about his CPAP use. Mark reported that he had used the machine a few times and he concluded that he does not need this treatment right now and he is not sure if he would benefit from it. The physician checked Mark's CPAP use and pointed out that Mark had used the machine only for a few days and told Mark that based on that it may be premature to conclude that the treatment is not useful for him. He also showed Mark that his AHI was low during the titration night as an evidence that the treatment works. He devoted time to patiently explain to Mark why he needs this treatment (he has severe OSA and high blood pressure) and how the treatment would benefit him (e.g., improve his tiredness and health). He made sure that the explanation was complete and accurate and understandable to a lay person using multiple examples and analogies to illustrate the main points. He also told Mark that he has an obligation to report to the Ministry of Transport if he has a sleepy patient who drives and he really hopes and trusts that Mark will use the device; otherwise, he will have to submit a report. He asked Mark to consult with the CPAP coordinator with any issues he may have with CPAP use. Mark felt furious and yelled at his wife at home when she told him that the doctor was right: it is time for him to finally start using the treatment that would stop his snoring so that she could also have better sleep. She said that she had enough of his constantly irritated mood and complaints about stress in his life and he really need to see a psychologist to deal with his problems.

6.1.1 Background

Motivational interviewing is a "collaborative conversation style for strengthening a person's own motivation and commitment to change", page 12 in [24]. In motivational interviewing, the clinician builds a collaborative partnership with the client in the spirit of acceptance of the inherent worth of the client as an autonomous person, relates to the client with empathy and compassion and actively affirms and evokes the knowledge, strengths and skills that the client already has.

Starting to use a PAP device requires behavioral changes. When a person comes to the sleep clinic with:

- A clear goal (My partner tells me that I stop breathing when I sleep. I would like to find out if I have a breathing issue in my sleep)
- High motivation for change (My health and my relationship with my partner are very important for me. If I need sleep treatment, I would like to start it as soon as possible) and
- Confidence in their skills in bringing about the change

then education about sleep apnea and CPAP will be enough to successfully start the treatment and is as effective as motivational interviewing [16]. In this situation, there is also a perfect match between the patients' and the clinician's agenda and therefore their relationship will likely be uncomplicated.

When clinicians comment on the patient's "low CPAP adherence", "non-compliance with CPAP treatment", and "problems with using CPAP", it may be that CPAP use is not currently a shared goal of the clinician and the patient. Motivational interviewing was specifically developed for situations when the clinician hopes for a behavioral change for a patient (e.g., starting PAP treatment or increasing CPAP use) that the patient is ambivalent about. In these situations, clinicians are facing a dilemma: if the clinicians do not address the issue of low adherence actively, the patient may stop using CPAP and if the health care providers push their agenda, they may arrive at a roadblock in their communication and relationship with the patient, which may result in the cessation of CPAP treatment. Motivational interviewing helps in these situations to facilitate behavioral change and at the same to avoid irreparable ruptures in the clinician-client relationship.

Motivational interviewing involves four processes:

1. *Engaging* – building a collaborative working relationship with the client in an equal partnership
2. *Focusing* – identifying and maintaining a focus for the interaction that leads to specifying change goals
3. *Evoking* – "bringing forth" the client' knowledge, ideas, and skills of how they will bring about the change
4. *Planning* – developing a commitment to change and formulating a specific action plan

Communication style that reflects the clinician's respect, acceptance, empathy, and compassion toward the patient as an equal partner in the dialogue and that strategically uses langue that evokes the person's own argument, skills, ability, and commitment to change underlies each of the motivational interviewing processes.

Notice the language when we talk about "CPAP nonadherence", "problems with CPAP use", or "the patient cannot get used to the CPAP": some of words are negative (e.g., problem), "all-or-nothing" (e.g., nonadherence, cannot) and reflect the clinician's viewpoint/agenda.

Mark was furious after his follow-up visit with the physician because he felt that he was not heard (the physician did not explore why he thought that the treatment is not timely and effective), that he was talked down to (his perception was that the physician gave a lecture about how CPAP would be useful for him without knowing anything about his life), he felt threatened (the physician told him that he would report him to the Ministry) and thought that his autonomy and his right to make choices were not respected. Accordingly, the physician's intention to help Mark use a treatment that would be the best choice from the medical perspective did not lead to the desired outcome.

Motivational interviewing involves a way of communication that includes "*OARS*":

*O*pen-ended questions (What may contribute to the tiredness you feel?)

*A*ffirming client's intentions for change, skills, strengths, and achievements (I am so happy that you came today! You kept the mask on for more than 1.5 h even though you felt frustrated. You have good stress tolerance skills. What helped you to keep the mask on for that long?)

*R*eflective listening (Client: There is this plastic thing under my nose and that ugly gray hose on my chest. Clinician: You feel unattractive when you are using CPAP)

*S*ummarizing (So you came to the sleep lab because you hoped that you would get help to feel less tired. You feel it was worth having a sleep study because it revealed that you have poor sleep quality and the same time, you feel disappointed because you were given a treatment that does not help you to fall asleep faster and you still feel tired during the day).

Sharing information with the client is an essential part of the sleep study follow-up appointment and using a "sandwich" method of "*E-P-E*" can help clients to feel accepted and stay engaged:

Elicit – ask for permission to provide information; ask about the client's knowledge of the topic so that you will not repeat what they already know; ask what they are most interested in to know

Provide – a few pieces of information at a time

Elicit – the client's understanding of and reaction to the information you provided

When clinicians are eager to help, they invertedly may use langue that restricts clients' autonomy to express their view and make choices (for example, telling what patients should do; trying to persuade with a logical argument; directing; cautioning or threatening). In response, the client's verbal behavior or actions will try to reinstate their autonomy, which may be labeled as "resistance". When clients are ambivalent about CPAP use, they already have a mental list of both pros and cons in relation to this treatment and have already engaged in internal dialogues about CPAP use. When their awareness highlights one side of the argument (I should use the CPAP machine to have a better sleep), it will be followed by thoughts that represent the other side of debate (Yes, but I will not be able to get used to it). Likewise, when the clinician argues for CPAP use during a medical visit, it automatically evokes the other side of the argument in a client's mind that is ambivalent about CPAP use (Fig. 6.1).

In situations where the patient is ambivalent about CPAP use, the patient-centered approach is to take time to curiously and empathetically explore the ambivalence with the client with full appreciation of the fact that the patients are experts of their own lives. During the discussion about ambivalence, the patient will verbalize their own argument for CPAP use. It is crucial that clinicians learn to notice this "change talk" (i.e., the patient's own argument for behavioral change) and learn how to elicit it while evoking hope and confidence in the patients' ability to make the behavioral changes necessary for increased CPAP use (for more detailed description, please refer to motivational interviewing text books). When the client is ready for CPAP use, the discussion shifts to developing a specific, behavioral plan for CPAP use, including, for example

- The steps I plan to take in increasing my CPAP use are…
- The ways other people can help me are…
- I know my plan is working if…
- Some things that could interfere with my plan are…
- If these things arise, what I will do is….

Fig. 6.1 The clinician's
argument for change evokes
the other side of argument
from the patient

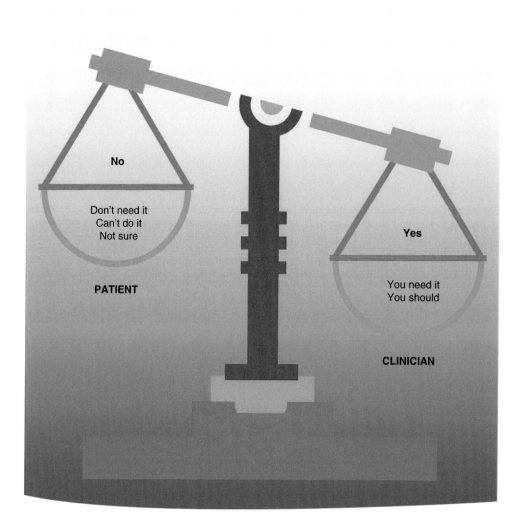

6.1.2 What Happened to Mark?

The psychologist started with building a collaborative relationship with Mark (engaging) and then focusing on the topics that mattered to Mark. Mark wanted to focus on improving his energy, his mood, and his relationship with his wife. They discussed Mark's values and the discrepancy between some of his values (e.g., health and fitness; care and self-care; love; forgiveness; perseverance) and his current actions. When it was clear that Mark was ready to set value-based goals, they agreed to do it in the framework of acceptance and commitment therapy that involved setting and pursuing value-based goals, while learning how to relate to internal experiences (thoughts, emotions, physical sensations) in an adaptive way. Mark and the psychologist returned to discussing CPAP use during the course of psychotherapy in relation to Mark's values. Mark

identified CPAP use as a personal value-based behavior (in line with his values of health and fitness, self-care, and care for his wife). Frustration and emotion-based actions previously interfered with Mark's CPAP use but at this point in therapy Mark's awareness in his ability of using the device had increased, because he had practiced techniques of how to "tame" his frustration and act based on his values instead of his anger. Mark set specific goals with regard to CPAP use and made a specific plan with the psychologist of what to do if challenges arise while they tracked his daily CPAP use. Fortunately, Mark was a sound sleeper and his average CPAP use was 6.5 h/night within three weeks after he started using the device. His CPAP use was positively reinforced by the improvement of his wife's sleep quality and her appreciative comments about this behavioral change (for more information about the role of partner support, see Chap. 10).

6.1.3 Research Evidence

Motivational enhancement (ME) therapy ("Motivating Adherence to Positive Airway Pressure") was developed as a short, structured program following the principles of motivational interviewing to help with CPAP use [25]. Evidence suggests that those who participate in ME adhere more to CPAP treatment than those who receive standard care [17–19, 21]. In a randomized control study comparing ME, education, and usual care, patients who were ambivalent about PAP use based on the hours of use during the first week (at least 2 but less than 6 h of average PAP use per night) benefited most from ME treatment compared to those who received standard care or education [16], which is not surprising, given that MI has been developed for clients who are ambivalent about behavioral change. Mark's example also illustrates the research finding that CPAP use correlates with improvement in bed partner's subjective sleep quality [26, 27].

6.2 When the Patient Has Insomnia: Treating Comorbid Chronic Insomnia to Help with CPAP Use

---

Box 2: Case Example (Steve)

Steve has been having difficulties with falling asleep since his late teenage years. He did not see this as being a problem until 6 years ago, when his first child was born and he had to get up early to help his wife in the mornings. He is now a father of two and he is responsible for preparing breakfast for his children and taking them to school. He describes that he has a successful business and he often works until late in the evening. He goes to bed soon after he finishes work and he spends 1.5–2 h awake in bed, reading the news on his cell phone and listening to podcasts because he is not able to fall asleep. He describes that he feels tired in the morning and during the day but he is still unable to fall asleep after he goes to bed. He requested a sleep assessment because he wanted to improve his ability to fall asleep and increase his energy level during the day.

The overnight laboratory PSG study showed increased sleep onset latency (91 min) and reduced sleep efficiency (77%). AHI was mildly increased in total sleep time (6/h) but moderately elevated in REM sleep (24/h) and in supine position (17/h) without significant oxygen desaturations. The PLM index was also high (19/h) during the recoded night. The sleep study also showed high arousal index (17/h) with predominantly spontaneous arousals.

Steve and his sleep physician discussed his treatment plan during the sleep study follow-up visit. They agreed that Steve would start using a CPAP machine ASAP and he also will be referred to a behavioral sleep specialist for the treatment of insomnia disorder.

On his first visit to the behavioral sleep specialist psychologist, Steve listed difficulty with falling asleep and feeling tired as his main sleep-related concerns. He reported that he had tried to use the CPAP every night but he gets frustrated when he is not able to fall asleep and removes the mask when he cannot fall asleep. There are also nights when he wakes up and he removes the mask so that he can go back to sleep faster.

6.2.1 Background

Approximately one-third to half of patients diagnosed with OSA report clinically significant symptoms of insomnia [28]. Despite its high prevalence, insomnia remains largely undiagnosed in this clinical group [29]. Individuals who have comorbid OSA and insomnia disorder (COMISA) report worse sleep, have more psychiatric comorbidities and pain, show more neurocognitive impairment, have worse daytime functioning and quality of life than those who have OSA as a stand-alone condition [28, 30]. When OSA causes sleep maintenance insomnia symptoms, the treatment of OSA may improve sleep continuity; however, when insomnia disorder is a comorbid condition, it requires specific treatment so as to achieve an optimal overall sleep treatment outcome, as well as daytime functioning and quality of life. Sleep laboratories with a primarily respiratory focus may emphasize OSA treatment but even in these settings effective treatment of insomnia is imperative since comorbid insomnia disorder predicts low adherence to CPAP treatment [29, 31–34]. Accordingly, it is imperative to include insomnia evaluation in the initial sleep assessment even when OSA risk factors and symptoms are clearly present and incorporate evidence-based insomnia management in the sleep treatment plan.

6.2.2 What Happened to Steve?

Steve and the psychologist discussed how insomnia and OSA are related to his main concerns (i.e., difficulty with falling asleep and feeling tired) and how the two sleep disorders may be functionally related. In addition, they discussed: (1) evidence-based treatment options for both conditions; (2) ways in which insomnia makes CPAP use challenging for Steve; and (3) how different evidence-based treatments for one condition may affect his experience with the other sleep disorder or with its treatment.

For insomnia treatment, Steve's first choice was CBT-I (cognitive behavioral therapy for insomnia); primarily because he did not want to take sleep-promoting medications. With regard to OSA treatment, he wanted to use CPAP because of its effectiveness and low cost in the jurisdiction where he lives (the cost of the device is largely covered by the local health plan and his extended work insurance). Steve and the behavioral sleep specialist weighed the options of either doing CBT-I first and re-initiating CPAP after the insomnia dissipates or doing the two treatments concurrently. Steve opted for the second option because he wanted to achieve the largest possible sleep improvement as soon as possible.

Accordingly, the psychologist and Steve included a CPAP use plan in the CBT-I treatment (for a description of CBT for insomnia, see Chap. 17). For example, they agreed that Steve would go to bed only when he is very sleepy and at a time that is in accordance with his chronotype (and they set an earliest bedtime taking these factors into account). This strategically planned earliest bedtime would help him to fall asleep with the mask on, which – they agreed – he will put on each night when he goes to bed. The implication of this is that one is maximizing the likelihood of a person falling asleep with the CPAP on if sleep attempt is at the peak of sleep propensity. If he wakes up during the night and notices that the mask came off, he would place it back on his face before he goes back to sleep. He would also leave the bedroom every time when he is awake during the night for more than 15–20 minutes instead of trying to rest in bed but would put the mask on again when he returns to bed with a strong feeling of sleepiness. They also practiced how to relax the body and disengage from thoughts that would fuel frustration when the mask is on while he is in bed. With implementing the CBT-I interventions, Steve's sleep onset latency reduced from 118 min (baseline) to 31 min within 2 weeks and his sleep efficiency increased from 72% (baseline) to 86% during the same period. He put on the mask every night and had it on 68% of his time in bed. Steve rated his sleep quality as "good" on most nights. He was still sleepy in the mornings but had higher energy during the day. He continued CBT with a slightly modified schedule to help with morning sleepiness and found that CPAP use became easier over the next several weeks even though he still did not like using the device. He was able to keep the CPAP on most nights for the duration of the whole night by the time he completed treatment.

6.2.3 Research Evidence

Cognitive behavioral therapy for insomnia (CBT-I) is the first-line recommended treatment for insomnia disorder [35–38]. Research has consistently shown that CBT-I can be safely implemented and is effective for the treatment of insomnia disorder even if patients have a comorbid, untreated OSA [39–41]. When patients participate in CBT-I before, concurrently or after the OSA treatment, they experience a significant improvement in their sleep [40, 42, 43]. The clinical intuition that treatment outcome is optimal when both conditions are treated is corroborated by research evidence [40, 42]. Given that a presence of comorbid insomnia disorder is a predictor of poor PAP adherence, providing CBT-I before the commencement of PAP therapy or soon after PAP treatment is initiated may enhance adherence to CPAP treatment. Indeed, research has demonstrated that those patients who received CBT-I before starting CPAP therapy had higher initial acceptance of CPAP treatment and an hour longer average CPAP use at 6 months follow-up than patients who did not receive CBT-I initially [40]. In another study, CBT-I combined with a behavioral CPAP adherence program led to greater long-term CPAP adherence than sleep education [42]. Conversely, a head-to-head comparison did not find a difference in CPAP adherence when CBT-I was provided before CPAP treatment; concurrently with CPAP treatment; or when patients received CPAP treatment only but insomnia symptoms improved only in the first two groups [43]. This underlies the importance of treating insomnia disorder in COMISA patients to achieve greater overall sleep improvement. The findings of this study also suggest that it may be necessary to focus both on insomnia and CPAP adherence in CBT with COMISA patients to alleviate insomnia and at the same time facilitate CPAP use. Research evidence suggests that CBT designed specifically to help CPAP use improved adherence with CPAP treatment [22]. For COMISA patients, this approach can be combined with CBT-I to alleviate insomnia and increase CPAP use [42]. Further research is needed to study optimal sequencing of CBT-I and PAP treatment. In clinical practice, patient preference is an important factor and decisions can be made collaboratively with clients, as the above case examples illustrate.

6.3 When the Patient Has Anxiety that Impedes CPAP Use

Box 3: Case Example (Catherine)

Catherine has recently been diagnosed with OSA. She and her sleep physician have discussed treatment options and agreed that she would use CPAP every night. Catherine is highly motivated to follow the treatment plan because excessive daytime sleepiness has been significantly impacting her life and interfering with her everyday functioning. She also has been feeling ashamed about her obesity and she is concerned that she will not find a partner and will develop health problems if she does not loose weight. She feels optimistic that if she uses CPAP, she will have more energy to exercise and finally "do something good for myself".

Catherine is in tears when she sees her friend 6 months after the CPAP was prescribed. She laments that she has been trying very hard to adhere to the treatment; yet, she has not been able to get used to the machine. She has told her sleep physician about not being able to use the machine and her sleep physician sent her back to the CPAP vendor in order to find out if there is a technical issue. The vendor offered her a different type of mask, which was mildly helpful but did not solve the problem of getting heart palpitations when she tried to use the device. The vendor suggested to Catherine that she gradually "gets used" to CPAP by practicing for short periods during the day. Catherine has tried diligently but the situation became worse: she felt her heart beating rapidly and she had difficulties with breathing when she tried to use the CPAP device and eventually, she stopped trying. She has asked for a second opinion from a respirologist who saw her when she was younger and he said that if she cannot get used to the CPAP, she could use a positional device (Catherine's AHI was worse in supine position). Catherine has been following his advice but she still feels sleepy during the day. Catherine's friend knows a psychologist who has experience with treating sleep issues. When they meet for the first time, Catherine says to the psychologist that "I came to see you out of desperation".

6.3.1 Background

Intense fear or anxiety during CPAP use or active avoidance of CPAP use due to anticipated fear or anxiety, may cause significant distress and impact treatment adherence. Questionnaire-based data suggest that one-third to two-thirds of patients who are prescribed CPAP report "claustrophobic tendencies", i.e., fear or anxiety about being closed in, trapped, or not getting enough air when they use CPAP [44]. Both retrospective and prospective studies demonstrate that "claustrophobic tendencies" in this population are associated with low CPAP use [44, 45]. CPAP related anxiety can also be nonphobic, for example, a person with a history of tension headaches may be worried that CPAP use will increase the frequency of headaches or someone with generalized anxiety may be worried that the sound of air from the CPAP will cause insomnia for their partner.

Fear/anxiety about CPAP use may develop via classical conditioning during the first time when someone has a fear response while the person is using CPAP. CPAP may also become a fear cue when the person already has a history of reacting with fear to harmless physical sensations (for example rapid heart rate), to worry thoughts, or in certain situations (for example closed spaces). Vicarious learning (for example having witnessed the spouse's anxiety reaction to CPAP) and negative information received from others about CPAP (for example that it is "horrible") can also contribute to having fear/anxiety about CPAP use. Independently of the etiology, fear and anxiety are maintained by maladaptive beliefs (overestimation of actual danger and underestimation of the ability cope), biased information processing, and safety behaviors (see Fig. 6.2) [46].

6.3.2 What Happened to Catherine?

Catherine went to the psychologist with high motivation to use CPAP and a goal of being able to use it with ease. At the same time, she reported that she felt helpless because her fear and physical discomfort with using the machine have increased over time despite all her efforts. During their first meeting, the psychologist conducted a functional behavioral analysis: she asked Catherine questions to elicit information about fear cues, maladaptive beliefs, and safety behaviors.

From their initial discussion, the psychologist learned that the maintaining factors of Catherine's anxiety are:

Fear cues:

1. Air flow from the CPAP
2. Heart palpitation while using CPAP

Feared consequences:

1. She will not be able to breathe against the air flow and will faint
2. She will get a heart attack and die

Safety Behaviors:

1. Removing the mask
2. Having her cell phone next to her in case of an emergency
3. Trying to sleep with the machine at her mother's place
4. Lately avoiding using the machine

The psychologist drew a model (similar to Fig. 6.2) on a white board as they were talking with Catherine and then used the model to provide education about what maintains (and escalates) Catherine's anxiety in the context of CPAP use. As they discussed the model, the psychologist used the

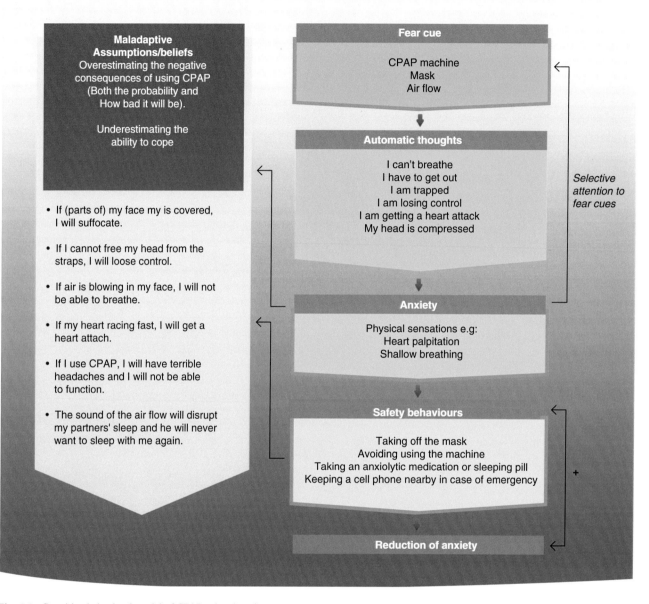

Fig. 6.2 Cognitive behavioral model of CPAP-related anxiety

Elicit-Provide-Elicit method (see in the motivational interviewing section of this chapter) to learn about Catherine's thoughts and feelings about the information she provided and created an opportunity for refining the model to describe Catherine's specific situation. Catherine was surprised to see that practicing for short periods and removing the mask when she felt uncomfortable increased her difficulties with using the device – the exact opposite of what she had hoped to achieve. The psychologist then used Socratic questioning to elicit Catherine's thoughts about where and how she could "break the anxiety cycle". By the end of the first meet-

ing, they agreed that they would do exposure therapy to provide opportunities for Catherine to feel the air flow and her heart beating fast while she is using the CPAP and discover what happens if she turns toward these experiences with curiosity and allows the physical sensation to be present without trying to stop them or escape from them.

Catherine and the psychologist created an exposure list, including situations that Catherine anticipated would lead to the negative outcomes she feared, including the worst outcome (getting a heart attack and dying). The psychologist consulted with the sleep physician about safe increase of pressure for specific exposure items and involved the respiratory therapist to help setting the pressure for these exposure items. The list included:

- Holding the mask close to the face so that Catherine feels that air flow but not as strongly as she feels it when the mask is on the face
- Using the CPAP device during the day in the psychologist's office (in session exposure)
- Using the CPAP machine during the day when she is alone at home, cell phone switched off
- Using the CPAP machine during the day while running on the spot, cell phone switched off
- Using the CPAP machine during the night while she is sleeping alone in her home, cell phone switched off
- Using the CPAP machine during the day with a higher pressure while the psychologist is present
- Using the CPAP machine during the day with a higher pressure while she is alone, cell phone switched off
- Using the CPAP machine during the night with a higher pressure while she is sleeping alone at home, cell phone switched off

Catherine and the psychologist agreed that they will use a scale of "subjective units of distress" to estimate Catherine's anticipated level of distress for each item on the list and quantitatively capture Catherine's level of stress before, during, and after the exposures. They discussed that Catherine can start with the exposure item to which she assigned the lowest rating and move up in a hierarchical order but the most effective method is to choose items randomly from the list. They also agreed that Catherine would record before and after each exposure what she anticipates would happen and what actually happened during the exposures. Catherine also listed all the safety behaviors that she would avoid while doing exposures. They discussed that the exposures would be prolonged, so that Catherine has the opportunity to experience various physical sensations with varying intensity as well as thoughts and urges that may arise. They also agreed that Catherine will do each exposure several times to create multiple opportunities for new learning.

Catherine completed items on her exposure list within 8 weeks. She became very comfortable with CPAP use, as she experienced that she could breathe well and did not faint even when the pressure was set temporarily higher than what had been prescribed. She also learned that heart palpitation does not lead to heart attacks even when she increases her heart rate with exercising with the CPAP on or when she had decreased self-awareness during sleep. Catherine described that she was very confident that she would be able to use the CPAP "under any circumstance".

She started regular gentle physical activity during the treatment period and was hopeful that she would increase and maintain regular exercise and will lose weight in the coming months.

6.3.3   Research Evidence

Exposure therapy as a stand-alone treatment or as part of cognitive behavioral therapy is a highly efficacious and effective treatment for anxiety disorders. It yields large effect sizes from pre- to post-treatment for specific phobia (including claustrophobia) and fear of harmless bodily sensations (panic disorder) compared to no treatment and outperforms control conditions, including wait list, placebo control, and other psychological interventions [47, 48]. Interestingly, clinical research studies focusing on exposure therapy for claustrophobia in the context of CPAP use are scarce [49].

6.4   When the Patient Has Mental Health Problems

There is a high prevalence of sleep disorders among people who experience chronic stress or symptoms of mental health problems. When people seek psychological help, the psychologist may be the first clinician who obtains detailed information about the client's sleep and recognize symptoms of OSA. This gives an opportunity to include the (possible) OSA in the clinical mental health case formulation and link it to the patient's concerns (for example tiredness, irritability, nonrefreshing sleep) and goals in treatment. In the author's experience, clients generally appreciate when a possible OSA diagnosis is discussed during the initial visit and a referral to a sleep laboratory is suggested. After clients receive an OSA diagnosis and a PAP machine, a PAP use plan can be incorporated in the psychology treatment plan. By the time this happens, there is a strong alliance between the psychologist and the client and the client may already be familiar with the theoretical framework that will also help with CPAP use, for example CBT. The strong alliance and trust that are established between the psychologist and the client during psychotherapy, the psychologist's knowledge of the individual and regular meetings during the course of psychotherapy create an optimal interpersonal environment for working on PAP treatment adherence.

Insomnia – a leading sleep disorder in mental health conditions – may already have been addressed in the psychology treatment by the time a PAP treatment is prescribed. Alternatively, the psychologist and the client may wait for the diagnostic sleep study results and implement a sleep improvement plan – including CBT-I and a PAP use – after the follow-up meeting with the sleep physician. For people with PTSD, imagery rehearsal therapy (IRT) can be incorporated into a psychological sleep treatment plan that may also include CBT-I and methods to facilitate PAP use. Essentially, the treatment of sleep disorders (e.g., OSA, insomnia, or nightmares) can be integrated into a psychological, case formulation-based mental health treatment plan so that clients receive treatment both for the mental health and the sleep disorder during the treatment period, with a potential to enhance both sleep and mental health treatment outcomes.

6.5 Chapter Summary

The behavioral sleep specialist psychologist uses a biopsychosocial, case formulation-based approach to conceptualize the challenges with CPAP treatment and select evidence-based methods to help clients use the PAP device. This opens avenues to flexibly work with clients who would otherwise be locked in categories as "non-adherent" or "does not tolerate CPAP" and give up CPAP use or being switched to a treatment modality that may not provide sufficient improvement in sleep quality or sleep-related quality of life. The knowledge and skillset of the behavioral sleep specialist psychologist are unique in a multidisciplinary sleep specialist team and complement the expertise of the physicians and respiratory therapists. Ideally, the psychologist is involved from the treatment planning phase with COMISA patients and comes on board soon after the sleep apnea is detected in patients without insomnia when the patient is ambivalent about CPAP use or has difficulties with using CPAP that goes beyond pure technical problems. Clinical experience and research evidence clearly shows that a biomedical approach alone is insufficient to help patients resolve ambiance about CPAP use or overcome challenges with PAP treatment. As client-centered, personalized, and multidisciplinary approaches are being advocated for the treatment of sleep apnea in the twenty-first century, behavioral sleep specialist psychologists have an essential and invaluable role as treatment providers in this field [50, 51].

References

1. Chai-Coetzer CL, Luo YM, Antic NA, Zhang XL, Chen BY, He QY, et al. Predictors of long-term adherence to continuous positive airway pressure therapy in patients with obstructive sleep apnea and cardiovascular disease in the SAVE study. Sleep. 2013;36(12):1929–37.
2. Worsnop CJ, Miseski S, Rochford PD. Routine use of humidification with nasal continuous positive airway pressure. Intern Med J. 2010;40(9):650–6.
3. Ruhle KH, Domanski U, Schroder M, Franke KJ, Nilius G. Heated humidification during CPAP with and without tube insulation. Pneumologie. 2010;64(5):316–9.
4. Gulati A, Oscroft N, Chadwick R, Ali M, Smith I. The impact of changing people with sleep apnea using CPAP less than 4 h per night to a Bi-level device. Respir Med. 2015;109(6):778–83.
5. Gillespie MB, Wylie PE, Lee-Chiong T, Rapoport DM. Effect of palatal implants on continuous positive airway pressure and compliance. Otolaryngol Head Neck Surg. 2011;144(2):230–6.
6. Bakker JP, Marshall NS. Flexible pressure delivery modification of continuous positive airway pressure for obstructive sleep apnea does not improve compliance with therapy: systematic review and meta-analysis. Chest. 2011;139(6):1322–30.
7. Bogan RK, Wells C. A randomized crossover trial of a pressure relief technology (SensAwake) in continuous positive airway pressure to treat obstructive sleep apnea. Sleep Disord. 2017;2017:3978073.
8. Smith I, Lasserson TJ. Pressure modification for improving usage of continuous positive airway pressure machines in adults with obstructive sleep apnoea. Cochrane Database Syst Rev. 2009;(4):CD003531.
9. Wallace DM, Shafazand S, Aloia MS, Wohlgemuth WK. The association of age, insomnia, and self-efficacy with continuous positive airway pressure adherence in black, white, and Hispanic U.S. Veterans. J Clin Sleep Med. 2013;9(9):885–95.
10. Stepnowsky CJ, Marler MR, Palau J, Annette BJ. Social-cognitive correlates of CPAP adherence in experienced users. Sleep Med. 2006;7(4):350–6.
11. Baron KG, Berg CA, Czajkowski LA, Smith TW, Gunn HE, Jones CR. Self-efficacy contributes to individual differences in subjective improvements using CPAP. Sleep Breath. 2011;15(3):599–606.
12. Sawyer AM, Canamucio A, Moriarty H, Weaver TE, Richards KC, Kuna ST. Do cognitive perceptions influence CPAP use? Patient Educ Couns. 2011;85(1):85–91.
13. Stepnowsky CJ Jr, Bardwell WA, Moore PJ, Ancoli-Israel S, Dimsdale JE. Psychologic correlates of compliance with continuous positive airway pressure. Sleep. 2002;25(7):758–62.
14. Sawyer AM, Deatrick JA, Kuna ST, Weaver TE. Differences in perceptions of the diagnosis and treatment of obstructive sleep apnea and continuous positive airway pressure therapy among adherers and nonadherers. Qual Health Res. 2010;20(7):873–92.
15. Philip P, Bioulac S, Altena E, Morin CM, Ghorayeb I, Coste O, et al. Specific insomnia symptoms and self-efficacy explain CPAP compliance in a sample of OSAS patients. PLoS One. 2018;13(4):e0195343.
16. Aloia MS, Arnedt JT, Strand M, Millman RP, Borrelli B. Motivational enhancement to improve adherence to positive airway pressure in patients with obstructive sleep apnea: a randomized controlled trial. Sleep. 2013;36(11):1655–62.
17. Olsen S, Smith SS, Oei TP, Douglas J. Motivational interviewing (MINT) improves continuous positive airway pressure (CPAP) acceptance and adherence: a randomized controlled trial. J Consult Clin Psychol. 2012;80(1):151–63.
18. Bakker JP, Wang R, Weng J, Aloia MS, Toth C, Morrical MG, et al. Motivational enhancement for increasing adherence to CPAP: a randomized controlled trial. Chest. 2016;150(2):337–45.
19. Lai AYK, Fong DYT, Lam JCM, Weaver TE, Ip MSM. The efficacy of a brief motivational enhancement education program on CPAP adherence in OSA: a randomized controlled trial. Chest. 2014;146(3):600–10.
20. Parthasarathy S, Wendel C, Haynes PL, Atwood C, Kuna S. A pilot study of CPAP adherence promotion by peer buddies with sleep apnea. J Clin Sleep Med. 2013;9(6):543–50.
21. Aloia MS, Smith K, Arnedt JT, Millman RP, Stanchina M, Carlisle C, et al. Brief behavioral therapies reduce early positive airway pressure discontinuation rates in sleep apnea syndrome: preliminary findings. Behav Sleep Med. 2007;5(2):89–104.
22. Richards D, Bartlett DJ, Wong K, Malouff J, Grunstein RR. Increased adherence to CPAP with a group cognitive behavioral treatment intervention: a randomized trial. Sleep. 2007;30(5):635–40.
23. Crawford MR, Espie CA, Bartlett DJ, Grunstein RR. Integrating psychology and medicine in CPAP adherence–new concepts? Sleep Med Rev. 2014;18(2):123–39.

24. Miller WR, Rollnick S. Motivational interviewing. 3rd ed. New York: Guilford Press; 2013.
25. Aloia MS, Arnedt JT, Riggs RL, Hecht J, Borrelli B. Clinical management of poor adherence to CPAP: motivational enhancement. Behav Sleep Med. 2004;2(4):205–22.
26. McArdle N, Kingshott R, Engleman HM, Mackay TW, Douglas NJ. Partners of patients with sleep apnoea/hypopnoea syndrome: effect of CPAP treatment on sleep quality and quality of life. Thorax. 2001;56(7):513–8.
27. Kiely JL, McNicholas WT. Bed partners' assessment of nasal continuous positive airway pressure therapy in obstructive sleep apnea. Chest. 1997;111(5):1261–5.
28. Sweetman A, Lack L, Bastien C. Co-Morbid Insomnia and Sleep Apnea (COMISA): prevalence, consequences, methodological considerations, and recent randomized controlled trials. Brain Sci. 2019;9(12):371.
29. Saaresranta T, Hedner J, Bonsignore MR, Riha RL, McNicholas WT, Penzel T, et al. Clinical phenotypes and comorbidity in european sleep apnoea patients. PLoS One. 2016;11(10):e0163439.
30. Sweetman AM, Lack LC, Catcheside PG, Antic NA, Chai-Coetzer CL, Smith SS, et al. Developing a successful treatment for co-morbid insomnia and sleep apnoea. Sleep Med Rev. 2017;33:28–38.
31. Wickwire EM, Smith MT, Birnbaum S, Collop NA. Sleep maintenance insomnia complaints predict poor CPAP adherence: a clinical case series. Sleep Med. 2010;11(8):772–6.
32. Pieh C, Bach M, Popp R, Jara C, Cronlein T, Hajak G, et al. Insomnia symptoms influence CPAP compliance. Sleep Breath. 2013;17(1):99–104.
33. Wallace DM, Vargas SS, Schwartz SJ, Aloia MS, Shafazand S. Determinants of continuous positive airway pressure adherence in a sleep clinic cohort of South Florida Hispanic veterans. Sleep Breath. 2013;17(1):351–63.
34. Wallace DM, Sawyer AM, Shafazand S. Comorbid insomnia symptoms predict lower 6-month adherence to CPAP in US veterans with obstructive sleep apnea. Sleep Breath. 2018;22(1):5–15.
35. Qaseem A, Kansagara D, Forciea MA, Cooke M, Denberg TD, Clinical Guidelines Committee of the American College of Physicians. Management of chronic insomnia disorder in adults: a clinical practice guideline from the American college of physicians. Ann Intern Med. 2016;165(2):125–33.
36. Wilson SJ, Nutt DJ, Alford C, Argyropoulos SV, Baldwin DS, Bateson AN, et al. British Association for Psychopharmacology consensus statement on evidence-based treatment of insomnia, parasomnias and circadian rhythm disorders. J Psychopharmacol. 2010;24(11):1577–601.
37. Riemann D, Baglioni C, Bassetti C, Bjorvatn B, Dolenc Groselj L, Ellis JG, et al. European guideline for the diagnosis and treatment of insomnia. J Sleep Res. 2017;26(6):675–700.
38. Edinger JD, Arnedt JT, Bertisch SM, Carney CE, Harrington JJ, Lichstein KL, et al. Behavioral and psychological treatments for chronic insomnia disorder in adults: an American Academy of Sleep Medicine clinical practice guideline. J Clin Sleep Med. 2021;17(2):255–62.
39. Sweetman A, Lack L, Lambert S, Gradisar M, Harris J. Does comorbid obstructive sleep apnea impair the effectiveness of cognitive and behavioral therapy for insomnia? Sleep Med. 2017;39:38–46.
40. Sweetman A, Lack L, Catcheside PG, Antic NA, Smith S, Chai-Coetzer CL, et al. Cognitive and behavioral therapy for insomnia increases the use of continuous positive airway pressure therapy in obstructive sleep apnea participants with comorbid insomnia: a randomized clinical trial. Sleep. 2019;42(12):zsz178.
41. Fung CH, Martin JL, Josephson K, Fiorentino L, Dzierzewski JM, Jouldjian S, et al. Efficacy of cognitive behavioral therapy for insomnia in older adults with occult sleep-disordered breathing. Psychosom Med. 2016;78(5):629–39.
42. Alessi CA, Fung CH, Dzierzewski JM, Fiorentino L, et al. Randomized controlled trial of an integrated approach to treating insomnia and improving use of positive airway pressure therapy in veterans with comorbid insomnia disorder and obstructive sleep apnea. Sleep. 2020;44(4):zsaa235.
43. Ong JC, Crawford MR, Dawson SC, Fogg LF, Turner AD, Wyatt JK, et al. A randomized controlled trial of CBT-I and PAP for obstructive sleep apnea and comorbid insomnia: main outcomes from the MATRICS study. Sleep. 2020;43(9):zsaa041.
44. Edmonds JC, Yang H, King TS, Sawyer DA, Rizzo A, Sawyer AM. Claustrophobic tendencies and continuous positive airway pressure therapy non-adherence in adults with obstructive sleep apnea. Heart Lung. 2015;44(2):100–6.
45. Chasens ER, Pack AI, Maislin G, Dinges DF, Weaver TE. Claustrophobia and adherence to CPAP treatment. West J Nurs Res. 2005;27(3):307–21.
46. Abramowitz JS, Deacon BJ, Whiteside SPH. Exposure therapy for anxiety, principles and prcatice. 2nd ed. New York: Guilford Press; 2019.
47. Wolitzky-Taylor KB, Horowitz JD, Powers MB, Telch MJ. Psychological approaches in treatment of specidic phobia: a meta-analysis. Clin Psychol Rev. 2008;28:1021–37.
48. Pompoli A, Furukawa TA, Imai H, Tajika A, Efthimiou O, Salanti G. Psychological therapies for panic disorder with or without agoraphobia in adults: a network meta-analysis. Cochrane Database Syst Rev. 2016;4:CD011004.
49. Means MK, Edinger JD. Graded exposure therapy for addressing claustrophobic reactions to continuous positive airway pressure: a case series report. Behav Sleep Med. 2007;5(2):105–16.
50. Pack AI. Application of personalized, predictive, preventative, and participatory (P4) medicine to obstructive sleep apnea. A roadmap for improving care? Ann Am Thorac Soc. 2016;13(9):1456–67.
51. Ong JC, Crisostomo MI. The more the merrier? Working towards multidisciplinary management of obstructive sleep apnea and comorbid insomnia. J Clin Psychol. 2013;69(10):1066–77.

Role of the Physician in CPAP Adherence and CPAP Trials

Laura H. Buckley and James R. Catterall

Abbreviations

AHI	Apnea-hypopnea index
ASV	Adaptive servo-ventilation
BMI	Body mass index
CBT-i	Cognitive behavioral therapy—insomnia
COMISA	Comorbid obstructive sleep apnea and insomnia
CPAP	Continuous positive airway pressure
EEG	Electroencephalogram
OSA	Obstructive sleep apnea
PLM	Periodic leg movement

7.1 Introduction

In many patients with obstructive sleep apnea (OSA), the benefits of CPAP are clear-cut, and the treatment brings about remarkable improvements in quality of life. However, in others, the benefits are uncertain, incomplete, or absent, or they are outweighed by the drawbacks and inconvenience of the treatment, even when technical problems have been resolved.

These patients need guidance. Some need further investigation, some should be encouraged to persevere with CPAP and given further help, a proportion of patients may benefit from an alternative treatment, and others need to be reassured that they do not need CPAP. The presence of OSA does not necessarily mean that it explains their symptoms. Those who do not need CPAP may need further explanation and/or exploration of their symptoms and a plan for further management of their condition. A negative CPAP trial (i.e., a lack of improvement in symptoms despite adequate usage) can be a useful and important step in the diagnostic process.

L. H. Buckley (✉) · J. R. Catterall
Department of Respiratory Medicine, University Hospitals Bristol, Bristol, UK
e-mail: Laura.Buckley@uhbw.nhs.uk

Many factors may need to be considered in formulating this guidance, including the severity of the sleep apnea, the reasons for presentation, the individual's expectations, and, in many cases, the patient's comorbidities and medication. A holistic approach is required, by a diagnostician. The physician is often the best-placed member of the team to provide this.

In this chapter, we attempt to describe our experience in managing these issues. The aim is to provide something that will be useful to practicing clinicians, especially those who are relatively new to the field. However, it is not a step-by-step guide. All patients are different and need to be managed as individuals. Also, different teams use different patient pathways and that may affect the precise way that things are done.

7.2 Threshold for CPAP Trials

One of the variations in patient pathways between different centers is the threshold for CPAP trials. Some centers offer CPAP mainly to patients who have proven severe or moderately severe OSA on polysomnography, thus reserving the treatment for those in whom there is greatest evidence of benefit [1]. In contrast, others place more emphasis on symptoms and offer CPAP trials to symptomatic patients with only mild or minimal abnormalities on polysomnography or on simpler tests such as overnight oximetry. Although full polysomnography is the gold standard investigation for detecting physiological abnormalities during sleep, the measurements made during polysomnography show only a limited correlation with symptomatic response to CPAP in symptomatic patients with a wide range of severity of sleep apnea-hypopnea. Furthermore, there is evidence that, of those measurements, improvement in sleepiness (subjective and objective) with CPAP is best predicted by simple measures such as the rate of 4% falls in arterial oxygen saturation or the frequency of body movements [2, 3].

In our practice, we have a relatively low threshold for CPAP trials in patients with clinically suspected OSA syndrome, even if oximetry is not diagnostic, and we reserve full polysomnography for those who are thought to have a different diagnosis, either before or after a CPAP trial. This is reflected in some of the examples described below. It is likely that negative CPAP trials are less common in those centers which have a higher threshold for trials of CPAP. However, whichever approach is used, a significant number of patients will not respond to CPAP in the way that they might have hoped, and the principles for managing these patients are the same.

7.3　Suboptimal Compliance Versus Lack of Effectiveness of CPAP

When a patient reports a negative or suboptimal response to CPAP, the first thing to establish is whether the difficulty lies mainly in compliance or whether the key problem is lack of effectiveness of CPAP in improving the patient's symptoms. The approaches to these problems are fundamentally different. This is shown schematically in Fig. 7.1.

The difference can usually be established easily by asking the patient to describe his or her experience with CPAP and by examining data from the CPAP machine. If there is overlap or uncertainty, it is usually best to deal with compliance first as it is obviously difficult to make a full assessment of effectiveness without reasonably good use of CPAP. However, there are patients, particularly those with mild OSA or minimal symptoms, whose low compliance reflects lack of benefit from CPAP, in which case continuing CPAP may not be in their best interests.

7.4　Strategies to Manage a Poor Response to CPAP

7.4.1　Poor Adherence

CPAP usage of more than 4 h per night, for at least 70% of nights, is accepted as adequate, although sleepiness improves in a linear response with increased CPAP usage [4]. Average CPAP usage is 4–5 h per night, but only 60–70% of patients use CPAP for more than 4 h per night on average, and approximately 30% of patients discontinue CPAP [4, 5]. Therefore, managing patients with poor adherence is a

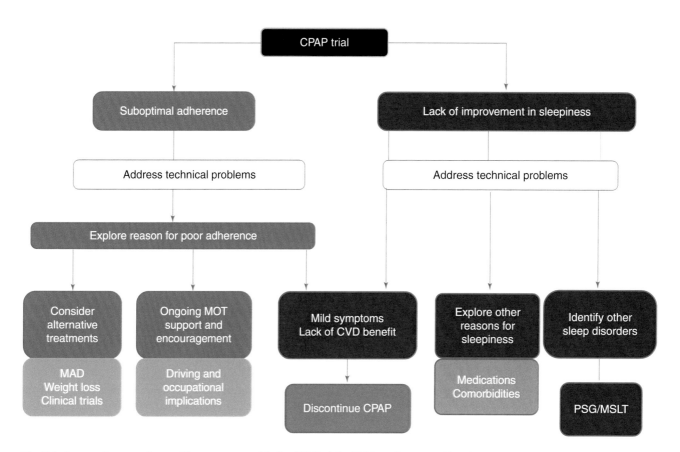

Fig. 7.1 Systematic approach to problems encountered during CPAP trials. CPAP continuous positive airway pressure, MAD mandibular advancement device, CVD cardiovascular disease, PSG/MSLT polysomnography/multiple sleep latency test

common scenario faced in the sleep clinic and the role of the physician is to determine which patients should persevere with CPAP, which may benefit from alternative therapies, and which can discontinue CPAP. This generally depends on severity of OSA and degree of symptoms.

7.4.1.1 Technical Factors

The first step if a patient has poor CPAP adherence is to address technical issues. Although the physician has an important role, this technical support is usually delivered by non-medics, usually sleep physiologists/technologists or respiratory care practitioners. Practical support and education are essential to achieve good CPAP compliance, and often poor compliance can be resolved by addressing practical issues, such as:

- Mask fit: often patients complain of discomfort from the mask, claustrophobia, or excessive leak which may be remedied by switching to a different style of mask (Box 7.1)
- Addition of humidification if the patient complains of a dry mouth
- Prescribing nasal decongestants for nasal blockage

Although practice varies across countries, follow-up after a period of a few weeks of CPAP is generally recommended to identify and address any problems, in addition to patients having open access to the CPAP provider so there is no delay in resolving practical problems. With advancing technology, newer CPAP machines can be accessed remotely to enable telemonitoring of CPAP data, including compliance, mask leak, and residual events, which allows early identification of issues. However, as yet intensive telemonitoring of patients has generally not resulted in significant improvements in CPAP adherence [6]. Nevertheless, there may be other benefits of telemonitoring, such as facilitating non-face-to-face consultations in areas where patients would need to travel long distances to clinic, or during the COVID-19 pandemic.

7.4.1.2 Poor Adherence after Technical Factors Have Been Addressed

Even once practical issues such as mask fit and humidification have been resolved, some patients still do not tolerate CPAP well and therefore do not gain the expected benefit. In patients with moderate-to-severe OSA and excessive daytime sleepiness, it is likely that CPAP will be the most effective treatment and generally we would recommend persevering with it. Reasons for failure to use CPAP adequately need to be explored: In addition to taking a thorough history, the CPAP download data should be reviewed and discussed with the patient. Although the headline figure on the CPAP download is average nightly usage, this may not tell the whole story. Other metrics, such as average usage on

nights used, and the pattern of usage over time should be reviewed (Box 7.1). For example:

- Some patients may use CPAP for an adequate amount of time on the nights they use it, but may not use it at all on other nights giving an overall lower average usage. This could be because of working patterns or intercurrent illness, for example.
- Some patients have good usage initially but it then tails off, which can be identified from the daily usage charts. In some cases, this can be due to a lack of understanding that CPAP is a long-term treatment, or an initial lack of improvement in symptoms leads to subsequent poor compliance.

Although evidence suggests that CPAP usage in the first week predicts CPAP usage after 30 days, and possibly longer, in our experience if patients are willing to persevere with CPAP, some improve their usage over time, with a corresponding improvement in symptoms [7]. Clearly though, the CPAP setup process is of paramount importance in order to achieve the best long-term results.

In some excessively sleepy patients with moderate-to-severe OSA, poor CPAP usage has major implications for driving or occupation (Box 7.1). In the United Kingdom, the Driving and Vehicle Licensing Agency requires there to be an improvement in sleepiness along with adequate CPAP compliance (generally regarded as an average nightly usage of 4 h, although the exact number is not specified) in order for these patients to be deemed fit to drive [8]. For occupational drivers, this also applies to those with mild OSA and excessive daytime sleepiness. Similarly, other occupations, such as airline pilots and air traffic controllers, require medical confirmation that their sleepiness is controlled, sometimes with criteria set by their own licensing bodies. Therefore, the physician may have the difficult role of making a decision regarding fitness to drive or work and needs to be clear about the implications of poor CPAP compliance to these patients which may in turn encourage them to increase CPAP usage. There may also need to be liaison with the patient's occupational physician.

Whatever the reasons for suboptimal CPAP usage, further education about the potential benefits of CPAP is needed alongside close monitoring and other support, with the aim of improving compliance and symptoms. Despite this, there are some patients who still do not tolerate CPAP but would benefit from treatment of OSA, and at some point, the patient and physician will need to decide that persisting with CPAP is not likely to be effective. Second-line therapy would typically be with an oral appliance. While these are recognized to be less effective at controlling OSA than CPAP, particularly in more severe OSA, this lack of efficacy may be offset by better compliance and therefore symptoms may still improve [9]. Alternative treatments, such as implanted or transcutaneous hypoglossal nerve stimulation, are generally only available for a few patients in trial settings [10, 11]. Surgery is indicated only very infrequently and appears to be most effective in patients who have OSA due to a severe, surgically correctable lesion or craniofacial abnormality causing obstruction of the upper airway [12].

Finally, there are patients with minimally symptomatic OSA, or mild disease, who do not experience much benefit from CPAP which is the reason for their low compliance. In these patients, the role of the physician is to decide whether it is worth continuing CPAP to try and increase usage, or whether there has been truly no sign of improvement, in which case CPAP can be discontinued. These patients will be discussed in more detail in the next section.

7.4.2 Lack of Effectiveness of CPAP

If patients achieve adequate CPAP compliance but report no benefit, in the first instance it must be ensured that CPAP is actually controlling the OSA. Secondly, the physician must assess the degree of symptoms and response to CPAP to decide with the patient whether CPAP can be discontinued, which may be the case in patients with mild OSA and/or minimal symptoms. Thirdly, if the patient still complains of sleep-related symptoms despite adequate control of OSA, then it is important to consider other causes of sleepiness.

7.4.2.1 Failure to Control OSA

Patients may be established on fixed-pressure CPAP following a polysomnogram in which the CPAP pressure is titrated, or on auto-CPAP, in which the CPAP machine automatically adjusts the CPAP pressure. However, in some patients, OSA is still not well controlled and information about residual apnea-hypopnea index (AHI) can be obtained from the CPAP download data. In practice, the most common reason for this is excessive mask leak, information that can also be obtained from the CPAP download and can usually be addressed easily.

In some patients, the CPAP pressure may be too low. In patients using fixed-pressure CPAP, the pressure may be increased empirically or following a further CPAP titration study. In patients using auto-CPAP, if the average pressure is toward the upper end of the range, increasing the minimum pressure may help control OSA.

If the AHI remains elevated despite these measures and the patient remains symptomatic, a further sleep study may be required. This may be either full polysomnography, i.e., with electroencephalogram (EEG), or limited polysomnography, without EEG. If polysomnography was completed before the CPAP trial, and the diagnosis of OSA is certain,

a sleep study on CPAP will usually be preferred, to distinguish between residual obstructive events and CPAP-emergent central sleep apnea. However, if the only investigation before the CPAP trial was overnight oximetry, a sleep study off CPAP may be more appropriate to confirm that apneas and hypopneas are obstructive, rather than central or mixed, as patients with central sleep apnea may require other forms of nocturnal respiratory support (Box 7.2). In addition, it may be important to exclude obesity hypoventilation (in conjunction with arterial or transcutaneous carbon dioxide measurement) as this may require bilevel ventilation.

7.4.2.2 Mild OSA

Severity of OSA does not necessarily correlate with degree of sleepiness or other symptoms, and it can sometimes be difficult to predict which patients will respond well to CPAP from the results of sleep studies [2, 3]. Because of this, patients with mild OSA and/or mild symptoms may be offered CPAP very much as a trial, on the understanding that it may or may not benefit them significantly. However, there is accumulating evidence that CPAP can be beneficial in patients with mild OSA, hence the rationale for a CPAP trial in these patients. Randomized trials assessing the efficacy of CPAP in mild OSA have generally shown small, statistically significant benefits in patients with mild-to-moderate OSA, although a more recent study of patients with mild OSA (AHI <15) showed clinically significant improvements in quality of life and sleepiness [13–15]. However, CPAP usage is generally lower in these patients, probably because they obtain less benefit overall than patients with more symptomatic, severe OSA.

Therefore, as the treating physician, it is important to judge whether ongoing treatment with CPAP is in the patient's best interests. If patients with mild OSA have experienced little or no benefit from CPAP, even if compliance has been suboptimal, then pursuing CPAP is probably not the right course for them and this should be considered a negative CPAP trial and CPAP discontinued. If they are still sleepy, then OSA is unlikely to be the cause (especially if they have had good CPAP compliance), and other reasons need to be explored.

7.4.2.3 Patients with Non-Classical OSA Symptoms

Patients are referred to sleep clinics for a range of different reasons: with sleep-related symptoms, for example; because of snoring and witnessed apneas noted by a partner; following screening prior to bariatric surgery; or by a cardiologist investigating causes of hypertension or atrial fibrillation. It is recognized that there is a range of clinical presentations of

OSA, or phenotypes. Cluster analyses have shown that in a large cohort of patients with moderate-to-severe OSA, approximately one-third have "classical" OSA characterized by excessive daytime sleepiness, one-third have symptoms of disturbed sleep (insomnia and frequent awakenings) but less daytime sleepiness, and one-third are minimally symptomatic [16].

So, should patients without excessive daytime sleepiness be offered a trial of CPAP? In a randomized trial, non-sleepy patients with cardiovascular disease and moderate-to-severe OSA treated with CPAP had greater improvements in sleepiness and quality of life than controls [17]. Furthermore, in another randomized trial, patients with mild-to-moderate OSA without significant sleepiness randomized to CPAP also had greater improvements in sleepiness and quality of life than controls, and 70% opted to continue CPAP at the end of the trial [18]. Therefore, it is reasonable to offer a CPAP trial to patients with mild symptoms as some benefit from CPAP even if their perception of symptoms was low.

However, the chance of CPAP success, defined as adherence of more than 4 h per night and improvement in symptoms, is 80% lower in patients with minimal symptoms, and about 50% lower in patients in the "disturbed sleep" group than in those with excessive daytime sleepiness [19]. At follow-up, these patients may have low CPAP compliance as well as no or little improvement in symptoms, and it can be challenging to decide whether to extend the CPAP trial in the hope that adherence and symptoms will improve, or whether to accept that CPAP is not going to be of benefit (Box 7.3). This is a decision that needs to be made on a case-by-case basis by the physician and the patient and depends on severity and type of symptoms, whether there has been any sign of improvement, degree of non-adherence, and willingness of the patient to continue CPAP.

If patients truly have minimal symptoms and either do not wish to try CPAP, or obtain no benefit, they may still be worried about leaving OSA untreated, and there has been long-standing concern regarding the adverse cardiovascular consequences of OSA, especially if severe. This is particularly true in at-risk populations, in whom OSA is highly prevalent yet patients are frequently asymptomatic [20]. For example, OSA has a prevalence of up to 80% in patients with refractory hypertension and approximately 50% in patients with heart failure and ischemic heart disease respectively, yet many of these patients are not sleepy and do not benefit symptomatically from CPAP, possibly because increased sympathetic drive maintains alertness [21].

Observational studies have shown that patients with untreated OSA are at increased risk of cardiovascular events compared with those without OSA, or treated OSA [22]. However, randomized trials have failed to show a decrease in the incidence of cardiovascular events or all-cause mortality when non-sleepy OSA patients are treated with CPAP [17, 23, 24]. Therefore, CPAP cannot be recommended solely for the prevention of cardiovascular events in asymptomatic patients. CPAP lowers blood pressure, but only by 1–2 mmHg, and therefore, anti-hypertensive medications are both more effective and tolerable [25, 26]. The only caveat would be in drug-resistant hypertension, where CPAP has greater effects on blood pressure and could be recommended to optimize blood pressure control if patients are already on maximal anti-hypertensive medications [27].

Therefore, if a patient referred to the sleep clinic is found to have severe OSA but is genuinely asymptomatic, it is reasonable not to offer a trial of CPAP, although many physicians will reach a joint decision with the patient after discussing the evidence (Box 7.4). Similarly, if such a patient with mild symptoms does not experience benefit from CPAP, it can be stopped, and the patient can be reassured that there is no evidence to support continuing treatment with regard to long-term cardiovascular benefits.

7.4.2.4 Persistent Sleepiness Despite Control of OSA

Although many patients have improvements in sleepiness with CPAP, approximately 10–20% experience persistent sleepiness despite adequate control of OSA with CPAP [28]. The role of the physician is to identify other causes. This will often necessitate a detailed sleep study (on or off CPAP), if the patient has not already had one, to exclude other sleep disorders. However, there is often not another primary sleep disorder. In these cases, the sleepiness may be explained by medication or comorbidities, although it may be idiopathic.

Coexistent Sleep Disorders

If a patient has not responded well to CPAP, the sleep history should be revisited in order to try and identify any coexistent sleep disorders. The physician should ask about:

- Sleep pattern, in conjunction with a sleep diary, to identify insomnia or lifestyle factors affecting sleep
- Symptoms of restless legs and periodic leg movement (PLM) syndromes
- Narcolepsy symptoms (cataplexy, sleep-related hallucinations, sleep fragmentation, and sleep paralysis)

The patient is likely to need a full polysomnogram to look for other sleep disorders. In cases where the diagnosis of OSA is certain, a polysomnogram on CPAP will be appropriate, as this will confirm that OSA is well controlled and allow other non-respiratory sleep disorders to be identified. However, depending on local practice, patients may have been offered a CPAP trial on the basis of symptoms despite having had a screening test such as oximetry that was non-diagnostic. In these patients, it is probably more useful to perform a polysomnogram off CPAP to establish whether the patient actually has OSA and to look for other sleep disorders. If there is clinical suspicion of narcolepsy, then a multiple sleep latency test should also be performed, as patients may have been misdiagnosed with OSA when the diagnosis is in fact narcolepsy, a much rarer condition [29].

Periodic Leg Movements

PLMs commonly coexist with OSA and are associated with worse sleep quality, although not more sleepiness [30]. However, the clinical significance of PLMs that coexist with OSA is uncertain and the OSA should be treated first (Box 7.5). Nevertheless, PLMs frequently persist even when patients are treated with CPAP, and if these patients complain of persistently poor sleep quality, further management of the periodic leg movements may be warranted.

Comorbid OSA and Insomnia (COMISA)

It is increasingly recognized that insomnia, characterized by difficulty initiating and/or maintaining sleep, commonly coexists with OSA [31]. Studies have shown that 30–60% of patients with OSA also have insomnia, and these patients experience more daytime impairment, poorer quality of life, and more coexistent psychiatric disorders than patients with either condition alone. Furthermore, patients with insomnia are less likely to tolerate CPAP, although, in some patients whose insomnia is mainly secondary to sleep disturbance from apneas, treatment with CPAP may improve both conditions. However, in other patients, insomnia may persist (Box 7.6). Such patients benefit from cognitive behavioral therapy (CBT-i), a proven non-pharmacological treatment that modifies the behavioral and psychological factors that perpetuate insomnia. In patients with COMISA, four sessions of CBT-i prior to commencing CPAP increased CPAP adherence and improved insomnia although not daytime sleepiness [32]. However, access to CBT-i is not widely available in some regions, and while online CBT-i may be a second-line option, it has lower efficacy than face-to-face CBT-i and has not been tested in COMISA patients [33].

Comorbidities and Medications

In many patients, medications and comorbidities account for residual sleepiness (Box 7.7). Medications associated with excessive daytime sleepiness include benzodiazepines, opiates, anti-histamines, antidepressants, anti-epileptics, gabapentinoids, and beta-blockers. Patients are often well established on these drugs and the benefit often outweighs the side effects. However, the sleep physician is well placed to recognize which drugs may be contributing to residual sleepiness, and liaise with the patient's primary care physician or specialist who may be able to adjust medications. Many comorbidities are associated with excessive daytime sleepiness, including neurological disorders, heart failure, rheumatological and endocrine disorders, as well as psychiatric disorders such as depression. In some patients, the sleep physician may be satisfied that residual sleepiness is secondary to comorbidities and medications. However, a proportion of patients will need further investigation to rule out other causes.

Idiopathic Persistent Sleepiness

It is estimated that once coexistent sleep disorders, comorbidities, and medications that could cause residual sleepiness are excluded, approximately 10% of patients with adequate CPAP adherence have residual sleepiness [28]. These patients have more fatigue, depressive symptoms, and lower health self-perception at baseline, symptoms which persist despite CPAP treatment. Residual sleepiness should be assessed objectively as it may not correlate with patient-reported sleepiness. In some patients, treatment with a stimulant drug may be warranted. Modafinil and armodafinil are approved in the USA, but not in Europe, for treatment of excessive daytime sleepiness in OSA patients. More recently, solriamfetol has been approved in both the USA and Europe and can be considered in patients in whom CPAP adherence is suboptimal [34]. Pitolisant, a histamine H3 receptor antagonist, is currently only approved for use in narcolepsy, but a recent randomized trial in sleepy OSA patients who refused CPAP showed that it reduced Epworth sleepiness score more than placebo [35].

7.5   Conclusion

The physician has an important role as part of the multidisciplinary sleep team in assessing patients whose adherence to CPAP is suboptimal or who have incomplete resolution of symptoms. Making these assessments can be a complex process and may need to take into account severity of OSA, symptoms, reason for presentation, medical and psychiatric history, patient wishes, and other factors. Although each patient must be assessed individually, a systematic approach can guide management. Once technical factors have been optimized, the physician can decide with the patient whether they should persevere with CPAP, switch to an alternative therapy, or discontinue CPAP in cases of mild OSA and/or minimal symptoms. In patients who have persistent sleepiness despite treatment of OSA, the physician can initiate further sleep studies as appropriate. Finally, it must be recognized that persistent sleepiness may not be due a sleep disorder, but to comorbidities and medication.

Box 7.1 Case 1: Exploring Patterns of CPAP Use

A 32-year-old long-haul truck driver was started on CPAP after being diagnosed with severe OSA syndrome (4% oxygen desaturation index of 42). He had had a near miss while driving his truck and had excessive daytime sleepiness with an Epworth score of 20. He had a small beard. He was instructed not to drive until it was confirmed that his use of CPAP was adequate and that his symptoms were controlled.

The CPAP was set up by a specialist sleep physiologist with appropriate education and support. The patient requested a full-face mask because he thought that he would have difficulty breathing through his nose.

After 10 days, he called to say that he could not tolerate the CPAP. He reported that the machine was noisy that he did not like the sensation of air blowing onto his face and that air was sometimes blowing into his eyes. He had also developed a congested nose. Data from the machine showed that he had tried to use the CPAP every night but that his average nightly use was less than 2 h. There was excess leak, and the sleep apnea was not controlled.

It was thought likely that the beard was preventing a good mask seal. He agreed to try a nasal mask and was prescribed a nasal steroid spray to prevent nasal congestion. He was reassured that he was making progress and that a solution would be found.

Four weeks later, his average use of CPAP over all nights was only 2.75 h. He was concerned that he was about to lose his job and asked to see a physician.

However, this time the pattern of CPAP use was different. He had used CPAP well on 16 of the 28 nights, with an average nightly use of 4.25 h and, within that, a pattern of gradually increasing use up to maximum of 5.5 h. On those nights, there had been no excess leak and the sleep apnea had been well controlled. He had also experienced much better sleep quality on those nights and had felt refreshed the next day.

On the other twelve nights, he had not used the CPAP at all. He explained that he had first had a major family shock as his father had been taken seriously ill and the stress had rendered him unable to cope with the new treatment, and just as he had been ready to restart CPAP, he had caught a cold from his young children and had found it impossible to use the CPAP for a week.

He was reassured that these were understandable reasons for not using CPAP and that he was continuing to make progress. However, it was also explained that he would not be able to resume driving until there was clear evidence of adequate use of CPAP every night over a substantial period. He was given a letter for his employer, who, fortunately, was able to provide him with temporary non-driving work.

He became well established on CPAP with an overall average nightly use of more than 7 h, and the daytime sleepiness did not recur. He was able to resume driving after a further few weeks. Annual checks confirmed continued good use of CPAP and continued control of his symptoms.

Comment: By analyzing the pattern of this man's CPAP use, and exploring the reasons for it, it was possible to help, support, and reassure him. However, it was also necessary to be firm with him about driving until consistent use of CPAP was verified.

Box 7.2 Case 2: Mixed Obstructive and Central Sleep Apnea

A 65-year-old man presented with poor quality sleep. There was a history of loud snoring and witnessed apneas and of waking with a choking sensation. He was a busy professional photographer and did not experience sleepiness except sometimes when relaxing in the evening. His Epworth score was 10. However, he was concerned about his sleep quality and also about the cardiovascular effects of sleep apnea, as he had a history of hypertension and his mother had had a stroke. His medication consisted of candesartan, bendroflumethiazide, atorvastatin, and amitriptyline. He drank half a bottle of wine each night. His body mass index (BMI) was 31. Overnight oximetry showed marked cyclical oxygen desaturation with a 4% oxygen desaturation index of 48 and 38 on two nights of study. A provisional diagnosis of OSA syndrome was made and he was started on a trial of auto-CPAP. He was also given lifestyle advice.

During the first month, he used CPAP on 87% of nights and his nightly use of CPAP averaged 4.6 h. However, his sleep quality did not improve. He found the ramps in pressure difficult to tolerate and switched the machine off repeatedly. There was no excess leak but the residual AHI was 18. In an attempt to reduce the pressure changes, the maximum CPAP pressure was capped at a level that it was thought he would tolerate, based on the CPAP download. However, this did not help. Further adjustments were made to the CPAP but his sleep quality remained poor, and the AHI remained high. The CPAP download also showed Cheyne-Stokes respiration.

This was confirmed on limited polysomnography, off CPAP. The study showed an AHI of 54, comprising 12 obstructive apneas 18 central apneas, 5 mixed apneas, and 19 hypopneas per hour. 25% of the night was spent in Cheyne-Stokes respiration.

Echocardiography showed normal left ventricular function. As he was symptomatic, he was offered a trial of adaptive servo-ventilation (ASV). After starting ASV, the AHI fell to 5 and his sleep quality improved significantly. Six years later, he remains asymptomatic and fully compliant with ASV, averaging 8 h of nightly use. His cardiac function also remains normal.

Comment: This man had mixed obstructive and central sleep apnea. The frequent pressure changes which he found intolerable were probably due to the auto-CPAP device ineffectively trying to compensate for the central apneas.

Cheyne-Stokes respiration, a form of central sleep apnea, is often seen on CPAP downloads (CPAP-emergent central sleep apnea) and is frequently an incidental finding which does not require treatment. However, in this case the central sleep apnea was primary, rather than secondary to CPAP. He was offered treatment because he had continued symptoms which had not responded to CPAP. ASV could only be considered once it had been established that left ventricular function was preserved because there is evidence that ASV is associated with increased mortality in patients with a left ventricular ejection fraction of 45% or less [36]. No underlying cause was found for this man's Cheyne-Stokes respiration. However, when a cause is found, such as heart failure, the underlying condition should be treated first.

Box 7.3 Case 3: CPAP Started during Hospital Admission

A 70-year-old man was admitted to hospital with leg cellulitis. He was drowsy. He had a history of chronic kidney disease and recurrent venous thromboembolism. His BMI was 36. He was treated with intravenous antibiotics, and his temperature settled. However, he slept a lot during the day. He was noted to snore and to have obstructive apneas during sleep. On direct questioning, he did not feel that he usually had a problem with daytime sleepiness, although his wife reported that he sometimes fell asleep when watching television. Overnight oximetry showed evidence of severe sleep apnea with a 4% oxygen desaturation index of 34. He used CPAP in hospital for the next two nights. The sleepiness improved and he was discharged home.

Shortly after discharge, he stopped using the CPAP. He found the treatment inconvenient and he was not convinced that it was helping him. When he was reviewed in the outpatient clinic, a month later he reported that the sleepiness had improved as he had resumed his usual activities. His Epworth score was 10. There was no history of sleepiness when driving. This was confirmed by his wife.

He was informed about the potential cardiovascular effects of OSA, and it was suggested that he restart the CPAP on a trial basis. He used the CPAP well for a trial period of 3 weeks but then stopped it because he did not experience any symptomatic benefit. At review, 5 weeks after stopping CPAP, his Epworth score was 4. It was concluded that he had OSA without daytime sleepiness and it was agreed that he did not need to use CPAP. He was advised to lose weight.

Comment: This gentleman's temporary drowsiness and sleepiness were due to intercurrent illness and probably the boredom of being in hospital. Although he had severe OSA, he did not wish to continue CPAP, and because he did not have persistent daytime sleepiness, he could be reassured that there was no clear evidence that CPAP would be beneficial to him.

Box 7.4 Case 4: Obstructive Sleep Apnea and Atrial Fibrillation

A 61-year-old man with hypertension presented with palpitations due to atrial fibrillation. He was referred to a cardiologist, who prescribed anticoagulant medication and a beta-blocker. Cardioversion was initially successful but the arrhythmia returned. On direct questioning, his wife reported apneas during sleep and loud snoring. However, there was no history of daytime sleepiness, and the patient felt that his sleep quality was good. His Epworth score was 1. Overnight oximetry showed evidence of severe sleep apnea with a 4% oxygen desaturation index of 32. He consented to a trial of CPAP.

He used the CPAP well for 4 weeks, and the CPAP controlled the sleep apnea. However, he did not experience any symptomatic benefit, and he found the treatment inconvenient.

The potential pros and cons of CPAP treatment were discussed with the patient so that he could make an informed decision. It was explained that, overall, there is no evidence that CPAP has a beneficial effect on mortality in patients with cardiovascular disease in non-sleepy patients with OSA. However, it was also pointed out that in patients with OSA there is observational evidence that CPAP can reduce the chance of recurrence of atrial fibrillation, including after catheter ablation [37]. He opted not to continue CPAP.

Comment: Having tried CPAP, and having had an opportunity to discuss the evidence for and against the potential medical benefits for him, the patient felt confident to make his own decision regarding CPAP.

Box 7.5 Case 5: Obstructive Sleep Apnea, Periodic Leg Movements, and Coexistent Fibromyalgia

A 48-year-old man with fibromyalgia presented with poor quality sleep, morning headaches, marked tiredness, and excessive daytime sleepiness. His Epworth score was 22. He worked as a carer for his wife, who had commented on his loud snoring and apneas during sleep. His BMI was 34. He drank no alcohol. He was taking codeine for musculoskeletal pains, citalopram for depression, together with a small dose of amitriptyline at night, and also iron supplements and a proton pump inhibitor because of mild iron deficiency attributed to esophagitis and gastroesophageal reflux.

Overnight oximetry showed cyclical oxygen desaturation typical of OSA, with a 4% oxygen desaturation index of 10 and a 3% desaturation index of 18. He agreed to a trial of CPAP.

During the first month, he used CPAP very little. He found it inconvenient and noisy, and there were problems with a damaged hose. Also, he reasoned that his sleep disturbance was caused by pains from the fibromyalgia. However, he was persuaded to try again. It was explained that the hole in the hose would have made the treatment less effective and that the hose needed to be replaced. It was also pointed out that improving sleep quality by treating coexisting OSA can reduce the symptoms of fibromyalgia [38].

A month later, he was using CPAP for an average of 4 h a night. His sleep quality had improved and, in particular, the morning headaches had resolved. However, he still felt tired, and his Epworth score was still 18.

Polysomnography was performed while he was using CPAP. This showed good control of the sleep apnea but increased leg movements, with a PLM index of 70.

However, by the time the results of the study were discussed with the patient, his nightly use of CPAP had increased to an average of 7.3 h and he was feeling significantly better. His Epworth score had fallen to 14. The musculoskeletal pains had improved and he had been able to discontinue the codeine.

The possible contribution of the PLMs to his symptoms was discussed and also the potential role of iron deficiency and antidepressant use in causing the leg movements. The potential benefits and risks of dopamine agonists in the treatment of PLMs were also mentioned. His primary care physician was informed. The ferritin level was optimized, with no obvious benefit. The amitriptyline was discontinued, after which he experienced a further small reduction in daytime tiredness.

Overall, he felt much improved and, in consultation with his primary care physician, it was decided to make no more changes.

Comment: This patient had both OSA and PLMs. His clinical improvement was mainly due to the use of CPAP, which increased gradually over several months, resulting in progressively longer periods of good quality sleep and improvement in the fibromyalgia symptoms.

Box 7.6 Case 6: Insomnia and Obstructive Sleep Apnea

A 62-year-old recently retired teacher presented with symptoms of both OSA syndrome and insomnia. She snored loudly, her sleep quality was poor, and she fell asleep easily when relaxing. Her Epworth score was 16. In addition, for many years she had been waking during the night at least once and had been unable to get back to sleep for 1–2 h each time, despite good sleep hygiene.

Overnight oximetry confirmed moderate OSA. After using CPAP for a month, she reported that her sleep quality had improved and that she was less tired and sleepy during the day. The CPAP download showed an average nightly use of 5 h, and good control of the OSA.

However, she was frustrated because there had been no improvement in the long periods that she spent awake during the night. She indicated that she had been hoping for a single solution and that she was considering looking for an alternative to CPAP. It was explained that she had both insomnia and OSA syndrome and that the two usually required different treatments. She was advised that the recommended treatment for insomnia is CBT-i. She was keen to try this. As we could not access face-to face CBT-I, we advised her how to access online therapy. She was very grateful for this advice, and she also continued to use CPAP.

Comment: Having first been disappointed with CPAP because it did not solve all her sleep problems, this patient became much happier once she understood that she had two sleep conditions, which could be treated independently. This motivated her to continue using CPAP.

Box 7.7 Case 7: Residual Daytime Sleepiness Due to Medications

A 44-year-old woman with fibromyalgia presented with severe daytime sleepiness. Her Epworth score was 23. She was unable to work because of the sleepiness. She had symptoms of OSA syndrome, with loud snoring and witnessed apneas. There was no history of restless legs or abnormal leg movements, and there were no features of narcolepsy. However, her sleep was also disturbed by musculoskeletal pain from fibromyalgia, for which she took several potentially sedating drugs including duloxetine, gabapentin, and tramadol.

Overnight oximetry showed evidence of moderate OSA, and a trial of CPAP was started. She used the CPAP well with an average nightly use of 6 h by the end of the first month. Her sleep quality improved and she experienced reduction in the musculoskeletal pain. She felt less sleepy than she had done but she still had excessive daytime sleepiness with an Epworth score of 17.

Further investigation with polysomnography was considered and discussed with the patient. However, it was explained that some of her medication was potentially sedating and that a better option would be try to reduce the medication. She was in strong agreement with this approach. She was advised to discuss this with her primary care physician.

The tramadol was discontinued, and over the next few months, the dose of gabapentin was gradually reduced then stopped. The daytime sleepiness improved markedly. The Epworth score fell to 11, and the patient felt much better. It was agreed that she should continue CPAP and that she did not need more detailed sleep studies.

Comment: In this case, the residual daytime sleepiness after starting CPAP treatment was due to the patient's medication, and by recognizing this, full polysomnography was not required, a worthwhile consideration as it may not be readily available in some centers.

References

1. National Institute for Health and Care Excellence. Continuous positive airways pressure for the treatment of obstructive sleep apnea/hypopnea syndrome. Technology appraisal guideline TA139. 2008. Available at https://www.niceorguk/guidance/TA139. Accessed 1 Sept 2020.
2. Bennett LS, Langford BA, Stradling JR, Davies RJ. Sleep fragmentation indices as predictors of daytime sleepiness and nCPAP response in obstructive sleep apnea. Am J Respir Crit Care Med. 1998;158(3):778–86.
3. Stradling JR, Davies RJ. Sleep. 1: obstructive sleep apnoea/hypopnoea syndrome: definitions, epidemiology, and natural history. Thorax. 2004;59(1):73–8.
4. Weaver TE, Maislin G, Dinges DF, Bloxham T, George CF, Greenberg H, et al. Relationship between hours of CPAP use and achieving normal levels of sleepiness and daily functioning. Sleep. 2007;30(6):711–9.
5. Rotenberg BW, Murariu D, Pang KP. Trends in CPAP adherence over twenty years of data collection: a flattened curve. J Otolaryngol Head Neck Surg. 2016;45(1):43.
6. Pepin JL, Tamisier R, Hwang D, Mereddy S, Parthasarathy S. Does remote monitoring change OSA management and CPAP adherence? Respirology. 2017;22(8):1508–17.

7. Budhiraja R, Parthasarathy S, Drake CL, Roth T, Sharief I, Budhiraja P, et al. Early CPAP use identifies subsequent adherence to CPAP therapy. Sleep. 2007;30(3):320–4.

8. Jenkins N, Lewis, N, Edgeworth, A, Stradling J, Gibbons G, on behalf of the British Thoracic Society. Position statement on driving and obstructive sleep apnoea (OSA) 2018.

9. Phillips CL, Grunstein RR, Darendeliler MA, Mihailidou AS, Srinivasan VK, Yee BJ, et al. Health outcomes of continuous positive airway pressure versus oral appliance treatment for obstructive sleep apnea: a randomized controlled trial. Am J Respir Crit Care Med. 2013;187(8):879–87.

10. Pengo MF, Xiao S, Ratneswaran C, Reed K, Shah N, Chen T, et al. Randomised sham-controlled trial of transcutaneous electrical stimulation in obstructive sleep apnoea. Thorax. 2016;71(10):923–31.

11. Strollo PJ Jr, Soose RJ, Maurer JT, de Vries N, Cornelius J, Froymovich O, et al. Upper-airway stimulation for obstructive sleep apnea. N Engl J Med. 2014;370(2):139–49.

12. Kryger M, Malhotra A. Management of obstructive sleep apnea in adults. In: UpToDate, Post TW (Ed). Waltham, MA: UpToDate Inc. https://www.UpToDate.com. Accessed 4 Sept 2020.

13. Wimms AJ, Kelly JL, Turnbull CD, McMillan A, Craig SE, O'Reilly JF, et al. Continuous positive airway pressure versus standard care for the treatment of people with mild obstructive sleep apnoea (MERGE): a multicentre, randomised controlled trial. Lancet Respir Med. 2020;8(4):349–58.

14. Marshall NS, Barnes M, Travier N, Campbell AJ, Pierce RJ, McEvoy RD, et al. Continuous positive airway pressure reduces daytime sleepiness in mild to moderate obstructive sleep apnoea: a meta-analysis. Thorax. 2006;61(5):430–4.

15. Weaver TE, Mancini C, Maislin G, Cater J, Staley B, Landis JR, et al. Continuous positive airway pressure treatment of sleepy patients with milder obstructive sleep apnea: results of the CPAP Apnea Trial North American Program (CATNAP) randomized clinical trial. Am J Respir Crit Care Med. 2012;186(7):677–83.

16. Ye L, Pien GW, Ratcliffe SJ, Bjornsdottir E, Arnardottir ES, Pack AI, et al. The different clinical faces of obstructive sleep apnoea: a cluster analysis. Eur Respir J. 2014;44(6):1600–7.

17. McEvoy RD, Antic NA, Heeley E, Luo Y, Ou Q, Zhang X, et al. CPAP for prevention of cardiovascular events in obstructive sleep apnea. N Engl J Med. 2016;375(10):919–31.

18. Craig SE, Kohler M, Nicoll D, Bratton DJ, Nunn A, Davies R, et al. Continuous positive airway pressure improves sleepiness but not calculated vascular risk in patients with minimally symptomatic obstructive sleep apnoea: the MOSAIC randomised controlled trial. Thorax. 2012;67(12):1090–6.

19. Gagnadoux F, Le Vaillant M, Paris A, Pigeanne T, Leclair-Visonneau L, Bizieux-Thaminy A, et al. Relationship between OSA clinical phenotypes and CPAP treatment outcomes. Chest. 2016;149(1):288–90.

20. Arzt M, Young T, Finn L, Skatrud JB, Ryan CM, Newton GE, et al. Sleepiness and sleep in patients with both systolic heart failure and obstructive sleep apnea. Arch Intern Med. 2006;166(16):1716–22.

21. Bradley TD, Floras JS. Obstructive sleep apnoea and its cardiovascular consequences. Lancet. 2009;373(9657):82–93.

22. Marin JM, Carrizo SJ, Vicente E, Agusti AG. Long-term cardiovascular outcomes in men with obstructive sleep apnoea-hypopnoea with or without treatment with continuous positive airway pressure: an observational study. Lancet. 2005;365(9464):1046–53.

23. Yu J, Zhou Z, McEvoy RD, Anderson CS, Rodgers A, Perkovic V, et al. Association of positive airway pressure with cardiovascular events and death in adults with sleep apnea: a systematic review and meta-analysis. JAMA. 2017;318(2):156–66.

24. Sanchez-de-la-Torre M, Sanchez-de-la-Torre A, Bertran S, Abad J, Duran-Cantolla J, Cabriada V, et al. Effect of obstructive sleep apnoea and its treatment with continuous positive airway pressure on the prevalence of cardiovascular events in patients with acute coronary syndrome (ISAACC study): a randomised controlled trial. Lancet Respir Med. 2020;8(4):359–67.

25. Pepin JL, Tamisier R, Barone-Rochette G, Launois SH, Levy P, Baguet JP. Comparison of continuous positive airway pressure and valsartan in hypertensive patients with sleep apnea. Am J Respir Crit Care Med. 2010;182(7):954–60.

26. Bakker JP, Edwards BA, Gautam SP, Montesi SB, Duran-Cantolla J, Barandiaran FA, et al. Blood pressure improvement with continuous positive airway pressure is independent of obstructive sleep apnea severity. J Clin Sleep Med. 2014;10(4):365–9.

27. Pedrosa RP, Drager LF, de Paula LK, Amaro AC, Bortolotto LA, Lorenzi-Filho G. Effects of OSA treatment on BP in patients with resistant hypertension: a randomized trial. Chest. 2013;144(5):1487–94.

28. Launois SH, Tamisier R, Levy P, Pepin JL. On treatment but still sleepy: cause and management of residual sleepiness in obstructive sleep apnea. Curr Opin Pulm Med. 2013;19(6):601–8.

29. Morse AM. Narcolepsy in children and adults: a guide to improved recognition, diagnosis and management. Med Sci (Basel). 2019;7(12):106.

30. Budhiraja R, Javaheri S, Pavlova MK, Epstein LJ, Omobomi O, Quan SF. Prevalence and correlates of periodic limb movements in OSA and the effect of CPAP therapy. Neurology. 2020;94(17):e1820–e7.

31. Sweetman AM, Lack LC, Catcheside PG, Antic NA, Chai-Coetzer CL, Smith SS, et al. Developing a successful treatment for co-morbid insomnia and sleep apnea. Sleep Med Rev. 2017;33:28–38.

32. Sweetman A, Lack L, Catcheside PG, Antic NA, Smith S, Chai-Coetzer CL, et al. Cognitive and behavioral therapy for insomnia increases the use of continuous positive airway pressure therapy in obstructive sleep apnea participants with comorbid insomnia: a randomized clinical trial. Sleep. 2019;42(12):zsz178.

33. van Straten A, van der Zweerde T, Kleiboer A, Cuijpers P, Morin CM, Lancee J. Cognitive and behavioral therapies in the treatment of insomnia: a meta-analysis. Sleep Med Rev. 2018;38:3–16.

34. Schweitzer PK, Rosenberg R, Zammit GK, Gotfried M, Chen D, Carter LP, et al. Solriamfetol for excessive sleepiness in obstructive sleep apnea (TONES 3). A randomized controlled trial. Am J Respir Crit Care Med. 2019;199(11):1421–31.

35. Dauvilliers Y, Verbraecken J, Partinen M, Hedner J, Saaresranta T, Georgiev O, et al. Pitolisant for daytime sleepiness in patients with obstructive sleep apnea who refuse continuous positive airway pressure treatment. A randomized trial. Am J Respir Crit Care Med. 2020;201(9):1135–45.

36. Cowie MR, Woehrle H, Wegscheider K, Angermann C, d'Ortho MP, Erdmann E, et al. Adaptive servo-ventilation for central sleep apnea in systolic heart failure. N Engl J Med. 2015;373(12):1095–105.

37. Li L, Wang ZW, Li J, Ge X, Guo LZ, Wang Y, et al. Efficacy of catheter ablation of atrial fibrillation in patients with obstructive sleep apnea with and without continuous positive airway pressure treatment: a meta-analysis of observational studies. Europace. 2014;16(9):1309–14.

38. Marvisi M, Balzarini L, Mancini C, Ramponi S, Marvisi C. Fibromyalgia is frequent in obstructive sleep apnea and responds to CPAP therapy. Eur J Intern Med. 2015;26(9):e49–50.

PAP Therapy for Sleep Breathing Disorders: Good Policies and Practices

8

Mubdiul Ali and Meir Kryger

8.1 Guiding Patients to Improve Adherence

Positive airway pressure (PAP) therapy introduced into clinical practice in the mid-1980s remains the treatment of choice for patients with sleep-disordered breathing (SDB) when used effectively. Adherence is the key, however, as the clinical benefits of PAP therapy fall off significantly if not routinely used. Initiation of successful PAP therapy involves a new habit formation, a difficult task for a significant portion of the adult target patient population. Over the years, PAP therapy as emerged as one of the most successful treatment modalities of various forms of SDB including obstructive sleep apnea (OSA). However, achieving adequate adherence to PAP therapy remains as one of the biggest challenges of SDB treatment. There are many reasons for non-adherence with PAP therapy. In this chapter, we will discuss some of the ways to improve PAP adherence in patients with SDB.

8.2 What Practice Guidelines Suggest

The American Academy of Sleep Medicine has published guidelines on the treatment of OSA with PAP [1]. This document made recommendations based on the strength of the published literature. These were the strong recommendations: use PAP, compared with no therapy, to treat OSA in adults with excessive sleepiness; PAP therapy be initiated using either APAP at home or in-laboratory PAP titration in adults with OSA and no significant comorbidities; use either CPAP or APAP for ongoing treatment of OSA in adults; and educational interventions be given with initiation of PAP therapy in adults with OSA. These were the conditional recommendations: use PAP, compared with no therapy, to treat OSA in adults with impaired sleep-related quality of life; use

PAP, compared with no therapy, to treat OSA in adults with comorbid hypertension; use CPAP or APAP over BPAP in the routine treatment of OSA in adults; behavioral and/or troubleshooting interventions be given during the initial period of PAP therapy in adults with OSA; and use telemonitoring-guided interventions during the initial period of PAP therapy in adults with OSA.

8.3 What Is Adherence?

The parameter for adequate PAP therapy adherence has largely been driven by third-party payers who are responsible for device reimbursement. A dose–response relationship between PAP usage and clinical outcomes in OSA has been well demonstrated in existing literature [2]. In clinical practice, even some use of PAP therapy is better than no therapy at all. In the medical literature, a (perhaps arbitrary) threshold of less than 4 h of nightly PAP use on 70% of nights has been adopted to define non-adherence [3]. In a cohort of 149 patients with severe OSA, Weaver et al. demonstrated that a 4 h of nightly continuous PAP (CPAP) use was associated with improvement in the Epworth Sleepiness Scale [2]. As for patients with hypertension, CPAP usage of more than 3.5 h was associated with greater reduction in 24-h diastolic blood pressure after 4 weeks of treatment [4]. Using a criterion of 4 h or less of nightly use, CPAP non-adherence has been estimated between 29% and 83% [5–7].

8.4 Strategies to Augment PAP Compliance

8.4.1 Match Patient to the Optimal Interface

One of the most common barriers to successful PAP initiation is poor mask fitting. Poor fit with leak, skin pressure and irritation, dry mouth, and nasal congestion make mask interface less tolerable. Fortunately, most of these common complaints

M. Ali · M. Kryger (✉)
Yale School of Medicine, Pulmonary Critical Care and Sleep Medicine, New Haven, CT, USA
e-mail: meir.kryger@yale.edu

have reasonable solutions. There are now a wide variety of interfaces available in the market that patients can choose from. Heated humidification was developed to try to minimize dryness of nose, mouth, and throat. Condensation in the tubing or rainout can be minimized using heated tubing or tube covers to reduce exposure of the tubing air to the cooler surrounding environment. These solutions are not expensive but do require multiple follow-ups either via in person visits or by phone calls to make sure patients' complaints are appropriately addressed. It is critical for a sleep clinic to have PAP follow-up visit available throughout the day where a dedicated sleep technician or respiratory therapist can address ongoing issues with mask interface with patients. Although choosing the right mask interface is important, there is no strong evidence that the PAP mask interface at treatment initiation significantly influences adherence [6].

Pressure-related discomfort has led to the development of expiratory pressure relief technologies, which reduce airway pressure during early expiration with a return to the prescribed pressure at the end of expiration to varying degrees. It too has not been shown to improve adherence reliably [8]. The ramp feature reduces the initial PAP level and then gradually increases the pressure over a set time period to the prescribed target, but no improvement in adherence has been shown with the addition of the ramp [3]. Again, studies comparing auto-titrating units to traditional PAP units have shown similar adherence [3]. In 62 OSA patients randomized to continuous PAP (CPAP) or bilevel PAP (BPAP), there was no significant difference between hourly use, the percentage of time that the device was running, and the prescribed pressure that was being delivered at 1 year. Thus, bilevel PAP cannot be routinely recommended as a strategy to improvement adherence in OSA [9].

8.4.2 Patient Education and Serial Follow-Up

Patient education is recognized as a standard of care in the treatment of SDB [10]. Unfortunately, there is no standardized approach of this education that has been shown to be effective. Knowledge and support are likely of greater importance in those with less educational background. Meurice et al. studied the effects of four educational strategies on CPAP compliance in 112 severe OSA patients in seven centers in the French ANTADIR homecare network [11]. Patients received either a simple oral explanation or an oral and written explanation of CPAP use. In addition, they received, from homecare technicians, either a single home visit at CPAP onset or repeated home visits at CPAP onset and at 1 week, 1 month, and 3 months after. There was no significant difference in adherence between all four education groups. In contrast, Lai et al. randomized 100 OSA patients to a brief motivational enhancement education program or usual care [12]. The intervention group received usual care plus a brief motivational education program directed at enhancing the subjects' knowledge, motivation, and self-efficacy to CPAP through the use of a 25-min video, a 20-min patient-centered interview, and a 10-min telephone follow-up. The intervention group had better CPAP use (higher daily CPAP usage by 2 h per day ($P < 0.001$)) and a fourfold increase in the number of patients using CPAP for $\geq 70\%$ of days with ≥ 4 h/day.

8.4.3 Frequent Telephone Follow-Up

The pattern of PAP usage is established early, typically during the first week of therapy, and has been shown to predict long-term use [13–15]. Therefore, it is imperative for sleep providers to set the expectations of their patients from the beginning and schedule frequent follow-up soon after receiving the PAP device. This will make sure patients would not have unrealistic treatment outcome expectations about the quality of their sleep after starting PAP therapy. Frequent early follow-up will also make sure all their mask interface-related questions are appropriately addressed as well as provide necessary troubleshooting and feedback. Early adoption of PAP use has been associated with long-term adherence and successful treatment of SDB in clinical setting.

8.4.4 Matching Patient and Treatment

Not every patient with SDB is a candidate for PAP therapy. For a relatively healthy patient with newly diagnosed OSA, relatively low apnea-hypopnea index (AHI), and minimal symptom burden, PAP is likely not the appropriate initial treatment modality. For such patients, adequate PAP compliance would be hard to achieve, especially when perceived benefits are so minimal. Patients with realistic treatment outcome expectations, and healthy coping mechanism handle PAP therapy better [16]. These psychological factors may be more important than any other patient characteristic in determining patterns of PAP use. Patients who self-initiate their referral have been shown to have greater PAP use [17]. Reporting problems after the first night of PAP has been shown to be an important predictor of ensuing CPAP use [18].

8.4.5 Familiarizing Patients with Their Medical Equipment Provider

It is imperative that every PAP user is familiar with the durable medical equipment (DME) supplier, the company responsible for supplying the necessary accessories for their PAP therapy. Each DME supplier should be the first line of resource to answering questions on PAP therapy. The contact information of the DME supplier should be placed on the equipment.

8.4.6 Scheduling In-Lab PAP Titration

PAP can be introduced both in-laboratory or at home using auto-titrating PAP technologies based on patient characteristics, preference. There is some evidence of greater comfort and improved adherence with auto-titrating PAP in patients requiring PAP levels higher than 10 cm H_2O and in patients reporting side effects on conventional PAP [19]. In relatively healthy patients, administration of home auto-titrating PAP with follow-up as needed may be sufficient. These patients can be followed remotely via cloud monitoring to ensure compliance. However, in patients with significant comorbidities, who may struggle with the interface or may not be able to follow instructions at home, scheduling in-lab PAP titration might be more beneficial.

8.4.7 Modifying the Definition of PAP Adherence

The Centers for Medicare and Medicaid Services (CMS) require that for continued PAP coverage beyond the first 3 months of therapy, the treating physician must conduct a face-to-face clinical re-evaluation no sooner than 31 days but no later than 91 days after initiating therapy [1]. Additionally, there must be documentation that the patient is benefiting from PAP therapy with objective evidence of PAP adherence based on download data showing >4 h of nightly use for >70% of nights monitored during a consecutive 30-day period. Such strict adherence guidelines create unnecessary pressure on the patient to make frequent in-person visits to the sleep clinic. Any level of PAP use was associated with some mortality benefit over no PAP use. Thus, patients are likely to benefit from some form of PAP therapy even if that is not adequate by CMS definition. Additionally, adherence usually improves over time, with one Big Data analysis showing up to 87% adherence using modern technology [20]. The patients who are not adherent during the first 90 days can become more adherent as they get more used to the idea of wearing mask [21]. While follow-up is absolutely necessary in ensuring treatment adherence, the frequency, intensity, and modality of follow-up to optimize adherence remain unknown.

8.4.8 Identify the Group of Patients with High Risk of Non-Compliance

Not every patient requires the same level of follow-up to ensure appropriate PAP adherence. Identifying patients at risk of poor compliance is helpful [39]. There is no single factor that has been consistently identified as a predictor of compliance. A multi-dimensional approach using education, behavioral, technological, and potentially pharmacological strategies is required to augment the complex behavior of PAP use [6]. A more convincing association has been observed between initial severity of daytime sleepiness and PAP use, and an Epworth Sleepiness score >10 was shown to be an independent predictor of long-term CPAP use in 1211 consecutive OSA patients [15]. Patients with AHI over 15 but with relatively lesser symptomatic burden will need more encouragement from the providers to maintain adequate PAP compliance. Some studies have suggested worse CPAP adherence in African Americans, although reasons for this disparity are unclear, but may be a function primarily of socioeconomic status [1]. In a sample of 126 New Zealand patients with OSA initiating CPAP therapy, 19.8% were Māori, a group that had significantly lower CPAP usage than non-Māori but in a multiple regression model including ethnicity, socioeconomic status, annual income, level of formal education, and eligibility for government-subsidized health care, only non-completion of tertiary education and socio-economic deprivation remained as significant independent predictors of CPAP non-adherence [22]. In a retrospective cohort of 260 veterans with newly diagnosed OSA, initial CPAP adherence was closely associated with higher neighborhood socio-economic factors [23]. CPAP users have been shown to have more years of education and be more likely to work in professional occupations [5]. On the other side, certain psychological traits and disposition have been liked to PAP non-compliance. The type D (distressed) personality, defined as a combination of negative affectivity and social inhibition, was found in 30% of 247 OSA patients treated with PAP for longer than 60 months. Brostrom et al. showed that this personality type significantly increased the perceived frequency and severity of a range of side effect and had lower objective PAP adherence compared with patients without type D personality [24]. Interestingly enough, depression and anxiety do not seem to influence PAP adherence significantly, and no association was demonstrated between the Hospital Anxiety and Depression Scale and PAP use [18]. (For more information on socioeconomic differences, personality disorders, and depression in relation to PAP use, see Chaps. 9, 11, and 19).

8.4.9 Ruling Out Claustrophobia

A 15-item subscale measuring claustrophobic tendencies was measured pre-CPAP and after 3 months of CPAP in a secondary analysis of data from a prospective study of 153 OSA participants that completed 3 months of CPAP therapy [25]. Poor CPAP adherence (<2 h per night) was more than two times higher in participants with a claustrophobia score of ≥25. Identification of patients with claustrophobic tendencies and targeted interventions designed to reduce the fear and intrusiveness of SDB therapies may be beneficial, see Chap. 6. With the advancement of mask interface technology, claustrophobia has been less of an issue in recent years than in the past few decades.

8.4.10 Cognitive Therapy

Cognitive behavioral or motivational strategies have been successful in improving PAP adherence [17]. In a meta-analysis assessing the effectiveness of educational, supportive, or behavioral strategies in encouraging PAP use, most studies incorporated elements of more than one intervention [26]. Low-to-moderate-quality evidence showed that all three types of interventions led to increased PAP usage in PAP-naive participants with moderate-to severe-OSA. Behavioral therapies led to improvement in average PAP usage by 1.44 h/night (95% CI: 0.43–2.45, n = 584, six studies: low-quality evidence) and increased the number of participants who used their machines for longer than 4 h per night from 28 to 47 per 100 (OR: 2.23, 95% CI: 1.45–3.45, n = 358, 3 studies, low-quality evidence) [27]. For more information on these psychological methods, see Chap. 6.

8.4.11 Social Support

Lewis et al. found that PAP use was higher in those living with someone as compared with those living alone [18]. Having a spouse does not always improve compliance since spousal pressure to use PAP has not been found to be beneficial for adherence [18]. Baron et al. found that perception of wives' support for PAP treatment predicted increased adherence, but only in patients with high disease severity [28]. For more information on the impact of partner and family support, see [40] and Chap. 10.

8.4.12 Convenient Referral Stream to Ear, Nose, and Throat (ENT) Specialists

PAP devices rely on delivery of pressurized air via flexible tubing connecting to an external mask that interfaced with the patient—a key to such air delivery is nasal patency. This is especially true for nasal mask interface. PAP use is lower in patients with smaller nasal passages, and nasal congestion has been associated with a decrease in mean daily PAP use [29, 30]. Patients should be referred to an otolaryngologist if there is any concern regarding nasal patency. If symptoms persist despite medical therapies, surgery may be required [31]. Surgical correction of severe nasal obstruction in 12 patients with severe OSA refractory to PAP treatment resulted in a significant decrease in nasal resistance and rendered all patients tolerant to CPAP [32]. According to some

otolaryngologists, nasal septoplasty to facilitate PAP adherence is the most common surgery for OSA [33].

8.4.13 Sedative-Hypnotic Use Early on

There is limited evidence for the efficacy sedative-hypnotic during PAP initiation in improving long-term PAP adherence. Both the approach of using a single sedative dose, typically a Z-hypnotic, prior to split-night or titration polysomnography and regular use of a sedative for the first 14 days of CPAP therapy have been studied, but again no consistent improvement in adherence has been shown [34–36].

8.4.14 Using Smartphone-Based Technologies to Improve Compliance

Microprocessors embedded within modern PAP units monitor cumulative time that PAP device is turned on at the effective pressure and can transmit these data to patients' smartphones. A motivated patient with basic smartphone knowledge can easily use these data to track their adherence and efficacy. This information can then be viewed by sleep providers using various transmission systems including smartcards, memory sticks, or wireless transmission. Malhotra et al. compared active patient engagement (APE) technology, a real-time Internet-based patient engagement tool, to usual care monitoring in a retrospective analysis of two cloud-based databases (AirView and myAir) [20]. In this study, APE was associated with more patients achieving adherence defined by US Medicare criteria compared with usual care with remote monitoring of PAP adherence (87.3% compared with 70.4%). Average therapy usage was 5.9 h in the APE group versus 4.9 h in the matched usual care group and patients 'struggling' with PAP therapy adherence had a 17.6% absolute improvement in adherence using APE compared with usual care. This is, however, not possible for oral appliances (without an integrated sensor to monitor adherence), where a provider still must rely on self-reporting to measure compliance. Of note, self-reported PAP use overestimates actual use by approximately 1 h [37].

8.4.15 The Importance of Patient Feedback

A key to PAP compliance is to continue frequent exchange of feedback between patients and their providers. In a four-arm randomized trial of 1455 patients, Hwang et al. showed PAP usage was significantly higher in the group with PAP telemonitoring with automated patient-messaging feedback by itself and mixed with web-based OSA education versus usual care but not for the group that only received web-based OSA education [38]. Similar to prior studies on education, this study found that even with a telemedicine platform, education alone had no significant influence on PAP use and it again suggested that accountability may be more effective at inducing changes in adherence behavior.

8.5 Conclusion

There is no one definitive way to achieve adherence to PAP therapy in patients with SDB. It is a habit-forming process that requires frequent feedback from the clinicians as well from the PAP supplier to keep the patients engaged and motivated. With the recent explosion of technological advances in the world of sleep medicine, tracking PAP compliance has become easier than ever. We strongly believe achieving PAP compliance is not an implausible goal as long as we all work together to ensure optimal management of SDB.

References

1. Patil SP, Ayappa IA, Caples SM, Kimoff RJ, Patel SR, Harrod CG. Treatment of adult obstructive sleep apnea with positive airway pressure: an American Academy of Sleep Medicine clinical practice guideline. J Clin Sleep Med. 2019;15(2):335–43.
2. Weaver TE, Maislin G, Dinges DF, Bloxham T, George CF, Greenberg H, Kader G, Mahowald M, Younger J, Pack AI. Relationship between hours of CPAP use and achieving normal levels of sleepiness and daily functioning. Sleep. 2007;30:711–9.
3. Sunwoo BY, Light M, Malhotra A. Strategies to augment adherence in the management of sleep-disordered breathing. Respirology. 2020;25:363–71.
4. Faccenda JF, Mackay TW, Boon NA, Douglas NJ. Randomized placebo-controlled trial of continuous positive airway pressure on blood pressure in the sleep apnea-hypopnea syndrome. Am J Respir Crit Care Med. 2001;163:344–8.
5. Kribbs NB, Pack AI, Kline LR, Smith PL, Schwartz AR, Schubert NM, Redline S, Henry JN, Getsy JE, Dinges DF. Objective measurement of patterns of nasal CPAP use by patients with obstructive sleep apnea. Am Rev Respir Dis. 1993;147:887–95.
6. Sawyer AM, Gooneratne NS, Marcus CL, Ofer D, Richards KC, Weaver TE. A systematic review of CPAP adherence across age groups: clinical and empiric insights for developing CPAP adherence interventions. Sleep Med Rev. 2011;15:343–56.
7. Weaver TE, Grunstein RR. Adherence to continuous positive airway pressure therapy: the challenge to effective treatment. Proc Am Thorac Soc. 2008;5:173–8.
8. Aloia MS, Stanchina M, Arnedt JT, Malhotra A, Millman RP. Treatment adherence and outcomes in flexible vs standard continuous positive airway pressure therapy. Chest. 2005;127:2085–93.
9. Reeves-Hoche MK, Hudgel DW, Meck R, Witteman R, Ross A, Zwillich CW. Continuous versus bilevel positive airway pressure for obstructive sleep apnea. Am J Respir Crit Care Med. 1995;151:443–9.
10. Epstein LJ, Kristo D, Strollo PJ Jr, Friedman N, Malhotra A, Patil SP, Ramar K, Rogers R, Schwab RJ, Weaver EM, et al. Adult Obstructive Sleep Apnea Task Force of the American Academy of Sleep Medicine. Clinical guideline for the evaluation, management and long-term care of obstructive sleep apnea in adults. J Clin Sleep Med. 2009;5:263–76.
11. Meurice JC, Ingrand P, Portier F, Arnulf I, Rakotonanahari D, Fournier E, Philip-Joet F, Veale D. ANTADIR Working Group "PPC", CMTS ANTADIR. A multicentre trial of education strategies at CPAP induction in the treatment of severe sleep apnoea-hypopnoea syndrome. Sleep Med. 2007;8:37–42.
12. Lai AYK, Fong DYT, Lam JCM, Weaver TE, Ip MSM. The efficacy of a brief motivational enhancement education program on CPAP adherence in OSA: a randomized controlled trial. Chest. 2014;146:600–10.
13. Budhiraja R, Parthasarathy S, Drake CL, Roth T, Sharief I, Budhiraja P, Saunders V, Hudgel DW. Early CPAP use identifies subsequent adherence to CPAP therapy. Sleep. 2007;30:320–4.
14. Krieger J. Long-term compliance with nasal continuous positive airway pressure (CPAP) in obstructive sleep apnea patients and nonapneic snorers. Sleep. 1992;15:S42–6.
15. McArdle N, Devereux G, Heidarnejad H, Engleman HM, Mackay TW, Douglas NJ. Long-term use of CPAP therapy for sleep apnea/hypopnea syndrome. Am J Respir Crit Care Med. 1999;159:1108–4.
16. Sawyer AM, Deatrick JA, Kuna ST, Weaver TE. Differences in perceptions of the diagnosis and treatment of obstructive sleep apnea and continuous positive airway pressure therapy among adherers and nonadherers. Qual Health Res. 2010;20:873–92.
17. Hoy CJVM, Kingshott R, Engleman HM, Douglas NJ. Can intensive support improve continuous positive airway pressure use in patients with the sleep apnea/hypopnea syndrome? Am J Respir Crit Care Med. 1999;159:1096–100.
18. Lewis KE, Seale L, Bartle IE, Watkins AJ, Ebden P. Early predictors of CPAP use for the treatment of obstructive sleep apnea. Sleep. 2004;27:134–8.
19. Hukins C. Comparative study of autotitrating and fixed-pressure CPAP in the home: a randomized, single-blind crossover trial. Sleep. 2004;27:1512–7.
20. Malhotra A, Crocker ME, Willes L, Kelly C, Lynch S, Benjafield AV. Patient engagement using new technology to improve adherence to positive airway pressure therapy: a retrospective analysis. Chest. 2018;153:843–50.
21. Naik S, Al-Halawani M, Kreinin I, Kryger M. Centers for Medicare and Medicaid Services Positive Airway Pressure Adherence Criteria May Limit Treatment to Many Medicare Beneficiaries. J Clin Sleep Med. 2019;15(2):245–51. https://doi.org/10.5664/jcsm.7626. PMID: 30736874; PMCID: PMC6374085.
22. Bakker JP, O'Keeffe KM, Neill AM, Campbell AJ. Ethnic disparities in CPAP adherence in New Zealand: effects of socioeconomic status, health literacy and self-efficacy. Sleep. 2011;34:1595–603.
23. Platt AB, Field SH, Asch DA, Chen Z, Patel NP, Gupta R, Roche DF, Gurubhagavatula I, Christie JD, Kuna ST. Neighborhood of residence is associated with daily adherence to CPAP therapy. Sleep. 2009;32:799–806.
24. Brostrom A, Stromberg A, Martensson J, Ulander M, Harder L, Svanborg E. Association of Type D personality to perceived side effects and adherence in CPAP-treated patients with OSAS. J Sleep Res. 2007;16:439–47.
25. Chasens ER, Pack AI, Maislin G, Dinges DF, Weaver TE. Claustrophobia and adherence to CPAP treatment. West J Nurs Res. 2005;27:307–21.
26. Wozniak DR, Lasserson TJ, Smith I. Educational, supportive and behavioural interventions to improve usage of continuous positive airway pressure machines in adults with obstructive sleep apnoea. Cochrane Database Syst Rev. 2014;(1):CD007736.
27. Crawford MR, Espie CA, Bartlett DJ, Grunstein RR. Integrating psychology and medicine in CPAP adherence - new concepts? Sleep Med Rev. 2014;18:123–39.

28. Baron KG, Smith TW, Berg CA, Czajkowski LA, Gunn H, Jones CR. Spousal involvement in CPAP adherence among patients with obstructive sleep apnea. Sleep Breath. 2011;15:525–34.

29. Budhiraja R, Kushida CA, Nichols DA, Walsh JK, Simon RD, Gottlieb DJ, Quan SF. Impact of randomization, clinic visits, and medical and psychiatric cormorbidities on continuous positive airway pressure adherence in obstructive sleep apnea. J Clin Sleep Med. 2016;12:333–41.

30. Li HY, Engleman H, Hsu CY, Izci B, Vennelle M, Cross M, Douglas NJ. Acoustic reflection for nasal airway measurement in patients with obstructive sleep apnea-hypopnea syndrome. Sleep. 2005;28:1554–9.

31. Fiorita A, Scarano E, Mastrapasqua R, Picciotti PM, Loperfido A, Rizzotto G, Paludetti G. Moderate OSAS and turbinate decongestion: surgical efficacy in improving the quality of life and compliance of CPAP using Epworth score and SNOT-20 score. Acta Otorhinolaryngol Ital. 2018;38:214–21.

32. Nakata S, Noda A, Yagi H, Yanagi E, Mimura T, Okada T, Misawa H, Nakashima T. Nasal resistance for determinant factor of nasal surgery in CPAP failure patients with obstructive sleep apnea syndrome. Rhinology. 2005;43:296–9.

33. Awad MI, Kacker A. Nasal Obstruction Considerations in Sleep Apnea. Otolaryngol Clin North Am. 2018;51(5):1003–9. https://doi.org/10.1016/j.otc.2018.05.012. Epub 2018 Jun 20. PMID: 29934201.

34. Bradshaw DA, Ruff GA, Murphy DP. An oral hypnotic medication does not improve continuous positive airway pressure compliance in men with obstructive sleep apnea. Chest. 2006;130:1369–76.

35. Lettieri CJ, Collen JF, Eliasson AH, Quast TM. Sedative use during continuous positive airway pressure titration improves subsequent compliance: a randomized, double-blind, placebo-controlled trial. Chest. 2009;136:1263–8.

36. Lettieri CJ, Shah AA, Holley AB, Kelly WF, Chang AS, Roop SA, CPAP Promotion and Prognosis-The Army Sleep Apnea Program Trial. Effects of a short course of eszopiclone on continuous positive airway pressure adherence: a randomized trial. Ann Intern Med. 2009;151:696–702.

37. Rauscher H, Formanek D, Popp W, Zwick H. Self-reported vs measured compliance with nasal CPAP for obstructive sleep apnea. Chest. 1993;103:1675–80.

38. Hwang D, Chang JW, Benjafield AV, Crocker ME, Kelly C, Becker KA, Kim JB, Woodrum RR, Liang J, Derose SF. Effect of telemedicine education and telemonitoring on continuous positive airway pressure adherence. The tele-OSA randomized trial. Am J Respir Crit Care Med. 2018;197:117–26.

39. Julie, Bros Caroline, Poulet Jonathan El, Methni Chrystèle, Deschaux Marc, Gandit Petrus J, Pauwels Marie, Charavel. Determination of risks of lower adherence to CPAP treatment before their first use by patients. J Health Psychology. 2022;27(1):223–35. https://doi.org/10.1177/1359105320942862.

40. Nazia Naz S, Khan David, Todem Shireesha, Bottu M. Safwan, Badr Adesuwa, Olomu. Impact of patient and family engagement in improving continuous positive airway pressure adherence in patients with obstructive sleep apnea: a randomized controlled trial. J Clin Sleep Med. 2022;18(1):181–91. https://doi.org/10.5664/jcsm.9534.

Socioeconomic Differences in CPAP Adherence

Martha E. Billings and Susan Redline

9.1 Introduction

Social determinants of health are the conditions under which people are born, grow up, live, work, and age. Shaped by the distribution of money, power, and resources, social determinants of health contribute to health inequities, i.e., unjust and avoidable differences in health status [1, 2]. Socioeconomic status (SES) strongly influences health outcomes across a wide range of conditions, from infant mortality to overall life expectancy [3]. Life experiences of individuals with low SES may include growing up in poverty, living in an urban slum, working in stressful and unhealthy environments, and aging on a fixed income with limited access to healthcare. Life experiences of chronic stress, deprivation, and high allostatic load (cumulative physiological effects of neuro-cortical activation) may contribute to health behaviors and altered hypothalamic pituitary cortisol response [4, 5]. Epidemiological studies consistently demonstrate a greater burden of cardiovascular disease (CVD), as well as diabetes, obesity, and hyperlipidemia [6] among individuals in lower socioeconomic positions [7, 8]. Additionally, lower SES has long been associated with worse health outcomes beyond CVD, with high rates of mortality from cancer and lung disease [3, 9]. Social determinants of health also contribute to sleep health disparities: lower SES is associated with shorter duration of sleep, more fragmented sleep, delayed sleep onset, and poor-quality sleep [10], in addition to circadian rhythm disturbances associated with increased sleep timing variability and shift work. Emerging data indicate that low SES also is a risk factor for obstructive sleep apnea (OSA) [11], with possible mechanisms including increased exposures to environmental pollutants, low neighborhood walkability and reduced physical activity, poor diet, and obesity [12–14]. As a social determinant of health, SES also likely impacts OSA outcomes, including delays in OSA recognition and diagnosis and, once identified, suboptimal treatment and long-term chronic disease management. A key aspect of effective OSA management relates to adherence to positive airway pressure (PAP) therapy.

PAP is the most efficacious therapy for OSA; however, its effectiveness is often limited by adherence. PAP adherence, empirically defined as 4 or more hours of use per night for 5 nights a week or 70% of days, is low across populations, with only 40–50% users adhering long term [15]. Data support a dose-response relationship, with greater clinical benefit with longer duration of PAP use, leading to resolution of sleepiness and improved daytime functioning [16, 17]. Observational studies have shown reduced risk of cardiovascular events in those with OSA on PAP treatment compared to controls [18, 19], but this has not been supported in larger randomized clinical trials [20]. However, secondary analyses of subgroups with higher adherence suggest improved outcomes [21, 22]. Longitudinal studies consistently show use of PAP improves sleep quality, excessive daytime sleepiness, and quality of life in those with OSA symptoms [17].

Socioeconomic status is associated with lower adherence to medications [23] and therapies in many other chronic diseases, such as HIV, asthma, COPD, hypertension, and diabetes [24, 25]. Socioeconomic status is also associated with PAP adherence. In this chapter, we review the evidence and the possible factors behind differences in adherence by socioeconomic status through a socioecological lens, examining the physical, social, and environmental factors that may influence sleep and adherence patterns.

M. E. Billings (✉)
Division of Pulmonary, Critical Care & Sleep Medicine,
Department of Medicine, University of Washington School of
Medicine, Seattle, WA, USA
e-mail: mebillin@uw.edu

S. Redline
Division of Sleep and Circadian Disorders, Department of
Medicine, Brigham and Women's Hospital, Harvard Medical
School, Boston, MA, USA

9.2 The Evidence for Differences in CPAP Adherence by SES

Though data are limited, poor adherence to PAP is more prevalent in those with lower socioeconomic position. Lower PAP adherence in low SES groups compared to upper SES groups has been observed in both observational cohort studies and clinical trials. A cohort study at a single center identified that neighborhood SES measured by median household income predicted 1-year PAP adherence [26]. An observational study from a single community sleep center with a diverse population identified education as an independent predictor of PAP adherence. Those with a college degree or more were six times more likely to meet PAP adherence thresholds than those with a high school or less education, in adjusted analyses for race/ethnicity. However, this study did not find differences in use by residential ZIP code SES or insurance status [27]. In an observational study of veterans, PAP adherence was associated with neighborhood SES, with only 34% using CPAP for ≥4 h among those residing in the lowest SES census block compared to 62% in the highest SES census [28]. In the HomePAP trial, a randomized multi-city trial comparing home study vs. full polysomnography diagnostic and treatment strategies in the USA, residing in the lowest 25% SES ZIP codes was associated with an average 50 fewer minutes of PAP use compared to those in higher SES ZIP codes, after adjustment for sleep apnea severity and study arm [29]. These differences were observed despite standardized support for PAP use for all study participants. In both of the latter two studies, participants did not have PAP equipment expenses or out of pocket costs to explain the differences, suggesting that behavioral change (i.e., regularly wearing PAP) may be influenced by a broad range of individual, household, and neighborhood level stressors and challenges not addressed by routine PAP support methods.

Differences in adherence by SES have also been observed utilizing large administrative databases. Using a random 5% sample of all Medicare claims data, a recent study identified a cohort of beneficiaries diagnosed with OSA who initiated CPAP between 2009 and 2011; the authors assessed adherence by CPAP equipment charges. Low SES, identified by proxy as Medicaid eligibility, was found to be a strong predictor of poor CPAP adherence [OR 1.48, 95% CI (1.24, 1.75)] among Medicare beneficiaries ≥65 years [30]. Another recent study utilized a large sample of PAP use data from the USA and geo-linked the participants by ZIP code to US census socioeconomic data. The researchers found that PAP users living in the lowest median household income ZIP codes had significantly lower adherence levels than those living in the highest, at 40% vs. 47%, respectively [31]. These studies reveal differences in PAP adherence by SES with real-world, modern big data.

Not surprisingly, SES has also been associated with CPAP acceptance, as those with less financial means are less likely to agree to PAP. In studies in Israel, India, and Canada, those with lower income and residing in lower SES areas were less likely to agree to purchase PAP [32–34]. Offers of financial incentives did off-set this PAP acceptance, but financial coverage did not improve adherence [35]. Thus, clearly, when PAP is not covered by insurance or national health service, the cost of the device and equipment may make uptake of PAP prohibitive to those in the lower SES strata. However, the persistent low adherence despite financial coverage further supports the need to identify additional factors that operate as barriers and facilitators to continued PAP usage.

Often confounding observed SES associations with adherence, especially in the United States, are race and ethnicity. Due to the consequences of systemic racism, white supremacy, and segregation, low SES is tightly associated with non-white race in the USA. Low SES neighborhoods have higher proportion of Black, Latin, and indigenous populations due to historical housing policies (so-called redlining) with higher rates of poverty, unemployment, and low home ownership in non-white communities [36]. Many adverse health outcomes more prevalent in non-white communities are linked with chronic economic and social deprivation, related to the consequences of structural and institutional racism [37]. Racism and discrimination can additionally adversely impact sleep [38]. Racial discrimination was recently identified as a strong mediator of insomnia severity among Black compared to non-Black groups [39]. Studies examining sleep apnea disparities observe differences by race/ethnicity and similar disparities by SES [29, 31]. Race and ethnicity are social constructs, reflecting cultural norms, ancestry, and shared social history often tied to political oppression and exploitation and hence patterned by SES [40]. Thus, many sleep health disparities, including sleep apnea and PAP therapy adherence, are associated with both race/ethnicity and SES.

9.3 Possible Explanatory Factors for Differences by SES

There are several possible factors contributing to this disparity in PAP adherence. One may be that individuals in low SES neighborhoods experience less and poorer quality of sleep than those living in high SES neighborhoods. Achieving optimal adherence not only relates to the ability and motivation to use PAP but also the ability to achieve sufficient sleep. Individuals who routinely sleep less than 6 h per night have a more limited time during the sleep period to achieve the minimal target of 4 h per night of PAP use. In addition, factors that prolong sleep latency may make nightly adjustment to PAP more challenging. Similarly, frequent nighttime awakenings may challenge the individual to readjust to PAP with each awakening, thus reducing the likelihood of continuing to use PAP throughout the night.

Neighborhood physical and social environmental features have been shown to impact aspects of sleep that may adversely affect PAP adherence. Living in disordered neighborhoods has been associated with difficulty falling asleep and more awakenings in the night [41]. People living in disadvantaged neighborhoods are more likely to report insufficient sleep, delayed onset, and poor quality sleep [10, 42]. Additionally, those residing in composite low SES neighborhoods have more insomnia symptoms [10, 43]. Shorter sleep duration and reduced continuity, measured objectively by actigraphy, is also associated with neighborhood disadvantage [44]. Disrupted, delayed sleep and difficulty getting to sleep may make adapting to PAP use more difficult and limit sustained use.

Deleterious ambient environment features that influence sleep are more prevalent in low SES residential areas. Aspects of the built environment such as housing quality and household and neighborhood density may negatively impact PAP adherence through adverse effects on the sleeping environment. Inopportune light and excess noise are common in dense, poor urban areas and may contribute to delayed and disturbed sleep [45, 46]. Individuals residing in low SES neighborhoods are also more likely to have poorer air quality and greater urban heat [47, 48], both of which can impact sleep quality. Furthermore, greater pollution has been associated with worse sleep apnea [14] and chronic rhinosinusitis [49]. This may make wearing PAP more challenging via more nasal congestion as well as contribute to adeno-tonsillar hypertrophy.

Additional potential factors influencing PAP adherence may be home, family, and work features that differ by SES. Those in lower SES may have more crowded homes and more shared sleeping spaces [50]; they may have less consistent access to electrical outlets and less comfortable sleeping environments to utilize PAP. However, there is limited research addressing these factors. Lack of dedicated bedroom, conflicting sleep schedule from bed partner, and uncomfortable room temperature were not shown to associate with PAP adherence in one survey study [27].

The social neighborhood environment, often deleterious to sleep in lower SES neighborhoods, may also contribute to reduced PAP use. Fear of crime, violence, and lack of social cohesion are more prevalent in low SES neighborhoods. These adversities heighten vigilance, negatively impact sleep quality, and are associated with more insomnia symptoms [51]. Using PAP may be more challenging when sleep is impacted by fears and external threats to the vulnerable sleeper. Longer sleep duration by objective measurements was observed in neighborhoods perceived to be safer and with greater social cohesion [52]. Less neighborhood trust and lower social capital were also associated with insomnia symptoms and differed by SES [53]. Reported longer sleep latency was associated with reduced PAP use in the HomePAP trial; those residing in the lowest SES ZIP codes reported longer sleep latency [54]. PAP may be perceived to be less beneficial when sleep remains disturbed by fear and hypervigilance related to the neighborhood social environment.

Early life home experiences and SES have also been associated with less sleep duration and longer latency [55]. Thus, poor sleep during childhood may impact sleep later in life and ability to utilize PAP successfully. Other potential factors include work schedules, with more night shifts, longer hours with less control, and irregular schedules impacting circadian rhythms, worsening sleepiness [56, 57]. Those in low SES employment positions often have more shift work requirements [58]. These work requirements may impair the ability to establish a routine for consistent PAP use and more difficult with PAP due to circadian misalignment.

Other hypothesized barriers to PAP use in lower SES groups include financial hardship, competing health burdens, and difficulty with access to care. The greater burden of costs of extra supplies (e.g., ability to try a different masks) to enable PAP tolerance may preclude use despite health insurance coverage of the device. Many observational studies additionally demonstrate more comorbidities in the OSA patients with lower SES [30, 59]. These competing health issues may negatively impact the ability to find the time and energy to prioritize PAP use. Comorbid insomnia and mental health issues such as anxiety may impact sleep and thus ability to use PAP, as seen in veterans [60]. Post-traumatic stress disorder, by heightening vigilance and claustrophobia, also may negatively influence ability to adjust to wearing a nasal/face mask [61]. Improving PAP tolerance, through gradual acclimation, behavioral change, cognitive therapy, and desensitization [62, 63], often requires extended time, particularly for under-resourced populations with additional contextual issues. With less job flexibility and competing child-care and elder-care needs, individuals in low SES employment may not have the time required to adapt to PAP. Modern telehealth innovations may improve adherence [64, 65], but their impact on lower SES populations is likely lower given the diminished Internet access, health literacy, and technical fluency compared to high SES population [66]. The digital divide may thus reduce the benefits of these emerging technologies in low SES PAP users.

9.4 Summary

PAP adherence is reported to be poorer in OSA patients with low socioeconomic position and among those residing in lower SES neighborhoods compared to those in the higher SES positions and neighborhoods. The factors that contribute to low PAP adherence are likely complex and multilevel, including suboptimal living and sleeping environments, adverse neighborhood conditions that hinder sleep, cost issues of the device and supplies, and competing demands at work and home as well as competing health and social concerns. Further research is needed to understand how these interrelated factors impact PAP adherence and identify multilevel interventions to mitigate these barriers while facilitating better PAP use in individuals from low SES communities. Implementation Science, which applies evidence-based approaches in real-world settings and practice, is an ultimate translational goal. Certainly, the burden of sleep apnea and effects on sleepiness and daytime functioning may be more profound in the low SES groups with additional life stressors, limited resources, and serious comorbid health issues. Thus, interventions that could enhance sleep quality and ability to utilize PAP low SES groups may have substantive impacts on quality of life and well-being.

References

 1. Braveman P, Gottlieb L. The social determinants of health: it's time to consider the causes of the causes. Public Health Rep. 2014;129:19–31.
 2. Organization WH. Social determinants of health; 2020. https://www.who.int/health-topics/social-determinants-of-health
 3. Stringhini S, Sabia S, Shipley M, Brunner E, Nabi H, Kivimaki M, Singh-Manoux A. Association of socioeconomic position with health behaviors and mortality. JAMA. 2010;303:1159–66.
 4. Matthews KA, Gallo LC. Psychological perspectives on pathways linking socioeconomic status and physical health. Annu Rev Psychol. 2011;62:501–30.
 5. McEwen BS, Stellar E. Stress and the individual: mechanisms leading to disease. Arch Intern Med. 1993;153:2093–101.
 6. Winkleby MA, Kraemer HC, Ahn DK, Varady AN. Ethnic and socioeconomic differences in cardiovascular disease risk factors: findings for women from the third National Health and Nutrition Examination Survey, 1988–1994. JAMA. 2015;280:356–62.
 7. Clark AM, DesMeules M, Luo W, Duncan AS, Wielgosz A. Socioeconomic status and cardiovascular disease: risks and implications for care. Nat Rev Cardiol. 2009;6:712–22.
 8. Schultz WM, Kelli HM, Lisko JC, Varghese T, Shen J, Sandesara P, Quyyumi AA, Taylor HA, Gulati M, Harold JG, Mieres JH, Ferdinand KC, Mensah GA, Sperling LS. Socioeconomic status and cardiovascular outcomes: challenges and interventions. Circulation. 2018;137:2166–78.
 9. Hegewald MJ, Crapo RO. Socioeconomic status and lung function. Chest. 2007;132:1608–14.
10. Grandner MA, Williams NJ, Knutson KL, Roberts D, Jean-Louis G. Sleep disparity, race/ethnicity, and socioeconomic position. Sleep Med. 2016;18:7–18.
11. Guglielmi O, Lanteri P, Garbarino S. Association between socioeconomic status, belonging to an ethnic minority and obstructive sleep apnea: a systematic review of the literature. Sleep Med. 2019;57:100–6.
12. Billings ME, Johnson DA, Simonelli G, Moore K, Patel SR, Diez Roux AV, Redline S. Neighborhood walking environment and

13. Reid M, Maras JE, Shea S, Wood AC, Castro-Diehl C, Johnson DA, Huang T, Jacobs DR Jr, Crawford A, St-Onge MP, Redline S. Association between diet quality and sleep apnea in the Multi-Ethnic Study of Atherosclerosis. Sleep. 2019;42(1):zsy194.
14. Billings ME, Gold D, Szpiro A, Aaron CP, Jorgensen N, Gassett A, Leary PJ, Kaufman JD, Redline SR. The association of ambient air pollution with sleep apnea: the multi-ethnic study of atherosclerosis. Ann Am Thorac Soc. 2018;16(3):363–70.
15. Baratta F, Pastori D, Bucci T, Fabiani M, Fabiani V, Brunori M, Loffredo L, Lillo R, Pannitteri G, Angelico F, Del Ben M. Long-term prediction of adherence to continuous positive air pressure therapy for the treatment of moderate/severe obstructive sleep apnea syndrome. Sleep Med. 2018;43:66–70.
16. Weaver TE, Maislin G, Dinges DF, Bloxham T, George CF, Greenberg H, Kader G, Mahowald M, Younger J, Pack AI. Relationship between hours of CPAP use and achieving normal levels of sleepiness and daily functioning. Sleep. 2007;30:711–9.
17. Weaver TE, Mancini C, Maislin G, Cater J, Staley B, Landis JR, Ferguson KA, George CF, Schulman DA, Greenberg H, Rapoport DM, Walsleben JA, Lee-Chiong T, Gurubhagavatula I, Kuna ST. Continuous positive airway pressure treatment of sleepy patients with milder obstructive sleep apnea: results of the CPAP Apnea Trial North American Program (CATNAP) randomized clinical trial. Am J Respir Crit Care Med. 2012;186:677–83.
18. Marin JM, Carrizo SJ, Vicente E, Agusti AG. Long-term cardiovascular outcomes in men with obstructive sleep apnoea-hypopnoea with or without treatment with continuous positive airway pressure: an observational study. Lancet. 2005;365:1046–53.
19. Campos-Rodriguez F, Martinez-Garcia MA, Reyes-Nuñez N, Caballero-Martinez I, Catalan-Serra P, Almeida-Gonzalez CV. Role of sleep apnea and continuous positive airway pressure therapy in the incidence of stroke or coronary heart disease in women. Am J Respir Crit Care Med. 2014;189:1544–50.
20. Yu J, Zhou Z, McEvoy RD, Anderson CS, Rodgers A, Perkovic V, Neal B. Association of positive airway pressure with cardiovascular events and death in adults with sleep apnea: a systematic review and meta-analysis. JAMA. 2017;318:156–66.
21. Peker Y, Glantz H, Eulenburg C, Wegscheider K, Herlitz J, Thunstrom E. Effect of positive airway pressure on cardiovascular outcomes in coronary artery disease patients with nonsleepy obstructive sleep apnea. The RICCADSA randomized controlled trial. Am J Respir Crit Care Med. 2016;194:613–20.
22. Marin JM, Agusti A, Villar I, Forner M, Nieto D, Carrizo SJ, Barbé F, Vicente E, Wei Y, Nieto FJ, Jelic S. Association between treated and untreated obstructive sleep apnea and risk of hypertension. JAMA. 2012;307:2169–76.
23. Oates GR, Juarez LD, Hansen B, Kiefe CI, Shikany JM. Social risk factors for medication nonadherence: findings from the CARDIA study. Am J Health Behav. 2020;44:232–43.
24. Cockerham WC, Hamby BW, Oates GR. The social determinants of chronic disease. Am J Prev Med. 2017;52:S5–S12.
25. Leslie KH, McCowan C, Pell JP. Adherence to cardiovascular medication: a review of systematic reviews. J Public Health (Oxf). 2019;41:e84–94.
26. Somers ML, Peterson E, Sharma S, Yaremchuk K. Continuous positive airway pressure adherence for obstructive sleep apnea. ISRN Otolaryngol. 2011;943586. https://doi.org/10.5402/2011/943586. PMID: 23724263; PMCID: PMC3658812.
27. Liou HYS, Kapur VK, Consens F, Billings ME. The effect of sleeping environment and sleeping location change on positive airway pressure adherence. J Clin Sleep Med. 2018;14(10):1645–52.
28. Platt AB, Field SH, Asch DA, Chen Z, Patel NP, Gupta R, Roche DF, Gurubhagavatula I, Christie JD, Kuna ST. Neighborhood of

residence is associated with daily adherence to CPAP therapy. Sleep. 2009;32:799–806.

29. Billings ME, Auckley D, Benca R, Foldvary-Schaefer N, Iber C, Redline S, Rosen CL, Zee P, Kapur VK. Race and residential socioeconomics as predictors of CPAP adherence. Sleep. 2011;34:1653–8.

30. Wickwire EM, Jobe SL, Oldstone LM, Scharf SM, Johnson AM, Albrecht JS. Lower socioeconomic status and co-morbid conditions are associated with reduced CPAP adherence use among older adult Medicare beneficiaries with obstructive sleep apnea. Sleep. 2020;43(12):zsaa122.

31. Pandey A, Mereddy S, Combs D, Shetty S, Patel SI, Mashaq S, Seixas A, Littlewood K, Jean-Luis G, Parthasarathy S. Socioeconomic inequities in adherence to positive airway pressure therapy in population-level analysis. J Clin Med. 2020;9(2):442.

32. Kendzerska T, Gershon AS, Tomlinson G, Leung RS. The effect of patient neighbourhood income level on the purchase of continuous positive airway pressure treatment among sleep apnea patients. Ann Am Thorac Soc. 2015;13(1):93–100.

33. Simon-Tuval T, Reuveni H, Greenberg-Dotan S, Oksenberg A, Tal A, Tarasiuk A. Low socioeconomic status is a risk factor for CPAP acceptance among adult OSAS patients requiring treatment. Sleep. 2009;32:545–52.

34. Goyal A, Agarwal N, Pakhare A. Barriers to CPAP use in India: an exploratory study. J Clin Sleep Med. 2017;13(12):1385–94.

35. Tarasiuk A, ea. Financial incentive increases CPAP acceptance in patients from low socioeconomic background. PLoS One. 2012;7:e33178.

36. Williams DR, Collins C. Racial residential segregation: a fundamental cause of racial disparities in health. Public Health Rep. 2001;116:404–16.

37. Bailey ZD, Krieger N, Agénor M, Graves J, Linos N, Bassett MT. Structural racism and health inequities in the USA: evidence and interventions. Lancet. 2017;389:1453–63.

38. Hicken MT, Lee H, Ailshire J, Burgard SA, Williams DR. "Every shut eye, ain't sleep"1: the role of racism-related vigilance in racial/ethnic disparities in sleep difficulty. Race Soc Probl. 2013;5:100–12.

39. Cheng P, Cuellar R, Johnson DA, Kalmbach DA, Joseph CL, Cuamatzi Castelan A, Sagong C, Casement MD, Drake CL. Racial discrimination as a mediator of racial disparities in insomnia disorder. Sleep Health. 2020;6(5):543–9.

40. Williams DR, Priest N, Anderson N. Understanding associations between race, socioeconomic status and health: patterns and prospects. Health Psychol. 2016;35:407–11.

41. Chen-Edinboro LP, Kaufmann CN, Augustinavicius JL, Mojtabai R, Parisi JM, Wennberg AM, Smith MT, Spira AP. Neighborhood physical disorder, social cohesion, and insomnia: results from participants over age 50 in the Health and Retirement Study. Int Psychogeriatr. 2015;27(2):289–96.

42. Chen X, Wang R, Zee P, Lutsey PL, Javaheri S, Alcantara C, Jackson CL, Williams MA, Redline S. Racial/ethnic differences in sleep disturbances: the Multi-Ethnic Study of Atherosclerosis (MESA). Sleep. 2015;38:877–88.

43. Simonelli G, Dudley KA, Weng J, Gallo LC, Perreira K, Shah NA, Alcantara C, Zee PC, Ramos AR, Llabre MM, Sotres-Alvarez D, Wang R, Patel SR. Neighborhood factors as predictors of poor sleep in the Sueno ancillary study of the Hispanic community health study/study of Latinos. Sleep. 2017;40:zsw025.

44. Troxel WM, DeSantis A, Richardson AS, Beckman R, Ghosh-Dastidar B, Nugroho A, Hale L, Buysse DJ, Buman MP, Dubowitz T. Neighborhood disadvantage is associated with actigraphy-assessed sleep continuity and short sleep duration. Sleep. 2018;41(10):zsy140.

45. Obayashi K, Saeki K, Kurumatani N. Association between light exposure at night and insomnia in the general elderly population: the HEIJO-KYO cohort. Chronobiol Int. 2014;31:976–82.

46. Hume KI, Brink M, Basner M. Effects of environmental noise on sleep. Noise Health. 2012;14:297–302.

47. Hajat A, Diez-Roux AV, Adar SD, Auchincloss AH, Lovasi GS, O'Neill MS, Sheppard L, Kaufman JD. Air pollution and individual and neighborhood socioeconomic status: evidence from the Multi-Ethnic Study of Atherosclerosis (MESA). Environ Health Perspect. 2013;121:1325–33.

48. Chakraborty T, Hsu A, Manya D, Sheriff G. Disproportionately higher exposure to urban heat in lower-income neighborhoods: a multi-city perspective. Environ Res Lett. 2019;14:105003.

49. Velasquez N, Moore JA, Boudreau RM, Mady LJ, Lee SE. Association of air pollutants, airborne occupational exposures, and chronic rhinosinusitis disease severity. Int Forum Allergy Rhinol. 2020;10:175–82.

50. Adler NE, Newman K. Socioeconomic disparities in health: pathways and policies. Health Aff. 2002;21:60–76.

51. Hill TD, Trinh HN, Wen M, Hale L. Perceived neighborhood safety and sleep quality: a global analysis of six countries. Sleep Med. 2016;18:56–60.

52. Johnson DA, Simonelli G, Moore K, Billings M, Mujahid MS, Rueschman M, Kawachi I, Redline S, Diez Roux AV, Patel SR. The neighborhood social environment and objective measures of sleep in the multi-ethnic study of atherosclerosis. Sleep. 2017;40(1):zsw016.

53. Robbins R, Jean-Louis G, Gallagher RA, Hale L, Branas CC, Gooneratne N, Alfonso-Miller P, Perlis M, Grandner MA. Examining social capital in relation to sleep duration, insomnia, and daytime sleepiness. Sleep Med. 2019;60:165–72.

54. Billings ME, Rosen CL, Wang R, Auckley D, Benca R, Foldvary-Schaefer N, Iber C, Zee P, Redline S, Kapur VK. Is the relationship between race and continuous positive airway pressure adherence mediated by sleep duration? Sleep. 2013;36:221–7.

55. Doane LD, Breitenstein RS, Beekman C, Clifford S, Smith TJ, Lemery-Chalfant K. Early life socioeconomic disparities in children's sleep: the mediating role of the current home environment. J Youth Adolesc. 2019;48:56–70.

56. Garbarino S, De Carli F, Nobili L, Mascialino B, Squarcia S, Penco MA, Beelke M, Ferrilla F. Sleepiness and sleep disorders in shift workers: a study on a group of Italian police officers. Sleep. 2002;25:648–53.

57. Kivimäki M, Virtanen M, Kawachi I, Nyberg ST, Alfredsson L, Batty GD, Bjorner JB, Borritz M, Brunner EJ, Burr H, Dragano N, Ferrie JE, Fransson EI, Hamer M, Heikkilä K, Knutsson A, Koskenvuo M, Madsen IEH, Nielsen ML, Nordin M, Oksanen T, Pejtersen JH, Pentti J, Rugulies R, Salo P, Siegrist J, Steptoe A, Suominen S, Theorell T, Vahtera J, Westerholm PJM, Westerlund H, Singh-Manoux A, Jokela M. Long working hours, socioeconomic status, and the risk of incident type 2 diabetes: a meta-analysis of published and unpublished data from 222 120 individuals. Lancet Diabetes Endocrinol. 2015;3:27–34.

58. Reid KJ, Weng J, Ramos AR, Zee PC, Daviglus M, Mossavar-Rahmani Y, Sotres-Alvarez D, Gallo LC, Chirinos DA, Patel SR. Impact of shift work schedules on actigraphy-based measures of sleep in Hispanic workers: results from the Hispanic Community Health Study/Study of Latinos ancillary Sueño study. Sleep. 2018;41(10):zsy131.

59. Joo MJ, Herdegen JJ. Sleep apnea in an urban public hospital: assessment of severity and treatment adherence. J Clin Sleep Med. 2007;3:285–8.

60. Wallace DM, Vargas SS, Schwartz SJ, Aloia MS, Shafazand S. Determinants of continuous positive airway pressure adherence in a sleep clinic cohort of South Florida Hispanic veterans. Sleep Breath. 2013;17:351–63.

61. El-Solh AA, Ayyar L, Akinnusi M, Relia S, Akinnusi O. Positive airway pressure adherence in veterans with posttraumatic stress disorder. Sleep. 2010;33:1495–500.

62. Bakker JP, Wang R, Weng J, Aloia MS, Toth C, Morrical MG, Gleason KJ, Rueschman M, Dorsey C, Patel SR, Ware JH, Mittleman MA, Redline S. Motivational enhancement for increasing adherence to CPAP: a randomized controlled trial. Chest. 2016;150:337–45.

63. Sawyer AM, Gooneratne NS, Marcus CL, Ofer D, Richards KC, Weaver TE. A systematic review of CPAP adherence across age groups: clinical and empiric insights for developing CPAP adherence interventions. Sleep Med Rev. 2011;15:343–56.

64. Hwang D, Chang JW, Benjafield AV, Crocker ME, Kelly C, Becker KA, Kim JB, Woodrum RR, Liang J, Derose SF. Effect of telemedicine education and Telemonitoring on continuous positive airway pressure adherence. The tele-OSA randomized trial. Am J Respir Crit Care Med. 2018;197:117–26.

65. Malhotra A, Crocker ME, Willes L, Kelly C, Lynch S, Benjafield AV. Patient engagement using new technology to improve adherence to positive airway pressure therapy: a retrospective analysis. Chest. 2018;153:843–50.

66. Estacio EV, Whittle R, Protheroe J. The digital divide: examining socio-demographic factors associated with health literacy, access and use of internet to seek health information. J Health Psychol. 2019;24:1668–75.

The Impact of Partner and Family Support in PAP Therapy

10

Faith S. Luyster and Daniel J. Buysse

Abbreviations

OSA Obstructive sleep apnea
PAP Positive airway pressure
PSG Polysomnography

10.1 Introduction

Positive airway pressure (PAP) therapy for obstructive sleep apnea (OSA) is a challenging treatment, and, consequently, acceptance and adherence to PAP therapy are often problematic. Maximum therapeutic benefits including reductions in symptoms of OSA (i.e., snoring, apneas) are achieved through consistent PAP use. For many patients, OSA and PAP therapy are not experienced in isolation: patients often have close family members who may be directly or indirectly affected by and invested in the health and well-being of the patient. This chapter will present data on the impact that untreated OSA and PAP treatment have on spouses/partners and family members as these effects are likely to contribute to the level and type of engagement of partners and family members in patients' acceptance and adherence to PAP treatment. It will also present data on the impact of partner and family involvement on PAP acceptance and adherence and highlight PAP adherence intervention studies that included partner or family involvement.

F. S. Luyster (✉)
University of Pittsburgh, School of Nursing, Pittsburgh, PA, USA
e-mail: luysterfs@upmc.edu

D. J. Buysse
University of Pittsburgh, School of Medicine, Department of Psychiatry, Pittsburgh, PA, USA

10.2 Impact of Untreated OSA on Partners and Family Members

In addition to its documented adverse effects on patients' health and quality of life [1–3], untreated OSA can have negative daytime and nighttime consequences for close family members [4, 5]. Although the majority of research has focused on the effect of untreated OSA on partners, family members other than the patient's partner may also be impacted. For instance, an OSA patient's interactions with other family members may be impaired by disruptions in sleep due to loud snoring or reduced engagement in daytime activities due to daytime sleepiness. In a qualitative study of 42 OSA patients experiencing excessive daytime sleepiness (52% male; mean age 51.4 years), participants reported that excessive daytime sleepiness interfered with their caregiving ability and ability to do general housework and chores as a result of needing to plan the day around their symptoms, made it difficult to take vacations with family, and negatively affected their relationship with family members [5].

OSA symptoms are primary causes of sleep disturbance among partners. Up to 66% of partners of patients with OSA reported moderate to severe sleep disturbance and poor sleep quality due to the patient's snoring, apneas, and restlessness [6, 7]. During qualitative interviews and focus groups, partners voiced being distressed by witnessing patients stop breathing during the night and feeling the need to monitor the patient's breathing throughout the night [8, 9]. Objective sleep data acquired by polysomnography (PSG) corroborated partners' reports of sleep difficulties. Wives of husbands with untreated OSA have more wake after sleep onset, a higher percentage of stage 1 sleep, and greater alpha power during slow wave sleep compared to wives of healthy husbands [10]. In a study of concurrent PSG of wives and husbands with suspected OSA sharing the same bed, wives had a median sleep efficacy of 71% and an arousal index of 21, and almost a third (32%) had an arousal within 1–3 s of a snore by the patient [11]. Various tactics for mitigating the disturbed sleep caused by patients' OSA symptoms have been reported by partners, including using earplugs and/or sleep medication, alternating sleep schedule with the patient, and sleeping in separate rooms [7–9, 12, 13]. For some partners, bed sharing is maintained in order to avoid social sigma and create the façade of a "happy" relationship [8]. Compared to partners who shared a bed with a patient with untreated OSA, partners who did not share a bed had worse quality of life and depression and anxiety symptoms [14].

In addition to sleep disturbance, partners often report frustration, exhaustion, interference with work, and relationship problems due to sleep loss [7, 9, 13]. Untreated OSA can also negatively impact the quality of life of partners [6, 14]. Prior to patients' initiation of PAP therapy, over 50% of partners reported anxiety symptoms, and 18% reported depressive symptoms [14]. Qualitative interviews conducted with 12 spouses to explore how they managed living with a patient with untreated OSA identified numerous approaches used by spouses to deal with their situation [15]. These approaches included sacrificing social activities, taking on more of the household workload, managing the everyday life for the patient, maintaining bed sharing despite sleep disturbance, ensuring that the patient sought medical treatment for his or her symptoms, and making diet and lifestyle changes, all of which often lead to relationship problems and feelings of being a caregiver or parent rather than a spouse. Some spouses approached the situation by feeling empathic toward the patient, thus making adaptions to daytime activities to accommodate patient's sleepiness, and generally trying to make the best out of the difficult situation.

The burden of untreated OSA on partners is a common impetus for patients to seek medical care for their symptoms. Semi-structured interviews with OSA patients who had received PAP treatment ($n = 16$) revealed that most would have remained unaware of their OSA symptoms if it hadn't been for a loved one or close friend bringing it to the patient's attention [16]. Patients also reported that partners' frustration with snoring and shared poor sleep initiated a collaborative team process aimed at improving the couple's sleep. On the other hand, most partners reported difficulty in getting the patient to take action in response to his or her OSA symptoms. Partners sometimes reported that bullying the patient about snoring was what enabled the patient to begin noticing OSA symptoms [16]. Similarly, couples participating in a joint interview noted that the partner played a key role in aiding in the diagnosis and treatment process. It often took repetitive discussions and, for some, years before the patient scheduled an appointment with a healthcare provider [17]. Partners identified disruptions to their own sleep and concern about the health of the patient as motivators for encouraging the patient to seek treatment. Although partner encouragement can incentivize treatment seeking, it can negatively influence patient's PAP use. Patients who reported seeking treatment due to their partner had lower PAP usage during the first 6 months of treatment (4.0 ± 0.4 h) compared to patients who self-referred (5.3 ± 0.4 h) [18].

10.3 Impact of PAP Treatment on Partners' Sleep and Daytime Functioning

PAP treatment has positive effects on partners' sleep. During an overnight diagnostic PSG study in which patients were treated with PAP, partners exhibited immediate increases in PSG-assessed sleep efficiency and percentage of rapid eye movement (REM) sleep and decreases in number of arousals and percentage of non-REM sleep [11]. Self-reported improvements in sleep quality are maintained for up to 1 year in partners of OSA patients treated with PAP [6, 19, 20]. However, spouses have reported sleep disturbance related to PAP use, primarily due to noise or cold air [6]. Inconsistent responses have been reported by partners regarding daytime sleepiness, quality of life, mood, and marital quality in response to PAP therapy [14, 19–22], which may be partially due to differences in assessments between studies and normal baseline values of these variables. Furthermore, adherence to PAP may also have influenced partners' outcomes, as consistent use is needed for improvement in patients' symptoms. Interestingly, qualitative data from spouses of patients treated with PAP revealed initial anxiety associated with not hearing the patient snoring during the night with PAP, although spouses soon adjusted to this "new normal" [9].

10.4 Impact of Partner and Family Involvement on PAP Adherence

10.4.1 Presence of Spouse or Live-in Partner

Having a spouse or living with a partner can positively influence patients' acceptance and adherence to PAP therapy. Among average- or high-income patients with OSA, those living with a partner were almost 9 times (OR = 8.82; 95% CI = 1.03–74.8) more likely to accept PAP treatment; however, living with a partner was not associated with PAP acceptance among low-income patients [23]. As compared to married patients with OSA, unmarried patients voiced having no support, less belief in their ability to use PAP, and fewer positive experiences within the first week of PAP treatment during semi-structured interviews [24]. During the first month of PAP treatment, patients living with a partner had higher average nightly hours of PAP use (5.0 h) compared those living alone (3.6 h) [25]. Among women with OSA in one small study, none of the unmarried or unpartnered patients ($n = 7$) were adherent to PAP-based Medicare criteria of ≥4 h of use on 70% of nights, whereas 40% of married or partnered patients ($n = 13$) were adherent based on this criterion [26]. In a study of 1141 OSA patients, being married or living with a partner was an independent predictor of long-term PAP adherence assessed over an average of 504 days following PAP initiation [27]. Conversely, studies have found no significant differences in marital status between adherent or consistent users of PAP and non-adherent or intermittent users during short-term follow-up (i.e., 9 weeks and 6 months) [28, 29]. A potential explanation for the inconsistencies in findings could be related to relationship quality. In a study of 23 married, male patients with OSA, patient-reported marital conflict, in particular negative emotions like anger and criticism, predicted lower average nightly PAP adherence over the first 3 months of treatment [30]. Likewise, relationship conflict was associated with lower PAP adherence in married or partnered women with OSA [26].

A recent study identified clusters of couples and their association with PAP adherence during the first 120 days of treatment among 290 newly diagnosed PAP-naïve OSA patients. Latent class analyses revealed three distinct clusters of couples: (1) older retired couples ($n = 86$; 88% married, 15% had children at home, 78% together >30 years, 97% both not working), (2) young working couples ($n = 128$; 70% married, 84% had children at home, 59% together 10–30 years, 75% both working), and (3) mature active couples ($n = 76$; 95% married, 44% had children at home, 65% together >30 years, 53% both working). PAP adherence at 120 days was significantly higher among the older retired couples (6.6 h; IQR 5.7–7.5) compared to the young working couples (5.9 h; IQR 4.9–6.6) and the mature active couples (5.9 h; IQR 4.9–7.3). Interestingly, there was no significant differences in spousal involvement in PAP therapy between the couple clusters. However, having a stable relationship exceeding 30 years has been shown to predict PAP adherence at 120 days [31]. These findings suggest that the effect of a spouse's or partner's presence on PAP adherence could be influenced by the quality and stability of the couple's relationship.

In addition to the presence of a spouse or live-in partner, frequency of bed sharing can also influence PAP acceptance and adherence. A partner's decision to sleep in a separate room quadrupled the odds (OR = 4.3; 95% CI 4.1–13.3) of a patient purchasing a PAP device, potentially with the intention of improving the relationship with their partner [32]. Utilizing data from wives' sleep logs kept during the first 2 weeks of PAP treatment, a greater number of nights the couple slept together was associated with a higher percentage of nights PAP was used and greater hours of PAP use [13]. A study of 119 sleep apnea patients examined the effect of sleeping environment on average PAP adherence over 30 days [33]. Although patients reporting a different sleep schedule than their bed partner had similar adherence as those with a compatible schedule, changing sleep location more than once per month, primarily due to spending a few nights per week at a significant other's residence, was associated with reduced PAP adherence, independent of sociodemographic factors.

10.4.2 Family Involvement

Few studies have investigated the role of family involvement in PAP adherence; however, available data suggests that family members can influence patients' use of PAP (Table 10.1). Positive experiences with PAP among family and/or friends predict PAP acceptance among PAP-naïve OSA patients [23, 32]. In a study examining the effect of family coping on PAP adherence among 107 OSA patients, poor PAP adherence over the first 6 months of treatment was related to families seeking less spiritual support and support from others and being less able to make stressful events more manageable through redefinition [34]. Family coping may impact PAP adherence through its influence on self-efficacy: how a family deals with stressful situations (i.e., OSA diagnosis and PAP treatment) may reinforce patients' perceived ability to use PAP consistently [35]. During motivational interviews conducted as part of an educational PAP intervention, patients' reported encouragement from their caregiver (i.e., spouse/partner, children, sister) was a primary driver of PAP use [36]. Some partners were currently using PAP, so their encouragement stemmed from their own experience with OSA and ability to attest to the benefits of PAP. Encouragement to use PAP also came from other family members and friends who were PAP users. The desire to live to foster close family ties, particularly with spouses and grandchildren, contributed to PAP adherence by patient report.

Qualitative interviews conducted with OSA patients who had personal knowledge of using PAP revealed that *becoming a team*, or the collaborative nature of close relationships with family members, contributed to their success in using PAP [16]. Patients reported receiving support with PAP from their families during travel and feeling like part of a collaborative team (with their partner) whose aim was to achieve good sleep by adapting sleep habits, changing sleeping positions if PAP machine bothered the partner, and maintaining night-time rituals. However, a couple of patients reported not feeling supported by their team due to annoyance by the PAP machine, letting the patient handle PAP him/herself, and unwillingness to understand the importance of PAP, all of which contributed to PAP non-adherence [16]. These findings support research in other disease states indicating that family support in disease self-management results in better patient outcomes [37].

Table 10.1 Overview of chapter findings

Authors	Key consistent findings	Unresolved issues
Impact of untreated OSA on partners and family members		
Waldman et al. (2020) [5] McArdle et al. (2001) [6] Virkkula et al. (2005) [7] Henry et al. (2013) [8] Luyster et al. (2016) [9] Smith et al. (2009) [10] Beninati et al. (1999) [11] Billman & Ware (2002) [12] Cartwright & Knight (1987) [13] Doherty et al. (2003) [14]	Patients' excessive daytime sleepiness interfered with caregiving ability and housework, made difficult to take family vacations, and affected relationships with family members OSA symptoms disrupt partners' sleep Partners are distressed by witnessing patients stop breathing Partners engaged in various tactics to mitigate disturbed sleep due to patients' OSA symptoms Partners experienced frustration, relationship problems, anxiety and depression symptoms, and poor quality of life	Bed sharing varied among couples
Impact of PAP treatment on partners' sleep and daytime functioning		
Beninati et al. (1999) [11] McArdle et al. (2001) [6] Kiely & McNicholas (1997) [19] Siccoli et al. (2008) [20] Acar et al. (2016) [21] Doherty et al. (2003) [14] Parish et al. (2003) [22]	PAP treatment improved partners' sleep PAP treatment can have negative effects such as noise or cold air disturbing sleep and initial anxiety due to ceasing of patients' snoring	Changes in daytime sleepiness, quality of life, mood, and marital quality associated with PAP treatment were inconsistent
Impact of partner and family involvement on PAP adherence		
Tarasiuk et al. (2012) [23] Lewis et al. (2004) [25] Baron et al. (2017) [26] Gagnadoux et al. (2011) [27] Russo-Magno et al. (2001) [28] Weaver et al. (1997) [29] Simon-Tuval et al. (2009) [32] Cartwright & Knight (1987) [13] Liou et al. (2018) [33] Sampaio et al. (2013) [34] Khan et al. (2019) [36] Ward et al. (2018) [16] Baron et al. (2011) [39] Baron et al. (2012) [40] Batool-Anwar et al. (2017) [41] Gentina et al. (2019) [31] Luyster et al. (2016) [9] Elfström et al. (2012) [43] Broström et al. (2010) [44] Ye et al. (2017) [17]	Infrequent bed sharing was associated with greater PAP acceptance and worse PAP adherence Most common positive partner and family behaviors that improved PAP adherence: general partner involvement in PAP treatment, encouragement to use PAP, assistance with PAP equipment, engagement in educational situations regarding OSA and PAP, sharing personal benefits from PAP treatment Most common negative partner and family behaviors that discouraged PAP adherence: no partner involvement in PAP treatment, unwillingness to understand importance of PAP treatment, inability to deal with noise or air coming from the PAP device	Comparison in PAP adherence between patients who were married/living with a partner versus unmarried or unpartnered/living alone were inconsistent The types of partner involvement that are most positively influential on PAP adherence remain unclear, although collaboration seems to be important Little is known about family involvement in PAP adherence

PAP Positive airway pressure, *OSA* obstructive sleep apnea

10.4.3 Partner Involvement

Limited quantitative and qualitative data suggest that partners can play a positive and negative role in PAP adherence (Table 10.1). Patients' perspectives on partner involvement in PAP initiation and adherence has primarily been reported in quantitative studies, whereas partners' reports of involvement have been captured more often in qualitative studies. Encouragement from their partner is a primary reason for OSA patients to purchase PAP [32, 38]. In a study of 31 male OSA patients, spouses' involvement and PAP adherence were assessed during a 10-day period shortly after starting treatment [39]. Support was the most frequent and highest

rated type of spousal involvement, with 94% reporting feeling supported by their spouse at least 1 day out of the 10 days. Collaboration and pressure were less frequently reported, and 13% of patients reported no spouse involvement during the 10 days. Support from a spouse was associated with increased next-day self-reported PAP adherence among patients with more severe OSA. Following nights with PAP problems, patients with lower relationship conflict reported greater next-day collaboration (e.g., helping with the PAP machine). Furthermore, patients with low support in the relationship reported increased daily support for PAP following nights with PAP problems. Perceived spousal pressure was not associated with increased PAP adherence [39]. Another study examining spousal involvement (i.e., collaborative, one-sided, positive, negative) in 23 male patients with OSA found both positive and negative involvement occurred roughly one to two times during the first week of PAP treatment [40]. Examples of positive involvement included "praise or compliment patient for using PAP," "gave patient space," "showed patience in order to get patient to use PAP," and "changed something at home or work to get patient to use PAP." On the other hand, negative involvement included telling the patient that he or she was unhappy the patient wasn't using PAP, withdrawal and silence to get patient to use PAP, and trying to make patient scared of the consequences of not using PAP. At 3-month follow-up, frequency of spousal involvement remained low, although negative involvement decreased. Collaborative spousal involvement (e.g., changed something at home or work to get patient to use PAP) was associated with higher PAP adherence at 3 months. Positive, negative, and one-sided involvement were not associated with adherence [40].

In a study of 194 patients (73% male) with predominately severe OSA, spousal involvement with patients' general health was associated with greater PAP adherence at 6-month follow-up but not longer-term adherence [41]. When analyses were stratified by sex, the association between spousal involvement and PAP adherence at 6-months was only significant for men, potentially suggesting limited or negative involvement from partners of female patients. Partner engagement (i.e., pressure to use PAP, emotional support, and collaboration in solving issues with PAP use) was assessed 45 days after PAP initiation among 290 OSA patients (77% male; all married or living with a partner) [31]. Structural equation modeling revealed that partner engagement was directly linked to greater PAP adherence and identified marital quality as a moderator of this relationship indicating that partner engagement improved PAP adherence only when marital quality was high. These results highlight the importance of the quality of the couple's relationship in PAP adherence as pressure to use PAP may not be beneficial in those with poor relationship quality. Interestingly, among women with OSA, general levels of perceived social support, rather than emotional support in the relationship, were associated with greater PAP adherence at 12-week follow-up [26].

A study of 92 married or cohabiting new OSA patients (63% male) examined the association of patients' perception of autonomy support from their partner, such as trying to understand how the patient sees his/her use of PAP before suggesting a new way to do things, with PAP adherence over the first 60 days of treatment [42]. Higher levels of perceived partner autonomy support predicted greater duration of PAP use at 60 days and increasing PAP use over time, independent of the effects of negative social control (i.e., partner negativity) and limited positive effects of partner responsive-

ness. These findings add to the literature examining spousal involvement in PAP adherence and suggest that partner autonomy support is another positive partner behavior that can influence PAP adherence. Acknowledging the patient's perspective, providing choices for how to manage PAP, encouraging self-initiation, and minimizing pressure may facilitate PAP use [42].

Qualitative studies help provide a more in-depth understanding of partner involvement and give insight from the partners' perspective. Focus groups conducted with 12 partners of PAP-treated OSA patients described motivating the patient to use his or her PAP by providing emotional support (e.g., encouragement) and instrumental support (e.g., verbal reminders, help with putting on mask) [9]. During semi-structured interviews with 25 partners of patients with OSA treated with PAP, partners revealed situations that influenced their support of the patient and strategies for managing these situations during the PAP initiation phase [43]. The following situations were identified as negatively influencing the partners' support: noise from the PAP disturbing their sleep, physical (e.g., mask leakage) and practical (e.g., limited sleeping positions, travel) problems associated with PAP experienced by the patient, patients' shame, and interference with intimacy. Positive situations that motivated partners to provide support included understanding the consequences of OSA, benefits of treatment, patients' positive attitude toward PAP, and receiving support from family, friends, and healthcare providers. Partners identified three management strategies: letting the patient handle treatment by himself/herself, handing the treatment together, and taking over the treatment by handling all practical aspects of the treatment [43].

By comparison, patients with OSA treated with PAP indicated that facilitators of PAP adherence were partner engagement in education provided during the diagnostic and treatment initiation phases and providing practical support such as helping adjust the mask during the night [44]. Barriers to adherence were noted as insufficient emotional and practical support from their partner. Female patients with OSA ($n = 7$) reported 1 week after PAP initiation varying types of involvement from their spouse or partner, with most reporting helpful support (e.g., problem-solving, asking about PAP, helping patient feel less self-conscious about it, and checking to see if patient was snoring at night) or encouragement to use PAP [26]. One patient reported no involvement from her husband, and two others reported unhelpful involvement such as repeatedly asking if it is working and making fun of the patient.

A qualitative study conducted joint interviews with 20 newly diagnosed OSA patients treated with PAP and their partners to explore facilitators and barriers to PAP use [17]. Couples identified working together as a key facilitator of PAP adherence in that they took a "we" or joint coping approach to addressing PAP problems and learning about the condition and treatment. Other facilitators of PAP use were perceived benefits of PAP for both the patient and partner in the areas of sleep, daytime functioning, and relationship quality, patients' motivation to use PAP for benefits of the partner, and partners' support, which included helping with the PAP machine and mask, going to appointments with the patient, verbal encouragement, and general acceptance of PAP. Barriers to PAP use voiced by couples were shared anxiety about PAP treatment initially, disruptions to sleep and bedtime routine caused by use of PAP equipment (e.g., noise, air blowing, interruptions to bedtime conversations), interruptions to intimacy, and patients' concern about their appearance when wearing PAP. When asked what they wished they had known prior to PAP treatment, couples highlighted the importance of negotiation, openness, and supportive communication as important factors for adjusting to PAP treatment.

10.5 Partner and Family Involvement in PAP Adherence Interventions

With the positive and negative influences that partners and families can have on patients' PAP adherence, involvement of partners and other family members in interventions aimed at improving acceptance and adherence to PAP treatment should be a consideration. Inclusion of partners was identified during focus groups with OSA patients and their partners as an important element of a new PAP user program [9]. Presence of a partner or family member has been incorporated into PAP adherence interventions, yet the engagement of the partner or family member is often limited. Several PAP adherence intervention studies reported having the patients' partners or family present but not actively engaged during pre-treatment and follow-up education and/or instructional sessions. These sessions included basic information about OSA and treatment options and benefits of adherence to treatment, patients' experiences and concerns with using PAP and their perceptions of their partner or family's concerns about PAP use, and demonstration of the PAP equipment, along with information about how to manage and clean the equipment [18, 45–48]. In a randomized controlled trial, 28 patients and their caregivers (24 spouses/partner, 2 son/daughter, 1 sister, and 1 friend) in the intervention arm participated in a group visit that involved an interactive educational session, peer coaching from a PAP user, hands-on experience with the PAP machine from a respiratory therapist, and a one-on-two semi-structured motivational interview that provided encouragement and offered advice to improve adherence [36]. Although the intervention provided specific examples of ways for the caregiver to provide support to the patient, there was no collaboration between the patient and caregiver to identify what types of support may be most beneficial in helping the patient use PAP.

Dyadic interventions for chronic illness that take a more collaborative approach to family involvement lead to improvements in both patients' and family members' health and functioning [37, 49, 50]. To date, only one study has taken a couple-oriented approach to improving PAP adherence [51]. In this pilot study, patients and partners in the couple-oriented education and support intervention attended two face-to-face sessions together and one telephone session individually [51]. The sessions provided information about OSA and benefits of PAP, hands-on demonstration of PAP equipment, and review of changes in both patient's and partner's sleep quality and mood and included shared discussions about PAP concerns and barriers to PAP use, collaborative strategizing to identify ways for the partner to support the patient's use of PAP, and goal setting. Both patients and partners in the couple-oriented intervention had improvements in sleep quality, daytime sleepiness, and daytime function during the first 3 months of PAP treatment. PAP adherence increased over the first month of treatment, but then declined. Results from this pilot study suggest that engaging the partner in interventions aimed at improving PAP adherence is likely to have beneficial effects on patients' and partners' health and PAP use.

10.6 Summary

Partners' involvement is interwoven in the diagnosis and treatment trajectories of OSA, and thus partners can have a profound impact on the health outcomes associated with OSA and its treatment (Table 10.1). Symptoms of OSA disturb partners' sleep which is a primary reason for patients seeking diagnosis and treatment of OSA. Once OSA is diagnosed and treatment is prescribed, partners play a pivotal role in patients' acceptance and adherence to PAP therapy. Partner support is likely to contribute to greater PAP acceptance and adherence, whereas partner undermining is likely to contribute to PAP nonacceptance and nonadherence. The path of partner support and associated PAP adherence can lead to improvement in health outcomes as adequate levels of PAP adherence are necessary for achieving treatment benefits. On the other hand, the path of partner undermining and accompanying inadequate PAP use may contribute to poor health outcomes. Thus, partners of patients with OSA are a key target for intervention efforts aimed at improving PAP adherence and, ultimately, improving the health and well-being of patients.

10.7   Conclusion

OSA is a shared problem that affects not only patients but their partners and other family members. Treatment with PAP can have beneficial effects of partners such as improving sleep, mood, and quality of life. Research is lacking on the effect of PAP treatment on other family members, although it could be hypothesized that these individuals also experience benefits. Partners and family members can positively and negatively influence patients' adoption and consistent use of PAP treatment. Positive involvement by partners and family members which includes encouragement and practical support, along with taking a collaborative approach to managing PAP treatment, is associated with greater patient acceptance and adherence to PAP therapy. Negative partner/family involvement, such as abstaining from providing support or encouragement potentially due to issues associated with PAP use like noise or interruption to intimacy, and an unwillingness to understand the importance of PAP therapy are associated with poor PAP adherence. Given the important role that partners and other family members have in patients' PAP adherence, engaging close family members in interventions promoting PAP adherence may be beneficial, particularly when intervention components promote open communication and advocate for collaborative problem-solving and planning. Further research, including intervention studies, is needed to explore partners and family members involvement in successful PAP management.

References

1. Dong J-Y, Zhang Y-H, Qin L-Q. Obstructive sleep apnea and cardiovascular risk: meta-analysis of prospective cohort studies. Atherosclerosis. 2013;229(2):489–95.
2. Ip MS, Lam B, Ng MM, Lam WK, Tsang KW, Lam KS. Obstructive sleep apnea is independently associated with insulin resistance. Am J Respir Crit Care Med. 2002;165(5):670–6.
3. Moyer CA, Sonnad SS, Garetz SL, Helman JI, Chervin RD. Quality of life in obstructive sleep apnea: a systematic review of the literature. Sleep Med. 2001;2(6):477–91.
4. Luyster FS. Impact of obstructive sleep apnea and its treatments on partners: a literature review. J Clin Sleep Med. 2017;13(03):467–77.
5. Waldman LT, Parthasarathy S, Villa KF, Bron M, Bujanover S, Brod M. Understanding the burden of illness of excessive daytime sleepiness associated with obstructive sleep apnea: a qualitative study. Health Qual Life Outcomes. 2020;18:1–14.
6. McArdle N, Kingshott R, Engleman H, Mackay T, Douglas N. Partners of patients with sleep apnoea/hypopnoea syndrome: effect of CPAP treatment on sleep quality and quality of life. Thorax. 2001;56(7):513–8.
7. Virkkula P, Bachour A, Hytönen M, Malmberg H, Salmi T, Maasilta P. Patient-and bed partner-reported symptoms, smoking, and nasal resistance in sleep-disordered breathing. Chest. 2005;128(4):2176–82.
8. Henry D, Rosenthal L. "Listening for his breath:" the significance of gender and partner reporting on the diagnosis, management, and treatment of obstructive sleep apnea. Sci Med. 2013;79:48–56.
9. Luyster FS, Dunbar-Jacob J, Aloia MS, Martire LM, Buysse DJ, Strollo PJ. Patient and partner experiences with obstructive sleep apnea and cpap treatment: a qualitative analysis. Behav Sleep Med. 2016;14(1):67–84.
10. Smith AKA, Togeiro SMG, Tufik S, Roizenblatt S. Disturbed sleep and musculoskeletal pain in the bed partner of patients with obstructive sleep apnea. Sleep Med. 2009;10(8):904–12.
11. Beninati W, Harris CD, Herold DL, Shepard JW Jr. The effect of snoring and obstructive sleep apnea on the sleep quality of bed partners. Mayo Clin Proc. 1999;74(10):955–8.
12. Billmann SJ, Ware JC. Marital satisfaction of wives of untreated sleep apneic men. Sleep Med. 2002;3(1):55–9.
13. Cartwright RD, Knight S. Silent partners: the wives of sleep apneic patients. Sleep. 1987;10(3):244–8.
14. Doherty LS, Kiely JL, Lawless G, McNicholas WT. Impact of nasal continuous positive airway pressure therapy on the quality of life of bed partners of patients with obstructive sleep apnea syndrome. Chest. 2003;124(6):2209–14.
15. Stålkrantz A, Broström A, Wiberg J, Svanborg E, Malm D. Everyday life for the spouses of patients with untreated OSA syndrome. Scand J Caring Sci. 2012;26(2):324–32.
16. Ward K, Gott M, Hoare K. Becoming a team: findings from a grounded theory study about living with CPAP. Collegian. 2018;25(1):81–8.
17. Ye L, Antonelli MT, Willis DG, Kayser K, Malhotra A, Patel SR. Couples' experiences with continuous positive airway pressure treatment: a dyadic perspective. Sleep Health. 2017;3(5):362–7.
18. Hoy CJ, Vennelle M, Kingshott RN, Engleman HM, Douglas NJ. Can intensive support improve continuous positive airway pressure use in patients with the sleep apnea/hypopnea syndrome? Am J Respir Crit Care Med. 1999;159(4):1096–100.
19. Kiely JL, McNicholas WT. Bed partners' assessment of nasal continuous positive airway pressure therapy in obstructive sleep apnea. Chest. 1997;111(5):1261–5.
20. Siccoli MM, Pepperell JC, Kohler M, Craig SE, Davies RJ, Stradling JR. Effects of continuous positive airway pressure on quality of life in patients with moderate to severe obstructive sleep apnea: data from a randomized controlled trial. Sleep. 2008;31(11):1551–8.
21. Acar M, Kaya C, Catli T, Hancı D, Bolluk O, Aydin Y. Effects of nasal continuous positive airway pressure therapy on partners' sexual lives. Eur Arch Otorhinolaryngol. 2016;273(1):133–7.
22. Parish JM, Lyng PJ. Quality of life in bed partners of patients with obstructive sleep apnea or hypopnea after treatment with continuous positive airway pressure. Chest. 2003;124(3):942–7.
23. Tarasiuk A, Reznor G, Greenberg-Dotan S, Reuveni H. Financial incentive increases CPAP acceptance in patients from low socioeconomic background. PLoS One. 2012;7(3):e33178.
24. Sawyer AM, Deatrick JA, Kuna ST, Weaver TE. Differences in perceptions of the diagnosis and treatment of obstructive sleep apnea and continuous positive airway pressure therapy among adherers and nonadherers. Qual Health Res. 2010;20:873–92.
25. Lewis KE, Seale L, Bartle IE, Watkins AJ, Ebden P. Early predictors of CPAP use for the treatment of obstructive sleep apnea. Sleep. 2004;27(1):134–8.
26. Baron KG, Gunn HE, Wolfe LF, Zee PC. Relationships and CPAP adherence among women with obstructive sleep apnea. Sleep Sci Pract. 2017;1(1):10.
27. Gagnadoux F, Le Vaillant M, Goupil F, Pigeanne T, Chollet S, Masson P, et al. Influence of marital status and employment status on long-term adherence with continuous positive airway pressure in sleep apnea patients. PLoS One. 2011;6(8):e22503.
28. Russo-Magno P, O'Brien A, Panciera T, Rounds S. Compliance with CPAP therapy in older men with obstructive sleep apnea. J Am Geriatr Soc. 2001;49(9):1205–11.
29. Weaver TE, Kribbs NB, Pack AI, Kline LR, Chugh DK, Maislin G, et al. Night-to-night variability in CPAP use over the first three months of treatment. Sleep. 1997;20(4):278–83.

30. Baron KG, Smith TW, Czajkowski LA, Gunn HE, Jones CR. Relationship quality and CPAP adherence in patients with obstructive sleep apnea. Behav Sleep Med. 2009;7(1):22–36.

31. Gentina T, Bailly S, Jounieaux F, Verkindre C, Broussier P-M, Guffroy D, et al. Marital quality, partner's engagement and continuous positive airway pressure adherence in obstructive sleep apnea. Sleep Med. 2019;55:56–61.

32. Simon-Tuval T, Reuveni H, Greenberg-Dotan S, Oksenberg A, Tal A, Tarasiuk A. Low socioeconomic status is a risk factor for CPAP acceptance among adult OSAS patients requiring treatment. Sleep. 2009;32(4):545–52.

33. Liou HYS, Kapur VK, Consens F, Billings ME. The effect of sleeping environment and sleeping location change on positive airway pressure adherence. J Clin Sleep Med. 2018;14(10):1645–52.

34. Sampaio R, Pereira MG, Winck JC. A new characterization of adherence patterns to auto-adjusting positive airway pressure in severe obstructive sleep apnea syndrome: clinical and psychological determinants. Sleep Breath. 2013;17(4):1145–58.

35. Sampaio R, Pereira MG, Winck JC. Obstructive sleep apnea representations, self-efficacy and family coping regarding APAP adherence: a longitudinal study. Psychol Health Med. 2014;19(1):59–69.

36. Khan NNS, Olomu AB, Bottu S, Roller MR, Smith RC. Semistructured motivational interviews of patients and caregivers to improve CPAP adherence: a qualitative analysis. J Clin Sleep Med. 2019;15(12):1721–30.

37. Martire LM, Lustig AP, Schulz R, Miller GE, Helgeson VS. Is it beneficial to involve a family member? A meta-analysis of psychosocial interventions for chronic illness. Health Psychol. 2004;23(6):599–611.

38. Brin YS, Haim Reuveni M, Sari Greenberg M, Tal A. Determinants affecting initiation of continuous positive airway pressure treatment. Isr Med Assoc J. 2005;7(1):13–8.

39. Baron KG, Smith TW, Berg CA, Czajkowski LA, Gunn H, Jones CR. Spousal involvement in CPAP adherence among patients with obstructive sleep apnea. Sleep Breath. 2011;15(3):525–34.

40. Baron KG, Gunn HE, Czajkowski LA, Smith TW, Jones CR. Spousal involvement in CPAP: does pressure help? J Clin Sleep Med. 2012;8(2):147–53.

41. Batool-Anwar S, Baldwin CM, Fass S, Quan SF. Role of spousal involvement in continuous positive airway pressure (CPAP) adherence in patients with obstructive sleep apnea (OSA). Southwest J Pulm Crit Care. 2017;14(5):213–27.

42. Baron CE, Smith TW, Baucom BR, Uchino BN, Williams PG, Sundar KM, et al. Relationship partner social behavior and continuous positive airway pressure adherence: the role of autonomy support. Health Psychol. 2020;39(4):325–34.

43. Elfström M, Karlsson S, Nilsen P, Fridlund B, Svanborg E, Broström A. Decisive situations affecting partners' support to continuous positive airway pressure–treated patients with obstructive sleep apnea syndrome: a critical incident technique analysis of the initial treatment phase. J Cardiovasc Nurs. 2012;27(3):228–39.

44. Broström A, Nilsen P, Johansson P, Ulander M, Strömberg A, Svanborg E, et al. Putative facilitators and barriers for adherence to CPAP treatment in patients with obstructive sleep apnea syndrome: a qualitative content analysis. Sleep Med. 2010;11(2):126–30.

45. Bouloukaki I, Giannadaki K, Mermigkis C, Tzanakis N, Mauroudi E, Moniaki V, et al. Intensive versus standard follow-up to improve continuous positive airway pressure compliance. Eur Respir J. 2014;44(5):1262–74.

46. Turino C, de Batlle J, Woehrle H, Mayoral A, Castro-Grattoni AL, Gómez S, et al. Management of continuous positive airway pressure treatment compliance using telemonitoring in obstructive sleep apnoea. Eur Respir J. 2017;49(2):1601128.

47. Sedkaoui K, Leseux L, Pontier S, Rossin N, Leophonte P, Fraysse J-L, et al. Efficiency of a phone coaching program on adherence to continuous positive airway pressure in sleep apnea hypopnea syndrome: a randomized trial. BMC Pulm Med. 2015;15(1):102.

48. Richards D, Bartlett DJ, Wong K, Malouff J, Grunstein RR. Increased adherence to CPAP with a group cognitive behavioral treatment intervention: a randomized trial. Sleep. 2007;30(5):635–40.

49. Martire LM, Helgeson VS. Close relationships and the management of chronic illness: associations and interventions. Am Psychol. 2017;72(6):601–12.

50. Martire LM, Hemphill RC, Polenick CA. Harnessing the power of the marital relationship to improve illness management: considerations for couple-based interventions. In: Bookwala J, editor. Couple relationships in the middle and later years: their nature, complexity, and role in health and illness. American Psychological Association; 2016. p. 325–44.

51. Luyster FS, Aloia MS, Buysse DJ, Dunbar-Jacob J, Martire LM, Sereika SM, et al. A couples-oriented intervention for positive airway pressure therapy adherence: a pilot study of obstructive sleep apnea patients and their partners. Behav Sleep Med. 2019;17(5):561–72.

Personality and Mental Health as Determinants of CPAP Use

11

Royi Gilad

11.1 Introduction

This chapter contains two halves. First, there is a theoretical introduction to the concept of personality which is not a familiar territory for most clinicians. The second half describes the potential ways in which personality may impact CPAP adherence. The chapter concludes with strategies on how to help patients whose personality traits pay a role in treatment non-adherence.

Mental disorders are a cause of immense burden, pain, and disability on the individual level, but also on the social and financial level. Mental disorders are very prevalent with an estimation that around 15% (970 million people) of the world's population were suffering in 2017 from mental disorders and substance use disorders [1]. According to the World Health Organization, one in four people in the world will be affected by mental or neurological disorders at some point in their lives [2], but only a third will seek medical assistance (due to stigma, lack of services, and other reasons), and in between 25% and 40% of countries, there are no available mental health services at all. The global burden of mental illness accounts for 32.4% of years lived with disability (YLDs) and 13.0% of disability-adjusted life-years (DALYs) [3].

While thinking about mental disorders, it is fairly easy to understand why a patient crippled by a major depressive episode might miss out on a follow-up appointment; why a patient suffering from an anxiety disorder might feel claustrophobic after using a CPAP, even after one night, and will cease their use completely; or why a patient grappling with substance use disorder, or gambling disorder, might decide not to allocate funds for purchasing a CPAP device. These are indeed prevalent mental disorders, and their impact on adherence to CPAP treatment is mostly intuitive (for more on these issues, see Chaps. 6, 19, and 20).

It is far more challenging to understand the impact of personality and patients suffering from personality disorders on obstructive sleep apnea therapy adherence.

In order to understand the concept of personality disorder, we first need to define the elusive concept of personality. Personality consists of enduring patterns of perceiving, relating to, and thinking about the environment and oneself that are exhibited across numerous social and personal contexts. A personality disorder is diagnosed when personality traits are so inflexible and maladaptive across a wide range of situations that they cause significant distress and impairment of social, occupational, and role functioning. Cognition, displays of emotion, impulsivity, and interpersonal behavior of the individual must deviate markedly from the expectations of the individual's culture in order to qualify as a personality disorder.

The estimated international prevalence of personality disorders in the community is 11% [4]. Personality disorders, in general, are significantly more common in males and the young, poorly educated, and unemployed, although individual personality disorders differ on gender and age. These disorders are highly comorbid with other, non-personality mental disorders.

The prevalence of personality disorders in clinical populations has been estimated to be over 64% [5]. Personality disorders were diagnosed by structured interview in 45.5% of 859 patients presenting for psychiatric outpatient treatment [6]. In comparison, the worldwide prevalence of anxiety disorders, depressive disorders, alcohol use disorder, and drug use disorder in adults was 3.76%, 3.44%, 1.4%, and 0.94%, respectively, in 2017 [1]. The prevalence of other well-known mental disorders such as schizophrenia or bipolar disorder is less than 1% [1].

One may wonder why personality disorders, which are much more prevalent than other well-known mental disorders in adults, pass almost unnoticed by healthcare providers? Some of the reasons lie in the fact that these disorders

R. Gilad (✉)
Department of Psychiatry, University of Toronto, Toronto, ON, Canada

Youthdale Child and Adolescent Sleep Centre, Toronto, ON, Canada

are ego-syntonic (experienced by the individuals as part of their being, and not as a disorder that inflicted them), and therefore, neither the patients nor their families will think of seeking medical assistance, until there is a crisis or a secondary mental disorder develops (e.g., depressive episode, suicide attempt, substance use, etc.), and the clinicians are faced with only the symptoms of the crisis that is fairly easy to diagnose, as opposed to the diagnosis of underlying personality disorder, which is far more complicated and time-consuming and requires special expertise.

11.2   Diagnosis of Personality Disorders

According to the *Diagnostic and Statistical Manual of Mental Disorders*, 5th Edition [7], in order to diagnose personality disorder, the following criteria must be met:

A. An enduring pattern of inner experience and behavior that deviates markedly from the expectations of the individual's culture. This pattern is manifested in two (or more) of the following areas:
   1. Cognition (i.e., ways of perceiving and interpreting self, other people, and events)
   2. Affectivity (i.e., the range, intensity, lability, and appropriateness of emotional response)
   3. Interpersonal functioning
   4. Impulse control
B. The enduring pattern is inflexible and pervasive across a broad range of personal and social situations.
C. The enduring pattern leads to clinically significant distress or impairment in social, occupational, or other important areas of functioning.
D. The pattern is stable and of long duration, and its onset can be traced back at least to adolescence or early adulthood.
E. The enduring pattern is not better explained as a manifestation or consequence of another mental disorder.
F. The enduring pattern is not attributable to the physiological effects of a substance (e.g., a drug of abuse, a medication) or another medical condition (e.g., head trauma).

The disorder is a consistent presence of certain behaviors and traits, with onset in middle to late adolescence, continuing into adult life, which might be characterized by [8]:

- Frequent mood swings
- Anger outbursts
- Social anxiety sufficient to cause difficulty making friends
- Need to be the center of attention
- Feeling of being widely cheated or taken advantage of
- Difficulty delaying gratification

- Not feeling there is anything wrong with one's behavior (ego-syntonic symptoms)
- Externalizing and blaming the world for one's behaviors and feelings

Adverse outcomes for patients with personality disorders include:

- Physical injury from fights and accidents due to impulsive and reckless behavior [9–11]
- Suicide attempts [12, 13]
- Unplanned pregnancy and high-risk sexual behavior [14, 15]
- Comorbid anxiety, mood, and/or substance use disorder [16, 17]
- Less favorable response to treatment for depression, anxiety disorder, or substance use disorder [18–22]
- Comorbid physical disorders, including cardiovascular disease, arthritis, diabetes, and gastrointestinal conditions; reduced life expectancy [23–25]
- Functional impairment (e.g., self-care, work, and interpersonal functioning) [18, 26]

The different personality disorders are subcategorized to three clusters [7]:

Cluster A
- *Paranoid* – Distrust and suspiciousness of others such that their motives are interpreted as malevolent
- *Schizoid* – Detachment from social relationships and a restricted range of expression of emotions in interpersonal settings
- *Schizotypal* – Social and interpersonal deficits marked by acute discomfort with, and reduced capacity for, close relationships as well as by cognitive or perceptual distortions and eccentric behavior

Cluster B
- *Antisocial* – Disregard for and violating the rights of others, lying, stealing, defaulting on debts, neglect of children or other dependents
- *Borderline* – Instability of interpersonal relationships, self-image, affects, and control over impulses
- *Histrionic* – Excessive emotionality and attention seeking
- *Narcissistic* – Grandiosity (in fantasy or behavior), need for admiration, and lack of empathy

Cluster C
- *Avoidant* – Social inhibition, feelings of inadequacy, and hypersensitivity to negative evaluation
- *Dependent* – Feelings of inadequacy, inability to make own decisions, submissiveness, avoidance of confrontation for fear of losing source of support

- *Obsessive-compulsive* – Preoccupation with perfectionism, mental and interpersonal control, and orderliness, at the expense of flexibility, openness, and efficiency

Avoidant personality disorder and obsessive-compulsive personality disorder are the most common in the community. Borderline personality disorder and avoidant personality disorder are the most common in clinical populations.

Despite the diagnostic manuals' (DSM and ICD) effort to characterize personality disorders into distinct subcategories, in clinical practice, the most prevalent personality disorder diagnosis by clinicians is "personality disorder unspecified." This demonstrates that most clinicians can diagnose a patient suffering from a personality disorder, but the subtleties of diagnosing a specific subcategory of personality disorder are less helpful in the clinical realm.

In the latest edition, the DSM also proposed an alternative method of conceptualizing the diagnosis of personality disorders, not in a categorical model but in a dimensional model. This model assesses personality not in the presence of pathology but as a spectrum of traits that are related to self (identity and self-direction) and interpersonal (empathy and intimacy).

Other diagnostic views also consider the personality as a continuum of traits that can fluctuate over time. One well-established model is the "NEO five factors" [27, 28] that measures the person's personality on the spectrum of five axes: Neuroticism, Extraversion, Openness to experience, Agreeableness, and Conscientiousness.

The main therapeutic value in understanding personality disorders derives from the psychotherapeutic literature. The first to address the concept of personality and personality disorders was psychoanalytic scholars such as Sigmund Freud, Anna Freud, Melanie Klein, Donald Winnicott, Heinz Kohut, and many others, but it was Otto F. Kernberg whose pivotal work in the field of personality disorders from the 1960s onwards laid out the foundations of current psychoanalytic understanding on the concept of personality and its disorders.

In his work, Kernberg describes the personality as a continuum which he named "personality organization" [29]. The more mature (developed) the personality organization, the more the self can be distinguished from objects, and reality testing is preserved (i.e., the person knows to distinguish between his thoughts and real signal from the outside world), the more the person will use mature defensive strategies and coping mechanisms, and the more able he/she will be in sustaining and coping with anxiety and difficult emotional situations.

In contrast, the less mature the personality organization is, the more it is prone to "glitches" in his reality testing with less ability to discern between outside real signal and one's own thoughts. Moreover, a person with a less mature personality organization will be more reliant on the use of immature defense mechanisms, such as projection, i.e., the attribution of one's own thoughts and feeling to the other (e.g., an employee that is resentful to his employer will not feel resentful but will be certain that his employer is resentful to him and is even contemplating on firing him); splitting, the inability to perceive an object (e.g., another person, a job) as having good and bad sides all together, and attributing only good or bad to anything; and idealization-devaluation, the tendency to treat someone else with blind admiration that can be flipped in a fraction of a second to total despise and hatred. The person with a low-level personality organization will be less able to sustain anxiety, uncertainty, and ambiguity. He will also display difficulties in maintaining sustained ego functions, and therefore, his ability to function will be unstable (e.g., he may organize his young child an extravagant birthday party with numerous participants, but immediately at its end, he will retire to lying in bed for weeks, neglecting his family, work, and his personal hygeine).

Thus, it is not surprising how after a pleasant first meeting between the patient and a physician, the patient might declare that he "met the greatest doctor on earth" only to be slandering the doctor next time stating "a doctors that needs to have his license revoked", after waiting too long in the waiting room.

Kernberg's early work was transformed to a therapeutic method for the treatment of personality disorders, called transference-focused psychotherapy (TFP). It is a modification of the classic psychodynamic treatment.

Other psychotherapeutic approaches conceptualized the understanding on personality disorders in a different way. As opposed to the psychoanalytic approach which attributed the arrest in emotional development to the relations between the child and his early caregivers (objects relations theories), other therapeutic approaches emphasized the presence of traumatic and real adverse events in the child's development that contribute to the development of a personality disorder (e.g., emotional, physical, and sexual abuse and neglect).

Marsha Linehan and colleagues developed the dialectical behavioral therapy (DBT) for borderline and other personality disorders [30]. The approach sees the development of personality disorders as a combination of inborn vulnerability of emotional dysregulation that was met with invalidating and often abusing parenting. In DBT, the patient, through a very intensive, validating, and empathic treatment (both individual psychotherapy and skill group learning), will be able to recognize, trust, and control his/her emotions and reactions, to himself/herself and others. The approach combines behavioral and cognitive techniques with mindfulness, emotional regulation, and social skills.

Jeffrey E. *Young* and colleagues developed schema focused therapy (SFT) [31]. This therapeutic approach for the treatment of personality disorders emphasizes the maladaptive cognitive schemes that developed during childhood and adolescent. The therapeutic process includes cognitive techniques aimed in unveiling the maladaptive automatic cognitive and emotional schemes (primarily forged during childhood) that drive the patient's cognition, affect, and behavioral reactions. After some degree of insight was achieved, the patient then practices, with the therapist's direction, how to "acquire" more "freedom" in making his/her choices, not by being unconsciously driven by the maladaptive schemes but by better acknowledging his/her emotions and thoughts and acting on his/her best adult interest.

Peter Fonagy and colleagues [30] developed the mentalization-based therapy (MBT). The approach tries to treat the patient suffering from a personality disorder with the ability, through therapy, to take notice the processes that are running through their head (i.e., mentalization). The therapist becomes a model to assess their own mental processes and reflecting them to the patient for the patient to start understanding how to be able to access the meta-cognition. The premise is that once the patients gain awareness to these thought and emotional processes, they might gain more ability to control them.

All the above therapeutic methods have proven efficiency in the treatment of patients with personality disorders, but are all lengthy (usually between 3 and 5 years of treatment) and require enormous dedication and motivation by the patients and their families in adhering to the treatment, which is emotionally painful. In most countries, these treatments are paid by the patients or their families, as unfortunately, although their impact on the patient's health, quality of life, and even life expectancy is paramount, they are not covered by public health insurances. This makes them out of reach for most patients who actually need them.

Pharmacological treatments (mainly antidepressants and mood stabilizers) are used in the treatment of patients suffering from personality disorders (with little to no evidence to support their efficiency) [30], mostly as a desperate attempt to help the patients gain some control over their mood, impulsivity, and aggression. If secondary mental disorders co-exist (e.g., mood disorder, substance use disorder, sleep, anxiety or trauma-related disorders), they are treated (usually pharmacologically) according to regular clinical guidelines.

11.3 Personality Disorders and Adherence to CPAP and Obstructive Sleep Apnea Therapies

There is a paucity of published data about the relationship between mental disorders and specifically personality disorders and adherence to CPAP and other obstructive sleep apnea therapies.

Sleep disorders (mainly insomnia disorder) are an integral feature of almost all psychiatric disorders (particularly mood and anxiety disorders, but also trauma-related disorders and substance use disorders) [30]. Even in mental disorders in which sleep disruption is not a part of the diagnostic criteria of the disorder (e.g., attention deficit hyperactivity disorder, obsessive-compulsive disorders, eating disorders, personality disorders, etc.), they are far more prevalent than in the general population [30]. Thus, it is highly likely that patients suffering from personality or other mental disorders will seek help for their insomnia in a sleep clinic setting and would also be diagnosed with obstructive sleep apnea. As most patients with personality disorders do not perceive their condition as a mental disorder or even a medical problem, it is likely that the sleep physician will encounter patients with personality disorders who seek relief for their sleep difficulties, before any mental health professional have even examined them in the past.

Patients suffering from personality disorders might vigorously reject any insinuation made by a healthcare professional to the fact that they might be suffering from psychiatric symptoms (or disorder), but as the diagnosis of obstructive sleep apnea (OSA) does not carry the stigma related to mental disorders and is mostly perceived in the public as a "general medical" condition, it is possible that patients displaying symptoms characteristic of personality disorder might be more receptive to the diagnosis of OSA and willing to go about possible treatment options.

It is well-known that being afflicted with a severe mental illness (SMI) increases the patient's risk for cardiovascular disease [32], obesity and metabolic disorders, COPD, and respiratory disease and decreases life expectancy by 10–20 years [30]. The excessive morbidity and mortality risk is attributed to pathological processes of the mental disorders (i.e., metabolic changes and microvascular pathology), but also to the metabolic effects of the pharmacological treatments and the patient's lifestyle (sedentary lifestyle, cigarette smoking, etc.).

In studies that examined CPAP adherence in the military veteran population, patients suffering from severe mental illness (SMI) (e.g., psychotic disorders, bipolar disorder, depressive disorder, post-traumatic stress disorder) [33, 34] had lower CPAP adherence than without a mental disorder, in both first 90-day use and subsequent long-term use.

Studies aimed at examining the relations between CPAP adherence and personality traits using different modalities of personality assessment have failed to demonstrated significant association between certain personality traits and CPAP adherence [35–37].

Adherence refers to the degree that an individual follows a recommended health or illness-related recommendation [38]. Patient adherence is dependent upon multiple economic, social, and psychological constraints [39].

Factor that were considered to be associated with CPAP adherence [40]:

- Treatment method issues surrounding use of the CPAP machine: the cumbersome lifestyle change, adverse side effects, and associated stigma
- Clinical, situational, cognitive, and personality factors of the patient
- Family: the influence of family, encouragement, and spousal satisfaction with treatment
- Physician: the physician's role in providing education, maintaining open communication, gaining patient commitment and involvement, and opportune scheduling of follow-up appointments
- Healthcare professionals: personal and program support that is offered by healthcare professionals
- Healthcare facility: concerning wait times, organization, and flexibility
- Governmental policies: issues surrounding the funding of CPAP machines, restricting nonadherent OSA patients from driving, and health coverage for repeat evaluations

Patients generally make the decision to adhere to CPAP therapy early during the first week of therapy [41–44]. Those who adhere generally increase their duration of nightly use gradually.

While considering the above factors determining CPAP adherence, it is reasonable to predict what could be the challenges to CPAP adherence in patients suffering from mental illness in general and personality disorders in particular.

Patients suffering personality disorders (and sometimes other severe mental disorders) will have difficulties in adhering to therapy for several reasons:

- Intrapsychic aspects: lethargy and low motivation or inability to sustain function for a prolonged period. These can lead to neglecting treatment for one's medical condition and non-adherence with physician appointments, medication regimen, and medical recommendations. A patient who suffers from a personality disorder might enthusiastically declare in the physician's office their immediate intention to "take care of themselves" (i.e., go purchase a CPAP machine that same day), while by the time they reach the clinic's door, this notion will completely evaporates from their mind, either due to internal or external distractions, and in the next follow-up visit, the physician will find out the patient had not started treatment. Another aspect that is an obstacle for adherence is the reduced, to the point of non-existing tolerability for anxiety and decision-making in an atmosphere of uncertainty. It is likely that in the face of anxiety stemming from the need to start new and potentially subjectively uncomfortable/intrusive treatment, while acknowledging its importance and the possible complications of not treating the OSA, the patient may unconsciously suppress the awareness of the illness and its ramifications all together

and will not start treatment. The difficulty of focusing on the many steps to become a functional user of CPAP might lead the patient to quickly abandon the exercise of filling out forms and applications for governmental or other financial help, even in the cost of not receiving treatment. If not contacted directly, it is unlikely that the patient will initiate contact with the clinic to reschedule a missed appointment or to renew a prescription.

- Medication and substance use aspects: Many patients with severe personality disorders or other mental disorders are often treated with medications that may cause sedation. Many such patients are also using unprescribed sedative medications (e.g., benzodiazepines, opioids, etc.), cannabis, and alcohol. All these agents may contribute to lethargy and reduced motivation to adhere to physician follow-up appointments and may cause patients to fall asleep in different locations in their house, other than their bed, and at different times during the day. This may cause patients not to wear their CPAP mask for much of their sleep, even when they have already obtained a machine.
- Familial, socioeconomic, and housing aspects: Patients suffering from severe mental illness and especially those suffering from personality disorders, and substance use disorders, are extremely socially isolated. Their childhood and upbringing have (in many cases) been in an abusive and emotionally detached family environment, or they may have been raised apart from their biological family (e.g., in foster or group homes); therefore, it comes as no surprise that many of them are completely estranged from their immediate family and relatives, or maintaining only minimal relations with their families. As their behavior might be impulsive and aggressive, or extremely avoidant, their ability to establish beneficial and long-standing prosperous intrapersonal relationships (either friendly or romantic) is heavily impaired. Therefore, it is unlikely that such patients will have the assistance of a spouse, friends, or family members in their CPAP use. As their intimate relationships are often short and emotionally explosive, being with a partner (as opposed to the general population) does not necessarily serve as a treatment promoting factor, and may even reduce adherence to treatment. The patient may not want to be perceived in a new relationship, as old or sick. For the same reason, such individuals mostly reside alone or with roommates, mostly in rented apartments. Often, they are forced to repeatedly move between houses, due to altercations with their neighbors or the inability to make rent payments. This compounds the problem of getting used to using a CPAP device regularly. In contrast to other severe mental disorders (such as schizophrenia or bipolar disorder) in which after hospitalization due to a psychotic, manic, or suicidal episodes, the society recognizes the individual as

someone who suffers from a severe mental health disorder, and might offer help in accommodation and housing, finance, and supportive care (e.g., case manager or personal support worker), patients suffering from personality disorders don't see themselves as in need of such help, and usually the social and medical establishments do not offer them any assistance aside from psychiatric follow-up. There is often a false perception (by the patients, their families, and the medical and social establishments) that these patients are able to provide their own needs. Thus, it is very unlikely that they would be given assistance from a support worker in their diagnostic process and treatment of obstructive sleep apnea. As their ability to maintain constant employment is also very low (due to inability to maintain continuous function and frequent anger outbursts directed at colleagues and employers), their financial situation is often grim, and they require governmental aid programs. Thus, all "out-of-pocket" financial expenditure is likely to create difficulties.

- The relationship between the patient and the medical establishment and physician-patient relationship: As many of these patients grow up in an abusive or neglecting and unsupportive environment, any form of authority, such as the medical establishment, can immediately evoke high emotional tone and expression. These responses often originate from the repetitive re-enactment of negative childhood experiences. This emotional hypervigilance might activate the unconscious automatic responses of defending oneself toward that is considered by the patient as aggressive and punitive authority (i.e., the physician or the clinic's staff), either by responding aggressively or by avoidance. This can cause enormous difficulties in establishing a good rapport and cause the patient to distrust the physician, with tension in the doctor-patient relationship, poor communication skills, dependency, or excessive demands. Patients run the risk of alienating healthcare providers with late night phone calls, angry outbursts, repeated visits or admissions, signing out against medical advice, or being otherwise non-compliant with recommended treatment. Often, they will complain about their caregivers and will frequently replace their treating physicians and clinics. Some patients might also discontinue prescribed medications in the personal belief that herbal therapy is more effective, lie about compliance with treatment, and misinterpret delay in the clinician returning a phone call, leading to a feeling of being rejected and acting out by stopping or overdosing on a medications. They may worry about unusual side effects from a prescribed medication, such as blocking the body from absorbing essential nutrients or vitamins, or believe that one is being tricked into taking something harmful.

11.4 Increasing Adherence to CPAP and Other Treatments

In order to try and increase CPAP adherence, there is a need to address the underlying impediments to adherence in this population of patients.

- Clinic organization: Try to make it a "one-stop shop." There is a higher chance that a patient who suffers from a personality disorder (or any severe mental disorder) will be able to transcend the diagnostic process and actually start using CPAP treatment. Incorporating in the clinic the full process of purchasing, mask fitting, and filling out all required forms and applications, with all instructions and technical support done at the same place, with the same team, on the same day when the diagnosis is presented to the patient, might yield benefits for both the patients and the clinical team.
- Physician-patient relationship: Try to be as empathic and direct as possible. It should be acknowledged by the physician (or any other member of the healthcare team) that treating patients with personality disorders is a task that puts a heavy emotional burden on the caregiver. Awareness of one's emotions and reactions toward patients and open discussion about it in the clinical team might reduce the tendency of "falling into the trap" of responding to the patient as the patient unconsciously provokes the physician (i.e., to either respond in an aggressive manner or to avoid interactions and become indifferent). The "trick" is to always keep in mind that the unpleasant reactions by the patient do not necessarily suggest maltreatment or that the physician is bad but reflect automatic and rigid reactions to authority figures from the past. The physician then can try and direct the conversation more toward the needs, thoughts, and concerns of the patient and less toward explaining what the treatment is for, and what could be the repercussions of non-adherence to treatment. For example, the patient might say "so you're forcing me to take this treatment…", and the physician might rephrase "I am not forcing you to do anything you don't want to; I am only recommending that you start treatment, but this decision is totally up to you. If you are interested, I can share with you what is my knowledge about other people's experiences who are using this treatment."
- Try to explain in detail what the next steps will include (e.g., how long it generally takes to get used to sleeping with a CPAP machine, the need for pressure titration sleep study, etc.). Reduce anxiety and uncertainty to the minimum possible.
- Support: Make every possible effort to connect the patient with any type of support (whether a person or organization). Explain to the patients that for no fault of their own,

it will be extremely hard for them to adhere to therapy without assistance. Assess with the patients whether there is someone in their environment (family relative, friend, neighbor) that might be willing to accompany them to purchase a machine and will help them install the machine at their home. If the patient comes up with a name, immediately call (or have one of the clinic's staff call) the person (after obtaining the patient's consent) "while the iron is hot." Explain the situation and the need for help, and set with the patient and the person who is willing to support them a precise schedule of when and how they will go to purchase a device and what would be the next steps in the treatment program. Encourage the person to accompany the patient to his next appointments.

- Other healthcare providers: Connect with the patient's other health providers (e.g., family physician, psychiatrist, social worker, etc.). If needed, directly call the patient's primary care provider (PCP), and explain the diagnosis and treatment plan. Even if the patient will not proceed with the treatment plan, there is a good chance he/she will contact their PCP for other reasons in the foreseeable future, and the informed PCP might ask them again about OSA treatment and might reignite the treatment. A CPAP coordinator (see Chap. 33) in a clinic can be an enormous boon. Refer to a psychologist if there is ambivalence or significant anxiety about CPAP use (see Chap. 6). It can only succeed as a team effort. Consult with the other providers on how they can support their treatment (e.g., by reducing sleep impairing medications, providing topical ointments to treat mask bruises, etc.).

11.5 Conclusion

Treating a patient suffering from severe mental illness and especially a personality disorder is no doubtebly a daunting and challenging task. It is sometimes made harder due to its emotional toll as compared to treating the most severe of medical conditions. Nevertheless, if one wishes to be successful and increase treatment adherence for OSA or any other medical condition, there is no escape from "diving" into the patients' intricate intrapsychic realm and addressing their responses and attitudes from a compassionate and emphatic point of view, that is, being able to "see" their anxiety and insecurity beyond their maladaptive and sometimes aggressive reactions, connecting with the patient on the emotional level. This is referred to as "forming a therapeutic alliance" [30]. As in most cases, success in OSA treatment stands almost entirely on the patient's cooperation. Cognizance of this point will allow one to take the sometime extraordinary measures that are required to get a patient with a personality disorder to be adherent with the recommended treatment.

References

1. Mental health – Our world in data [Internet]. Available from: https://ourworldindata.org/mental-health
2. WHO | Mental disorders affect one in four people [Internet]. Available from: https://www.who.int/whr/2001/media_centre/press_release/en/
3. Vigo D, Thornicroft G, Atun R. Estimating the true global burden of mental illness. Lancet Psychiatry. 2016;3:171–8. Available from: https://pubmed.ncbi.nlm.nih.gov/26851330/
4. Torgersen S. In: Oldham JM, Skodol AE, editors. American Psychiatric Publishing textbook of personality disorders. 2nd ed. Arlington: American Psychiatric Publishing; 2014. p. 109.
5. Widiger TA, editor. The oxford handbook of personality disorders. Oxford University Press; 2012. https://doi.org/10.1093/oxfordhb/9780199735013.001.0001.
6. Zimmerman M, Rothschild L, Chelminski I. The prevalence of DSM-IV personality disorders in psychiatric outpatients. Am J Psychiatry. 2005;162(10):1911–8. https://doi.org/10.1176/appi.ajp.162.10.1911.
7. American Psychiatric Association. Diagnostic and statistical manual of mental disorders, fifth edition (DSM-5). 5th ed. Arlington: American Psychiatric Association; 2013.
8. Langbehn DR, Pfohl BM, Reynolds S, Clark LA, Battaglia M, Bellodi L, et al. The Iowa personality disorder screen: development and preliminary validation of a brief screening interview. J Personal Disord. 1999;13(1):75–89. https://doi.org/10.1521/pedi.1999.13.1.75.
9. Dumais A, Lesage AD, Boyer R, Lalovic A, Chawky N, Ménard-Buteau C, et al. Psychiatric risk factors for motor vehicle fatalities in young men. Can J Psychiatr. 2005;50(13):838–44. https://doi.org/10.1177/070674370505001306.
10. Cadoret RJ, Leve LD, Devor E. Genetics of aggressive and violent behavior. Psychiatr Clin North Am. 1997;20(2):301–22. https://doi.org/10.1016/s0193-953x(05)70314-2.
11. Caspi A, Begg D, Dickson N, Harrington H, Langley J, Moffitt TE, et al. Personality differences predict health-risk behaviors in young adulthood: evidence from a longitudinal study. J Pers Soc Psychol. 1997;73(5):1052–63. https://doi.org/10.1037/0022-3514.73.5.1052.
12. Soloff PH, Fabio A. Prospective predictors of suicide attempts in borderline personality disorder at one, two, and two-to-five year follow-up. J Personal Disord. 2008;22(2):123–34. https://doi.org/10.1521/pedi.2008.22.2.123.
13. Kessler RC, Borges G, Walters EE. Prevalence of and risk factors for lifetime suicide attempts in the National Comorbidity Survey. Arch Gen Psychiatry. 1999;56(7):617. https://doi.org/10.1001/archpsyc.56.7.617.
14. Zanarini MC, Parachini EA, Frankenburg FR, Holman JB, Hennen J, Reich DB, et al. Sexual relationship difficulties among borderline patients and axis ii comparison subjects. J Nerv Ment Dis. 2003;191(7):479–82. https://doi.org/10.1097/01.nmd.0000081628.93982.1d.
15. Daley SE, Burge D, Hammen C. Borderline personality disorder symptoms as predictors of 4-year romantic relationship dysfunction in young women: addressing issues of specificity. J Abnorm Psychol. 2000;109(3):451–60. https://doi.org/10.1037/0021-843x.109.3.451.
16. Hasin DS, Stinson FS, Ogburn E, Grant BF. Prevalence, correlates, disability, and comorbidity of DSM-IV alcohol abuse and dependence in the United States. Arch Gen Psychiatry. 2007;64(7):830. https://doi.org/10.1001/archpsyc.64.7.830.
17. Huang Y, Kotov R, de Girolamo G, Preti A, Angermeyer M, Benjet C, et al. DSM-IV personality disorders in the WHO World Mental Health Surveys. Br J Psychiatry. 2009;195(1):46–53. Available from: https://pubmed.ncbi.nlm.nih.gov/19567896

18. Newton-Howes G, Tyrer P, Johnson T. Personality disorder and the outcome of depression: meta-analysis of published studies. Br J Psychiatry. 2006;188(1):13–20. https://doi.org/10.1192/bjp.188.1.13.

19. Hansen B, Vogel PA, Stiles TC, Gunnar GK. Influence of co-morbid generalized anxiety disorder, panic disorder and personality disorders on the outcome of cognitive behavioural treatment of obsessive-compulsive disorder. Cogn Behav Ther. 2007;36(3):145–55. https://doi.org/10.1080/16506070701259374.

20. Jansson I, Hesse M, Fridell M. Personality disorder features as predictors of symptoms five years post-treatment. Am J Addict. 2008;17(3):172–5. https://doi.org/10.1080/10550490802019725.

21. Gabbard GO, Simonsen E. The impact of personality and personality disorders on the treatment of depression. Personal Ment Health. 2007;1(2):161–75. https://doi.org/10.1002/pmh.21.

22. Bieling PJ, Green SM, Macqueen G. The impact of personality disorders on treatment outcome in bipolar disorder: a review. Personal Ment Health. 2007;1(1):2–13. https://doi.org/10.1002/pmh.13.

23. Quirk SE, El-Gabalawy R, Brennan SL, Bolton JM, Sareen J, Berk M, et al. Personality disorders and physical comorbidities in adults from the United States: data from the National Epidemiologic Survey on Alcohol and Related Conditions. Soc Psychiatry Psychiatr Epidemiol. 2014;50(5):807–20. https://doi.org/10.1007/s00127-014-0974-1.

24. Quirk SE, Berk M, Chanen AM, Koivumaa-Honkanen H, Brennan-Olsen SL, Pasco JA, et al. Population prevalence of personality disorder and associations with physical health comorbidities and health care service utilization: a review. Personal Disord Theory Res Treat. 2016;7(2):136–46. https://doi.org/10.1037/per0000148.

25. Fok ML-Y, Hayes RD, Chang C-K, Stewart R, Callard FJ, Moran P. Life expectancy at birth and all-cause mortality among people with personality disorder. J Psychosom Res. 2012;73(2):104–7. https://doi.org/10.1016/j.jpsychores.2012.05.001.

26. Skodol AE. Impact of personality pathology on psychosocial functioning. Curr Opin Psychol. 2018;21:33–8. https://doi.org/10.1016/j.copsyc.2017.09.006.

27. Costa PT, McCrae RR. Normal personality assessment in clinical practice: the NEO personality inventory. Psychol Assess. 1992;4(1):5–13. Available from: /record/1992-25763-001

28. Briggs SR. The optimal level of measurement for personality constructs. In: Personality psychology. Springer; 1989. p. 246–60.

29. Kernberg O. Borderline personality organization. J Am Psychoanal Assoc. 1967;15(3):641–85.

30. Sadock BJ, Sadock VA, Ruiz P, editors. Kaplan and Sadock's comprehensive textbook of psychiatry. 10th ed. Lippincott Williams & Wilkins (LWW); 2017.

31. Young JE, Klosko JS, Weishaar ME. Schema therapy: a practitioner's guide. Guilford Press; 2006. Available from: https://www.guilford.com/books/Schema-Therapy/Young-Klosko-Weishaar/9781593853723

32. Newcomer JW, Hennekens CH. Severe mental illness and risk of cardiovascular disease. JAMA. 2007;298:1794–6.

33. El-Solh AA, Ayyar L, Akinnusi M, Relia S, Akinnusi O. Positive airway pressure adherence in veterans with posttraumatic stress disorder. Sleep. 2010;33(11):1495–500. Available from: /pmc/articles/PMC2954699/?report=abstract

34. May AM, Gandotra K, Jaskiw GE. 1106 associations between severe mental illness and positive airway adherence in a veteran cohort. Sleep. 2020;43(Supplement_1):A420–1. Available from: https://academic.oup.com/sleep/article/43/Supplement_1/A420/5847358

35. Wild MR. Can psychological factors help us to determine adherence to CPAP? A prospective study. Eur Respir J. 2004;24(3):461–5. https://doi.org/10.1183/09031936.04.00114603.

36. Poulet C, Veale D, Arnol N, Lévy P, Pepin JL, Tyrrell J. Psychological variables as predictors of adherence to treatment by continuous positive airway pressure. Sleep Med. 2009;10(9):993–9. https://doi.org/10.1016/j.sleep.2009.01.007.

37. Edinger JD, Carwile S, Miller P, Hope V, Mayti C. Psychological status, syndromatic measures, and compliance with nasal CPAP therapy for sleep apnea. Percept Mot Skills. 1994;78(3_suppl):1116–8. https://doi.org/10.2466/pms.1994.78.3c.1116.

38. Taylor SE. Health psychology. 10th ed. Columbia University Press; 1991. p. 444.

39. Lutfey KE, Wishner WJ. Beyond "compliance" is "adherence". Improving the prospect of diabetes care. Diabetes Care. 1999;22(4):635–9. https://doi.org/10.2337/diacare.22.4.635.

40. Shapiro GK, Shapiro CM. Factors that influence CPAP adherence: an overview. Sleep Breath. 2010;14:323–35.

41. Sawyer AM, Gooneratne NS, Marcus CL, Ofer D, Richards KC, Weaver TE. A systematic review of CPAP adherence across age groups: clinical and empiric insights for developing CPAP adherence interventions. Sleep Med Rev. 2011;15:343–56.

42. Aloia MS, Arnedt JT, Stanchina M, Millman RP. How early in treatment is PAP adherence established? Revisiting night-to-night variability. Behav Sleep Med. 2007;5(3):229–40.

43. Rosenthal L, Gerhardstein R, Lumley A, et al. CPAP therapy in patients with mild OSA: implementation and treatment outcome. Sleep Med. 2000;1(3):215–20. Available from: http://www.ncbi.nlm.nih.gov/pubmed/10828432

44. Budhiraja R, Parthasarathy S, Drake CL, Roth T, Sharief I, Budhiraja P, Saunders V, Hudgel DW. Early CPAP use identifies subsequent adherence to CPAP therapy. Sleep. 2007;30(3):320–4. https://doi.org/10.1093/sleep/30.3.320.

John O'Reilly

Abbreviations

AAA	American Automobile Association
CPAP	Continuous positive airway pressure
CVD	Cardiovascular disease
EDS	Excessive daytime sleepiness
FN-PSG	Full-night polysomnography
ICER	Incremental cost-effectiveness ratio
MVAs	Motor vehicle accidents
OHS	Obesity hypoventilation syndrome
OSA	Obsructive sleep apnoea
OSAS	Obsructive sleep apnoea syndrome
PAP	Positive airway pressure
QALY	Quality-adjusted life year
QOL	Quality of life
SES	Socioeconomic status
SN-PSG	Single night polysomnography
UPHM	Unmonitored portable home monitoring

12.1 Prevalence of OSA

It is estimated that almost one billion people suffer from OSA worldwide, with prevalence exceeding 50% in some countries [1]. Most cases of OSA remain undiagnosed and untreated, even in developed countries [2].

It has been estimated that 936 million (95% CI 903–970) adults aged 30–69 years (men and women) have mild-to-severe OSA and 425 million (range 399–450) adults aged 30–69 years have moderate-to-severe obstructive sleep apnoea globally. The number of affected individuals was highest in China, followed by the USA, Brazil and India [1].

The landmark US Wisconsin Sleep Cohort Study evaluated the prevalence of sleep apnea in state employees and

demonstrated that 24% of men and 9% of women have mild-to-severe OSAS (AHI > 5) [3]. Another study showed that 17% of men and 9% of women aged 50–70 years have at least moderate-to-severe OSA [4]. A more recent Swiss epidemiological study in an adult general poplation showed that 49.7% of men and 23.4% of women have moderate-to-severe OSA defined as an apnoea-hypopnoea index (AHI) $\geq$ 15/h [5].

OSA prevalence is higher in older adults; males; minority races; people with high body mass index, large neck circumference, craniofacial abnormalities, and menopausal status; smokers; and among people who consume alcohol [6]. In addition, prevalence is higher in certain medical populations, including those with coronary artery disease (moderate-to-severe OSAS in 55% of patients) and diabetes mellitus (37% of patients) [7].

12.2 Burden of Untreated OSA

12.2.1 Clinical Burden of Untreated OSA

The consequences of untreated OSA are considered to represent a great threat to individual and global health [8]. Untreated OSA patients are at a significantly increased risk of developing daytime sleepiness and have reduced quality life (QOL), as well as cardiovascular, metabolic and neurocognitive diseases, anxiety and depression, motor vehicle accidents (MVAs), work accidents and all-cause mortality [9–12]

Individuals with asthma who are high risk for OSA were 2.87 times more likely to have insufficient asthma control than those at risk for OSA [13]. OSA has been associated with an increased risk for cancer and mortality in OSA patients, particularly for those with severe OSA (AHI > 30) [7]. Perioperative complications including need for prolonged intubation, need for re-intubation, pneumonias, aspiration, arrhythmias and cardiac arrest are more prevalent in those with untreated OSA than individuals without OSA [7].

J. O'Reilly (✉)
Aintree University Hospital, Liverpool, UK

London Sleep Centre, London, UK

© The Author(s), under exclusive license to Springer Nature Switzerland AG 2022
C. M. Shapiro et al. (eds.), *CPAP Adherence*, https://doi.org/10.1007/978-3-030-93146-9_12

12.2.2 Societal and Economic Burden of Untreated OSA

OSA leads to high usage of healthcare resources [14, 15]. Case-control studies have consistently shown that OSA patients use more physician services and are admitted to hospital at greater rates in years prior to diagnosis compared with individuals without OSA [16].

OSA has predictable effects in decreasing economic outcomes [3, 17]. Determination of the economic consequences of OSA, and the effects of treatment and treatment adherence, is complex and requires assessment of disease severity and patient clinical and socioeconomic factors including occupation and driving risk, as well as geographical factors [16]. Direct economic costs can include comorbidities such as high blood pressure or diabetes, motor vehicle or workplace accidents and compensating behaviors such as substance abuse of pills, tobacco and alcohol. Indirect economic costs can include decreased productivity at work, reduced quality of life and stress in interpersonal relationships. Direct costs associated with comorbidities include increased medical expenses due to emergency room visits, hospital inpatient visits, medication use as well as increased mortality rates. In 2015, the cost of diagnosing and treating obstructive sleep apnoea in the USA was approximately US$12·4 billion [18].

Untreated OSA can lead to about a twofold increase in medical expenses because of cardiovascular disease (CVD) morbidity [16]. Healthcare costs are not normally distributed, such that the costliest and the sickest upper third of patients consume 65–82% of all medical costs. There are limited numbers of studies exploring the effect of CPAP on medical costs, and this important area requires further investigation. Identifying barriers to CPAP adherence will enable the development of effective interventions tailored to improve treatment, especially in the costliest and sickest at-risk populations that consume the most medical resources [16, 19].

The medical costs of undiagnosed OSA patients are about twice those of controls [15, 16, 19]. Frost and Sullivan's analysis of only the most well-understood comorbidities linked to OSA indicated that costs among the undiagnosed OSA population were approximately $30 billion in the USA in 2015. This model considered only medication and healthcare utilization costs, and only the portion of overall comorbidity costs that could be potentially avoided if OSA were treated [18].

Accurate diagnosis and appropriate treatment will reduce direct and indirect costs related to CVD, occupational and driving risks, but diagnostic procedures, treatment and management costs of OSA add to direct costs whether or not patients maintain long-term adherence to treatment. Active patient engagement in their care leads to better health outcomes and measurable cost savings [16].

12.2.3 Patient Factors in Socioeconomic Burden of OSA

Patient factors that can affect healthcare utilization include not only illness level (perceived health state, symptoms and diagnosis) but also predisposing factors (demographics, social structure and beliefs) and enabling factors (income, insurance type and family characteristics) [20].

Independent determinants of costs have been identified as hyperlipidemia (adjusting for age, AHI and BMI) for 'most costly' young adult male OSA patients, and as age, BMI, CVD, hypertension supplied psychoactive drugs, and hyperlipidaemia and diabetes (adjusting for AHI) for 'most costly' middle-aged adults, and as CVD and supplied psychoactive drugs in older adults [21, 22].

Excessive daytime sleepiness (EDS) is associated with increased societal burden, which may have an impact on healthcare utilization and costs. Several studies indicate an association between EDS in OSA and indirect economic burden, including motor vehicle accidents (MVAs), near misses, work productivity, mood and QOL [23].

Low socioeconomic status (SES) is an independent risk factor for CVD among adult OSA patients requiring treatment. Patients with OSA incur a significant socioeconomic burden because their lower employment rates and the lower earning potential among those who are employed exceed the direct costs of the disease [24]. Patients with OSA and people with low low socioeconomic status (SES) have higher rates of obesity, glucose intolerance and cigarette smoking [16, 25]. Low SES may lead to a lack of effective functioning in self-care, particularly in chronic illnesses, due to poor health literacy, knowledge, skill and confidence. OSA patients with low SES were the sickest patients, and they had the lowest referral rate to sleep diagnosis services because of poor awareness and knowledge [16].

12.2.4 Geographic Factors in Socioeconomic Burden of OSA

Healthcare utilization and costs vary by geographic setting, and healthcare utilization is difficult to compare among different health systems that have more than one payer, as in the USA [16].

A cross-sectional study in the USA in 1999 found that, in the year prior to the diagnosis of OSA, mean annual medical cost per patient was $2720, versus $1384 for age-matched and sex-matched controls [19]. Regression analysis showed that the apnoea hypopnea index (AHI) among cases was significantly related to annual medical costs after adjusting for age, sex and BMI. This study estimated the annual cost of treating the medical consequences of OSA in 1999 at $3.4 billion in the USA [19].

Data from the Danish National Patient Registry found that OSA was associated with about 2.8-fold greater direct health costs from general practitioner care, in-hospital services and medication used up to 12 years before OSA diagnosis [24]. In this study, snoring, and especially OSA and obesity hypoventilation syndrome (OHS), were associated with significantly higher rates of health-related contact, medication use and unemployment and accounted for increased socioeconomic costs (especially indirect costs). These effects increased with the severity of OSA, and patients with OHS had the lowest employment rates. The income level of patients with OSA and OHS who were employed was lower than that of employed control subjects. The annual excess total direct and indirect costs for patients who snore and with OSA and OHS were €705, €3860 and €11,320, respectively. Patients with snoring episodes, OSA and OHS received an annual mean excess social transfer income of €147, €879 and €3263, respectively. These socioeconomic consequences were present up to 8 years prior to the first diagnosis in patients with SA and OHS and further increased with disease advancement.

12.2.5 Motor Vehicle Accidents (MVA) in Socioeconomic Burden of OSA

OSA is a source of motor vehicle accidents, leading to predictable effects in decreasing economic outcomes [3, 17]. EDS and impaired vigilance due to OSA are associated with a two- or threefold increase in motor vehicle accident rates, especially those associated with personal injury [2, 26].

The costs specifically related to OSAS-related motor vehicle crashes are significant. In 2004, it was estimated that 810,000 motor vehicle crashes a year are attributable to OSAS, resulting in 1400 fatalities and costing roughly $15.9 billion [27]. This study concluded that treating the same OSAS sufferers with CPAP, assuming 70% adherence, would prevent roughly 500,000 collisions, save 1000 lives and reduce cost by $11.1 billion. The cost of CPAP was factored into the dollars saved [27]. Another study estimated that treatment with CPAP reduces the 10-year risk of MVCs (fatal and non-fatal) by 52%, the 10-year expected number of myocardial infarctions by 49% and the 10-year risk of stroke by 31% [28]. A report in 2016 described that the total economic impact of all motor vehicle accidents in the USA where undiagnosed OSA was a contributing factor estimated at $26.2 billion in 2015, and included vehicular damages, lost wages from corresponding absenteeism, property damage, rising insurance premiums and medical expenses for accidents involving drowsiness [18]. In the USA, a report by the American Automobile Association (AAA) reported that drowsy driving caused nearly 29% of 328,000 crashes, resulting in 1090 injuries and 6400 fatalities each year [18].

12.2.6 Workplace Accidents and OSA in Socioeconomic Burden of OSA

Untreated OSA patients are at significantly increased risk of non-vehicular work accidents [29, 30]. The costs for these accidents due to undiagnosed and untreated OSA totalled $6.5 billion in 2015 [18]. Another study found that people with OSA were nearly twice as likely to be hurt on the job [31]. For individuals severely injured, returning to work may not be an option due to physical or mental constraints.

12.2.7 Work Productivity in Socioeconomic Burden of OSA

EDS with OSA (OSAS) may affect work productivity in a broad range of occupations. Productivity, absenteeism, presenteeism, risk of occupational injury, changes in job duties, opportunities for job promotions and other aspects may also be negatively affected [2].

The impact of SDB on work capability is considerable as patients already have a significantly reduced employment status and a higher level of direct and indirect costs before the diagnosis is established and further reductions occurred after the diagnosis is made [25]. Loss of productivity includes absenteeism, underperformance and negative workplace behaviour. OSA was found to contribute to both work disability and decreased productivity with a cost of $86.9 billion because of lost workplace productivity representing 77.4% of the total US cost burden of OSA [4, 32].

12.3 Benefits of OSA Treatment

12.3.1 Societal and Health Economic Benefits of OSA Treatment

A systematic review found that four studies in different geographic settings showed PAP adherence to enhance economic outcomes, while one study detected no relationship between adherence and outcomes [33]. Aggregated study data indicate that PAP treatment reduced outpatient visits and that relative to no treatment, PAP was associated with favourable economic outcomes, including increased cost-effectiveness, reduced healthcare utilization (HCU), improved workplace productivity and reduced days missed from work [15, 16]. Non-PAP therapies including oral appliances and surgical approaches might also be cost-effective, but data are limited and equivocal such that future studies are warranted.

Although some retrospective analysis of claims showed that CPAP users had significantly lower hospitalization risks and all-cause US healthcare costs [34, 35], one Danish observational study and meta-analysis of two RCTs did not demonstrate a significant reduction in hospitalizations, or in ambulatory, or drug costs associated with PAP therapy compared with control conditions [9, 24].

Frost and Sullivan's 2016 survey showed that absences of employed OSA patients declined by 1.8 days per year and productivity on the job increased by 17.3% on average [18].

12.3.2 Benefits of CPAP in Mild OSA

A number of trials have shown QOL benefits from use of CPAP in mild OSA with good treatment adherence [36–40], although some studies have shown that the beneficial effects of CPAP on HrQOL are diminished among patients with mild disease [33].

Despite the positive association between AHI and symptoms such as sleepiness, patients with very high AHIs may however report little if any daytime impact of OSA and vice versa. It is generally agreed that a trial of CPAP may be warranted in symptomatic patients with objectively mild OSA [11, 41].

12.4　Costs of OSA Diagnosis and Treatment

Treatment of OSA is an investment in long-term health, and healthcare utilization and financial costs can be reduced by reducing the impact of OSA symptoms, comorbidities, and accidents. Conversely, non-adherence will prevent patients and society from achieving those savings.

Frost and Sullivan estimated that, in 2015, approximately $12.4 billion was spent in diagnosing and treating OSA for the 5.9 million US adults with OSA and a larger and more significant investment of approximately $49.5 billion would be necessary every year to care for the 23.5 million individuals with OSA who are undiagnosed today [18]. The direct upfront costs of diagnosis and treatment are substantially lower than the costs of leaving the condition untreated [18].

Diagnostic costs are variable due to differing diagnostic protocols which vary in complexity [28]. Comparisons of diagnostic modalities indicated that full-night polysomnography (FN-PSG) was cost-effective and preferred over other diagnostic modalities in almost all of the investigated populations and scenarios. In terms of prevention of MVCs and reduction in CVS events, Pietzsch et al. calculated that the preferred diagnostic strategy was FN-PSG. At pretest probabilities of 20% and 50% FN-PSG, which is initially more expensive with an incremental cost-effectiveness (ICER) of

$17,131 per quality-adjusted life year (QALY) gained, costs less and provides more QALYs than single night polysomnography (SN-PSG) and unmonitored portable home monitoring (UPHM) over the lifetime of the patient.

Over the lifetime horizon, SN-PSG and UPHM proved more expensive than FN-PSG because they are less specific tests and therefore result in more false-positive diagnoses. Even though FN-PSG was the most expensive technology at diagnosis requiring patients to undergo two overnight in-lab assessments (one for diagnosis and the other for titration), the superior diagnostic accuracy of this technology resulted in it costing less and providing more health benefits than any other approach to diagnosis in the long term.

Diagnosis with type IV unattended portable home monitoring devices costs more overall and provided fewer QALYs than type III devices [28].

From a health-economic perspective, UPHM, FN-PSG and SN-PSG have very similar outcomes in populations with a high pretest probability of OSA (patients with several clinical indicators highly suggestive of having OSA). This is important, as it indicates that UPHM, despite its lower sensitivity and specificity, can be a cost-effective diagnostic approach (incremental cost-effectiveness ratio of $19,707 per QALY gained compared to no diagnosis) in situations where FN-PSG or SN-PSG is not available, where there are substantial wait times for in-lab diagnosis or when patients are not willing or able to undergo evaluation in a sleep lab [28].

The costs of OSA diagnosis and treatment and impact on healthcare and workplace economics have been assessed in the United States in 2015 [1, 18] (Fig. 12.1). Approximately 7% of costs were from physician office visits and testing necessary for diagnosis and management. Another 50% was generated from the sale and rental of PAP machines

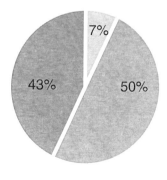

■ Physician Office visits ░ PAP costs ▨ Surgical costs

Fig. 12.1 Costs of sleep apnoea diagnosis and treatment. (Adapted with permission from Frost and Sullivan 2016)

and their accessories, as well as customized oral appliances in a small proportion of population use. Surgical costs for treating OSA condition were estimated to account for the remaining 43% of costs. Costs per OSA patient averaged $2105 per person per year. Most OSA patients do not require surgery, so when removing those costs, the average dropped to $1190.

In Spain, Mar et al. calculated diagnostic costs in 2003, including consultations with conventional testing (€111), cardiorespiratory polygraphy (€98) and polysomnography (€243) (Table 12.1) [42]. The diagnostic cost incurred in the population in order to treat one patient with CPAP was were €1028. This figure included the 10% dropout rate from treatment. The impact of diagnostic costs on the economic efficiency of treatment of OSA was quite low, as the key factor in the overall cost is the cost of the CPAP device. The cost of CPAP differs greatly from one country to another, depending mainly on whether the device is bought or rented. Mar et al. noted that the cost is the aggregate value of the resources needed to provide a health or clinical intervention, such that what varies is not cost but charges. In Spain, the annual cost of CPAP treatment in 2001 was calculated at €251, and at €1256 over 5 years including all supplies and maintenance. Other costs associated with CPAP treatment included in-home technical maintenance twice a year (€82) and medical follow-up once a year (€25) (Table 12.1). Across Europe, CPAP device prices are similar, with the main charge difference apparently due to National Health Services renting devices, usually at higher charges [42].

Mar et al. noted that these results are very sensitive to time horizon. Over a time horizon of 5 years, the purchase and maintenance costs of CPAP were responsible for 61% of the overall incremental cost, increasing to 86% over the whole life of the patient (Table 12.2) [42].

In the UK, Weatherley et al. calculated in 2009 that, for a hypothetical 50-year-old man, total costs were £8140 for lifestyle advice, £8797 for dental devices, and £9301 for CPAP [43] (Table 12.3). The increased costs of CPAP were due to higher treatment costs, while the non-treatment costs were lower than those for the other strategies.

Table 12.1 Management costs of OSA treatment (Spain)

	€
Consultation	111
Resp PG	98
PSG	243
Treatment cost per patient	1028
Annual cost of CPAP	251
Annual CPAP maintenance	82
Annual medical follow-up	25

Reproduced with permission from Mar et al. (2003)

Table 12.2 Disaggregated incremental costs in 50-year-old males treated with nCPAP in two time horizons

	Diagnostic cost		Treatment cost	
Horizon	€	%	€	%
5 years	1028	39	1636	61
Lifespan	1028	14	6238	86

Reproduced with permission from Mar et al. (2003)

Table 12.3 Management costs of OSA treatment (UK)

	UK (GBP)
Lifestyle advice	8140
Dental	8797
CPAP	9301

Reproduced with permission from Weatherley et al. (2009)

12.5 Cost-Effectiveness and Socioeconomic Impact of OSA Treatment

12.5.1 Cost-Effectiveness and Socioeconomic Impact of CPAP Treatment

A number of guidelines reflect studies which have demonstrated cost-effectiveness of CPAP therapy in OSA, enabling assessment of costs of non-adherence to CPAP [9, 44, 45].

Treatment of OSAS is both economical and effective. A number of studies have supported the economic benefits of treating OSAS, particularly when comparing the incremental costs of treatment with CPAP per quality-adjusted life years. When quality of life, costs of therapy and motor vehicle outcomes are considered, CPAP therapy for patients with OSAS is attractive for both economic and health benefits [43, 46, 47].

There is no clear consensus in the health economics literature regarding the value of an incremental cost-effectiveness ratio below which a treatment should be regarded as efficient [42]. A Canadian study found it to lie in the range of 20,000–100,000 Canadian dollars/QALY [48]. An ICER of less than $50,000 per QALY gained is generally considered cost-effective, but some evidence suggests this value should be higher [49–51]. By comparison, a review of the cost-effectiveness of 500 life-saving interventions by Tengs et al. found that the median cost per life year saved was US$19,000 in the health sector [52]. An assessment of the cost-effectiveness of cardiovascular prevention programmes in Spain showed figures ranging between US$ 3000 and $100,000 [53].

An analysis of ICERs by Mohit and Cohen demonstrated that interventions for OSA would increase costs but would also improve health by increasing QALYs [54]. The majority indicated that intervention represents good value in accruing QALYs at a relatively low cost with a value below $50,000 per QALY gained in the USA and in other settings.

The literature regarding utility gain in OSAS patients reveals widely varying figures, with mean utility gain obtained using nCPAP ranging from 0.23 to 0.05 [44, 55–57].

Cost-effectiveness analyses conducted in Canada, the UK, Spain, the USA and France have demonstrated that CPAP is cost-effective from the payer perspective, with costs per quality-adjusted life year (QALY) gained, well below societal cutoffs (typically $50,000 per QALY in the USA) [29, 43, 44, 47–49, 55, 57–61] (Table 12.4).

In Canada, a study in 1992 showed that the ICER for CPAP lies in the range of Can $20,000–100,000/QALY [48]. In a further study in 1994, the mean utility and the standard deviation obtained with the standard gamble method were 0.87 ± 0.17 on CPAP treatment and 0.63 ± 0.29 pretreatment [55]. This resulted in an average gain of 5.4 QALYs and a cost-utility ratio between Can $3397 and Can $9792 per QALY added. These costs were relatively small when compared to the cost per QALY for many other clinical interventions. Tan et al. calculated that 1 year of CPAP treatment increased the health utility score from 0.611 ± 0.112 to 0.710 ± 0.121 ($P < 0.01$) [59]. Therefore, CPAP resulted in a mean gain of 0.092 QALY/patient [59]. Studies from Manitoba concluded that the treatment of OSA with CPAP reversed the trend of increasing healthcare utilization seen prior to diagnosis. CPAP results in a long-term health benefit, as measured by the use of healthcare services [62, 63]. In a later study, Pietzsch et al. demonstrated an incremental cost-effectiveness ratio (ICER) of CDN$15,915 per quality-adjusted life year (QALY) gained for the life-time horizon with CPAP therapy [28]. Over the lifetime horizon in a population with 50% prevalence of OSAS, full-night polysomnography in conjunction with CPAP therapy was considered the most economically efficient strategy at any willingness-to-pay greater than $17,131 per QALY gained, because it dominates all other strategies in comparative analysis [28, 29].

In the UK, the Trent Report provided a cost-utility analysis which compared nCPAP with a 'do nothing' alternative for the treatment of patients with OSAS [58]. QALY gain after 1 year was 0.10 (CI 0.07 0.12). Cost per QALY gained at 1 month was £99,000, at 1 year £8300, 2 years £5200 and 5 years £3200 (Table 12.5). All estimates of cost-effectiveness over 1 year were <£16,000 per QALY gained. In another UK study in 2002, severely impaired health status at baseline improved by 23% (0.32–0.55) in utility by the standard gamble approach, adding 8 QALYs in the CPAP group compared to a 4% improvement (0.31–0.35) with 4.7 QALYs added in the lifestyle group [57]. Utility measured by EQ-5D showed a marginal change with CPAP (0.73–0.77) but did not demonstrate any improvement with lifestyle, suggesting that

Table 12.5 Baseline cost per QALY gained in the UK Trent report (Chilcott et al. 2000)

Time horizon	Cost per QALY gained
1 month	£99,000
1 year	£8300
2 years	£5200
5 years	£3200

Adapted with permission from Wetherley et al. (2009)

Table 12.4 Cost-effectiveness analysis in OSA treatment

Country	QALYs gained (CPAP)	Cost per QALY (CPAP)	ICER/QALY (CPAP)	QALYs gained (dental devices)	Cost per QALY (CPAP over dental device)
Canada (Laupacis et al. 1992)			Can $20,000–$100,000		
Canada (Tousignant et al. 1994)	5.4	Can $3397–$9792			
UK (Chakravorty et al. 2002)	8				
Spain (Mar et al. 2003)		€ 5000	<€6000		
USA (Ayas et al. 2006)	0.75		$3354		
Canada (Tan et al. 2008)	0.092				
UK (Guest et al. 2008)		>£20,000 (2 years) <10,000 (13 years)			
UK (Weatherley et al. 2009)	12.39		£4413 (severe OSA) to £20,585 (mild OSA)	12.26	£3899
UK (McDaid et al. 2009)		£2500		12.26	£3900
Canada (Pietzch et al. 2011)			Can $15,915		
Brazil (Rizzi et al. 2014)	0.093				
France (Pouillie et al. 2016)	0.62		€10,128 (high CVS risk)		

poor CPAP adherence leads to significant cost in terms of quality of life.

A later UK study in 2008 showed that treatment with CPAP for a period of 1 year was found not to be a cost-effective option, since the cost per quality-adjusted life year (QALY) gained is expected to be >£20,000, but after 2 years of treatment, the cost per QALY gained is expected to be £10,000 or less, and after 13 years of treatment, CPAP becomes a dominant treatment (i.e., more effective than no treatment for less cost) [60]. Within the limitations of the model, CPAP was found to be clinically more effective than no treatment and, from the perspective of the UK's NHS, a cost-effective strategy after a minimum of 2 years of treatment.

From a UK National Health Service perspective in 2009, CPAP was found to be a cost-effective alternative to dental devices and lifestyle advice, especially in patients with more severe disease [43]. Estimated QALYs were 11.93 with lifestyle advice, 12.26 with dental devices and 12.39 with CPAP. The incremental cost per QALY gained with CPAP over dental devices was £3899. The probability of CPAP being more cost-effective than its comparators, at a cost-effectiveness threshold of £20,000 per QALY, was 0.78 for men and 0.80 for women. The cost-effectiveness of CPAP improved in patients with more severe symptoms. The ICER for CPAP therapy compared to dental devices or lifestyle advice ranged from £4413 to £20,585 depending on the OSA severity [43].

The UK economic review by McDaid et al. in 2009 demonstrated that continuous positive airway pressure devices reduce symptoms of sleepiness and are cost-effective for obstructive sleep apnoea-hypopnoea syndrome [47]. Cost-effectiveness of CPAP, based on a hypothetical cohort of men aged 50 years, using a lifetime time horizon, and including costs for treatment, cardiovascular disease events and traffic accidents, was estimated at £2500 per quality-adjusted life year (QALY) compared with usual care and £3900 per QALY compared with dental devices.

In the USA, a study by Ayas et al. in 2006 calculated that CPAP therapy was more effective but more costly than no CPAP [49]. Non-compliant patients were assumed to use the CPAP machine for 3 months, incurring rental costs of the machine and humidifier, and costs associated with the mask, tubing, headgear and one physician visit. Patients were assumed not to benefit from CPAP for this period of 3 months. From the perspective of third-party payor, considering only direct costs, CPAP was associated with a mean gain of 0.75 QALY (2.22 QALYs vs 1.47 QALYs [95% CI, 0.28–3.08] in the CPAP and no-CPAP groups, respectively, resulting in an ICER of $3354 per QALY gained. From the perspective of society, the CPAP strategy was more costly ($7123 [95% CI, $4324–$11,906] vs $6887 [95% CI, $3113–$14,843] for the no-CPAP strategy) as well as more

effective, implying an incremental cost-effectiveness of $314 (95% CI, cost saving to $6114).

The most influential factor was analytical perspective (i.e., third-party payer vs societal), leading to a more than tenfold difference in ICER estimates. The second most influential factor was choice of utilities values. When EQ-5D utilities were used instead of standard gamble utilities, the ICER estimate increased more than 5 times. Using the value of society's willingness to pay for a QALY of $50,000, 100% of the Monte Carlo simulations favoured the cost-effectiveness of CPAP therapy. The results were described as conservative, with benefits of CPAP likely greater, as some potential benefits were not calculated including improvements in work productivity, reduction in occupational injuries, reduced use of antihypertensive medications and improvements in bed-partner quality of life [49].

In the USA, Wickwire et al. published a systematic review of published literature regarding the impact of treatment for OSA on monetized health economic outcomes [34]. Although study methodologies varied widely, evidence consistently suggested that treatment of OSA was associated with favourable economic outcomes, including QALYs, within accepted ranges of cost-effectiveness, reduced HCU and reduced monetized costs.

Long-term CPAP therapy may reduce healthcare utilization and hospitalization costs in some patients with cardiac and pulmonary comorbidity [64].

In Spain, cost-effectiveness of CPAP was found to be €7861 for the base case, €4938/QALY at a time horizon of 5 years, and only in the least favourable scenario rose above €20,000 per QALY [44]. Improvements in QOL account for 98% of the incremental effectiveness of CPAP over a time horizon of 5 years changes and 84% over the whole life of the patient (Table 12.6).

CPAP represented an incremental cost <6.000 euros/QALY, and in a disaggregated analysis, 84% of the incremental effectiveness was attributed to the improved QOL. By comparison an assessment of the cost-effectiveness of cardiovascular prevention programmes showed figures ranging US$3000–$100,000 [53].

In Brazil, Rizzi et al. used the SF-6D questionnaire and showed that 1 year of CPAP treatment increased the health utility score from 0.611 ± 0.112 to 0.710 ± 0.121

Table 12.6 Cost-effectiveness and ICER for the base case and two time horizons in male

Horizon €/ QALY	Cost €		Effectiveness QALY		
	No treatment	nCPAP	No treatment	nCPAP	ICER
5 years	55	2719	3.39	3.73	7861
Life span	591	7902	12.90	14.38	4938

Reproduced with permission from Mar et al. (2003)

($P < 0.01$) and resulted in a mean net gain of 0.0929 QALY/patient [65].

Long-term CPAP treatment results in QALY gains similar to other chronic disorders, such as hypertension (0.54), depression (0.055), diabetes (0.07), insomnia (0.006831) and COPD (0.009) [65].

Comorbidities associated with OSA such as hypertension and diabetes are a significant and increasing financial burden. In the survey by Frost and Sullivan in 2016, approximately 3% of hypertensive patients with OSA were able to stop medication, and another 17% were able to decrease medication after receiving treatment [18]. For diabetics treating OSA, hospital visits were cut from 2.8 to 1.5 annually. They estimated that the overall reduction in medication use and annual hospital visits saved patients millions of dollars each year and that approximately 78% of survey respondents stated that OSA treatment was a good investment.

A review of economic studies found that non-treated patients with OSAS consume significantly more health resources and present with decreased work performance which creates deficits that extend beyond health resources, affecting other areas of economic functioning. CPAP treatment has the potential to decrease these costs and the direct costs with health [65].

In professional drivers with OSA, CPAP treatment led to a 73% reduction in preventable driving accidents [66]. Frost and Sullivan noted that a large commercial truck crash can cost up to $9 million, but if drivers were screened and subsequently treated for OSA, up to $11 billion annually could be saved [18].

12.5.2 Cost-Effectiveness of CPAP Treatment in Mild OSA

Incremental cost-effectiveness ratios related to rapid introduction of treatment are significantly lower in the patients with more severe OSAS and provide serious medical and economic arguments in favour of early management of the patients with more severe OSAS [67]. McDaid et al. found that the clinical treatment effect of CPAP on the Epworth sleepiness scale, relative to conservative therapy, was greater in patients with greater baseline severity of OSAHS. In terms of cost-effectiveness of CPAP in separate severity groups, the ICER (probability of being cost-effective at a threshold of £20,000 per QALY) varied between £20,585 (0.43) and £4413 (0.98) in patients with mild and severe disease, respectively [47].

As quality of life is a major factor in cost-effectiveness, current guidelines state that there appear to be clinical and health economic arguments in favour of offering treatment to patients with mild OSA associated with symptoms or CVS

comorbidities, and a potential cost saving in reducing non-adherence [1].

Nevertheless, although QOL is improved by CPAP in mild OSA, and is a major factor in cost-effectiveness, further research is needed to establish whether there is a potential health economic as well as clinical benefit in offering treatment to patients with mild OSA, and to assess the potential cost in CPAP non-adherence in this patient group [37, 38, 40, 41].

12.5.3 Cost-Effectiveness of OAT and Surgery

In addition to PAP, oral appliance (OA) therapy has been found to be cost-effective. OAs are preferred by many patients and are an accepted treatment alternative for patients with mild-to-moderate OSA or who are unable to tolerate PAP [68, 69] (See Chap. 28).

As previously noted, CPAP was found to be a cost-effective alternative to dental devices and lifestyle advice from the perspective of the UK NHS, especially in patients with more severe disease [43]. Estimated QALYs were 11.93 with lifestyle advice, 12.26 with dental devices and 12.39 with CPAP. The incremental cost per QALY gained with CPAP over dental devices was £3899. The ICER for CPAP therapy compared to dental devices or lifestyle advice that ranged from £4413 to £20,585 depending on the OSA severity [43].

In France, one study has assessed the cost-effective efficiency of different treatments (i.e., CPAP, dental devices, lifestyle advice and no treatment) for patients with mild-to-moderate OSAHS, with low or high CV comorbidities at baseline [61]. For patients with low CV risk, the ICER of dental devices versus no treatment varied between 32,976 EUR (moderate OSAHS) and 45,579 EUR (mild OSAHS) per QALY, and for CPAP versus dental devices, above 256,000 EUR/QALY. For patients with high CV risk, CPAP was associated with a gain of 0.62 QALY compared with no treatment, resulting in an ICER of 10,128 EUR/QALY. The analysis suggested that it is economically efficient to treat all OSAHS patients with high CV risk with CPAP and that dental devices are more efficient than CPAP for mild-to-moderate OSAHS with low CV risk. By assuming an efficacy of dental devices up to 1.56 times less than that of CPAP on the prevention of CV events, the cost-effectiveness of dental devices would be the same as that for CPAP. Making an assumption of similar effectiveness based on an extrapolation of results reported by Anandam et al., the cost-effectiveness of dental devices becomes far superior to that of CPAP [61, 70]. For mild-to-moderate OSAHS with low CV risk, dental devices appeared more efficient than CPAP, but patient out-of-pocket costs were much higher for dental devices than for CPAP because of mainly non-refundable orthodontic treatment in France [61].

These results are difficult to compare with those of UK studies due to different integration of CV comorbidities and assessment of treatment effect by different methods (ESS and AHI) [43, 47].

The health economics of OA and surgical approaches have been less frequently studied, and results are more equivocal when compared with results with PAP. Non-PAP therapies might also be cost-effective, but data are limited, and future studies are warranted.

Surgical approaches were associated with a positive health economic outcome in two paediatric studies and found treatment to reduce outpatient visits, hospitalizations, emergency department visits and costs [3, 71]. One study reported a negative economic outcome at 2 years, but uvulo-palatoplasty was included, and adherence was not assessed [15]. Uvulo-palatoplasty is considered an expensive procedure that does not reliably normalize the apnea-hypopnea index [19].

Bariatric surgery appears to be a definitive treatment for OSA and markedly more efficient than usual care in the prevention of type 2 diabetes leading to higher rates of diabetes remission, lower risk of CVD and other adverse health outcomes, and with related medication cost savings [72–75].

12.6   CPAP Non-adherence

12.6.1   Prevalence of Non-adherence to CPAP

Poor CPAP adherence is widely recognized as a critical problem in the treatment of OSAHS [76–79]. The outcomes of adherence to PAP therapy, sleepiness and side effects are critical for clinical and health-economic decision-making [9].

A wide range of prevalence of adherence is quoted in the literature. When adherence is defined as greater than 4 h of nightly use, 29–83% of patients with OSAHS have been reported to be non-adherent to treatment [78].

The average daily use of those who use CPAP every night is approximately 6 h, and those who routinely skip nights use it on average for 3 hours [80]. Those patients who are non-adherent during early treatment generally remain non-adherent over the long term [80, 81]. The return of symptoms and other manifestations of OSA with even one night of non-use underscores the critical nature of adherence to CPAP [82, 83].

A 2004 quantitative review found that, compared to other chronic conditions, adherence to therapy for sleep disorders was the lowest of the 17 conditions studied, including HIV, cancer, cardiovascular disease, renal disease and diabetes mellitus [84].

Later studies showed that, on a long-term basis, 20–25% of OSAS patients have been found to discontinue CPAP treatment although CPAP adherence is crucial to improve symptoms and cardiometabolic outcomes with a dose-effect relationship [76, 85].

In other reviews, long-term empiric assessment of PAP compliance or adherence is quoted at 30–60% and has frequently remained inadequate and persistently low over 20 years of published data [79, 86]. 5–89% of patients will reject CPAP as a treatment immediately, and 25–50% of patients who commence treatment will fail to continue [87]. 50% will discontinue CPAP treatment within 1 year [88], and 25% will terminate CPAP treatment within 3 years [89].

Although CPAP is sometimes singled out as a therapy with particularly poor adherence, it is worth noting that it is one of the few therapies in which detailed, objective, daily adherence monitoring is standard clinical practice and that optimal use of CPAP requires a level of patient engagement that exceeds what is needed to follow a pill-based regimen [11].

Bollig reported non-adherence rates to be similar to other populations with health concerns, where roughly 20–40% of individuals with acute illness, 30–60% with chronic illness and 50–80% of those using preventative care are non-adherent to their prescribed medical treatment [88]. Only 30–50% of asthma patients adhere to therapy; 8% do not even collect their first prescription, while 68–83% of patients adhere to antihypertensives.

12.6.2   Clinical Factors Associated with Non-adherence to CPAP

Factors that are likely to influence CPAP adherence have been evaluated and can be arbitrarily separated into three domains of general patient characteristics, sleep apnoea severity and technical aspects of CPAP treatment including delivery interfaces and side effects [76, 79, 85].

No consistent association has been found between non-adherence and age, gender or BMI [67, 76, 90–92].

No single factor has been consistently identified as predictive of CPAP adherence, although studies demonstrate that overweight, obesity, comorbid conditions, smoking, low socioeconomic status, ethnicity, marital status, employment and financial coverage for CPAP treatment are factors that are associated with low CPAP adherence [11, 16, 93–96].

The evidence suggests that early experiences with CPAP, combined with patients' perceptions and beliefs about OSA and CPAP, and the balance of their sociostructural facilitators and barriers, are critical factors that influence patients' decisions to use CPAP over the long term [97].

The most consistent predictive factors for adherence include early PAP adherence, self-reported daytime sleepiness and certain psychological traits such as self-efficacy [93, 98]. Type D personality, associated with unhealthy lifestyle and a reluctance to consult or follow medical advice, increases non-compliance and poor treatment outcomes [87]. Claustrophobic tendencies have been associated with lower overall adherence [83, 99].

The balance between symptom severity pre-treatment and post-treatment symptom relief and sleep quality on CPAP treatment seems among the strongest predictors of CPAP compliance, although clearly not predictive prior to treatment [95].

Disease severity, as measured by the apnea-hypopnea index (AHI) and nocturnal hypoxemia, has been shown to have an inconsistent predictive relationship with CPAP adherence [11, 67, 92, 95, 100, 101].

In other studies, severity of sleep disordered breathing assessed as number of oxygen desaturation events, was the only clinical condition associated with long-term adherence [91, 102].

Treatments for OSA, such as CPAP and oral appliances, are frequently underused or rejected by patients due to discomfort, insurance, perceptions of efficacy and other issues [2].

12.6.3 Socioeconomic Factors Associated with Non-adherence to CPAP

There are also factors at play that go far beyond patient demographic characteristics and disease characteristics, such as cultural considerations, fragmented care and policies related to diagnosis and treatment reimbursement and delivery [11, 76, 94, 103, 104].

Technological aspects associated with polysomnography and treatment delivery are less important in promoting adherence than a supportive environment and first impressions of ease of use and benefit of therapy, and technical aspects such as CPAP mode, humidification or interface are likely to be modified during treatment follow-up [76, 79].

Meta-analysis demonstrated similar levels of PAP adherence in adults with OSA with PAP initiation by either home APAP or in-laboratory titration [9]. There is little evidence that adherence is affected by PAP mode or pressure modification, although patients have shown a preference for APAP over fixed pressure CPAP [105, 106].

Side effects of the treatment have not been shown to be predictive of adherence to CPAP, and it has been shown that those who reported mask side effects were in fact those patients who used CPAP regularly [80].

Oronasal masks have a negative impact on CPAP adherence, and meta-analysis has demonstrated clinically significant improvements in adherence in adults with OSA with nasal interfaces compared to oronasal interfaces [1, 85, 107]. Regardless of the type of interface, mask leaks have been shown as being associated with a higher risk of non-adherence [85]. Non-intentional leaks are more frequent with oronasal masks than with nasal masks [90, 108–110].

Meta-analysis has demonstrated no clinically significant difference in PAP usage, self-reported sleepiness or QOL in adults with OSA with the addition of humidification [1].

12.7 Costs of OSA Treatment Non-adherence

12.7.1 Clinical Costs of OSA Treatment Non-adherence

The costs of non-adherence can be considered in terms of personal medical burden; the costs of diagnosis and treatment, usually involving CPAP purchase, loan or rental, and the societal economic burden of illness.

OSA is linked to preventable causes of readmissions which include congestive heart failure, ischaemic cardiomyopathy, obstructive lung disease and diabetes [111]. 30-day hospital readmissions are used as a key quality indicator to help reduce healthcare costs [112].

Non-adherence to CPAP is associated with increased 30-day all-cause and cardiovascular-cause readmission in patients with OSA, such that ensuring CPAP adherence is considered crucial in addressing general and cardiovascular-related healthcare utilization and morbidity in patients with OSA [113]. Non-adherence to CPAP has been associated with increased chronic obstructive pulmonary disease (COPD) exacerbations, worsened insulin resistance, psychiatric illnesses and lower urinary tract symptoms [113]. A single-centre study demonstrated that congestive heart failure patients with OSA who were adherent to CPAP had lower 6-month readmissions and emergency department visits than patients who were non-adherent [114]. Furthermore, inpatient OSA screening, diagnosis and treatment initiation resulted in decreased 30-day cardiac readmissions in hospitalized cardiac patients [115].

Non-adherence to treatment will clearly lead to persistence of the clinical burden of OSA and related risks in about 50% of treated patients, including daytime sleepiness and reduced QOL cardiovascular, metabolic and neurocognitive diseases, anxiety and depression, increased risk of motor vehicle (MVAs), work accidents, and all-cause mortality [9, 11].

12.7.2 Socioeconomic Costs of Non-adherence to OSA Treatment

Non-adherence to CPAP is considered expensive, as effective OSA management improves individual health and promotes public safety while producing significant cost savings for payors, employers and patients [116].

Treating OSA is seen as an investment in long-term health. Patients are able to reduce their healthcare utilization and save money by reducing the impact of OSA symptoms, comorbidities and accidents [18]. Conversely, non-adherence will prevent patients and society from achieving those savings. Furthermore, costs of diagnosis and initial treatment provision will be wasted in patients non-adherent to treatment.

Tarasiuk et al. reported in 2013 that untreated OSA can lead to about a twofold increase in medical expenses because of CVD morbidity [16]. The costliest patients are also the sickest OSA patients in each population stratum, and these sub-groups of patients consume 65–82% of all OSA patient costs. As healthcare markets are characterized by limited resources, it was proposed that the 'most costly' should become the main target for decision-makers, to better allocate scarce resources and to focus on early diagnosis and treatment of these groups.

On the other hand, Pietschz et al. considered that treatment compliance did not have a substantial effect on the cost-effectiveness of CPAP therapy in any population. Perfect compliance with CPAP would not be substantially more cost-effective, with an ICER of $15,769 per QALY gained. This increased marginally to $16,112 per QALY gained in a worst-case compliance scenario in which double the number of patients refused therapy immediately when offered and twice the number of patients discontinued treatment each month [28].

Frost and Sullivan considered that while the vast majority of costs are related to comorbidities, the occupational sector is also affected as it results in lost productivity, market increases in healthcare utilization and increased absenteeism [18].

Current US Medicare policy restricts long-term CPAP coverage to those demonstrating adherence during a 90-day trial defined as CPAP use ≥ 4 h a night, for 70% of days within a 30 consecutive day period. Billings et al. reported that this policy denies coverage to those unlikely to use CPAP long term and prevent wasted resources. Although more costly than a clinic-only programme, with an additional cost of $30,544 more per QALY, it results in greater adherence with higher net utility [94].

Patel et al. calculated an incremental cost of about $2000 per percent adherence gained over 5 years [117]. The incremental cost of one quality of life adjusted year, as assessed by the EQ-5D, was below societal thresholds at $30,000/

QALY. If utilities were derived from the standard gamble method instead, the ICER was much lower at $6872 per QALY. If the impact of CPAP on quality of life is greater than assessed by the EQ-5D and better reflected by the standard gamble-derived utilities, the current CMS policy would be more cost-effective. Varying the cost by 20% of the PSG and CPAP rental, which may have been projected drivers of cost, had minimal impact on the ICER. CPAP accessory refill patterns had the largest impact on the ICER, making the current CMS policy not cost-effective if maximal refills were routinely obtained. But literature suggests that minimal refill rates are more the norm. A larger decline in long-term adherence, considered likely more consistent with real-world observations, suggested that the current CMS policy is even less cost-effective with higher ICERs. The base model assumed only a 4% decline in adherence which may falsely elevate the incremental benefit in adherence and utility over 5 years. If adherence declines precipitously over the years, the current CMS policy is not cost-effective [117].

Future Directions

OSA provides a good model for designing and testing feasible, scalable and affordable interventions to manage non-adherence to treatment. Given that adherence to therapy for chronic disease in developed nations is estimated to be approximately 50% and that 10% of annual healthcare costs in the USA are attributable to medication non-adherence, sleep healthcare professionals are in a good position to tackle this widespread and important problem [11].

However, no integrated, end-to-end assessment comprehensively evaluating the overall impact of OSA diagnosis and therapy, including long-term patient outcomes and associated costs, has been conducted to date [28].

OSA and other important sleep disorders still lack baseline heath economic measurements, highlighting the need for further research in this area including measurement of QALYs to establish health utility weights. Future studies aimed at establishing baseline utility measures for more sleep disorders will pave the way for more advanced burden of disease studies, as well as for measuring the economic impact of interventions and treatments [54].

Direct costs of EDS and indirect costs of OSA have not yet been fully established, and further studies exploring the effect of CPAP on medical costs are essential [23]. Future studies should examine the direct costs of EDS in OSA, quantify the cost associated with MVAs and lost work productivity and detail QOL and social impacts of the condition [23]. Future studies should also examine the linear dose-response relationship between PAP use and cost-effectiveness.

Existing studies do not address the potential benefits of future medical cost savings due to improved health status and reduction of comorbidities. Cost analyses are needed to assess cost-effectiveness regarding PAP therapy and outcomes related to blood pressure as resource use may be substantial [9].

Further studies should be designed to better address work-related barriers to CPAP adherence. Active employment might reflect numerous competing interests which take precedence over regular CPAP use. CPAP machines are often considered to be bulky, which can contribute to limit CPAP adherence in patients travelling for work. Furthermore, conflicting demands imposed by work schedules may compromise long-term CPAP follow-up visit attendance. Greater insight into the employer perspective is essential because roughly one-half of OSA indirect costs are associated with lost workplace productivity (i.e., absenteeism) and workplace accident and injury risk [16]. Assessment of the cost-benefit ratio of treating OSA is likely to be of particular interest to the increasing number of large (*N* > 1000) self-insured employers [16].

For countries with well-resourced healthcare systems, there is a need to evaluate delivery models whereby many patients can receive high-quality care without the need for multiple office visits with subspecialists, along with alternative payment models [1, 118]. Primary care physicians and nurse practitioners can achieve good outcomes in management of OSA under appropriate supervision [119].

The magnitude of any costs savings related to routine use of APAP rather than fixed pressure CPAP remains to be studied, as over the long term, APAP therapy may reduce costs due to reduced need for patient visits and in-laboratory titrations as pressure requirements change over time.

Future studies should seek to evaluate interventions to improve CPAP adherence among older adults of lower socioeconomic status, including financial incentives as a policy to encourage CPAP acceptance, mainly among vulnerable populations [63, 96].

In the USA, current Medicare policy denies funding of long-term CPAP long term in non-compliant patients to prevent wasted resources. Future studies are needed to measure long-term adherence in an elderly population with and without current adherence requirements to verify the cost-effectiveness of a policy change [94].

The potential mechanisms and financial incentives for increased adherence and cost-effectiveness of tele-monitoring in CPAP use have yet to be fully evaluated and may include access to real-time assistance from a clinical provider and increased motivation from daily monitoring to increase patient engagement and increase sense of accountability for their care or to their healthcare provider [9, 11, 120].

In light of the rapidly expanding number of alternate OSA treatment modalities, comparative effectiveness analyses between PAP and other OSA treatments will allow stakeholders to make evidence-based decisions regarding allocation of scarce healthcare resources [16].

Glossary

Obstructive Sleep Apnoea and Obstructive Sleep Apnoea Syndrome

Obstructive sleep apnoea (OSA) refers to a physiological condition defined by documented apnoeas and hypopnoeas and may be asymptomatic. Obstructive sleep apnoea syndrome (OSAS) refers to symptomatic OSA, usually presenting as excessive daytime sleepiness. The terms are sometimes used interchangeably in the literature.

CPAP Compliance and Adherence

CPAP compliance is a term which is often used interchangeably with adherence, but more strictly reflects initial acceptance and usage after treatment setup.

CPAP adherence reflects longer-term satisfactory use of treatment in terms of nightly hours of use of CPAP, and duration of use in the longer term, usually considered to be at least 3 months for health economic assessment. Some patients may refuse treatment without even initiating it, and some eventually abandon therapy [93].

Cost-Effectiveness Analysis in OSA Treatment

Cost-effectiveness analysis measures the economic value of an intervention in terms of its incremental cost-effectiveness ratio (ICER) [54]. An ICER is a ratio of an intervention's incremental cost (the difference in the financial resource cost of the intervention and its comparator) divided by its incremental health benefits. The comparator for an intervention may be another intervention or the current standard of care. The ICER can be thought of as a unit 'price'. Large ICER values indicate a high cost for each incremental gain in health and vice versa.

Quality-adjusted life years (QALYs) are used to express health benefits and used in the calculation of ICERs. QALYs are the sum of the durations of health states multiplied by the mean utility of each of the health states [121]. A QALY is a year of life scaled by a utility preference weight associated with a variety of health states, and which ranges from 0 to 1, where a utility weight of 1 corresponds to a hypothetical state of perfect health and 0 corresponds to a state equivalent in preference to being dead.

Utility is a parameter that refers to subjective satisfaction that people derive from consuming goods and services such that utility weights between 0 and 1 indicate greater or lesser morbidity, with weights closer to 1 corresponding to less severe, more preferred states and weights closer to 0 corresponding to more severe, less preferred states [54]. Utility results can be derived using the 'standard gamble' as the standard of care [122, 123]. EQ-5D is a preference-based measure which can map to QALYs and provide standardized utility weights that are comparable across health states and can be combined to estimate quality adjusted survival [124].

References

1. Benjafield AV, Eastwood PR, Heinzer R, Ip MSM, Morrell MJ, Nunez CM, Patel SR, Penzel T, Pépin J-LD, Peppard PE. Estimation of the global prevalence and burden of obstructive sleep apnoea: a literature-based analysis. Lancet Respir Med. 2019;7(8):687–98.

2. Waldman LT, Parthasarathy S, Kathleen F, Villa KF, Bron M, Bujanover S, Brod M. Understanding the burden of illness of excessive daytime sleepiness associated with obstructive sleep apnea: a qualitative study. Health Qual Life Outcomes. 2020;18:128.

3. Young T, Peppard PE, Gottlieb DJ. Epidemiology of obstructive sleep apnea: a population health perspective. Am J Respir Crit Care Med. 2002;165(9):1217–39.

4. Peppard PE, Young T, Barnet JH, Palta M, Hagen EW, Hla KM. Increased prevalence of sleep-disordered breathing in adults. Am J Epidemiol. 2013;177(9):1006–14.

5. Heinzer R, Vat S, Marques-Vidal P, Marti-Soler H, Andries D, Tobback N, Mooser V, Preisig M, Malhotra A, Waeber G, Vollenweider P, Tafti M, Haba-Rubio J, J. Prevalence of sleep-disordered breathing in the general population: the HypnoLaus study. Lancet. Respir Med. 2015;3(4):310–8.

6. Punjabi N. The epidemiology of adult obstructive sleep apnea. Proc Am Thoracic Soc. 2008;5(2):136–43.

7. Knauert M, Sreelatha Naik S, Gillespie MB, Kryger M. Clinical consequences and economic costs of untreated obstructive sleep apnea syndrome. World J Otorhinolaryngol Head Neck Surg. 2015;1:17–27.

8. Lyons M, Bhatt NY, Pack AI, Magalang UJ. Global burden of sleep-disordered breathing and its implications. Respirology. 2020;25:690–702.

9. Patil SP, Ayappa IA, Caples SM, Kimoff RJ, Patel SR, Harrod CG. Treatment of adult obstructive sleep apnea with positive airway pressure: an American Academy of Sleep Medicine systematic review, meta-analysis, and GRADE assessment. J Clin Sleep Med. 2019;15(2):301–34.

10. Tarasiuk A, Reuveni H. The economic impact of obstructive sleep apnea. Curr Opin Pulm Med. 2013;19:639–44.

11. Bakker JP, Weaver TE, Parthasarathy S, Aloia MS. Adherence to CPAP what should we be aiming for, and how can we get there? Chest. 2019;155(6):1272–87.

12. Jennum P, Tonnesen P, Ibsen R, Kjellberg J. All-cause mortality from obstructive sleep apnea in male and female patients with and without continuous positive airway pressure treatment: a registry study with 10 years of follow-up. Nat Sci Sleep. 2015;7:43–50.

13. Teodorescu M, Polomis DA, Hall SV, Teodorescu MC, Gangnon RE, Peterson AG, Xie A, Sorkness CA, Jarjour NN. Association of obstructive sleep apnea risk with asthma control in adults. Chest. 2010;138(3):543–50.

14. Albarrak M, Banno K, Sabbagh AA, et al. Utilization of healthcare resources in obstructive sleep apnea syndrome: a 5-year follow-up study in men using CPAP. Sleep. 2005;28:1306–11.

15. Léger D, Bayon V, Laaban JP, Philip P. Impact of sleep apnea on economics. Sleep Med Rev. 2012;16:455–62.

16. WHO. Adherence to long-term therapies – Evidence for action. World Health Organization; 2003. Website: http://www.who.int/chp/knowledge/publications/adherence_full_report.pdf

17. Aurora RN, Casey KR, Kristo D, et al. Practice parameters for the surgical modifications of the upper airway for obstructive sleep apnea in adults. Sleep. 2010;33(10):1408–13.

18. Frost & Sullivan. Hidden health crisis costing America billions. Underdiagnosing and undertreating obstructive sleep apnea draining healthcare system. Darien: American Academy of Sleep Medicine; 2016. https://aasm.org/advocacy/initiatives/economic-impact-obstructive-sleep-apnea/

19. Kapur V, Blough DK, Sandblom RE, Hert R, de Maine JB, Sullivan SD, Psaty BM. The medical cost of undiagnosed sleep apnea. Sleep. 1999;22(6):749–55.

20. Andersen R, Newman JF. Societal and individual determinants of medical care utilization in the United States. Milbank Q. 2005;83:4.

21. Reuveni H, Greenberg-Dotan S, Simon-Tuval T, et al. Elevated healthcare utilisation in young adult males with obstructive sleep apnoea. Eur Respir J. 2008;31:273–9.

22. Tarasiuk A, Greenberg-Dotan S, Simon-Tuval T, et al. The effect of obstructive sleep apnea on morbidity and healthcare utilization of middle-aged and older adults. J Am Geriatr Soc. 2008;56:247–54.

23. Léger D, Stepnowsky C. The economic and societal burden of excessive daytime sleepiness in patients with obstructive sleep apnea. Sleep Med Rev. 2020;51:1–11.

24. Jennum P, Kjellberg J. Health, social and economical consequences of sleep disordered breathing: a controlled national study. Thorax. 2011;66(7):560–6.

25. Tarasiuk A, Greenberg-Dotan S, Simon T, et al. Low socioeconomic status is a risk factor for cardiovascular disease among adult OSAS patients requiringtreatment. Chest. 2006;130:766–73.

26. Mulgrew AT, Nasvadi G, Butt A, Cheema R, Fox N, Fleetham JA, Ryan CF, Cooper P, Ayas NT. Risk and severity of motor vehicle crashes in patients with obstructive sleep apnoea-hypopnoea. Thorax. 2008;63(6):536–41.

27. Sassani A, Findley LJ, Kryger M, et al. Reducing motor-vehicle collisions, costs, and fatalities by treating obstructive sleep apnea syndrome. Sleep. 2004;27:453–8.

28. Pietzsch JB, Garner A, Cipriano LE, Linehan JH. An integrated healtheconomic analysis of diagnostic and therapeutic strategies in the treatment of moderate-to-severe obstructive sleep apnea. Sleep. 2011;34(6):695–709.

29. Toraldo DM, Passali D, De Benedetto M. Cost-effectiveness strategies in OSAS management: a short review. Acta Otorhinolaryngol Ital. 2017;37:447–53.

30. Sanna A. Obstructive sleep apnoea, motor vehicle accidents, and work performance. Chron Respir Dis. 2013;10:29–33.

31. Hirsch Allen AJ, Bansback N, Ayas NT. The effect of OSA on work disability and work-related injuries. Chest. 2015;147:1422–8.

32. Omachi TA, Claman DM, Blanc PD, Eisner MD. Obstructive sleep apnea: a risk factor for work disability. Sleep. 2009;32:791–8.

33. Wickwire EM, Albrecht JS, Towe MM, Abariga SA, Diaz-Abad M, Shipper AG, Cooper LM, Samson Z, Assefa SZ, Tom SE, Scharf SM. The impact of treatments for OSA on monetized health economic outcomes. A systematic review. Chest. 2019;155(5):947–61.

34. Aloia MS, Knoepke CE, Lee-Chiong T. The new local coverage determination criteria for adherence to positive airway pressure treatment: testing the limits? Chest. 2010;138:875–9.

35. Potts KJ, Butterfield DT, Sims P, et al. Cost savings associated with an education campaign on the diagnosis and management of sleep-disordered breathing: a retrospective, claims-based US study. Popul Health Manag. 2013;16:7–13.

36. Monasterio C, Vidal S, Duran J, et al. Effectiveness of continuous positive airway pressure in mild sleep apnea-hypopnea syndrome. Am J Respir Crit Care Med. 2001;164(6):939–43.

37. Barnes M, Houston D, Worsnop CJ, et al. A randomized controlled trial of continuous positive airway pressure in mild obstructive sleep apnea. Am J Respir Crit Care Med. 2002;165(6):773–80.

38. Barnes M, McEvoy RD, Banks S, et al. Efficacy of positive airway pressure and oral appliance in mild to moderate obstructive sleep apnea. Am J Respir Crit Care Med. 2004;170(6):656–64.

39. Marshall NS, Barnes M, Travier N, et al. Continuous positive airway pressure reduces daytime sleepiness in mild to moderate obstructive sleep apnoea: a meta-analysis. Thorax. 2006;61(5):430–4.

40. Wimms A, Kelly JL, Turnbull CD, McMillan A, Craig SE, O'Reilly JF, et al. Continuous positive airway pressure versus standard care for the treatment of people with mild obstructive sleep apnoea (MERGE): a multicentre, randomised controlled trial. Lancet Respir Med. 2019;8(4):349–58.

41. Epstein LJ, Kristo D, Strollo PJ Jr, et al. Clinical guideline for the evaluation, management and long-term care of obstructive sleep apnea in adults. J Clin Sleep Med. 2009;5(3):263–76.

42. Mar J, Rueda JR, Durán-Cantolla J, Schechter C, Chilcott J. The cost effectiveness of nCPAP treatment in patients with moderate-to-severe obstructive sleep apnoea. Eur Respir J. 2003;21:515–22.

43. Weatherly HL, Griffin SC, Mc Daid C, et al. An economic analysis of continuous positive airway pressure for the treatment of obstructive sleep apnea-hypopnea syndrome. Int J Technol Assess Health Care. 2009;25(1):26–34.

44. NICE TA139. Continuous positive airway pressure for the treatment of obstructive sleep apnoea/hypopnoea syndrome. National Institute of Clinical Excellence; 2008.

45. Canadian Agency for Drugs and Technologies in Health. CPAP treatment for adults with obstructive sleep apnea: review of the clinical and cost-effectiveness and guidelines. Ottawa: Canadian Agency for Drugs and Technologies in Health; 2013.

46. Krishnan V. The economic burden of medical care in general and sleep apnea syndrome in particular. Sleep Breath. 2009;13:315–6.

47. McDaid C, Griffin S, Weatherly H, Duree K, Van der Burgt M, Van Hout S, Akers J, Davies RJ, Sculpher M, Westwood M. Continuous positive airway pressure devices for the treatment of obstructive sleep apnoea–hypopnoea syndrome: a systematic review and economic analysis. Health Technol Assess. 2009;13(4):3–5.

48. Laupacis A, Feeny D, Detsky AS, Tugwell PX. How attractive does a new technology have to be to warrant adoption and utilization? Tentative guidelines for using clinical and economic evaluation. Can Med Assoc J. 1992;146:473–81.

49. Ayas NT, FitzGerald JM, Fleetham JA, et al. Cost-effectiveness of continuous positive airway pressure therapy for moderate to severe obstructive sleep apnea/hypopnea. Arch Intern Med. 2006;166:977–84.

50. Hirth RA, Chernew ME, Miller E, et al. Willingness to pay for a quality-adjusted life year: in search of a standard. Med Decis Mak. 2000;20:332–42.

51. Ubel PA, Hirth RA, Chernew ME, Fendrick AM. What is the price of life and why doesn't it increase at the rate of inflation? Arch Intern Med. 2003;163:1637–41.

52. Tengs OT, Adams ME, Pliskin JS, et al. Five-hundred life-saving interventions and their cost-effectiveness. Risk Anal. 1995;15:369–90.

53. Plans-Rubio P. Cost-effectiveness of cardiovascular prevention programs in Spain. Int J Technol Assess Health Care. 1998;14:320–30.

54. Mohit B, Cohen J. Trends of cost-effectiveness studies in sleep medicine. Sleep Med. 2019;53:176–80.

55. Tousignant P, Cosio MG, Levy RD, Groome PA. Quality adjusted life years added by treatment of obstructive sleep apnea. Sleep. 1994;17(1):52–60.

56. Jenkinson C, Stradling J, Petersen S. How should we evaluate health status? A comparison of three methods inpatients presenting with obstructive sleep apnoea. Qual Life Res. 1998;7:95–100.

57. Chakravorty I, Cayton RM, Szczepura A. Health utilities in evaluating intervention in the sleep apnoea/hypopneoea syndrome. Eur Respir J. 2002;20:1233–8.

58. Chilcott J, Clayton E, Chada N, Hanning CD, Kinnear W, Waterhouse JC. Nasal continuous positive airways pressure in the management of sleep apnoea. Leicester: Trent Institute for Health Services Research; 2000.

59. Tan MC, Ayas NT, Mulgrew A, et al. Cost-effectiveness of continuous positive airway pressure therapy in patients with obstructive sleep apnea-hypopnea in British Columbia. Can Respir J. 2008;15:159–65.

60. Guest JF, Helter MT, Morgan A, Stradling JR. Cost-effectiveness of using continuous positive airway pressure in the treatment of severe obstructive sleep apnoea/hypopnoea syndrome in the UK. Thorax. 2008;63:860–5.

61. Poullie A-I, Spath H-M, Cognet M, Perrier L, Gauthier A, Clementz M, Druais S, Scemama O, Pichon CR, Jean-Luc Harousseau J-L. Cost-effectiveness of treatments for mild-to-moderate obstructive sleep apnea in france. Int J Technol Assess Health Care. 2016;32:37–45.

62. Bahammam A, Delaive K, Ronald J, Manfreda J, Roos L, Kryger MH. Health care utilization in males with obstructive sleep apnea syndrome two years after diagnosis and treatment. Sleep. 1999;22(6):740–7.

63. Tarasiuk A, Reznor G, Greenberg-Dotan S, Reuveni H. Financial incentive increases CPAP acceptance in patients from low socio-economic background. PLoS One. 2012;7:e33178.

64. Peker Y, Hedner J, Johansson Å, Bende M. Reduced hospitalization with cardiovascular and pulmonary disease inobstructive sleep apnea patients on nasal CPAP treatment. Sleep. 1997;20(8):645–53.

65. Rizzi CF, Ferraz MB, Poyares D, Tufik S. Quality-adjusted life-years gain and health status in patients with OSAS after one year of continuous positive airway pressure use OSAS after one year of continuous positive airway pressure use. Sleep. 2014;37:1963–8.

66. Berger MB, Sullivan W, Owen R, Wu C, Precision Pulmonary Diagnostics, Inc., Schneider National, Inc., and Definity Health Corp. A corporate driven sleep apnea detection and treatment program: results and challenges. Sleep Apnea Detection and Disordered Breathing Treatment Program; 2006.

67. Pelletier-Fleury N, Meslier N, Gagnadoux F, Person C, Rakotonanahary D, Ouksel H, Fleury B, Racineux J-L. Economic arguments for the immediate management of moderate-to-severe obstructive sleep apnoea syndrome. Eur Respir J. 2004;23:53–60.

68. Ramar K, Dort LC, Katz SG, et al. Clinical practice guideline for the treatment of obstructive sleep apnea and snoring with oral appliance therapy: an update for 2015. J Clin Sleep Med. 2015;11(7):773–827.

69. Quinnell TG, Bennett M, Jordan J, et al. A crossover randomised controlled trial of oral mandibular advancement devices for obstructive sleep apnoea-hypopnoea (TOMADO). Thorax. 2014;69(10):938–45.

70. Anandam A, Patil M, Akinnusi M, et al. Cardio-vascular mortality in obstructive sleep apnea treated with continuous positive airway pressure or oral appliance: an observational study. Respirology. 2013;18:1184–90.

71. Tripathi A, Jerrell JM, Stallworth JR. Cost-effectiveness of adeno-tonsillectomy in reducing obstructive sleep apnea, cerebrovascular ischemia, vaso-occlusive pain, and ACS episodes in pediatric sickle cell disease. Ann Hematol. 2011;90(2):145–50.

72. Sarkhosh K, Switzer NJ, El-Hadi M, et al. The impact of bariatric surgery onobstructive sleep apnea: a systematic review. Obes Surg. 2013;23:414–23.

73. Carlsson LM, Peltonen M, Ahlin S, et al. Bariatric surgery and prevention of type 2 diabetes in Swedish obese subjects. N Engl J Med. 2012;367:695–704.

74. Adams TD, Davidson LE, Litwin SE, et al. Health benefits of gastric bypass surgery after 6 years. JAMA. 2012;308:1122–31.

75. Neovius M, Narbro K, Keating C, et al. Healthcare use during 20 years following bariatric surgery. JAMA. 2012;308:1132–41.

76. Gagnadoux F, Le Vaillant M, Goupil F, Pigeanne T, Chollet S, et al. Influence of marital status and employment status on long-term adherence with continuous positive airway pressure in sleep apnea patients. PLoS One. 2011;6(8):e22503.

77. Haniffa M, Lasserson TJ, Smith I. Interventions to improve compliance with continuous positive airway pressure for obstructive sleep apnoea. Cochrane Database Syst Rev. 2004;(4):CD003531.

78. Weaver TE, Grunstein RR. Adherence to continuous positive airway pressure therapy: the challenge to effective treatment. Proc Am Thorac Soc. 2008;5:173–8.

79. Weaver TE, Sawyer AM. Adherence to continuous positive airway pressure treatment for obstructive sleep apnoea: implications for future interventions. Indian J Med Res. 2010;131:245–58.

80. Weaver TE, Kribbs NB, Pack AI, Kline LR, Chugh DK, Maislin G, et al. Night-to-night variability in CPAP use over first three months of treatment. Sleep. 1997;20:278–83.

81. Aloia MS, Arnedt JT, Stanchina M, Millman RP. How early in treatment is PAP adherence established? Revisiting night-to-night variability. Behav Sleep Med. 2007;5:229–40.

82. Grunstein RR, Stewart DA, Lloyd H, Akinci M, Cheng N, Sullivan CE. Acute withdrawal of nasal CPAP in obstructive sleep apnea does not cause a rise in stress hormones. Sleep. 1996;19:774–82.

83. Kribbs NB, Pack AI, Kline LR, Smith PL, Schwartz AR, Schubert NM, et al. Objective measurement of patterns of nasal CPAP use by patients with obstructive sleep apnea. Am Rev Respir Dis. 1993;147:887–95.

84. DiMatteo MR. Variations in patients' adherence to medical recommendations: a quantitative review of 50 years of research. Med Care. 2004;42(3):200–9.

85. Borel JC, Tamisier R, Sonia Dias-Domingos S, Sapene M, Martin F, Stach B, Grillet Y, Muir J-F, Levy P, Frederic Series F, Pepin J-L. on behalf of the Scientific Council of The Sleep Registry of the French Federation of Pneumology (OSFP) 10. PLoS One. 2013;8(5):e64382.

86. Rotenberg BW, Murariu D, Pang KP. Trends in CPAP adherence over twenty years of data collection: a flattened curve. J Otolaryngol Head Neck Surg. 2016;45:43.

87. Maschauer EL, Fairley DM, Riha RL. Does personality play a role in continuous positive airway pressure compliance? Breathe (Sheff). 2017;13:32–43.

88. Bollig SM. Encouraging CPAP adherence: it is everyone's job. Respir Care. 2010;55:1230–9.

89. Olsen S, Smith S, Oei TP. Adherence to continuous positive airway pressure therapy in obstructive sleep apnoea sufferers: a theoretical approach to treatment adherence and intervention. Clin Psychol Rev. 2008;28:1355–71.

90. Boyaci H, Baris SA, Basyigit I, Yildiz F, Gacar K. Positive airway pressure device compliance of the patients with obstructive sleep apnea syndrome. Adv Clin Exp Med. 2013;22:809–15.

91. Kohler M, Smith D, Tippett V, Stradling JR. Predictors of long-term compliance with continuous positive airway pressure. Thorax. 2010;65:829–32.

92. McArdle N, Devereux G, Heidarnejad H, Engleman HM, Mackay TW, et al. Long-term use of CPAP therapy for sleep apnea/hypopnea syndrome. Am J Respir Crit Care Med. 1999;159:1108–14.

93. Shapiro GK, Shapiro CM. Factors that influence CPAP adherence: an overview. Sleep Breath. 2010;14:323–35.

94. Billings ME, Kapur VK. Medicare long-term CPAP coverage policy: a cost-utility analysis. J Clin Sleep Med. 2013;9(10):1023–102.

95. Baratta F, Pastori D, Bucci T, Fabiani M, Fabiani V, Brunori M, Loffredo L, Lillo R, Pannitteri G, Angelico F, Del Ben M. Long-term prediction of adherence to continuous positive air pressure therapy for the treatment of moderate/severe obstructive sleep apnea syndrome. Sleep Med. 2018;43:66–70.

96. Wickwire EM, Jobe SL, Oldstone LM, Scharf SM, Johnson AM, Albrecht JS. Lower socioeconomic status and co-morbid conditions are associated with reduced continuous positive airway pressure adherence among older adult medicare beneficiaries with obstructive sleep apnea. Sleep. 2020;43(12):zsaa122. https://doi.org/10.1093/sleep/zsaa122.

97. Sawyer A, Deatrick JA, Kuna ST, Weaver TE. Differences in perceptions of the diagnosis and treatment of obstructive sleep apnea and continuous positive airway pressure therapy among adherers and nonadherers. Qual Health Res. 2010;20(7):873–92.

98. May AM, Gharibeh T, Wang L, Hurley A, Walia H, Strohl KP, Mehra R. CPAP adherence predictors in a randomized trial of moderate-to-severe OSA enriched with women and minorities. Chest. 2018;154(3):567–78. McDaid C, Griffin S, Weatherly H, Duree K, van der Burgt M, et al. Continuous positive airway pressure devices for the treatment of obstructive sleep apnoea-hypopnoea syndrome: a systematic review and economic analysis. Health Technol Assess. 2009; 13: iii–iv, xi–xiv, 1–119, 143–274.

99. Chasens E, Pack A, Maislin G, Dinges D, Weaver T. Claustrophobia and adherence to CPAP treatment. West J Nurs Res. 2005;27:307–21.

100. Gay P, Weaver T, Loube D, Iber C. Evaluation of positive airway pressure treatment for sleep related breathing disorders in adults. Sleep. 2006;29:381–401.

101. Campos-Rodriguez F, Martinez-Garcia MA, de la Cruz-Moron I, Almeida-Gonzalez C, Catalan-Serra P, Montserrat JM. Cardiovascular mortality in women with obstructive sleep apnea with or without continuous positive airway pressure treatment: a cohort study. Ann Intern Med. 2012;156(2):115–22.

102. Palm A, Theorell-Haglow J, Janson C, Lindberg E, Midgren B. Factors influencing compliance to continuous positive airway pressure treatment in obstructive sleep apnea and mortality associated with treatment failure. Sleep Med. 2018;51:85–91.

103. Redline S, Baker-Goodwin S, Bakker JP, et al. Patient partnerships transforming sleep medicine research and clinical care: perspectives from the Sleep Apnea Patient-Centered Outcomes Network. J Clin Sleep Med. 2016;12(7):1053–8.

104. Afsharpaiman S, Shahverdi E, Vahedi E, Aqaee H. Continuous positive airway pressure compliance in patients with obstructive sleep apnea. Tanaffos. 2016;15(1):25–30.

105. Smith I, Lasserson TJ. Pressure modification for improving usage of continuous positive airway pressure machines in adults with obstructive sleepapnoea. Cochrane Database Syst Rev. 2009;(4):CD003531.

106. Bakker JP, Marshall NS. Flexible pressure delivery modification of continuous positive airway pressure for obstructive sleep apnea does not improve compliance with therapy: systematic review and meta-analysis. Chest. 2011;139(6):1322–30.

107. Chai CL, Pathinathan A, Smith B. Continuous positive airway pressure delivery interfaces for obstructive sleep apnoea. Cochrane Database Syst Rev. 2006;(4):CD005308.

108. Teo M, Amis T, Lee S, Falland K, Lambert S, et al. Equivalence of nasal and oronasal masks during initial CPAP titration for obstructive sleep apnea syndrome. Sleep. 2011;34:951–5.

109. Bakker JP, Neill AM, Campbell AJ. Nasal versus oronasal continuous positive airway pressure masks for obstructive sleep apnea: a pilot investigation of pressure requirement, residual disease, and leak. Sleep Breath. 2012;16:709–16.

110. Ebben MR, Oyegbile T, Pollak CP. The efficacy of three different mask styles on a PAP titration night. Sleep Med. 2012;13:645–9.

111. Rico F, Liu Y, Martinez DA, Huang S, Zayas-Castro JL, Fabri PJ. Preventable readmission risk factors for patients with chronic conditions. J Healthc Qual. 2016;38(3):127–42.

112. McIlvennan CK, Eapen ZJ, Allen LA. Hospital readmissions reductionprogram. Circulation. 2015;131(20):1796–803.

113. Truong KK, De Jardin R, Massoudi N, Hashemzadeh M, Jafari B. Nonadherence to CPAP associated with increased 30-day hospital readmissions. J Clin Sleep Med. 2018;14:183–9.

114. Sharma S, Mather P, Gupta A, et al. Effect of early intervention with positive airway pressure therapy for sleep disordered breathing on six-month readmission rates in hospitalized patients with heart failure. Am J Cardiol. 2016;117(6):940–5.

115. Kauta SR, Keenan BT, Goldberg L, Schwab RJ. Diagnosis and treatment of sleep disordered breathing in hospitalized cardiac patients: a reduction in 30-day hospital readmission rates. J Clin Sleep Med. 2014;10(10):1051–9.

116. Watson NF. Health care savings: the economic value of diagnostic and therapeutic care for obstructive sleep apnea. J Clin Sleep Med. 2016;12:1075–7. [PubMed: 27448424]

117. Patel N, Sam A, Valentin A, Quan SF, Parthasarathy S. Refill rates of accessories for positive airway pressure therapy as a surrogate measure of long-term adherence. J Clin Sleep Med. 2012;8:169–75.

118. Freedman N. Doing it better for less: incorporating OSA management into alternative payment models. Chest. 2019;155:227–33.

119. Antic NA, Catcheside P, Buchan C, Hensley M, Naughton MT, et al. The effect of CPAP in normalizing daytime sleepiness, quality of life, and neurocognitive function in patients with moderate to severe OSA. Sleep. 2011;34:111–9.

120. Malhotra A, Crocker ME, Willes L, Kelly C, Lynch S, Benjafield AV. Patient engagement using new technology toimprove adherence to positive airway pressure therapy: a retrospective analysis. Chest. 2018;153(4):843–50.

121. Gold MR, Siegel JE, Russell LB, Weinstein MC, editors. Cost-effectiveness in health and medicine. New York: Oxford University Press Inc; 1996.

122. Drummond MF, O'Brien B, Stoddart GL, Torrance GW, editors. Methods for the economic evaluation of health care programmes. 2nd ed. Oxford: Oxford Medical Publications; 1997.

123. Neumann PJ, Goldie SJ, Weinstein MC. Preference-based measures in economic evaluation in health care. Annu Rev Public Health. 2000;21:587–611.

124. Brooks RG. EuroQoL—the current state of play. Health Policy. 1996;37:53–72.

Meenakshi Gupta

13.1 Factors Affecting CPAP Adherence

Obstructive sleep apnea (OSA) is a common sleep-related breathing disorder, characterized by transient interruption of ventilation during sleep caused by complete or partial collapse of the upper airway. This disease may affect 26% of the population [1].

Severity of sleep apnea is based on the apnea-hypopnea Index (AHI) which is the number of apneas or hypopneas recorded during the sleep study per hour of sleep. Based on the AHI, the severity of OSA [2] is classified as follows:

- None/minimal: AHI <5 per hour
- Mild: AHI ≥5, but <15 per hour
- Moderate: AHI ≥15, but <30 per hour
- Severe: AHI ≥30 per hour

Excessive daytime sleepiness which negatively affects patients' quality of life and inability to sustain attention to different tasks is one of the main complaints. This condition is also associated with an increased risk of having motor vehicle accidents [3], cerebrovascular [4] and other cardiovascular diseases, and increased mortality [5].

CPAP has been found to be an effective modality for treatment of sleep apnea. However, the effectiveness of CPAP treatment strongly depends on patient adherence to therapy. Satisfactory adherence has been considered to be achieved when the usage rate is ≥4 h/day. Less than 4 h is used as a general metric for low adherence, since several studies have shown that normalization of daytime sleepiness, quality of life, and neurocognitive function improve with 4 or more hours of use [6–9]. Improvements in cardiovascular disease conditions and diabetes have also been greater in those using CPAP for greater than 4 h [10–12]. Studies have used 4 h as the cutoff point differentiating adherence and nonadherence to the treatment, and consequently insurers have also adopted this cutoff. It is possible that the field has been blighted by this early rule of thumb, and if a higher bar had been set, perhaps we would now think that the impact of CPAP is greater than what we now perceive. This is also demonstrated in another study which suggested that use of CPAP for longer than 6 h decreases sleepiness, improves daily functioning, reduces the risk of cardiovascular disease to the level among people who do not have OSA, and restores memory to normal levels [13]. For purposes of this paper, use of CPAP for a minimum of 4 h has been used to describe adherence.

A number of studies have demonstrated that patient adherence to therapy varies widely [6–9]. It has been noted that 46–83% of patients with obstructive sleep apnea have been reported to be nonadherent to treatment [7]. Adherence to CPAP treatment is crucial to patients with sleep apnea as the condition manifests rapidly when treatment is stopped. Even one night without CPAP may impact on the benefits of CPAP therapy, which include fewer apneas and hypopneas, reduced daytime sleepiness, and improvements in sleep architecture, daily activity, quality of life, hypertension, and neurobehavioral performance [14–18].

The impact of discontinuation of CPAP therapy was illustrated by a trial that included 41 patients with OSA who had been using CPAP successfully for at least 1 year without subjective daytime sleepiness [19]. After four nights of not using CPAP, the frequency of oxyhemoglobin desaturation events (defined as a decrease in the oxyhemoglobin saturation exceeding 4 percentage points of saturation) increased during sleep, indicating recurrence of OSA. The patients were then randomly assigned to a CPAP withdrawal group (i.e., sub-therapeutic CPAP) or a CPAP group (i.e., therapeutic CPAP) for 2 weeks. CPAP withdrawal led to recurrence of abnormal respiratory events (mean AHI >25 events per hour) within one night, increased morning and evening blood pressure within 2 weeks, and increased morning heart rate within 2 weeks. Subjective daytime sleepiness measured by the Epworth sleepiness scale also increased within 2 weeks,

M. Gupta (✉)
University of Saskatchewan, North Battleford, SK, Canada

Maple Leaf Medical Clinic, Toronto, ON, Canada

although the sleepiness score remained less than ten (i.e., considered within normal range). CPAP withdrawal for 2 weeks was not associated with deterioration of psychomotor performance.

Another small, randomized trial showed that after just 2 weeks without CPAP, hourly arousal events had more than tripled. Additionally, AHI had increased 17-fold [20]. Although objective measures of sleepiness did not significantly change, subjective sleepiness and OSA returned within days of ending CPAP treatment. By the study's end, morning heart rate, blood pressure, and urinary catecholamines increased significantly, and endothelial function had significantly decreased compared to people on CPAP.

The adherence of patients to CPAP therapy significantly improves their quality of life and daytime sleepiness. In addition, CPAP is effective in controlling a range of aspects associated with cardiovascular risk, morbidity, and mortality. Higher levels of CPAP adherence are also associated with significant improvements in vigilance [21].

Factors That Have Been Studied with Regard to CPAP Adherence

These can be divided into three broad categories (Table 13.1):

A. Patient-related factors
B. Therapy- and medication-related factors
C. Health professional-related factors

A. *Patient-Related Factors*
  1. *Use in First Week*

     Patients generally make the decision to use CPAP therapy early during the first week of therapy, usually by the second to fourth day [6, 22–24]. Those who adhere generally increase their duration of nightly use gradually in the following weeks. Initial problems have been shown to be associated with poorer adherence to CPAP [25].

     Decreased CPAP use in the first week has been shown to be associated with being black, less intimacy with partners, and higher residual AHI, accounting for 25 percent of the variance in use [24–27]. Additionally, self-efficacy (defined as one's motivation, volition, and confidence to engage in a healthy behavior) in the first week, but not prior to treatment, was also related to use in the first week [26].

  2. *Self-Efficacy and Perspective Regarding CPAP Therapy*

     OSA-specific transtheoretical model (TTM) and social cognitive theory (SCT) describe participant's readiness for treatment, his or her weighing of the pros and cons of treatment (decisional balance), and his or her confidence (self-efficacy) that he or she can

Table 13.1 Factors Relevant to CPAP Adherence

Patient-related factors	Therapy- and medication-related factors	Health professional-related factors
Failure to understand the importance of the therapy	Complexity of therapy, in device use, or medication dosing	Poor relationship with patient
Failure to understand instructions concerning the therapy	Increased rate of adverse reactions (Device use has complications, and the provider needs to meet with the patient periodically to determine adverse events and help address these issues.)	Expression of doubt concerning therapeutic potential
Concomitant self-administration of prescription or nonprescription medications or alcohol	Characteristics of illness; long-term or chronic illnesses are a problem, as compliance decreases over time	Unwillingness to educate patients
Social isolation, thus lack of social support (Patients with supportive families have been shown to be more compliant with prescription drugs – data not available for CPAP use.)	Expensive therapy (only a problem when a patient must pay out of pocket or has not met the deductible)	Lack of knowledge of medications the patient is taking or has access to (Sedatives and alcohol can compound OSA, and their use should be evaluated.)
Feeling ill, or being too tired to use the therapy	Lack of efficacy.	
Physical limitations, including vision, hearing, and hand coordination		

Source: UpToDate
CPAP Continuous positive airway pressure, *OSA* obstructive sleep apnea

use treatment effectively. Recent work has shown that OSA-specific scales measuring the TTM constructs of readiness and decisional balance and the SCT construct of self-efficacy account for 24% and 31% of the variance in CPAP adherence at 1 week, respectively, over and above the variance accounted for by subjective sleepiness and CPAP pressure [28]. At 1 month post-treatment, these variables accounted for 33% and 40% of the variance. These predictors account for significantly more of the variance in CPAP use than demographic, disease, and CPAP-focused predictors [28–31].

  3. Patient demographic characteristics such as *sex, marital and socioeconomic status, and race* have consistently been associated with CPAP use [26]. For example, a large retrospective study found that that long-term adherence was related to race, income,

body mass index, sex, or time spent with oxygen saturation of less than 90% [27].

Studies have shown a small but consistently reduced level of adherence in women compared with men across all ages, but this difference is magnified at extremes of age. Interestingly, the time course of the sex disparity also varies by age. In those younger than age 30, women have rates of use nearly identical to those of men during the first week, but their usage declines much more steeply than that for men over time. This steeper decline is associated with a larger proportion of young women abandoning CPAP use. This is different from women older than 70 years who substantially reduce their usage of CPAP in the first week compared to men. Reasons for the sex disparity include the fact that OSA is viewed as a male disease; thus, women may have greater reluctance to admit they have the disease and so may be less accepting of treatment. Societal expectations that place a greater emphasis on the appearance of women also may adversely impact the decisional balance for women such that they are less accepting of a treatment that may be viewed as unattractive [15]. Specific challenges related to CPAP use such as claustrophobia may be more common in women than men [16]. Another possibility is that the symptoms more commonly associated with OSA in women, such as insomnia and fatigue, may be less responsive to CPAP therapy, preventing the positive feedback from symptom resolution.

With regard to marital status, it has been found that married participants had a relatively higher CPAP use than those who were not married. It is likely that married participants have overall higher social support, which has been linked to a better adherence to medical treatment [32]. However, intimacy with partners has also been identified as an independent predictor for reduced CPAP use. Therefore, the nature of spousal involvement in CPAP use may be complicated and cannot be simply represented by marital status.

The issue of why race plays a role in adherence to CPAP remains to be determined. It may be related to multiple factors, including internal (e.g., patient knowledge, beliefs, motivation, health literacy) and external (e.g., socioeconomic status, social support, insurance or medical coverage, barriers to care) factors [33]. Mean daily CPAP use in blacks has been noted to be less than other patient groups. In a study done among US veterans with different ethnicity, it was noted that mean daily CPAP use in blacks was 1 h less than whites after adjusting for covariates. No CPAP adherence differences were noted between whites and Hispanics [33].

The relationship between age and CPAP adherence is unclear. For example, Sin et al. found that CPAP was used more by older patients [34], but others [6] have found that older patients used their machines less. There may be a bimodal distribution, with the youngest and oldest being less adherent to CPAP treatment. Further research is needed to explore the relationship between age and CPAP use.

4. Emerging evidence suggest that *increased nasal resistance* affects CPAP use and initial acceptance of this treatment [35–37]. Li and associates [35] employed acoustic rhinometry to measure the internal dimensions of the airway; those patients with smaller nasal cross-sectional area and reduced volume were much less likely to be adherent. Further, they found that minimum cross-sectional area was an independent predictor of adherence, accounting for 16% of the variance. Interestingly, self-reported nasal stuffiness was not associated with nasal dimensions. Nasal resistance/obstruction also seems to influence the initial acceptance of CPAP treatment, with increased nasal pressure resulting in a 50% greater chance of rejecting CPAP as a treatment [36, 37]. Two studies examined the influence of nasal resistance on the initial acceptance of CPAP. In the study by Sugiura [37] and colleagues, of 77 patients who had an AHI of more than 20, those who rejected CPAP as a therapy after initial exposure (brief nap and titration night; 27%) had higher nasal resistance than those who accepted this treatment. In those with nasal resistance, every increase in nasal pressure of 0.1 Pa/cm^3/s resulted in a 50% greater chance of rejecting CPAP as a treatment [38].

5. *Failure to understand the importance of the therapy and the instructions concerning the therapy and concomitant self-administration of prescription or nonprescription medications or alcohol* are also factors associated with poor adherence to CPAP treatment [36].

6. *Social isolation, thus lack of social support.* Patients with supportive families have been shown to be more adherent to CPAP treatment [7, 14, 38].

Patients who experience a *major stressful life event* (e.g., death of a spouse, hospital admission) within 6 months of initiating CPAP have been noted to have significantly lower CPAP use than those who do not have any recent life events [6, 7, 38]. It is likely that life events have a direct adverse effect on machine use due to concurrent stress. However, pretreatment anxiety and depression scores are not correlated with machine use over the first month of treatment [6].

7. *Claustrophobia.* One study reported that a feeling of claustrophobia, retrospectively reported after a mean

of 106 days use, was the only problem identified significantly more often by patients who used their CPAP less regularly [32]. Poor CPAP adherence (<2 h per night) has been noted to be more than two times higher in participants with a claustrophobia score > or = 25 [39].

8. *Ability to overcome obstacles and problem-solve.* Objectively measured average daily compliance is significantly associated with a measure of coping strategies. Active ways of coping account for a significant amount of variance in CPAP compliance.

9. Other factors associated with poor adherence include feeling ill, or being too tired for therapy or physical limitations, including vision, hearing, and hand coordination.

B. *Disease-Related Factors*

1. OSA During Rapid Eye Movement (REM) Sleep

In a prospective observational cohort study, patients were divided into the following two groups: (I) REM-predominantly OSA [AHI of ≥5, with a REM-AHI/NREM-AHI of >2, an NREM-AHI of <15, and a minimum of 15 min of REM-sleep duration] and (II) non-stage specific OSA. Follow-up was performed at 1, 6, and 12 months after the initiation of CPAP therapy. At 12 months, the number of hours used per day was 3.8 ± 1.8 and 5.1 ± 2.1 h in the REM-only and non-stage specific OSA groups, respectively. Thus, CPAP adherence was lower among patients with REM-only OSA compared to patients with non-stage specific OSA [40].

2. Subjective Excessive Daytime Sleepiness

The evidence shows that the degree of self-reported daytime sleepiness as measured by the Epworth sleepiness scale – especially a score of more than 10 – in combination with more severe OSA is associated with long-term use [27, 41]. Various studies have shown that adherence increased in the patients who experienced more severe daytime sleepiness [41–43]. Perceived improvement in symptoms after CPAP use has been shown to be related to better adherence [34].

In one study, 42 patients with OSA on polysomnography and symptoms of excessive daytime sleepiness were randomized in two equal groups. Good compliance to CPAP was seen in 52% and poor compliance in 48%. Epworth sleepiness scale (ESS) score >12, first night use of CPAP > 4 h, and usage of auto CPAP unit were statistically significant predictors of compliance. Usage of CPAP was low among patients with severe sleep apnea but little sleepiness [43]. Data for adherence in non-sleepy obstructive sleep apnea patients is scarce.

A German study showed that "positive early subjective statements" predicted acceptance of CPAP

therapy in a small group of 14 patients at 4 months [44].

3. Comorbid insomnia – it has been noted that pretreatment nocturnal insomnia symptoms and sleep dissatisfaction predicted poorer 6-month CPAP use [33, 45].

4. Disease severity, as measured by AHI, does not appear to play a major role in determining adherence relationship based on most [14, 24, 38] but not all studies [46]. Likewise, the number of respiratory events and the severity of intermittent hypoxemia (assessed by the ODI) have been found to not be relevant to treatment adherence [40].

High residual AHI was noted to be a significant predictor for poor CPAP use during the first week. Unresolved sleep apnea from residual events may lead patients to believe that the treatment is ineffective, resulting in low use or abandoning treatment. This finding underscores the need for close follow-up within the first few days of treatment with evaluation for the presence of residual events and the need for re-titration.

In another study, multivariate analysis showed that interactions between the AHI and the percentage of nighttime spent with an O_2 saturation of <90% (TC90) and between the AHI and hypertension at baseline predicted long-term compliance with CPAP. Good CPAP adherence was predicted by greater OSA severity as measured by both the AHI and TC90 and by the presence of hypertension at baseline in patients with higher AHI levels [47]. Another study revealed that the severity of sleep-disordered breathing rather than sleepiness determines long-term adherence to CPAP therapy.

However, other studies [14, 48] have only shown a weak relationship with CPAP adherence. There is a lack of evidence indicating that level of nocturnal hypoxemia is instrumental in determining CPAP adherence [2, 15, 24, 49, 50]. In contrast, there is stronger support for symptomatic severity to influence adherence.

5. Although side effects would seem central to discontinuing treatment, they do not appear to be important in some studies [51, 52] but are cited as being important in others [53, 54].

6. It is uncertain whether the routine application of heated humidification predicts adherence since the evidence is conflicting. While some studies indicate that heated humidification enhances adherence [55–57], other studies do not [56–60]. It has been suggested that humidification affects adherence only in those who experience nasal congestion [55, 58].

C. *Health Professional-Related Factors*

7. Some of the factors associated with poor adherence include [26]:
   (a) Poor relationship with patient
   (b) Expression of doubt concerning therapeutic potential
   (c) Unwillingness to educate patients
   (d) Lack of knowledge of medications the patient is taking or has access to (Sedatives and alcohol can compound OSA, and their use should be evaluated.)

In summary, the following factors have been associated with long-term nonadherence with CPAP therapy [26, 38, 61–65]:

- Nightly CPAP use <4 h/night during the first 1–2 weeks of therapy and problems encountered during the first night of use.
- Lack of a positive perspective regarding the benefit of CPAP therapy.
- Low self-efficacy.
- Demographic characteristics (sex, age, marital status, and race).
- Claustrophobic tendencies.
- Ability to overcome obstacles and problem-solve.
- It was the partner's idea, and not the patient's, to seek medical attention.
- Less severity of oxyhemoglobin desaturation during sleep on diagnostic polysomnography and poor sleep efficiency during CPAP titration.
- Small nasal volume and high nasal resistance.
- Moderate-to-severe OSA (i.e., an apnea hypopnea index >15 events per hour of sleep; controversial weak relationship) [9, 14, 61–65]

13.2 Phenotypes of Sleep Apnea in Regard to Adherence

Current strategies for the management of OSA reflect a one-size-fits-all approach. Diagnosis and severity of OSA are based on the AHI and treatment initiated with CPAP, followed by trials of alternatives (e.g., oral appliances) if CPAP "fails." This approach does not consider the heterogeneity of individuals with OSA, reflected by varying risk factors, pathophysiological causes, clinical manifestations, and consequences.

OSA is increasingly recognized as a complex and heterogeneous disorder [66]. The AHI is insufficient to capture clinical heterogeneity of patients with OSA and should not be used in isolation for management of patients. To help classify patients into relevant prognostic and therapeutic categories, an OSA phenotype can be identified.

A phenotype can be defined as "a category of patients with OSA distinguished from others by a single or combination of disease features, in relation to clinically meaningful attributes (symptoms, response to therapy, health outcomes, quality of life)" [66]. Identifying meaningful phenotypes of OSA can be accomplished by anchoring them to relevant patient outcomes.

Identifying clinical phenotypes may aid in guiding treatment and thus improve clinical outcomes as well as CPAP adherence.

Characterizing the heterogeneity of OSA into various well-defined phenotypes is challenging because there are sparse prospective data and long-term validation.

13.3 Phenotyping Approaches

Phenotyping strategies can be grouped by features (e.g., clinical vs. molecular) and by experimental approaches (e.g., supervised vs. unsupervised).

Clinical phenotyping focuses on identifying unique patient categories based on measures such as signs, symptoms, demographics, comorbidities, physiological and anatomic measures, or treatment responsiveness. Molecular phenotyping aims to classify individuals based on molecular features: DNA, RNA, mRNA, miRNA, proteins, metabolites, and other biological products. Additionally, the number of features considered in the approach can vary from one (e.g., sex) to thousands (e.g., single nucleotide polymorphisms) [66].

Complementary to molecular phenotyping, clinical phenotyping may serve as an intermediate step toward personalized medicine in OSA. Potential clinical phenotypes identified are discussed below.

1. *Excessive Daytime Sleepiness Phenotype*

The most common clinical phenotype (OSA subtype) is a patient with OSA and excessive sleepiness (EDS). Up to 60% of OSA patients can be excessively sleepy [67] and report higher rates of impaired concentration, mood lability, and other neurocognitive difficulties [68]. Epidemiologic studies demonstrate that EDS modifies the relationship between AHI and incidence of hypertension [69], glucose metabolism [70], inflammatory markers, cardiovascular comorbidities [70], and mortality [71]. Compared to those without sleepiness, treatment of patients with EDS has also been shown to reduce blood pressure and vascular risk and improve quality of life [66, 72]. Thus, it has been proposed that OSA with EDS is a unique phenotype [73]. The lack of awareness of this phenotypic distinction when in the early days of treating OSA most patients were sleepy has led to a mantra of not seeing any purpose in doing MSLT in patients being evaluated for OSA. This may have stunted the field and unnecessarily restricted the field from making more nuanced assessments.

A study from Andaku et al. [74] evaluated patients with metabolic syndrome and OSA. The authors compared patients with and without EDS. These were also compared to a control group with metabolic syndrome but without OSA and without daytime sleepiness. The authors described higher inflammatory markers (e.g., CRP) in participants with OSA and daytime sleepiness compared to the other groups adjusting for waist circumference, and triglycerides, without differences in oxidative stress markers.

2. Age-Related Phenotypes

Age, gender, and race ethnicity are increasingly recognized as factors impacting OSA presentation and implications [66, 75–77].

For example, compared to younger patients with the same AHI, OSA in older patients is associated with less sleepiness and often presents with enuresis, cognitive dysfunction, and mood impairments [66, 77]. The frequency of OSA increases with aging with a plateau after 65 years. Additionally, with increasing age, there is increased upper airway collapsibility, reduced airway caliber due to preferential deposition of fat around the pharynx, decreased lung volume, and ventilatory chemosensitivity, making the aging population anatomically susceptible to OSA. The genioglossal responsiveness to negative intra-pharyngeal pressure appears to deteriorate with age. Older adults apparently have an increased frequency of spontaneous arousals suggestive of a lower arousal threshold. However, the aging process desensitizes the ventilatory control system and lowers the loop gain. Hence, airway anatomy/collapsibility plays a greater role in older adults, whereas a sensitive ventilatory control system is a prominent trait in younger adults with OSA. These observations have led to the suggestion that OSA in the elderly may represent distinct physiological phenotype.

Supporting this claim is a consistent lack of association between OSA and increased risk of hypertension [78] or atrial fibrillation [79] among older adults. Conflicting results exist, however, about risk for coronary artery disease [80, 81], cognitive impairment [82–84], and death [85]. The potential reasons for such variability are many, including differing definitions of OSA used in these studies and differing measures employed to characterize OSA severity (AHI, oxygen desaturation index [ODI], time spent below 90% oxygen saturation).

Distinction must be made between adult and pediatric OSA. Pediatric sleep disordered breathing may affect up to 3% of school-aged children, with consequences similar to those for adults [77]. The most common cause of OSA in children is related to enlargement of the tonsillar and adenoidal tissue, with surgical removal usually resulting in significant improvement. The role of obesity is somewhat controversial in childhood OSA [77].

3. Gender-Related Phenotypes

Males are 2–3 times more likely to have OSA than females with longer periods of apnea and more significant oxygen desaturations, despite a lower body mass index (BMI) [76, 86]. Women tend to have longer sleep latency and more slow wave sleep [76]. Overall, their AHIs are lower, especially during NREM (non-rapid eye movement) sleep, and respiratory events tend to cluster in REM sleep [76]. Such findings suggest that OSA in women is a separate phenotype, further supported by differences in predisposing factors for OSA.

The male predisposition to OSA appears to be anatomically based with increased fat deposition around the pharyngeal airway [86]. The length of the vulnerable pharyngeal airway is greater in males compared with females. The android pattern of fat deposition around the abdomen contributes to reduced lung volume in males and increases the susceptibility to upper airway collapsibility as a result of loss of longitudinal caudal traction on the trachea [87].

4. OSA and Menopause

OSA is less prevalent among premenopausal women, but postmenopausal women have a similar risk to that of men. The odds ratio for the presence of OSA was 1.1 in perimenopausal and 3.5 in postmenopausal women [86, 88]. Menopause, pregnancy, and polycystic ovarian syndrome increase the risk for OSA in women. After menopause, the worsening severity of OSA predominantly occurs during the NREM sleep versus younger women with a predominantly REM-associated OSA. The pharyngeal airway is longer in postmenopausal versus premenopausal women [86]. Female sex hormones such as estrogen and progesterone have a protective effect on upper airway patency and ventilatory drive [86].

5. OSA in Various Ethnic Populations

The relative importance of the anatomical determinants of OSA varies between ethnicities. Asian OSA populations are found to primarily display features of craniofacial skeletal restriction, African Americans display more obesity and enlarged upper airway soft tissues, and Caucasians show evidence of both bony and soft tissue abnormalities [86]. Craniofacial restriction and central fat deposition favor a greater predisposition to OSA in Asians, despite a lower overall BMI compared with other populations. Brachycephaly, which is a disproportionately short and broad head, is associated with a higher AHI in Caucasians but not in African Americans [89–97].

6. *Supine Position-Related OSA*

Supine position-related OSA is a dominant phenotype of OSA with a prevalence of 20% to 60% in the general population [93]. Reports suggest that over 50% of those referred for OSA evaluation exhibit supine AHI that is at least twice that in non-supine position [66]. It may be attributable to unfavorable upper airway anatomy, reduced lung volume, and inability of airway dilator muscles to compensate for the airway collapse in the supine position. A consistent finding is that pharyngeal collapsibility (Pcrit) markedly improves in lateral position, suggesting that smaller lateral wall size, decreased fat content, and lower facial height are associated with velopharyngeal patency while lateral [66, 86]. Patients with positional (supine-predominant) OSA tend to be younger and have lower body mass indices (BMI) and lower AHIs compared to their non-positional counterparts.

7. *REM-Related OSA*

In addition to position, distribution of respiratory disturbance within sleep stages has been used to categorize OSA, with REM-predominant OSA being most studied. Hypopneas and apneas are known to be longer in duration and cause an increase in the severity of hypoxemia during REM compared with non-REM sleep in patients with OSA. The prevalence of REM-related OSA ranges from 10% to 36% of the patient population with OSA undergoing PSG. The female preponderance of patients experiencing REM sleep-specific obstruction is well established.

Patients with REM-predominant OSA tend to be younger women and have reduced sleep time, sleep efficiency, and REM duration. Decreased genioglossal muscle activity in REM, lower respiratory drive, longer duration events, and more severe hypoxia combined with increased sympathetic activity during REM sleep have led to hypotheses that events during this stage may have unique clinical implications [68]. Despite the physiological and polysomnographic differences, large cross-sectional analyses comparing REM-predominant to NREM (or stage independent) OSA have failed to show differences in sleepiness, functional outcomes, PAP adherence, or quality of life [95–97].

REM sleep is associated with greater sympathetic activity and cardiovascular instability in healthy individuals and OSA patients versus NREM sleep. REM-related OSA has been found to be associated with an increased risk of hypertension.

8. *Congenital Abnormalities and Craniofacial Morphology*

OSA is also associated with craniofacial abnormalities, with jaw abnormalities being more important in thinner OSA patients. Morphological features associated with sleep disordered breathing include cranial base dimensions being more obtuse, inferior displacement of the hyoid bone, macroglossia, adenotonsillar hypertrophy, increase in lower facial height, a retroposed maxilla, and a short mandible [66, 86, 98].

Growth of the craniofacial skeleton continues throughout adulthood, and there is also significant sexual dimorphism. For instance, women have increased growth of the craniofacial skeleton with pregnancy and other hormonal changes; mandibular orientation and occlusal relationships also change throughout the life cycle.

Environmental mechanisms play a strong role in determining cranio-skeletal growth. These include bad habits such as thumb-sucking and abnormal tongue posturing, nasopharyngeal disease, disturbed respiratory function (e.g., mouth breathing), tumors, loss of teeth, malnutrition, and endocrinopathy. Thus, environmental influences can significantly alter the skeleton, thereby altering phenotypic expression. Postnatal growth, head shape, and facial profile also possess certain characteristics that can affect breathing. On reviewing the current knowledge in this area, mandibular position and size were found to play the greatest role in determining facial alignment and predisposition to sleep disordered breathing.

Reduced nasal patency, due to congestion or anatomical defects, as well as respiratory allergies, can also significantly contribute to OSA. Overall, it has been suggested that hereditary factors invoke 40% of the variance in the occurrence of OSA in the population, with the rest attributable to environmental factors.

Additionally, certain congenital conditions, such as Marfan's syndrome, Down syndrome, and the Pierre Robin sequence, predispose to the development of OSA, as do acquired conditions, such as acromegaly, hypothyroidism, and menopause.

9. *Drug Use*

Alcohol ingestion exacerbates OSA by reducing the activity of the genioglossus muscle, thereby leading to upper airway collapse. Exacerbation of the condition can also occur as a result of sedative use, sleep deprivation, tobacco use, and sleeping in the supine posture [98].

10. *OSA and Insomnia*

A phenotype characterized by symptoms and/or signs of insomnia accounts for a higher prevalence of cardiometabolic disease among patients with mild OSA.

This was noted in a prospective follow-up cohort of 3947 adult patients with mild OSA (AHI of 5–15/h). Patients were divided into four clinical phenotypes based on the presence of excessive daytime sleepiness (EDS) and/or symptoms and signs of insomnia: (1) EDS (daytime+/nighttime−), (2) EDS/ insomnia (daytime+/nighttime+), (3) non-EDS/non insomnia (daytime−/nighttime−), and (4) insomnia (daytime−/nighttime+) phenotype.

It was noted that although the severity of sleep apnea (AHI) or the oxygen desaturation index (ODI) did not differ significantly between groups, the insomnia phenotype patients were older, more frequently female, and current smokers. Additionally, cardiovascular comorbidity was more common in the insomnia phenotype compared with the EDS and EDS-insomnia phenotypes. Metabolic, pulmonary, and psychiatric comorbidities were more prevalent in the insomnia phenotype [45].

Clinically relevant phenotypes of OSA are described above. Continuous positive airway pressure (CPAP) therapy is the treatment of choice for most patients with OSA, but tolerance and adherence can be a problem. Patient-centered individualized approaches to OSA management by understanding the various phenotypes will help develop potential treatment options that will thereby help decrease the disease burden and improve treatment effectiveness.

13.4 Summary

OSA is increasingly recognized as a complex and heterogeneous syndrome. Categorizing such conditions into smaller, more homogeneous categories ("phenotypes") can help advance understanding of pathophysiology, develop targeted treatments, and improve both prognostication and risk stratification. Adhering to treatment is important; however, various factors play a role including patient-related factors (such as demographics, nightly CPAP use <4 h/night during the first 1–2 weeks of therapy and problems encountered during the first night of use, lack of a positive perspective regarding the benefit of CPAP therapy, low self-efficacy), disease- and therapy-related factors, and finally healthcare provider-related factors.

The recognition is that some patients who are adherent in their CPAP use but continue to have an EDS may need a secondary intervention (e.g., an alerting medication). This emphasizes the need to characterize phenotypes and to apply appropriate management to the phenotype specific features for each patient.

References

1. Villar I, Izuel M, Carrizo S, Vicente E, Marin JM. Medication adherence and persistence in severe obstructive sleep apnea. Sleep. 2009;32(5):623–8. https://doi.org/10.1093/sleep/32.5.623.
2. Understanding the Results. (n.d.). Retrieved from http://healthysleep.med.harvard.edu/sleep-apnea/diagnosing-osa/understanding-results
3. Terán-Santos J, Jiménez-Gómez A, Cordero-Guevara J, Cooperative Group Burgos-Santander. The association between sleep apnea and the risk of traffic accidents. N Engl J Med. 1999;340:847–51. [PubMed] [Google Scholar]
4. Yaggi HK, Concato J, Kernan WN, Lichtman JH, Brass LM, Mohsenin V. Obstructive sleep apnea as a risk factor for stroke and death. N Engl J Med. 2005;353:2034–41. [PubMed] [Google Scholar]
5. Shahar E, Whitney CW, Redline S, et al. Sleep-disordered breathing and cardiovascular disease: cross-sectional results of the Sleep Heart Health Study. Am J Respir Crit Care Med. 2001;163:19–25. [PubMed] [Google Scholar]
6. Sawyer AM, Gooneratne NS, Marcus CL, et al. A systematic review of CPAP adherence across age groups: clinical and empiric insights for developing CPAP adherence interventions. Sleep Med Rev. 2011;15:343.
7. Weaver TE, Maislin G, Dinges DF, et al. Relationship between hours of CPAP use and achieving normal levels of sleepiness and daily functioning. Sleep. 2007;30:711.
8. Zimmerman ME, Arnedt JT, Stanchina M, et al. Normalization of memory performance and positive airway pressure adherence in memory-impaired patients with obstructive sleep apnea. Chest. 2006;130:1772.
9. Antic NA, Catcheside P, Buchan C, et al. The effect of CPAP in normalizing daytime sleepiness, quality of life, and neurocognitive function in patients with moderate to severe OSA. Sleep. 2011;34:111.
10. Barbé F, Durán-Cantolla J, Sánchez-de-la-Torre M, et al. Effect of continuous positive airway pressure on the incidence of hypertension and cardiovascular events in nonsleepy patients with obstructive sleep apnea: a randomized controlled trial. JAMA. 2012;307:2161.
11. Bratton DJ, Stradling JR, Barbé F, Kohler M. Effect of CPAP on blood pressure in patients with minimally symptomatic obstructive sleep apnoea: a meta-analysis using individual patient data from four randomised controlled trials. Thorax. 2014;69:1128.
12. Craig SE, Kohler M, Nicoll D, et al. Continuous positive airway pressure improves sleepiness but not calculated vascular risk in patients with minimally symptomatic obstructive sleep apnoea: the MOSAIC randomised controlled trial. Thorax. 2012;67:1090.
13. Marin JM, Carrizo SJ, Vicente E, Agusti AGN. Long-term cardiovascular outcomes in men with obstructive sleep apnoea-hypopnoea with or without treatment with continuous positive airway pressure: an observational study. Lancet. 2005;365:1046–53. [PubMed] [Google Scholar]
14. Gay P, Weaver T, Loube D, et al. Evaluation of positive airway pressure treatment for sleep related breathing disorders in adults. Sleep. 2006;29:381.
15. Kribbs NB, Pack AI, Kline LR, et al. Effects of one night without nasal CPAP treatment on sleep and sleepiness in patients with obstructive sleep apnea. Am Rev Respir Dis. 1993;147:1162.
16. Grunstein RR, Stewart DA, Lloyd H, et al. Acute withdrawal of nasal CPAP in obstructive sleep apnea does not cause a rise in stress hormones. Sleep. 1996;19:774.
17. Giles TL, Lasserson TJ, Smith BH, et al. Continuous positive airways pressure for obstructive sleep apnoea in adults. Cochrane Database Syst Rev. 2006;(1):CD001106.
18. Young LR, Taxin ZH, Norman RG, et al. Response to CPAP withdrawal in patients with mild versus severe obstructive sleep apnea/hypopnea syndrome. Sleep. 2013;36:405.
19. Kohler M, Stoewhas AC, Ayers L, et al. Effects of continuous positive airway pressure therapy withdrawal in patients with obstructive sleep apnea: a randomized controlled trial. Am J Respir Crit Care Med. 2011;184:1192.
20. Bankhead C. Sleep apnea returns rapidly when CPAP stopped 2011. Retrieved from https://www.medpagetoday.org/pulmonology/sleepdisorders/28026

21. Deering S, Liu L, Zamora T, Hamilton J, Stepnowsky C. CPAP adherence is associated with attentional improvements in a group of primarily male patients with moderate to severe OSA. J Clin Sleep Med. 2017;13(12):1423–8. https://doi.org/10.5664/jcsm.6838.

22. Aloia MS, Arnedt JT, Stanchina M, Millman RP. How early in treatment is PAP adherence established? Revisiting night-to-night variability. Behav Sleep Med. 2007;5:229.

23. Rosenthal L, Gerhardstein R, Lumley A, et al. CPAP therapy in patients with mild OSA: implementation and treatment outcome. Sleep Med. 2000;1:215.

24. Budhiraja R, Parthasarathy S, Drake CL, et al. Early CPAP use identifies subsequent adherence to CPAP therapy. Sleep. 2007;30:320.

25. Pengo MF, Czaban M, Berry MP, et al. The effect of positive and negative message framing on short term continuous positive airway pressure compliance in patients with obstructive sleep apnea. J Thorac Dis. 2018;10:S160.

26. UpToDate. 2021. Retrieved 2 March 2021, from https://www.uptodate.com/contents/assessing-and-managing-nonadherence-with-continuous-positive-airway-pressure-cpap-for-adults-with-obstructive-sleep-apnea

27. Russo-Magno P, O'Brien A, Panciera T, Rounds S. Compliance with CPAP therapy in older men with obstructive sleep apnea. J Am Geriatr Soc. 2001;49:1205–11. [PubMed] [Google Scholar]

28. Aloia M, Arnedt J, Stepnowsky C, Hecht J, Borrelli B. Predicting treatment adherence in obstructive sleep apnea using principles of behavior change. J Clin Sleep Med. 2005;01(04):346–53. https://doi.org/10.5664/jcsm.26359.

29. Kribbs NB, Pack AI, Kline LR, et al. Objective measurement of patterns of nasal CPAP use by patients with obstructive sleep apnea. Am Rev Respir Dis. 1993;147:887–95.

30. Prochaska JO, Redding CA, Evers KE. The transtheoretical model and stages of change. In: Glanz K, Lewis FM, Rimer BK, editors. Health behavior and health education. San Francisco: Jossey-Bass Publishers; 1997. p. 60–84.

31. Bandura A. Social foundations of thought and action. A social cognitive theory. Englewood Cliffs: Prentice Hall; 1986.

32. Dimatteo MR. Social support and patient adherence to medical treatment: a meta-analysis. Health Psychol. 2004;23:207–18.

33. Wallace DM, Shafazand S, Aloia MS, Wohlgemuth WK. The association of age, insomnia, and self-efficacy with continuous positive airway pressure adherence in black, white, and Hispanic U.S. Veterans. J Clin Sleep Med. 2013;9(9):885–95. https://doi.org/10.5664/jcsm.2988.

34. Sin DD, Mayers I, Man GC, Pawluk L. Long-term compliance rates to continuous positive airway pressure in obstructive sleep apnea: a population-based study. Chest. 2002;121:430–5. [PubMed] [Google Scholar]

35. Li HY, Engleman H, Hsu CY, Izci B, Vennelle M, Cross M, Douglas NJ. Acoustic reflection for nasal airway measurement in patients with obstructive sleep apnea-hypopnea syndrome. Sleep. 2005;28:1554–9. [PubMed] [Google Scholar]

36. Nakata S, Noda A, Yagi H, Yanagi E, Mimura T, Okada T, Misawa H, Nakashima T. Nasal resistance for determinant factor of nasal surgery in CPAP failure patients with obstructive sleep apnea syndrome. Rhinology. 2005;43:296–9. [PubMed] [Google Scholar]

37. Sugiura T, Noda A, Nakata S, Yasuda Y, Soga T, Miyata S, Nakai S, Koike Y. Influence of nasal resistance on initial acceptance of continuous positive airway pressure in treatment for obstructive sleep apnea syndrome. Respiration. 2007;74:56–60. [PubMed] [Google Scholar]

38. Weaver TE. Adherence to positive airway pressure therapy. Curr Opin Pulm Med. 2006;12(6):409–13. https://doi.org/10.1097/01.mcp.0000245715.97256.32.

39. Chasens ER, Pack AI, Maislin G, Dinges DF, Weaver TE. Claustrophobia and adherence to CPAP treat-

ment. West J Nurs Res. 2005;27(3):307–21. https://doi.org/10.1177/0193945904273283. PMID: 15781905.

40. Almeneessier AS, Almousa Y, Hammad O, Olaish AH, Alanbay ET, Bahammam AS. Long-term adherence to continuous positive airway pressure in patients with rapid eye movement-only obstructive sleep apnea: a prospective cohort study. J Thorac Dis. 2017;9(10):3755–65. https://doi.org/10.21037/jtd.2017.09.57.

41. McArdle N, Devereux G, Heidarnejad H, Engleman HM, Mackay TW, Douglas NJ. Long-term use of CPAP therapy for sleep apnea/hypopnea syndrome. Am J Respir Crit Care Med. 1999;159:1108–14. [PubMed] [Google Scholar]

42. Jurado-Gamez B, Bardwell WA, Cordova-Pacheco LJ, García-Amores M, Feu-Collado N, Buela-Casal G. A basic intervention improves CPAP adherence in sleep apnoea patients: a controlled trial. Sleep Breath. 2014;19(2):509–14. https://doi.org/10.1007/s11325-014-1038-1.

43. Barbe F, Mayoralas LR, Duran J, Masa JF, Maimo A, Montserrat JM, Monasterio C, Bosch M, Ladaria A, Rubio M, et al. Treatment with continuous positive airway pressure is not effective in patients with sleep apnea but no daytime sleepiness. A randomized, controlled trial. Ann Intern Med. 2001;134:1015–23. [PubMed] [Google Scholar]

44. Broderick A, Christl M, Kolpeck A, Spiessl H. Compliance with nCPAP therapy: is pre-diction possible? Wien Med Wochenschr. 1995;145:504–5.

45. Wallace DM, Sawyer AM, Shafazand S. Comorbid insomnia symptoms predict lower 6-month adherence to CPAP in US veterans with obstructive sleep apnea. Sleep Breath. 2018 Mar;22(1):5–15. https://doi.org/10.1007/s11325-017-1605-3.

46. Jacobsen AR, Eriksen F, Hansen RW, Erlandsen M, Thorup L, Damgård MB, Kirkegaard MG, Hansen KW. Determinants for adherence to continuous positive airway pressure therapy in obstructive sleep apnea. PLoS One. 2017;12(12):e0189614. https://doi.org/10.1371/journal.pone.0189614.

47. Campos-Rodriguez F, Martinez-Alonso M, Sanchez-De-La-Torre M, Barbe F. Long-term adherence to continuous positive airway pressure therapy in non-sleepy sleep apnea patients. Sleep Med. 2016;17:1–6. https://doi.org/10.1016/j.sleep.2015.07.038.

48. Kohler M, Smith D, Tippett V, Stradling JR. Predictors of long-term compliance with continuous positive airway pressure. Thorax. 2010;65(9):829–32. https://doi.org/10.1136/thx.2010.135848. PMID: 20805182.

49. Krieger J. Long-term compliance with nasal continuous positive airway pressure (CPAP) in obstructive sleep apnea patients and nonapneic snorers. Sleep. 1992;15(6, Suppl):S42–6. [PubMed] [Google Scholar]

50. Reeves-Hoche MK, Meck R, Zwillich CW. Nasal CPAP: an objective evaluation of patient compliance. Am J Respir Crit Care Med. 1994;149:149–54. [PubMed] [Google Scholar]

51. Hohenhaus-Beer A, Gleixner M, Fichter J. Long term follow-up of CPAP therapy inpatients with OSA. Wien Med Wochenschr. 1995;145:512.

52. Meurice JC, Dore P, Paquereau J, et al. Predictive factors of long-term compliance within CPAP treatment in sleep apnoea syndrome. Chest. 1994;105:429–33.

53. Lewis K, Seale L, Bartle I, Watkins A, Ebden P. Early predictors of CPAP use for the treatment of obstructive sleep apnea. Sleep. 2004;27(1):134–8. https://doi.org/10.1093/sleep/27.1.134.

54. Kaplan V, Bingisser R, Li Y, Hess T, Russi EW, Bloch KE. Compliance with nCPAP in obstructive sleep apnoea. Schweiz Med Wochenschr. 1996;126:15–21.

55. Neill AM, Wai HS, Bannan SP, et al. Humidified nasal continuous positive airway pressure in obstructive sleep apnoea. Eur Respir J. 2003;22:258.

56. Olsen S, Smith SS, Oei TP, Douglas J. Motivational interviewing (MINT) improves continuous positive airway pressure (CPAP)

acceptance and adherence: a randomized controlled trial. J Consult Clin Psychol. 2012;80:151.

57. Kreivi HR, Maasilta P, Bachour A. Persistence of upper-airway symptoms during CPAP compromises adherence at 1 year. Respir Care. 2016;61:652.

58. Mador MJ, Krauza M, Pervez A, et al. Effect of heated humidification on compliance and quality of life in patients with sleep apnea using nasal continuous positive airway pressure. Chest. 2005;128:2151.

59. Worsnop CJ, Miseski S, Rochford PD. Routine use of humidification with nasal continuous positive airway pressure. Intern Med J. 2010;40:650.

60. Ryan S, Doherty LS, Nolan GM, McNicholas WT. Effects of heated humidification and topical steroids on compliance, nasal symptoms, and quality of life in patients with obstructive sleep apnea syndrome using nasal continuous positive airway pressure. J Clin Sleep Med. 2009;5:422.

61. Shapiro GK, Shapiro CM. Factors that influence CPAP adherence: an overview. Sleep Breath. 2010;14:323.

62. Weaver TE, Grunstein RR. Adherence to continuous positive airway pressure therapy: the challenge to effective treatment. Proc Am Thorac Soc. 2008;5:173.

63. Engleman HM, Wild MR. Improving CPAP use by patients with the sleep apnoea/hypopnoea syndrome (SAHS). Sleep Med Rev. 2003;7:81.

64. Ye L, Pack AI, Maislin G, et al. Predictors of continuous positive airway pressure use during the first week of treatment. J Sleep Res. 2012;21:419.

65. Palm A, Midgren B, Theorell-Haglöw J, et al. Factors influencing adherence to continuous positive airway pressure treatment in obstructive sleep apnea and mortality associated with treatment failure - a national registry-based cohort study. Sleep Med. 2018;51:85.

66. Zinchuk AV, Gentry MJ, Concato J, Yaggi HK. Phenotypes in obstructive sleep apnea: a definition, examples and evolution of approaches. Sleep Med Rev. 2017;35:113–23. https://doi. org/10.1016/j.smrv.2016.10.002.

67. Bjorvatn B, Lehmann S, Gulati S, Aurlien H, Pallesen S, Saxvig IW. Prevalence of excessive sleepiness is higher whereas insomnia is lower with greater severity of obstructive sleep apnea. Sleep Breath. 2015;19(4):1387–93.

68. Vaessen TJ, Overeem S, Sitskoorn MM. Cognitive complaints in obstructive sleep apnea. Sleep Med Rev. 2015;19:51–8. [PubMed] [Google Scholar]

69. Kapur VK, Resnick HE, Gottlieb DJ, Sleep Heart Health Study G. Sleep disordered breathing and hypertension: does self-reported sleepiness modify the association? Sleep. 2008;31(8):1127–32. [PMC free article] [PubMed] [Google Scholar]

70. Barcelo A, Barbe F, de la Pena M, Martinez P, Soriano JB, Pierola J, et al. Insulin resistance and daytime sleepiness in patients with sleep apnoea. Thorax. 2008;63(11):946–50. [PubMed] [Google Scholar]

71. Gooneratne NS, Richards KC, Joffe M, Lam RW, Pack F, Staley B, et al. Sleep disordered breathing with excessive daytime sleepiness is a risk factor for mortality in older adults. Sleep. 2011;34(4):435–42. [PMC free article] [PubMed] [Google Scholar]

72. Weaver TE, Mancini C, Maislin G, Cater J, Staley B, Landis JR, et al. Continuous positive airway pressure treatment of sleepy patients with milder obstructive sleep apnea: results of the CPAP Apnea Trial North American Program (CATNAP) randomized clinical trial. Am J Respir Crit Care Med. 2012;186(7):677–83. [PMC free article] [PubMed] [Google Scholar]

73. Wang Q, Zhang C, Jia P, Zhang J, Feng L, Wei S, et al. The association between the phenotype of excessive daytime sleepiness and blood pressure in patients with obstructive sleep apnea-hypopnea syndrome. Int J Med Sci. 2014;11(7):713–20.

74. Andaku DK, D'Almeida V, Carneiro G, Hix S, Tufik S, Togeiro SM. Sleepiness, inflammation and oxidative stress markers in middle-aged males with obstructive sleep apnea without metabolic syndrome: a cross-sectional study. Respir Res. 2015;16:3. https:// doi.org/10.1186/s12931-015-0166-x.

75. Dudley KA, Patel SR. Disparities and genetic risk factors in obstructive sleep apnea. Sleep Med. 2015;18:96–102. [PMC free article] [PubMed] [Google Scholar]

76. Lin CM, Davidson TM, Ancoli-Israel S. Gender differences in obstructive sleep apnea and treatment implications. Sleep Med Rev. 2008;12(6):481–96.

77. Ramos A, Figueredo P, Shafazand S, Chediak A, Abreu A, Dib S, et al. Obstructive sleep apnea phenotypes and markers of vascular disease: a review 2017. Retrieved December 07, 2020, from https:// www.ncbi.nlm.nih.gov/pubmed/29259576

78. Haas DC, Foster GL, Nieto FJ, Redline S, Resnick HE, Robbins JA, et al. Age-dependent associations between sleep-disordered breathing and hypertension: importance of discriminating between systolic/diastolic hypertension and isolated systolic hypertension in the Sleep Heart Health Study. Circulation. 2005;111(5):614–21. [PubMed] [Google Scholar]

79. Lin GM, Colangelo LA, Lloyd-Jones DM, Redline S, Yeboah J, Heckbert SR, et al. Association of sleep apnea and snoring with incident atrial fibrillation in the multi-ethnic study of atherosclerosis. Am J Epidemiol. 2015;182(1):49–57. [PMC free article] [PubMed] [Google Scholar]

80. Gottlieb DJ, Yenokyan G, Newman AB, O'Connor GT, Punjabi NM, Quan SF, et al. Prospective study of obstructive sleep apnea and incident coronary heart disease and heart failure: the sleep heart health study. Circulation. 2010;122(4):352–60. [PMC free article] [PubMed] [Google Scholar]

81. Martinez-Garcia MA, Campos-Rodriguez F, Catalan-Serra P, Soler-Cataluna JJ, Almeida-Gonzalez C, De la Cruz MI, et al. Cardiovascular mortality in obstructive sleep apnea in the elderly: role of long-term continuous positive airway pressure treatment: a prospective observational study. Am J Respir Crit Care Med. 2012;186(9):909–16. [PubMed] [Google Scholar]

82. Foley DJ, Masaki K, White L, Larkin EK, Monjan A, Redline S. Sleep-disordered breathing and cognitive impairment in elderly Japanese-American men. Sleep. 2003;26(5):596–9. [PubMed] [Google Scholar]

83. Zamora LM, Garcia MA, Chiner E, Blasco L, Cortes J, Catalan P, et al. Obstructive sleep apnea (OSA) in elderly patients. Role of continuos positive airway pressure (CPAP) treatment. A multicenter randomized controlled clinical trial. Eur Respir J. 2014;44(Suppl 58):142–51. [Google Scholar]

84. Blackwell T, Yaffe K, Laffan A, Redline S, Ancoli-Israel S, Ensrud KE, et al. Associations between sleep-disordered breathing, nocturnal hypoxemia, and subsequent cognitive decline in older community-dwelling men: the Osteoporotic Fractures in Men Sleep Study. J Am Geriatr Soc. 2015;63(3):453–61. [PMC free article] [PubMed] [Google Scholar]

85. Punjabi NM, Caffo BS, Goodwin JL, Gottlieb DJ, Newman AB, O'Connor GT, et al. Sleep-disordered breathing and mortality: a prospective cohort study. PLoS Med. 2009;6(8):e1000132. [PMC free article] [PubMed] [Google Scholar]

86. Subramani Y, Singh M, Wong J, Kushida CA, Malhotra A, Chung F. Understanding phenotypes of obstructive sleep apnea: applications in anesthesia, surgery, and perioperative medicine. Anesth Analg. 2017;124(1):179–91. https://doi.org/10.1213/ ANE.0000000000001546.

87. Malhotra A, Huang Y, Fogel RB, et al. The male predisposition to pharyngeal collapse: importance of airway length. Am J Respir Crit Care Med. 2002;166:1388–95.

88. Young T, Finn L, Austin D, Peterson A. Menopausal status and sleep-disordered breathing in the Wisconsin Sleep Cohort Study. Am J Respir Crit Care Med. 2003;167:1181–5.

89. Lee RW, Vasudavan S, Hui DS, et al. Differences in craniofacial structures and obesity in Caucasian and Chinese patients with obstructive sleep apnea. Sleep. 2010;33:1075–80. [PMC free article] [PubMed] [Google Scholar]
90. James WP. The epidemiology of obesity: the size of the problem. J Intern Med. 2008;263:336–52. [PubMed] [Google Scholar]
91. Ip MS, Lam B, Tang LC, Lauder IJ, Ip TY, Lam WK. A community study of sleep-disordered breathing in middle-aged Chinese women in Hong Kong: prevalence and gender differences. Chest. 2004;125:127–34. [PubMed] [Google Scholar]
92. Young T, Peppard PE, Taheri S. Excess weight and sleep-disordered breathing. J Appl Physiol. 2005;99:1592–9. [PubMed] [Google Scholar]
93. Cakirer B, Hans MG, Graham G, Aylor J, Tishler PV, Redline S. The relationship between craniofacial morphology and obstructive sleep apnea in whites and in African-Americans. Am J Respir Crit Care Med. 2001;163:947–50.
94. Dieltjens M, Braem MJ, Van de Heyning PH, Wouters K, Vanderveken OM. Prevalence and clinical significance of supine-dependent obstructive sleep apnea in patients using oral appliance therapy. J Clin Sleep Med. 2014;10:959–64.
95. Chami HA, Baldwin CM, Silverman A, Zhang Y, Rapoport D, Punjabi NM, et al. Sleepiness, quality of life, and sleep maintenance in REM versus non-REM sleep-disordered breathing. Am J Respir Crit Care Med. 2010;181(9):997–1002. [PMC free article] [PubMed] [Google Scholar]
96. Khan A, Harrison SL, Kezirian EJ, Ancoli-Israel S, O'Hearn D, Orwoll E, et al. Obstructive sleep apnea during rapid eye movement sleep, daytime sleepiness, and quality of life in older men in Osteoporotic Fractures in Men (MrOS) Sleep Study. J Clin Sleep Med. 2013;9(3):191–8. [PMC free article] [PubMed] [Google Scholar]
97. Su CS, Liu KT, Panjapornpon K, Andrews N, Foldvary-Schaefer N. Functional outcomes in patients with REM-related obstructive sleep apnea treated with positive airway pressure therapy. J Clin Sleep Med. 2012;8(3):243–7.
98. Riha R, Gislasson T, Diefenbach K. The phenotype and genotype of adult obstructive sleep apnoea/hypopnoea syndrome. Eur Respir J. 2009;33(3):646–55. https://doi.org/10.1183/09031936.00151008.

Part III

PAP Adherence in Medical Conditions

PAP Adherence in Neurology Patients

14

Anne Marie Morse and Sreelatha Naik

14.1 Introduction

It has been suggested that in patients with complex neurological conditions, PAP adherence may be even poorer than the general population. In neurology patients requiring positive airway pressure (PAP) support to treat sleep disordered breathing, there are unique challenges that may be encountered. Improved troubleshooting and optimization of adherence to PAP therapy in this population will positively impact sleep disordered breathing, but this benefit may also extend to optimizing management of the patient's neurologic disease.

14.2 Attention Deficit Hyperactivity Disorder

ADHD is a neurobehavioral disorder of self-regulation whose impact extends across the 24-hour period [1, 2] with sleep disturbances being one of the most common comorbidities. In both European and US guidelines, it is recommended to assess sleep during evaluation of an individual for suspected ADHD and before initiation of pharmacotherapy [3, 4]. Sleep disordered breathing is much more prevalent in children with ADHD than in the general pediatric population (25–30% versus 1–3%). Surgical treatment of OSA and treatment with CPAP have both demonstrated significant improvement in ADHD-like symptoms, and not uncommonly can result in the ability to discontinue ADHD medications [5–7].

14.3 Challenges of Individuals with ADHD Requiring PAP Therapy

Hyperactivity and Distractibility: Settling Down for Sleep and Remembering to Use PAP

A regular structured bedtime routine is critical for any patient with a SWD, but with individuals with ADHD, a bedtime routine is critical for overcoming both the hyperactivity and inattentiveness that may interfere with successful PAP therapy. It is important to review the bedtime routine and include conversation incorporating getting the PAP ready and putting the mask on as part of the routine. In some patients, a scheduled alarm or reminder to put the PAP mask on may be necessary. Additionally, PAP data apps (Table 14.1) can provide positive reinforcement for continued use. These apps provide on-demand access to usage, leakage, and average treatment AHI for review, as well as some that also include coaching for encouragement and goal reminders.

Organization: Keeping the PAP Clean, Ordering New Supplies

The patient should also have a next day routine that outlines plans to clean the PAP and evaluate for need for replacement parts. Auto-replenishment of additional supplies should be established for all patients. A scheduled reminder for some may be necessary. In this case, check the model of the patients' PAP device as some devices have a reminder menu option capable of providing these types of reminders for the patient. In addition, as mentioned above, some PAP data apps also include options to help with patient organization.

14.4 Epilepsy

There is an intimate relationship between sleep and epilepsy. Most focus on either sleep deprivation as a provoking agent for seizure or that some seizures are more common during sleep. However, it is important to recognize that patients with epilepsy have multifactorial reasons for being higher risk for

A. M. Morse (✉)
Pediatric Neurology and Pediatric Sleep Medicine, Department of Pediatrics, Janet Weis Children's Hospital, Geisinger, Danville, PA, USA
e-mail: amorse@geisinger.edu

S. Naik
Division of Sleep Medicine, Department of Pulmonary and Critical Care, Geisinger Medical Center, Danville, PA, USA

C. M. Shapiro et al. (eds.), *CPAP Adherence*, https://doi.org/10.1007/978-3-030-93146-9_14

Table 14.1 Patient accessible PAP therapy monitoring

Company	Respironics	ResMed	MonitAir	Fisher & Paykel	Drive DeVilbiss Healthcare	Breas Medical Inc	3B Medical Inc
Mobile app name	DreamMapper	myAir	MonitAir	Sleep Style	DelVibiss Smartlink App	Nitelog	3B Luna QR
PAP device compatibility	DreamStation, DreamStation Go, one 50 & 60 series	All Air10 devices	All ResMed Air10, AirMini; All Respironics DreamStation, DreamStation Go	SleepStyle	DV6 CPAPs (Bluetooth), DV5 (SmartCodes)	Z1 CPAP, Z1 Auto	Luna, Luna II
In-app summary							
AHI	X	X	X	X	X	X	X
CAI	X		X		X	X	X
Pressure setting or trends	X		X				X
Usage hours	X	X	X	X	X	X	X
Mask leaks	X	X	X	X	X	X	X
Other	Hypopnea count, Obstructive apnea count, comfort settings	1-100 daily MyAir score, mask seal, mask on/off events	Adherence, risk stratification, NIV parameters and I:E ratios (where applicable), Monthly trends		Adherence score, usage AHI		Snore index, leak %, best 30 days
In-app notifications							
Low usage	X	X	X		X		
High leak	X	X			X		
No data received	X		X		X		
Resupply soon		X			X		
Other	Goal achievement, coaching messages, **clean equipment reminders**	30-day trends, myAir score	Adherence, risk stratification, monthly trends				
In-app educational material	Videos, guides content (defined by equipment used)	Personalized videos/guides cover mask fit and cleaning (defined by equipment used) maintenance and comfort settings, and adjusting to therapy. Full FAQ	None	Fitting My Simplus	Educational videos	None	None
Care team access	App connected to EncoreAnywhere/Care Orchestrator, (allows EMR connectivity)	AirView, U-Sleep, or third-party data providers if integrated with ResMed.	Patient can communicate with healthcare team via text, call, or video	Patient emails data or screenshots to team	SmartLink Desktop or My SmartLink Cloud.	Patient emails data or screenshots to team	Healthcare team can access

AHI apnea hypopnea index, *CAI* central apnea index

sleep disorders. Seizures during sleep negatively impact amount of REM sleep and sleep efficiency [8]. For instance, individuals with epilepsy, who had sleep complaints, and were evaluated with polysomnography revealed an association between worse seizure control and significantly lower sleep efficiency, higher arousal index, and a higher prevalence of sleep disordered breathing [9]. In addition to the disease itself, the treatment can also impact sleep quality and risk for sleep disordered breathing. Anti-seizure medications can influence sleep architecture and sleep quality [10], and vagus nerve stimulators (VNS) have been suggested to increase risk for sleep disordered breathing [11].

OSA is twice as common in adults with epilepsy than in age-matched control subjects [12]. Treatment of the OSA with either adenotonsillectomy or PAP therapy use often leads to seizure reduction [13] and improvement in overall well-being [13, 14] and may potentially decrease risk for sudden unexpected death in epilepsy (SUDEP) [15]. However, when evaluated, individuals with epilepsy were less likely to be adherent to PAP therapy during the first month of treatment as compared to peers without epilepsy [16].

14.5   Challenges of Individuals with Epilepsy Requiring PAP Therapy

Inadequate Response to PAP
Patients with epilepsy may continue to have greater residual AHI despite adequate PAP adherence. In fact, one study demonstrated that they were five times more likely than controls to have residual AHI ≥ 5 events/hour at 3 months and 1 year despite adequate use [16]. Close follow-up for PAP adherence is critical for all OSA patients, but detailed evaluation of the adherence report to monitor for persistent pathologic AHI is essential for patients with epilepsy. One explanation that needs to be evaluated is the potential for ictal apneic events [17] that may confound co-existing OSA. A second explanation can be related to anti-seizure treatments that may increase risk for worsened sleep disordered breathing, such as with barbiturates, benzodiazepines, or vagal nerve stimulator.

Patients with epilepsy and sleep disordered breathing should have diagnostic and PAP titration studies with an expanded EEG montage to evaluate for seizure related respiratory events. Collaborative management with the neurologist managing the patient's epilepsy may be beneficial, especially if there is concern of ictal related respiratory events or treatment-induced worsening of SDB. Respiratory events may be reduced with changes in the VNS operational parameters [11] or attention to anti-seizure medication selection, dosing, and timing.

Persistent EDS
Excessive daytimes sleepiness in patients with epilepsy can be multifactorial. The presence or persistence of EDS may discourage a patient from continued adherent use of PAP therapy, due to perception of lack of effectiveness. Characterizing baseline EDS with both a standardized tool, such as the Epworth sleepiness scale (ESS), and patient's perceived disability related to sleepiness is critical for expectation setting and evaluating response to treatment. It is also critical to consider anti-seizure medication regimen and seizure frequency and control as contributors to symptoms of EDS. Collaborative management with neurologist managing epilepsy may be beneficial if there is concern of timing or dosing of anti-seizure medication contributing to severity of EDS.

14.6   Neurodevelopmental Disorders

Neurodevelopmental disorders (NDD) are characterized by abnormal development of the brain, resulting in deficits related to language, cognition, motor, behavior, and other functional domains. Autism spectrum disorder (ASD) is a NDD specifically with persistent deficits beginning in early childhood of social communication and interaction and restricted and repetitive behaviors, interests, or activities, and cannot be better explained by intellectual disability or global developmental delay. Sleep difficulties are almost universally characteristic of children with both NDD and ASD. The most common being sleep onset and maintenance insomnia. However, sleep disordered breathing occurs at a higher frequency than the general population [18, 19] and may be related to differences in body habitus, increased medical comorbidity, oral motor apraxia craniofacial proportions, or hypotonia.

14.7   Challenges of Individuals with Neurodevelopmental Disorders Requiring PAP Therapy

Sensory Disorders
Sensory processing disorders are common in neurodevelopmental disorders and autism. Partnering with a sleep psychologist or behavioral specialist to aid in desensitization techniques is generally advantageous. Frequently, these professionals have already been engaged to aid in preparation for the successful completion of polysomnography. Sensory defensiveness, which is a phrase used to describe the situation when unfamiliar textures, pressures, smell, and sounds provoke a "fight or flight" or defensive reaction to get away from the source of the stimulus, may cause severe aversion to PAP use. Implementation of cognitive behavioral therapy (CBT) for improved PAP adherence can help overcome these difficulties [20].

Anxiety
History of sensory processing disorders can predict development of anxiety [21]. Anxiety may limit PAP use and may also require partnering with a sleep psychologist or behavioral specialist. It is possible for a patient to experience panic or panic attacks related to wearing the mask. This may be more likely in those patients with preexisting anxiety, post-traumatic stress disorder, and/or sensory processing disorders. CBT for PAP desensitization and adherence may provide benefit. Pharmacologic intervention as needed for anxiety can be considered and may require co-management with psychiatry. In these situations, it may be necessary to provide a letter to insurance that there will be a delay in achieving sustained adherence due to desensitization training to avoid having the equipment taken back due to non-adherence.

Inadequate or Irregular Sleep Time
Reduced total sleep time or irregular sleep times may limit PAP use and even reflect as PAP non-adherence due to total sleep time being less than required when using PAP. Behavioral interventions directed at consolidating sleep and regular sleep scheduling are recommended. Consistent PAP use is critical

when first employing these behavioral interventions to optimize sleep consolidation and scheduling. This strategy may allow for a more successful transition.

14.8 Neurodegenerative Disorders

Parkinson's

Parkinson's disease (PD) is a neurodegenerative disorder characterized by deterioration of the dopaminergic system primarily impairing coordination and movement. Secondary insults include sleep-wake dysfunction, major non-motor feature of PD, with up to 96% of patients impacted [22]. Sleep disturbances can develop at any time during the course of PD but tend to increase in prevalence with disease progression.

REM behavior disorder (RBD) is the most commonly depicted sleep disorder when discussing PD; however, the spectrum of sleep disturbances is much more diverse. In fact, other sleep disorders, such as OSA, occur more frequently in patients with PD than in the general elderly population [23]. Although studies evaluating the impact of treatment of sleep disorders on motor and non-motor symptoms in PD have offered mixed results, data on the treatment of moderate-to-severe OSA does demonstrate reduced symptoms of excessive daytime sleepiness, consolidated nighttime sleep, and improved cognition [23, 24]. In addition, there is emerging evidence to suggest that OSA treatment with PAP therapy conferred a protective effect from OSA-related exacerbation of PD motor impairment [25].

14.9 Challenges of Individuals with Parkinson's Requiring PAP Therapy

14.9.1 Movement-Related Difficulties

Nocturnal akinesia is a common challenge for PD patients. Treatment with short-acting levodopa/carbidopa or dopamine agonists frequently leads to this rigid "off" states as dopaminergic medications are metabolized until the next morning's dose. Inability to assume a position of comfort with the PAP mask or be able to manipulate the mask as needed during sleep may lead to reduced use. Optimization of dopaminergic therapies, either with bedtime redosing or long-acting medications, may improve nocturnal akinesia and reduce the experience of muscle cramps, paresthesias, and uncomfortable limb positioning [26]. Continuous, non-oral dopaminergic treatments (such as rotigotine patch and intrajejunal levodopa) may offer better relief of nighttime motor and nonmotor symptoms including turning in bed, insomnia, muscle cramps, distressing dreams, and daytime sleepiness [27, 28].

14.9.2 REM Behavior Disorder

RBD can occur independently or as a consequence of sleep apnea fragmenting REM sleep. In either case, ensure patient (and bed partner) safety by removing anything that can be used as a weapon and limiting ability for elopement. When RBD co-occurs with SDB, high-dose melatonin, 10–15 mg, should be considered first for the treatment of RBD. About 70% of patients will have a positive response. If there is continued difficulty, clonazepam should be tried. Once a therapeutic (usually very low) dose of clonazepam has been established, it is critical to evaluate the patient for worsening of sleep disordered breathing related to the use of benzodiazepine. Repeat PAP titration may be warranted.

14.9.3 Excessive Daytime Sleepiness

The presence or persistence of EDS may discourage a patient from continued adherent use of PAP therapy due to the perception of inadequate response to treatment. Characterizing baseline EDS with both a standardized tool, such as the ESS, and patient's perceived disability related to sleepiness is critical for expectation setting and evaluating response to treatment. In some patients, the use of wake-promoting agents, such as modafinil, armodafinil, or solriamfetol, may allow for improved symptoms of EDS and provide encouragement for continued use of PAP therapy (see Chap. 29).

Alzheimer's

Alzheimer's disease (AD) is the most common form of dementia in the United States affecting one in ten adults [29, 30]. Hallmark symptoms of AD are typically progressive deterioration of memory, language, and intellect. However, sleep-wake disturbances are now being recognized as a common and challenging behavioral symptom associated with AD [31]. There is no cure, only treatments aimed at slowing progression. Sleep optimization, including improved sleep disordered breathing, has become a key component of AD treatment regimens based on the causal and bidirectional relationship between cognitive decline and sleep disturbance [30].

Microarchitectural sleep alterations are significantly increased in those with mild cognitive impairment (MCI), AD, and high-risk older adults (i.e., carriers of the APOE4 allele) relative to cognitively normal older adults [32–34]. However, primary sleep disorders can be responsible for these symptoms and are present in approximately 60% of AD patients, with obstructive sleep apnea and insomnia being the most common.

Therapeutic intervention of sleep pathology has been shown to improve outcomes in AD. The most striking benefit is seen in the treatment of OSA with PAP therapy, which has demonstrated a significant improvement of subjective daytime sleepiness, as well as performance on neuropsychological testing [35, 36].

14.10 Challenges of Individuals with Alzheimer's Requiring PAP Therapy

14.10.1 Inadequate or Irregular Sleep Time

Treatment of insomnia and circadian rhythm disorders with melatonin and bright light therapy has shown mixed results, but with no significant side effects recorded. Therefore, melatonin and bright light therapy and behavioral therapy are recommended. Improving the consistency of night to night sleep scheduling is likely to also prove beneficial for improving nightly use of PAP. On the other hand, use of pharmacological agents, such as sedatives or hypnotics, has not been demonstrated in controlled trials with sleep-disturbed AD patients [37] and may augment severity of SDB. Drug therapy should be considered only after behavioral approaches have failed and reversible medical/environmental causes have been excluded.

14.10.2 Sundowning

Sundowning frequently refers to the phenomena of the emergence or worsening of neuropsychiatric symptoms in the late afternoon or early evening in patients with dementia syndromes [38]. Sundowning can be exacerbated by comorbid circadian rhythm disorders or insomnia. These neuropsychiatric features can be prohibitive to successful PAP therapy. Tailored, preferably non-pharmacologic, care regimens are recommended. As was suggested above, melatonin and bright light therapy may also provide benefit against sundowning. Attempt a gradual transition from natural daylight to artificial lighting as this may reduce behavioral deterioration [38]. Consider deferring PAP therapy in patients with active neuropsychiatric features, who are resisting treatment, as this can result in harm to the patient and/or caregiver. Once consistent improvement in sundowning is achieved, re-introduce PAP therapy.

14.11 Neuromuscular Disease

Amyotrophic Lateral Sclerosis, Muscular Dystrophies, Myotonic Dystrophy, Congenital and Metabolic Myopathies, Myasthenia Gravis, Peripheral Neuropathies (CMT, FD), Post-polio Syndrome, Spinal Cord Injuries

Individuals with neuromuscular disease (NMD) may experience a variety of sleep breathing disorders including obstructive sleep apnea, central sleep apnea, or hypoventilation. There are multiple contributing mechanisms related to the underlying NMD including diaphragmatic weakness, altered chest wall and lung compliance, altered hypercapnic and hypoxic ventilatory response, direct involvement of the respiratory centers, pharyngeal wall weakness, and restrictive lung disease [39]. Medical comorbidity such as obesity, medications that increase weight or impact respiration (steroids, opioids, or muscle relaxers), cerebral abnormalities, and physical deconditioning may further increase risk for sleep disordered breathing. The prevalence of the type of sleep breathing disorder can vary over time depending on the disorder [40]. For example, with Duchenne muscular dystrophy, OSA is often seen early on with hypoventilation predominating. Myasthenia gravis often occurs later on in life. Baseline risk of OSA may be variable depending on family history, anatomy, and body mass index, but hypoventilation may predominate during disease course, particularly during flares. Steroids used to treat myasthenia may lead to weight gain and can lead to development of OSA after disease remission.

Abnormalities during sleep are the earliest indicator of respiratory disturbance in this population. Nocturnal desaturation to less than 90% for 1 minute is a more sensitive indicator of nocturnal hypoventilation than vital capacity or maximal inspiratory pressure testing [41]. Nocturnal hypoxemia may also predict mortality in patients with certain conditions [42]. One of the earliest breathing abnormalities found in NMD is hypoventilation with a sawtooth pattern of desaturations during phasic REM sleep indicating early respiratory muscle involvement [43]. While central events during REM sleep have been described in patients with neuromuscular weakness, these events are now recognized as "pseudocentrals" as they do not share the pathophysiology of reduced central nervous system output seen with true central apneas as seen with Cheyne-Stokes respiration or Biot's respiration. These events appear to have reduced respiratory effort as the diaphragm is simply unable to generate a breath due to weakness, particularly in phasic REM when all other respiratory supportive muscles are paralyzed [40]. Elevated transcutaneous carbon dioxide level during sleep is the most sensitive indicator of hypoventilation, a common problem in NMD [44].

Given the sensitivity of sleep testing, an attended in-lab polysomnography of these patients is desirable, especially when obstructive sleep apnea is suspected. However, it is often difficult for patients with neuromuscular disease to travel to, and sleep in, a sleep center due to the limited mobility and intensity of care they require. Reimbursement-driven guidelines may also limit the value of polysomnography alone in obtaining NIV (noninvasive ventilation). Home nocturnal oximetry, which is widely available, and home end-tidal or transcutaneous capnography, which is frequently less available, are therefore often utilized to diagnose these patients with hypoventilation when daytime measures of carbon dioxide, vital capacity, or maximal inspiratory pressure are inconclusive. Noninvasive ventilation is a form of PAP therapy that is initiated without the utilization of polysomnography. The advent of remote monitoring of PAP devices and NIV can be extremely useful in evaluating factors such as dyssynchrony to optimize adherence to therapy and achieving therapeutic targets.

Identification and optimization of sleep disordered breathing reduces mortality risk by improving symptoms associated with sudden death. For example, sudden death risk is reduced with the treatment using PAP or tracheostomy in ALS patients with vocal cord paralysis. Treatment of sleep apnea has been shown to improve both quality of life and survival [45, 46].

Yearly polysomnography or repeat titrations may be useful in NMD.

Bilevel PAP (BPAP) therapy or NIV is generally the mainstay of treatment for sleep disordered breathing in patients with neuromuscular disease, as opposed to other patients who generally receive CPAP. Reduced pressure during expiration is easier to use for patients with NMD baseline weakness with exhalation. Inspiratory muscle training should be considered as an effective adjuvant [47]. Central apnea is also treated with BPAP. Servo-ventilator PAP may be more optimal than BPAP in patients with obstructive and central apneas.

In addition, future studies evaluating the impact of OSA treatment on comorbidities seen in neuromuscular diseases, such as cardiomyopathy and weight problems, are still needed. There is limited data available about other sleep disorders' relationship with neuromuscular disease, which suggests further exploration is needed.

14.12 Challenges of Individuals with Neuromuscular Disorders Requiring PAP Therapy for OSA

14.12.1 Insufficient Improvement or Progression in Sleep Disordered Breathing

Patients with NMD need close follow-up of their sleep breathing as the type of sleep breathing disorder they have may vary with time, and the degree of support needed may vary with time, with varying rates, depending on the underlying disorder. The following are the main treatment outcomes targeted in NMD: (1) AHI (apnea hypopnea index), (2) adequate Vt (tidal volume), (3) adequate oxygenation, (4) adequate ventilation, and (5) ventilatory rest.

14.12.2 High Residual AHI

A high residual AHI with may be due to numerous factors including mask leak, oronasal mask use in some neuromuscular patients (as opposed to nasal), worsening upper airway obstruction, or due to varying degrees of neuromuscular weakness. Excess mask leak may lead to leak of pressure as in other patients with SBD and result in suboptimal treatment. Remote monitoring systems are often able to provide leak-related information during therapy. Therefore, mask fitting should be addressed first. Oronasal masks may lead to worsening upper airway obstruction, particularly in individuals with NMD; nasal interface should therefore be considered [48, 49]. High residual obstructive events may be seen even after adjustments in EPAP if there is changing weight or other factors that may influence a further narrowing airway over time. Consideration should be given to utilization of setting a range if on CPAP or a range of EPAP if on bilevel or more advanced NIV. If able, the patient could be titrated in the sleep lab to determine optimum range of pressures, keeping in mind that if the disease is in flux, they will still require constant monitoring. Patients on bilevel PAP that may achieve disease remission (such as myasthenia) may have high residual AHI with high CAI as they may have resolution of neuromuscular weakness and no longer require NIV. These patients may require reevaluation of daytime metrics of respiratory strength, such as vital capacity, maximal inspiratory pressure, and arterial blood gas, as well as repeat sleep oximetry and/or capnography off PAP therapy.

14.12.3 Inadequate Tidal Volume and Ventilatory Rest

Vt with NIV is typically 8 milliliters (mL) per kilogram (kg) of ideal body weight (IBW). Cloud systems for tracking NIV report Vt (Fig. 14.1). When evaluating adequacy of tidal volume, it is important to also ensure that Vt is adequate to provide ventilatory rest. In the example patient's case, she is still relatively tachypneic at 21 breaths/minute (Fig. 14.1). Increasing the IPAP (inspiratory PAP) may help increase the Vt and thereby decrease the respiratory rate.

14.12.4 Inadequate Ventilation

Hypercapnia is associated with decline in respiratory muscle function and may result in increased daytime sleepiness, pulmonary hypertension, and poor quality of life. Normalization of hypercapnia is therefore a therapeutic target of NIV. Wake carbon dioxide can be measured utilizing arterial blood

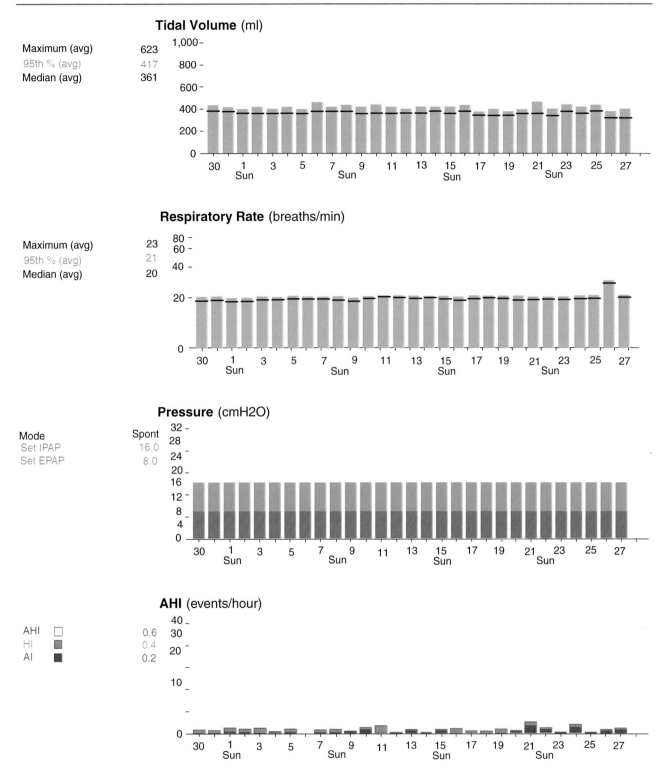

Fig. 14.1 Example download from Cloud systems for tracking NIV report Vt for a patient on BPAP 16/8. Patient's height is 61 inches. Vt is 417 mL, and her respiratory rate is 21 on average. 8 mL/kg for her height would be 380 mL, and the patient exceeds this goal

gases, and sleep capnography at home or in the sleep lab can also be evaluated to ensure improvement and/or resolution of hypercapnia. The patient described above had an arterial blood gas showing pH of 7.33 and carbon dioxide of 54, suggesting insufficient ventilation to normalize hypercapnia even 3 months on therapy. Increase in IPAP may therefore help with both ventilatory rest and improving her hypercarbia.

14.12.5 Inadequate Oxygenation

Adequate oxygenation on PAP can be assessed by obtaining home sleep oximetry. Caution is advised when evaluating oxygenation in patients with neuromuscular disease as hypoventilation may be the primary cause of hypoxemia in the absence of lung pathology or abdominal obesity. Adding supplemental oxygen alone would be insufficient if hypoxemia is due to hypoventilation. For this reason, sleep oximetry with concurrent capnography would be ideal in identifying etiology of hypoxemia.

14.13 Stroke

Sleep disordered breathing both impacts risk for stroke, stroke experience, and recovery from stroke. OSA promotes metabolic syndrome through increased insulin resistance and negative effects on leptin and ghrelin resulting in increased food-seeking behavior and reduced satiety. OSA can also lead to cardiac dysrhythmias leading to cardioembolic and arrhythmic events resulting in stroke. Patients with OSA and stroke can have early neurologic worsening and higher blood pressures in the acute setting. Post-stroke sleep disordered breathing has been associated with a negative impact on short-term and long-term neurologic recovery, as well as increased mortality and stroke recurrence risk [50–52].

Acute stroke outcomes are improved with CPAP use. PAP therapy may help reduce recurrent cardiovascular events, improve 5-year mortality, and reduce nighttime blood pressure [53]. Thus, adequate treatment of sleep disordered breathing in patients both at risk for and with history of stroke is imperative.

14.14 Challenges of Individuals with Stroke Requiring PAP Therapy

14.14.1 Difficulty with Putting on and Taking off Mask

Some patients may experience frustration due to increased time or effort required to set up or maintain their devices [54] related to disability from prior stroke. Anticipatory guidance that this may occur combined with more frequent check-ins for troubleshooting encouragement may reduce frustration. In some patients, scheduling an in-person or telehealth visit with the sleep technician to review the patient's process may aid in identifying ways to reduce excessive effort needed.

Weakness can impair ability to easily apply and secure the PAP headgear [54]. Learning how to put on a PAP mask with only one hand may be necessary, if there is no one to assist the patient at home. Strategies to aid in lifting the headgear overhead or fastening is required. Instead of placing the mask of the face first, instruct the patient to first assemble the mask and headgear and place the headgear onto the back of the head and then pull the mask down with non-paretic hand over the forehead and eyes. The patient should practice this technique with the sleep technician or DME company until demonstrating success. In some cases, consideration for a home health aide to assist with bedtime preparation may be needed.

14.14.2 Headaches

Sleep disturbances can be viewed as comorbid, predisposing, and even prognostic for headache development or persistence. The relationship between headache and sleep may be based in shared structural and neurotransmitters pathways [55–57]. Headache can be a symptom of sleep apnea [58, 59]. Headache frequency reported in OSA varies ranging from 15% to 50% [59–62]. Chronic morning headache is not specific to SDB but may also indicate severe depression or insomnia disorders [63]. However, OSA should be strongly considered in patients having headache during the night or exclusively in the morning [59, 64, 65].

14.15 Challenges of Individuals with Headache Requiring PAP Therapy

14.15.1 Headache Exacerbated by PAP Therapy/Head Gear

Patients complaining of exacerbation of headaches related to PAP use could have these issues as a result of multiple factors. The most common cause is overtightening the PAP mask. To avoid this, instruct the patient to work in one direction around the mask, making small adjustments until the mask is securely in place, but not overly tight. This approach helps prevent uneven adjustment with one side pulling more than the other. Remind the patient that the PAP mask should only be tightened enough to create a seal. Additional factors to consider for enhanced comfort and seal include use of mask strap pads or gels that are soft coverings to improve comfort. Instruct the patient to clean the mask cushion, nasal pillows, and nasal prongs daily as this will provide a more sustained seal.

14.15.2 Sinus Complaints

In patients with chronic sinus issues, PAP use can exacerbate sinus problems. In these patients, a full-face mask may be a preferred option over nasal mask or pillows. Independent of type of mask, partnering with an ENT to optimize nasal breathing and/or using over-the-counter medications may provide benefit. PAP heated humidifiers can contribute to a more optimal sinus environment and should be suggested.

If the PAP use is causing nasal irritation, in addition to a heated humidifier, recommend nasal saline, wash, and gel to maintain moist membranes. Nasal irritation can be cumulative and develop over time. This can result in increased susceptibility to infection due to dry, cracked, and even bleeding nasal passage.

14.15.3 Bruxism

Bruxism is a common comorbidity of sleep apnea. Despite adequate PAP titration, bruxism can still persist. Patient may experience persistent temporal mandibular pain and mistake it for pain due to PAP headgear. Evaluate for clinical and historical features of bruxism, and if present consider referring to a dentist for bite guards which can help alleviate the pain and misalignment from bruxism. Over-the-counter bite guards can also be used but generally have a shorter lifespan and are bulkier than tailor-made devices from the dentist.

14.15.4 Demyelinating Disease

Multiple sclerosis (MS) is a neurodegenerative autoimmune disorder of the central nervous system that affects about 2.5 million people in the world. Clinical symptoms, progression of disease, and response to treatment can be variable. Up to 90% of patients complain of fatigue, which is a poorly defined entity and distinct from excessive daytime sleepiness (EDS). Excessive daytime sleepiness is clearly defined as persistent sleepiness, even after adequate nighttime sleep. Fatigue, on the other hand, has been suggested to possibly be a direct result of demyelination and axonal loss or immunologic consequence versus a result of comorbidities found in MS, such as depression, medication side effects, pain, or sleep disturbance [66].

Sleep disorders are three times more likely to occur in patients with MS versus the general population [66]. It is not uncommon for the sleep disorder to be a symptom of a white matter lesion, such as cervical lesions causing RLS, focal hypothalamic lesions causing narcolepsy, and dorsal pontine lesions causing RBD [67, 68]. Sleep apnea can be central or obstructive and related to inactivity due to disability, brainstem lesions affecting the respiratory centers, or symptomatic medications that relax muscle tone in the pharynx. Treatment of these disorders can provide symptomatic improvement in sleepiness and fatigue, but it is yet to be determined if there is benefit in disease stability and reduced progression.

14.16 Challenges of Individuals with Demyelinating Disease Requiring PAP Therapy

14.16.1 Neurologic Deficits

As described in the section on stroke, some patients may experience frustration due to increased time or effort required to set up or maintain their devices [54] related to disability from demyelinating disease. Anticipatory guidance that this may occur combined with more frequent check-ins for troubleshooting encouragement may reduce frustration. This is especially important in individuals who have not achieved remission and continue to have progressive deficits.

Weakness, but perhaps more frequently encountered spasticity, can impair ability to easily apply and secure the PAP headgear [54]. As in the stroke recommendations, learning how to put on a PAP mask with only one hand may be necessary if there is no one to assist the patient at home (see stroke recommendations for one handed strategy to apply mask). In addition to weakness and spasticity, vision impairment can negatively impact the ability to operate the machine controls, replace the filters, or pour water into the water chambers [54]. Recommend discussion with a neurologist or an ophthalmologist to evaluate if patient would be eligible for use of either handheld or wearable technologies that can improve visual abilities to complete these tasks. In patients with significant or progressive disability, consideration for a home health aide to assist with bedtime preparation may be needed.

14.16.2 Persistent EDS

The presence or persistence of fatigue or EDS may discourage a patient from continued adherent use of PAP therapy. It is important to qualify that although these represent distinct symptoms, patients may perceive or endorse them similarly. In addition, there may be the expectation that these symptoms will resolve with PAP use. It is important to evaluate for and characterize the symptoms at baseline and periodically after PAP treatment initiation. If the features are more suggestive of EDS, ensure adequate PAP use and therapeutic AHI are being achieved. Patients with demyelinating disease are at risk for progression in both obstructive and centrally mediated sleep disordered breathing.

If these are stable, re-evaluate for symptoms of other reasons for EDS, such as medications, restless leg syndrome, or insufficient or irregular sleep patterns. If there are no alternative etiology for EDS, consider a central disorder of hypersomnolence, and evaluate the patient with a repeat PSG (while on CPAP) and next day multiple sleep latency test. If there is evidence of a hypersomnia disorder, patients may benefit from wake-promoting agents, stimulants, or oxybate preparations. If using an oxybate preparation, repeat PAP titration once at therapeutic dosing, as clinically significant desaturations or central apneas can emerge [69].

14.17 Conclusions

Optimal sleep disordered breathing management in patients with neurologic disease requires consideration of the patients' neurologic status. Close collaboration with their managing neurologist may allow a more nuanced understanding of the patients' functional limitations. As described within this chapter, patients with neurologic disease have unique barriers to optimal PAP therapy. These barriers are not uniform across diseases and, even within the same patient, do not remain static over time. Enhanced knowledge of these barriers, as well as improved understanding as to when to consider them, is critical. Appropriate due diligence addressing these barriers and revisiting them at future visits for emergence or regression will likely enhance PAP adherence.

References

1. Weiss MD, Craig SG, Davies G, Schibuk L, Stein M. New research on the complex interaction of sleep and ADHD. Curr Sleep Med Rep. 2015;1(2):114–21.
2. Stein MA, Weiss M, Hlavaty L. ADHD treatments, sleep, and sleep problems: complex associations. Neurotherapeutics. 2012;9(3):509–17.
3. Graham J, Banaschewski T, Buitelaar J, Coghill D, Danckaerts M, Dittmann R, et al. European guidelines on managing adverse effects of medication for ADHD. Eur Child Adolesc Psychiatry. 2011;20(1):17–37.
4. Subcommittee on Attention-Deficit/Hyperactivity Disorder, Steering Committee on Quality Improvement and Management, Wolraich M, Brown L, Brown RT, DuPaul G, et al. ADHD: clinical practice guideline for the diagnosis, evaluation, and treatment of attention-deficit/hyperactivity disorder in children and adolescents. Pediatrics. 2011;128(5):1007–22.
5. Soylu E, Soylu N, Yıldırım YS, Sakallıoğlu Ö, Polat C, Orhan İ. Psychiatric disorders and symptoms severity in patients with adenotonsillar hypertrophy before and after adenotonsillectomy. Int J Pediatr Otorhinolaryngol. 2013;77(10):1775–81.
6. Beebe DW. Neurobehavioral morbidity associated with disordered breathing during sleep in children: a comprehensive review. Sleep. 2006;29(9):1115–34.
7. Chervin RD, Ruzicka DL, Giordani BJ, Weatherly RA, Dillon JE, Hodges EK, et al. Sleep-disordered breathing, behavior, and cognition in children before and after adenotonsillectomy. Pediatrics. 2006;117(4):e769–78.
8. Touchon J, Baldy-Moulinier M, Billiard M, Besset A, Cadilhac J. Sleep organization and epilepsy. Epilepsy Res Suppl. 1991;2:73–81.
9. Kaleyias J, Cruz M, Goraya JS, Valencia I, Khurana DS, Legido A, et al. Spectrum of polysomnographic abnormalities in children with epilepsy. Pediatr Neurol. 2008;39(3):170–6.
10. Jain SV, Glauser TA. Effects of epilepsy treatments on sleep architecture and daytime sleepiness: an evidence-based review of objective sleep metrics. Epilepsia. 2014;55(1):26–37.
11. Parhizgar F, Nugent K, Raj R. Obstructive sleep apnea and respiratory complications associated with vagus nerve stimulators. J Clin Sleep Med. 2011;7(4):401–7.
12. Lin Z, Si Q, Xiaoyi Z. Obstructive sleep apnoea in patients with epilepsy: a meta-analysis. Sleep Breath. 2017;21(2):263–70.
13. Segal E, Vendrame M, Gregas M, Loddenkemper T, Kothare SV. Effect of treatment of obstructive sleep apnea on seizure outcomes in children with epilepsy. Pediatr Neurol. 2012;46(6):359–62.
14. Pornsriniyom D, won Kim H, Bena J, Andrews ND, Moul D, Foldvary-Schaefer N. Effect of positive airway pressure therapy on seizure control in patients with epilepsy and obstructive sleep apnea. Epilepsy Behav. 2014;37:270–5.
15. McCarter AR, Timm PC, Shepard PW, Sandness DJ, Luu T, McCarter SJ, et al. Obstructive sleep apnea in refractory epilepsy: a pilot study investigating frequency, clinical features, and association with risk of sudden unexpected death in epilepsy. Epilepsia. 2018;59(10):1973–81.
16. Latreille V, Bubrick EJ, Pavlova M. Positive airway pressure therapy is challenging for patients with epilepsy. J Clin Sleep Med. 2018;14(7):1153–9.
17. Dlouhy BJ, Gehlbach BK, Kreple CJ, Kawasaki H, Oya H, Buzza C, et al. Breathing inhibited when seizures spread to the amygdala and upon amygdala stimulation. J Neurosci. 2015;35(28):10281–9.
18. Tomkies A, Johnson RF, Shah G, Caraballo M, Evans P, Mitchell RB. Obstructive sleep apnea in children with autism. J Clin Sleep Med. 2019;15(10):1469–76.
19. Hirata I, Mohri I, Kato-Nishimura K, Tachibana M, Kuwada A, Kagitani-Shimono K, et al. Sleep problems are more frequent and associated with problematic behaviors in preschoolers with autism spectrum disorder. Res Dev Disabil. 2016;49:86–99.
20. Richards D, Bartlett DJ, Wong K, Malouff J, Grunstein RR. Increased adherence to CPAP with a group cognitive behavioral treatment intervention: a randomized trial. Sleep. 2007;30(5):635–40.
21. McMahon K, Anand D, Morris-Jones M, Rosenthal MZ. A path from childhood sensory processing disorder to anxiety disorders: the mediating role of emotion dysregulation and adult sensory processing disorder symptoms. Front Integr Neurosci. 2019;13:22.
22. Prudon B, Duncan GW, Khoo TK, Yarnall AJ, Burn DJ, Anderson KN. Primary sleep disorder prevalence in patients with newly diagnosed Parkinson's disease. Mov Disord. 2014;29(2):259–62.
23. Neikrug AB, Maglione JE, Liu L, Natarajan L, Avanzino JA, Corey-Bloom J, et al. Effects of sleep disorders on the non-motor symptoms of Parkinson disease. J Clin Sleep Med. 2013;9(11):1119–29.
24. Suzuki K, Miyamoto M, Miyamoto T, Hirata K. Parkinson's disease and sleep/wake disturbances. Curr Neurol Neurosci Rep. 2015;15(3):1–11.
25. Meng L, Benedetti A, Lafontaine A, Mery V, Robinson AR, Kimoff J, et al. Obstructive sleep apnea, CPAP therapy and Parkinson's disease motor function: a longitudinal study. Parkinsonism Relat Disord. 2020;70:45–50.
26. Albers JA, Chand P, Anch AM. Multifactorial sleep disturbance in Parkinson's disease. Sleep Med. 2017;35:41–8.
27. Van Wamelen DJ, Grigoriou S, Chaudhuri K, Odin P. Continuous drug delivery aiming continuous dopaminergic stimulation in Parkinson's disease. J Parkinsons Dis. 2018;8(s1):S65–72.
28. Trenkwalder C, Kies B, Rudzinska M, Fine J, Nikl J, Honczarenko K, et al. Rotigotine effects on early morning motor function and sleep in Parkinson's disease: a double-blind, randomized, placebo-controlled study (RECOVER). Mov Disord. 2011;26(1):90–9.
29. Alzheimer's Association. 2015 Alzheimer's disease facts and figures. Alzheimers Dement. 2015;11(3):332–84.

30. Mander BA, Winer JR, Jagust WJ, Walker MP. Sleep: a novel mechanistic pathway, biomarker, and treatment target in the pathology of Alzheimer's disease? Trends Neurosci. 2016;39(8):552–66.
31. Peter-Derex L, Yammine P, Bastuji H, Croisile B. Sleep and Alzheimer's disease. Sleep Med Rev. 2015;19:29–38.
32. Westerberg CE, Mander BA, Florczak SM, Weintraub S, Mesulam M, Zee PC, et al. Concurrent impairments in sleep and memory in amnestic mild cognitive impairment. J Int Neuropsychol Soc. 2012;18(03):490–500.
33. Prinz PN, Vitaliano PP, Vitiello MV, Bokan J, Raskind M, Peskind E, et al. Sleep, EEG and mental function changes in senile dementia of the Alzheimer's type. Neurobiol Aging. 1983;3(4):361–70.
34. Hita-Yanez E, Atienza M, Gil-Neciga EL, Cantero J. Disturbed sleep patterns in elders with mild cognitive impairment: the role of memory decline and ApoE ε4 genotype. Curr Alzheimer Res. 2012;9(3):290–7.
35. Ancoli-Israel S, Palmer BW, Cooke JR, Corey-Bloom J, Fiorentino L, Natarajan L, et al. Cognitive effects of treating obstructive sleep apnea in Alzheimer's disease: a randomized controlled study. J Am Geriatr Soc. 2008;56(11):2076–81.
36. Chong MS, Ayalon L, Marler M, Loredo JS, Corey-Bloom J, Palmer BW, et al. Continuous positive airway pressure reduces subjective daytime sleepiness in patients with mild to moderate Alzheimer's disease with sleep disordered breathing. J Am Geriatr Soc. 2006;54(5):777–81.
37. McCurry SM, Reynolds CF, Ancoli-Israel S, Teri L, Vitiello MV. Treatment of sleep disturbance in Alzheimer's disease. Sleep Med Rev. 2000;4(6):603–28.
38. Canevelli M, Valletta M, Trebbastoni A, Sarli G, D'Antonio F, Tariciotti L, et al. Sundowning in dementia: clinical relevance, pathophysiological determinants, and therapeutic approaches. Front Med. 2016;3:73.
39. Aboussouan LS. Sleep-disordered breathing in neuromuscular disease. Am J Respir Crit Care Med. 2015;191(9):979–89.
40. Aboussouan LS, Mireles-Cabodevila E. Sleep-disordered breathing in neuromuscular disease: diagnostic and therapeutic challenges. Chest. 2017;152(4):880–92.
41. Jackson C, Rosenfeld J, Moore D, Bryan W, Barohn R, Wrench M, et al. A preliminary evaluation of a prospective study of pulmonary function studies and symptoms of hypoventilation in ALS/MND patients. J Neurol Sci. 2001;191(1–2):75–8.
42. Velasco R, Salachas F, Munerati E, Le Forestier N, Pradat PF, Lacomblez L, et al. Nocturnal oxymetry in patients with amyotrophic lateral sclerosis: role in predicting survival. Rev Neurol (Paris). 2002;158(5 Pt 1):575–8.
43. Weinberg J, Klefbeck B, Borg J, Svanborg E. Polysomnography in chronic neuromuscular disease. Respiration. 2003;70(4):349–54.
44. Georges M, Nguyen-Baranoff D, Griffon L, Foignot C, Bonniaud P, Camus P, et al. Usefulness of transcutaneous PCO2 to assess nocturnal hypoventilation in restrictive lung disorders. Respirology. 2016;21(7):1300–6.
45. Pinto A, Evangelista T, Carvalho M, Alves MA, Luis MS. Respiratory assistance with a non-invasive ventilator (Bipap) in MND/ALS patients: survival rates in a controlled trial. J Neurol Sci. 1995;129:19–26.
46. Simonds AK. Recent advances in respiratory care for neuromuscular disease. Chest J. 2006;130(6):1879–86.
47. Gozal D, Thiriet P. Respiratory muscle training in neuromuscular disease: long-term effects on strength and load perception. Med Sci Sports Exerc. 1999;31(11):1522–7.
48. Vrijsen B, Buyse B, Belge C, Testelmans D. Upper airway obstruction during noninvasive ventilation induced by the use of an oronasal mask. J Clin Sleep Med. 2014;10(9):1033–5.
49. Schellhas V, Glatz C, Beecken I, Okegwo A, Heidbreder A, Young P, et al. Upper airway obstruction induced by non-invasive ventilation using an oronasal interface. Sleep Breath. 2018;22(3):781–8.
50. Young T, Finn L, Peppard PE, Szklo-Coxe M, Austin D, Nieto FJ, et al. Sleep disordered breathing and mortality: eighteen-year follow-up of the Wisconsin sleep cohort. Sleep. 2008;31(8):1071–8.
51. Yan-fang S, Yu-ping W. Sleep-disordered breathing: impact on functional outcome of ischemic stroke patients. Sleep Med. 2009;10(7):717–9.
52. Iranzo A, Santamaria J, Berenguer J, Sanchez M, Chamorro A. Prevalence and clinical importance of sleep apnea in the first night after cerebral infarction. Neurology. 2002;58(6):911–6.
53. Martínez-García MÁ, Soler-Cataluña JJ, Ejarque-Martínez L, Soriano Y, Román-Sánchez P, Illa FB, et al. Continuous positive airway pressure treatment reduces mortality in patients with ischemic stroke and obstructive sleep apnea: a 5-year follow-up study. Am J Respir Crit Care Med. 2009;180(1):36–41.
54. Fung CH, Igodan U, Alessi C, Martin JL, Dzierzewski JM, Josephson K, et al. Human factors/usability barriers to home medical devices among individuals with disabling conditions: in-depth interviews with positive airway pressure device users. Disabil Health J. 2015;8(1):86–92.
55. Evers S. Sleep and headache: the biological basis. Headache. 2010;50(7):1246–51.
56. Mascia A, Afra J, Schoenen J. Dopamine and migraine: a review of pharmacological, biochemical, neurophysiological, and therapeutic data. Cephalalgia. 1998;18(4):174–82.
57. Akerman S, Goadsby P. Dopamine and migraine: biology and clinical implications. Cephalalgia. 2007;27(11):1308–14.
58. Dexter JD. Headache as a presenting complaint 30 of the sleep-apnea syndrome. Headache. 1984;24:171.
59. Ulfberg J, Carter N, Talbäck M, Edling C. Headache, snoring and sleep apnoea. J Neurol. 1996;243(9):621–5.
60. Aldrich MS, Chauncey JB. Are morning headaches part of obstructive sleep apnea syndrome? Arch Intern Med. 1990;150(6):1265–7.
61. Guilleminault C, Eldridge FL, Tilkian A, Simmons FB, Dement WC. Sleep apnea syndrome due to upper airway obstruction: a review of 25 cases. Arch Intern Med. 1977;137(3):296–300.
62. Poceta JS, Dalessio DJ. Identification and treatment of sleep apnea in patients with chronic headache. Headache. 1995;35(10):586–9.
63. Ohayon MM. Prevalence and risk factors of morning headaches in the general population. Arch Intern Med. 2004;164(1):97–102.
64. Kirsch DB, Jozefowicz RF. Neurologic complications of respiratory disease. Neurol Clin. 2002;20(1):247–64, viii.
65. Paiva T, Farinha A, Martins A, Batista A, Guilleminault C. Chronic headaches and sleep disorders. Arch Intern Med. 1997;157(15):1701–5.
66. Strober LB. Fatigue in multiple sclerosis: a look at the role of poor sleep. Front Neurol. 2015;6:21.
67. Fleming WE, Pollak CP. Sleep disorders in multiple sclerosis. Semin Neurol. 2005;25:64–8.
68. Moreira N, Damasceno R, Medeiros C, De Bruin P, Teixeira C, Horta W, et al. Restless leg syndrome, sleep quality and fatigue in multiple sclerosis patients. Braz J Med Biol Res. 2008;41(10):932–7.
69. George CF, Feldman J, Inhaber N, Steininger TL, Grzeschik SM, Lai C, et al. A safety trial of sodium oxybate in patients with obstructive sleep apnea: acute effects on sleep-disordered breathing. Sleep Med. 2010;11(1):38–42.
70. Roy S. PAP therapy management mobile apps comparison guide. Sleep Reviews. 2018 (November/December).

Obstructive Sleep Apnea, CPAP, and Impact on Cognitive Function

15

Miqdad Hussain Bohra
and Mohammad Payman Hajiazim

Abbreviations

AHI — Apnea hypopnea index
CPAP — Continuous positive airway pressure
EDS — Excessive daytime sleepiness (or daytime sleepiness)
EEG — Electroencephalogram
MCI — Mild cognitive impairment
MRI — Magnetic resonance imaging
MSLT — Multiple sleep latency test
MWT — Maintenance of wakefulness test
NCF — Neurocognitive function (or cognitive function)
OSA — Obstructive sleep apnea (or sleep apnea)

15.1 Introduction

Obstructive sleep apnea (OSA) is a common sleep disorder, and it is characterized by repetitive obstruction in the upper airway during sleep which in turn fragments sleep quality and causes intermittent oxygen desaturation [1]. This manifests in a variety of systemic effects including affecting different aspects of neurocognitive function (NCF) and excessive daytime sleepiness (EDS) [2]. This effect on neurocognitive functioning and daytime sleepiness is however not a universal finding, and many individuals with OSA will not develop EDS or other NCF deficits [3–5] EDS is an important contributor to NCF considering that it is seen as a potential cause of cognitive problems [6].

M. H. Bohra (✉)
Department of Psychiatry, Faculty of Medicine, University of Toronto, Toronto, ON, Canada

Youthdale Child and Adolscent Sleep Center, Toronto, ON, Canada
e-mail: miqdad@youthdalesleepcenter.ca

M. P. Hajiazim
Psychiatry and Sleep Medicine, Cumming School of Medicine, University of Calgary, Calgary, AB, Canada

Hotchkiss Brain Institute, University of Calgary, Calgary, AB, Canada

15.2 Neurocognitive Testing

Impact on neurocognitive function due to any cause can be studied objectively using neuropsychological tests and subjectively using self-reported tests or questionnaires. Excessive daytime sleepiness can be measured subjectively using the Epworth sleepiness scale where a score of $\geq 10/24$ indicates subjective excessive daytime sleepiness as measured across a full day or the Stanford sleepiness scale which measures sleepiness at a specific moment in time [7, 8]. The gold-standard objective measure for daytime sleepiness is the multiple sleep latency test (MSLT). The maintenance of wakefulness test (MWT) measures a related concept, i.e., alertness [9].

Various aspects of NCF have been evaluated and are known to be impacted by OSA. These include aspects of memory including short-term verbal and visual memory and long-term semantic and declarative memory, executive functioning including working memory, and different aspects of attention including alertness, vigilance, and divided attention [3]. Some examples of tests measuring NCF in OSA patients include the psychomotor vigilance task and sustained working memory test [3].

The real-world translation of results of objectively measured cognitive functioning is limited in comparison to the real-world applicability of subjective cognitive dysfunction in both the healthy and morbid population [10–12]. This difference between subjective and objective tests makes it important to understand neurocognitive function both from a subjective and an objective viewpoint.

15.3 Subjective NCF in OSA

Subjective cognitive complaints are often associated with EDS, and among cognitive complaints, concentration appears to be the most affected [13]. Excessive daytime sleepiness is an important concern reported by individuals that is reported to be a function of disturbed sleep architecture [14]. It is among the most common symptoms in individuals with sleep disordered breathing and impacts occupational performance and quality of life in addition to directly being associated with other neurocognitive function parameters, including concentration, memory, and executive function [14, 15].

Studies have shown that there is a wide range of neurocognitive deficits observed in those who have OSA with EDS, but this does not necessarily extend to those who have obstructive sleep apnea without excessive daytime sleepiness [3]. Why some with OSA experience EDS and others with OSA do not remains a debated topic. Several factors are noted to play a part including severity of the apnea hypopnea index (AHI), disturbance in sleep architecture, intermittent arterial oxygen desaturation, sleep deprivation, chronicity of the condition, gender, and medical comorbidities such as obesity and psychiatric illness, indicating that the pathogenesis of daytime sleepiness in OSA is multifactorial [3].

15.4 Objective NCF in OSA

Objectively, OSA affects various spheres of NCF including intellectual function, executive function, memory, and attention. Each of these aspects of NCF has its own components as noted above [3]. Most research in the area of NCF in OSA supports the notion that there is a deficit in attention, aspects of memory (i.e., Delayed long-term verbal and visual memory), visuospatial/constructional abilities, and executive function, that there may not be a significant impact on language and psychomotor function, and that the effect on working memory, short-term memory, and global cognitive function is equivocal as concluded in a meta-review [16]. This is in contrast to more recent studies supporting an impairment in psychomotor function and working memory [17].

Studies exploring the effects of OSA on objectively measured NCF have yielded conflicting results, and no one factor has been found to consistently predict cognitive impairment indicating that this too has multifactorial causation. Whether it is related to EDS resulting in poor performance on objective cognitive measures [18] or the result of structural and functional changes in the brain that may result from sleep fragmentation or intermittent hypoxia remains debated [19]. Wang et al. have proposed that overall cerebrovascular health may perhaps be an important consideration when the impact of OSA on cognitive functioning is being assessed [20].

15.5 OSA Severity and NCF

It remains debated as to whether there is an association between the severity spectrum of OSA with measured NCF deficits and EDS. Some studies have shown that severity of OSA in terms of the apnea hypopnea index is a vital factor in predicting EDS [21, 22]. Those with severe OSA may have greater objective daytime sleepiness as compared to those with mild-to-moderate disease, despite no difference in subjective sleepiness [23]. On the other hand, other studies have emphasized that there is no robust relationship between severity of OSA and EDS [24, 25]. More recently, it has been proposed that other markers of OSA severity such as the severity of the individual respiratory events, e.g., desaturation events or the duration of the apneas/hypopneas itself rather than the AHI, are a stronger marker of daytime somnolence. [26]

Many studies have shown that impairment in neurocognitive function is reliant on sleep fragmentation, daytime sleepiness, and/or intermittent hypoxemia resulting from sleep apnea and not just related to the apnea hypopnea index itself [27–32]. Some on the other hand have suggested that sleep deprivation and EDS may be the reason behind impaired NCF rather than hypoxia [18]. It is possible that separate aspects impact separate domains of cognitive functioning. For example, sleep fragmentation and sleepiness may cause inattention, whereas intermittent hypoxia may cause executive dysfunction. [16, 33, 34]

The mechanisms involved in the OSA-related pathogenesis in Alzheimer's and ageing OSA could impact cognition via different pathways. OSA could fragment sleep and hence decrease slow wave sleep and REM sleep which hinders neuronal plasticity, a mechanism required for optimal cognitive function [35]. OSA-induced hypoxia could also lead to hypoxic injuries to different systems in the body, including causing oxidative stress, interfering with metabolic pathways, and also injury to the vessel walls; all could contribute to the formation of beta-amyloids and Tau protein [36]. On the other hand, the pathogenesis of Alzheimer's disease (AD) is accepted to be mainly due to the production of the β-amyloid peptide and its deposition. Tau protein function is also to promote the assembly of microtubules and stabilize its structure, which contributes to the proper function of neurons. Changes in the amount of tau protein and/or changes in its structure can affect its function as a stabilizer of microtubules as well as some of the processes in which it is implicated [37]. Another proposed mechanism includes impairment of CSF-ISF exchange in the brain which could hinder the removal of toxins from nervous system tissue during sleep [36]. This is the consequence of intrathoracic pressure swings following repetitive occlusion of the upper airway in OSA [36]. There are studies showing that using CPAP in OSA patients and also mild cognitive impairment could delay the progression of cognitive deficits [36, 38].

Familial aggregation for sleep apnea has been seen and replicated in different studies [39, 40]. The E4 isoform of apolipoprotein E (ApoE4) is strongly associated with an increased risk of early-onset Alzheimer's disease [41]. The association between Apo E4 and OSA has also been reported [42]. This could also explain why the cognitive changes seen in OSA may not only be related to the impact of OSA i.e. hypoxia and sleep fragmentation related to apnea events; but also that OSA and cognitive changes may have common genes which predispose the person to manifest both conditions. Further detail on genetic associations is beyond the scope of this chapter.

The occurrence of neurocognitive dysfunction in OSA patients and the clinical observation that in a significant portion of individuals with OSA, NCF and somnolence do not completely resolve on treatment suggests that certain physiological or structural changes are occurring in the brain, some of which might be irreversible, or alternatively, comorbid conditions may play a part on this [43, 44]. Functional MRI studies have shown reduction in activity in specific brain areas such as the prefrontal cortex and in the cingulate, frontal, and parietal areas of the brain correlating with impairment in executive functions and reduction in attention, respectively [45, 46]. Based on a review of studies on resting-state functional MRI in OSA, *Khazai* et al. have proposed that disruption of the functional connectivity in parts of the default mode network (ventromedial prefrontal cortex, hippocampal formation, and posterior cingulate cortex) may be a potential biomarker in OSA considering that the default mode network is an important area related to cognitive functioning [47].

In summary, OSA causes subjective and objective cognitive impairment; not all patients with OSA develop these impairments, and in those who do, the nature of these impairments varies, and the underlying mechanisms are multifactorial (Fig. 15.1).

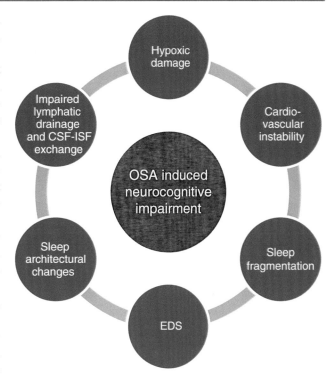

Fig. 15.1 OSA-induced systemic effects that contribute to neurocognitive dysfunction

15.6 Continuous Positive Airway Pressure Therapy (CPAP) for OSA

Among the different treatment options for OSA, CPAP therapy is considered the first-line choice of treatment since its introduction in the early 1980s [48]. CPAP works by reducing instability in the upper airway and helps stabilize breathing pattern during sleep which in turn addresses obstructive sleep disordered breathing, and this could improve daytime functioning by reducing sleep fragmentation, improving oxygenation, and reducing inflammation [49–52].

The effects of CPAP treatment on NCF have been noted from the early years of introduction of this treatment. Since then, over 300 papers have been published which discuss the impact of CPAP on different aspects of cognition including attention and vigilance, psychomotor processing, executive functioning, episodic memory, and intellectual ability [53].

Among its many effects on NCF, CPAP has been shown to improve daytime sleepiness and alertness in OSA, two separate functions that are a result of separate but dynamically interacting neurological processes [9]. Meta-analyses have shown that CPAP pressure improves subjective and objective EDS as measured with the Epworth sleepiness scale and MSLT and objective daytime alertness as measured with the MWT across the entire spectrum of severity of OSA [49, 50].

Varying degrees of positive effects of CPAP use on cognitive performance have been demonstrated with various possible underlying mechanisms (Fig. 15.2). This may be due, in part, to variability in study design and sampling methodology across studies [34]. It could also be related to the possibility that some of the cognitive changes related to OSA may not be fully reversible with CPAP treatment, but it may prevent further deterioration of NCF, as part of the changes are related to the vascular system [54]. This is similar to findings in chronic conditions such as diabetes mellitus and its impact on the peripheral and central nervous system. For example, there is less evidence on the reversibility of the ophthalmic changes in diabetes even after tight glucose regulations although further deterioration may be slowed indicating that existing damage because of diabetes may not be reversible but further damage may be slowed or prevented [54, 55].

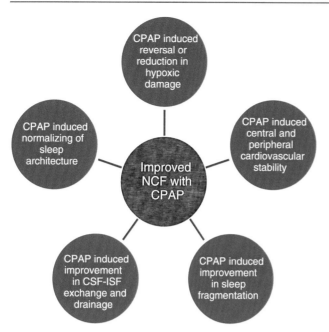

Fig. 15.2 Effects of CPAP therapy that contribute to improved neuro-cognitive functioning

15.7 Measuring Change in NCF with CPAP

Research has focused on neuroimaging findings of the NCF improvement in patients using CPAP, in parallel with looking into the neuroimaging findings of the impact of OSA. Some research has focused on the neuropsychological findings of cognitive improvements in patients using CPAP, in parallel with looking into the neuropsychological findings of the impact of OSA.

CPAP therapy in moderate-to-severe OSA has shown reduction in EDS and improvement NCF including parameters such as verbal memory and executive functioning but not necessarily in vigilance despite adequate adherence [56]. However to the contrary, a meta-analysis of 13 studies from 1994 to 2012 studying the effect of CPAP therapy on cognition in middle-aged adults with OSA showed a statistically significant improvement only in vigilance, whereas other cognitive functions such as attention, working memory, verbal fluency, visuo-constructive skills, and processing speed did not show statistically significant improvements [57]. Neither did the researchers observe a significant effect size difference based on duration of CPAP therapy or the AHI. Limitations included classifying disease severity on basis of AHI and, not considering other parameters, collection of data over a long period which may have affected the diagnosis of OSA due to change in scoring criteria and confounders introduced by the methodology of the initial studies included in the meta-analysis. The APPLES study concluded that those on CPAP therapy were less sleepy with more severe OSA individuals having a greater response and that

CPAP therapy benefitted executive functioning modestly. This led them to conclude that the relationship between OSA and NCF is complex, and when managing patients with CPAP, individual differences, disease severity, and sleepiness all should be taken into account [58].

More recently, CPAP therapy in mild-to-moderate OSA has shown to improve neurobehavioral functions such as verbal fluency, psychomotor functioning, and information processing speed along with an improvement in mood and quality of life measures [17]. However, this improvement in the same population was not associated with a similar degree of improvement in working memory, and neither was there a normalization of subjective or objective daytime alertness *post* treatment with CPAP despite a significant improvement in subjective daytime sleepiness as compared to baseline [17]. This improvement was noted particularly in those with adequate CPAP adherence defined as >4 hours/night of use, 70% of the nights. This is an arbitrary parameter determined by consensus rather than robust evidence [59]. This might impact the results of the studies that have evaluated the impact of CPAP on NCF, depending on how they define adherence.

In clinical practice, CPAP therapy is more likely to be prescribed in moderate to severe OSA or in those individuals with mild OSA who have co-morbidities or associated EDS. Cognitive impairment and daytime sleepiness, and the effects of CPAP therapy on these parameters, are also more commonly evaluated in severe OSA as compared to milder forms of OSA. This could be because of the assumption that less severe OSA is less likely to be associated with significant cognitive impairment due to the greater ability to compensate for the deficits, or it could be because minor changes are more difficult to measure or because milder sleep disordered breathing might not have as much of an impact on these parameters [60]. There is also the controversy of whether using CPAP in less severe OSA is worthwhile considering questionable improvement in quality of life, the cost implications of ongoing CPAP therapy, and sleep disturbance introduced by the use of CPAP therapy itself [61, 62].

15.8 Neurophysiological and Imaging Aspects of Effects of CPAP on NCF

Studies have investigated the effect of sleep apnea and CPAP on brain EEG activity. Selected 2-s electroencephalogram (EEG)-epochs were processed by LORETA (low-resolution electromagnetic tomography) to determine EEG sources for seven frequency bands, delta (1.5–6 Hz), theta (6.5–8 Hz), alpha1 (8.5–10 Hz), alpha2 (10.5–12 Hz), beta1 (12.5–18 Hz), beta2 (18.5–21 Hz), and beta3 (21.5–30 Hz) with reference to an earlier study [63]. Increase in the portion of delta and theta bands during the day could denote deviation from the normal function the same as reductions in the alpha and beta band portions. In the group of patients with moderate sleep apnea, significant changes were found in the posterior cingulate cortex (changes in the amount alpha2 band) as well as in the right posterior parietal cortex and the left supramarginal gyrus (in the beta1band in both regions). In the group of patients with severe sleep apnea, significant changes were found in the posterior cingulate cortex (changes in the theta and alpha1 bands). Following CPAP treatment, these significant differences disappeared in the severe group. In the group of patients who were dealing with moderate sleep apnea, the activity was significantly decreased in the right fusiform gyrus (in the beta3 band). These findings potentially suggest a normalizing effect of CPAP therapy on EEG background activity in both groups (moderate and severe groups) of OSA syndrome patients. Successful memory functioning, also the emotional perception, and the DMN, and fear network could be disrupted by chronic intermittent hypoxia, as evidenced by the alterations of brain electrical activity in the associated regions. This could possibly be reversed with the use of CPAP therapy [64].

Overall, in comparing moderate OSA groups to healthy controls, significantly increased activity was observed in alpha2 band bilaterally in the posterior cingulate cortex and in the beta1 band in the right posterior parietal cortex and left supramarginal gyrus. Following CPAP therapy, the patients experienced modified activity in the right fusiform gyrus (significantly decreased activity was detected associated with the beta3 band). In comparing the group of patients with severe sleep apnea and the control group, the patients with untreated severe sleep apnea had significantly increased activity in the theta and also alpha1 bands bilaterally in the posterior cingulate cortex prior to starting CPAP therapy. Notably, following CPAP therapy, this characteristic difference was normalized [64]. They also found that the changes are reversible following using CPAP in the group of patients with moderate OSA compared to those with severe OSA [64].

Research looking at regional blood flow in different areas of the brain in individuals with OSA before and 6 months after treatment with CPAP has shown a partial to complete reversal of decreased cerebral blood flow in areas of the brain that are associated with executive function, affect regulation, and memory such as the limbic and prefrontal areas, cerebellum, medial orbitofrontal, and angular cortex [65, 66]. Furthermore, there is evidence to support an improvement in cerebral vasoreactivity and cerebral blood flow, suggesting an improvement in cerebral vasodilator reserve and reduction in carotid intima media thickness, a proxy marker of atherosclerosis [67]. These findings point toward the possible reduction in the risk of cerebrovascular events [67].

Untreated younger and middle-aged adults with severe OSA have been noted to have significant impairment in objectively tested memory and executive cognitive functions and structural changes in the form of reduced gray matter in parts of the brain that are associated with these functions [68]. These deficits and structural changes were shown to respond to CPAP therapy over a 3-month period, and a direct relationship between improvements in gray matter volume and NCF was also observed [68]. Similarly, in individuals ≥65 years, with severe OSA, CPAP therapy has been shown to improve objective NCF including aspects of memory and executive functioning and positive structural changes such as improved neural connectivity in the right middle frontal gyrus in those using CPAP therapy as compared to those on conservative or no treatment [69, 70]. The partial recovery in structure and function reported above can be attributed to the sensitivity of the hippocampus to damage by intermittent hypoxia arising from untreated OSA, and the ability of the hippocampus to regenerate neurons [68, 71, 72]. This is particularly important as OSA is considered a modifiable risk factor for age-related hippocampal atrophy [73].

15.9 Comorbidity, NCF, and CPAP Treatment

CPAP therapy has been shown to improve NCF in addition to other parameters in stroke rehabilitation in individuals with comorbid OSA, with improvements in aspects of attention and executive function [74–76]. These changes may improve outcomes not only due to direct reduction in neural injury but also indirectly due to improved participation in the rehabilitation program by improved NCF and reduction in depressive symptoms and drowsiness [75]. It has been suggested that long-term CPAP therapy can improve survival and reduce the recurrence of stroke [77].

Richards et al. evaluated NCF in individuals with an AHI of ≥10/h and baseline mild cognitive impairment (MCI) who used CPAP at 1 year in comparison to matched controls with MCI and OSA who did not use CPAP [78]. They noted statistically significant improvements in cognitive processing speed, psychomotor function, daytime sleepiness, and possible protective effects on memory favoring the CPAP group. They also reported a possible subjective improvement in the CPAP group in comparison, although this improvement was not statistically significant. Similar improvements were also noted in individuals with MCI and mild OSA [79]. Although these studies are pilots and have low power statistically, their findings point toward an important place for CPAP therapy across the spectrum of OSA in individuals with pre-dementia.

Chronic kidney disease and sleep disordered breathing share a bidirectional relationship, and the prevalence of OSA in chronic kidney disease is significantly higher as compared to OSA in the general population [80]. This increase in prevalence is attributed directly to the underlying renal dysfunction [80]. Cognitive impairment is significantly higher in the chronic kidney disease population, reaching as high as 40% [81–83]. Although it is unclear at present whether there is a shared pathophysiology for cognitive impairment arising in OSA and that arising in chronic kidney disease, a synergistic effect of each condition and hence a complex relationship cannot be ignored considering that both these conditions have profound systemic effects. Although there are limited studies to our knowledge looking into the effect of CPAP therapy in individuals with chronic kidney disease and OSA, a case report has recently alluded to the beneficial effects of long-term CPAP therapy in end-stage renal disease on subjective cognitive function, quality of life, and EDS [84].

The positive effect of CPAP on mood has been well established, a factor which could improve cognitive function in those who have comorbid depression as well [85, 86]. This comorbidity exists in 20–40% of patients with OSA which could worsen the impact of OSA on one's cognitive functioning [85, 86]. Studies have shown that the CPAP treatment could improve depression in this population and also their cognitive dysfunction subsequently [87]. For more information on CPAP and depression, see Chap. 19.

15.10 Other Considerations for CPAP Therapy and Its Effects on NCF

Although there is building evidence supporting improvement in NCF with CPAP therapy, it still remains debated. This raises the question of why CPAP treatment addressing nocturnal hypoxia and sleep fragmentation only has a modest impact on some and not all aspects of NCF. To understand this issue better, using the analogy of the benefits of statins in preventing a heart attack may be helpful. Different studies have shown that the number needed to treat for the statins varies from 50 to 100 (90) [88]. In other words, up to 100 patients with hypercholesterolemia should be treated with statins on a regular basis, in order to prevent one heart attack. This suggests that hypercholesterolemia by itself is not the sole contributor to a cardiac ischemic event. Likewise, nocturnal hypoxia and sleep fragmentation may not be the primary (or sole) causes of impairment in NCF in people who live with OSA (see Fig. 15.1). It may be that other factors also have a significant impact on NCF, and identifying and addressing those factors in treatment may have better yield in protecting NCF, for example, addressing comorbid conditions.

Addressing comorbid conditions may also be vital in achieving stronger results with continuous positive airway pressure treatment and its effect on NCF. A significant portion of sleep apnea cases have comorbid diabetes, and obesity, conditions which also have their own share in the cognitive symptoms and deficits observed in those with sleep apnea [89]. OSA and chronic obstructive pulmonary disease are both accompanied by deficits in attention, memory, executive function, psychomotor function, and language abilities, suggesting that hypoxia/hypercarbia may be an important determinant of deficits in these domains in OSA [90].

Another issue which merits attention is the role of adjunct treatment to CPAP to observe more desirable effects. For example, it has been observed that pulmonary rehabilitation and the oropharyngeal exercises could be used as an adjunct therapy in OSA [91, 92]. In a clinical trial done to assess the effectiveness of CPAP and other adjunct treatment modalities, it was noted that although OSA severity was controlled with CPAP treatment in both groups, a significant reduction of neck, waist, and hip circumferences and body mass index and improvement of pulmonary function were achieved only in the CPAP and pulmonary rehabilitation group after treatment in comparison to the CPAP-only group [91]. One may speculate that cognitive functions might also benefit more from a multicomponent treatment. However, to our knowledge, there is no published research in the area of enhancement of the effect of CPAP on NCF by the aforementioned treatments and interventions.

Other adjunct treatments to CPAP in OSA include alerting agents. The safety and efficacy of adding modafinil/armodafinil to CPAP therapy continues to be debated although these agents are utilized clinically and recommended by guidelines to be used as adjuncts particularly to address residual daytime alertnes [93]. A recently published systematic review has shown that the effectiveness of CPAP on NCF can be augmented by these alertness-promoting agents [94]. The authors found clinically significant change in the MWT and also subjective changes recorded by Epworth sleepiness scale, along with minimal and tolerable side effects. For more information on wake-promoting medications in patients on CPAP therapy, see Chap. 29.

Another important issue to consider when evaluating cognitive changes in patients treated with CPAP is that other comorbid sleep disorders, including insomnia, could have its own impact on NCF [94, 95]. Insomnia is a common comorbidity in patients with OSA. Insomnia is known to impact the attention, memory, and executive functioning [94, 95]. A study on the phenotypic causes of OSA also showed how the hyperarousal state of the brain cortex, which plays a role in the pathogenesis of insomnia, could also play a role in the pathogenesis of sleep apnea [95]. They found that 37% of the population they studied had a low arousal threshold in their cortex [95]. Hence, treatment of comorbid insomnia could be helpful in an individual with OSA who is dealing with cognitive issues, especially when you are considering optimizing the treatment outcomes, including the positive effects of

Fig. 15.3 Optimizing NCF
in individuals with OSA

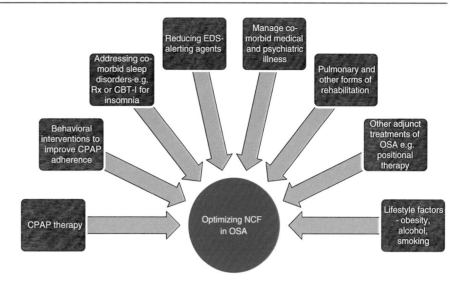

CPAP on NCF. In other words, CPAP treatment will address the critical pressure of the upper airway, but it may not be able to address hyperarousal state of the brain cortex, which plays a role in the pathogenesis of insomnia, at least for the first few months of treatment, until the patient is acclimatized to the treatment and reversible physiologic changes could take place in different systems including the brain cortex. For more information on insomnia treatment in patients with OSA, see Chaps. 6, 17, and 18.

15.11 Summary

In summary, OSA is a common condition that is associated with intermittent hypoxia, fragmentation in the sleep architecture, and increased chronic inflammation. Among its many systemic effects are its impact on NCF, daytime alertness, and sleepiness. These effects are not consistent across the population and have multifactorial causation resulting in a difficult to predict picture. CPAP is considered to be the most effective treatment of OSA and has been an important treatment not only for moderate-to-severe OSA but also in milder OSA where there are other comorbidities or there is noted improvement in quality of life. CPAP has been shown in various studies to positively influence NCF and reduce EDS, but these effects are not universal and difficult to predict due to numerous factors. These include, but are not limited to, multifactorial causation of neurocognitive deficits, reversible and irreversible reasons behind the neurocognitive dysfunction, comorbid disease states, and variability in adherence to CPAP.

Optimizing NCF in individuals with OSA likely requires a multimodal approach that takes into consideration addressing adherence, treating co-existing sleep disorders, treating comorbid medical and psychiatric conditions, rehabilitation, and lifestyle and behavioral changes (Fig. 15.3).

Research is lacking on the study of the impact of CPAP therapy on neurocognitive functioning in individuals with other comorbid conditions. Because comorbidities play a significant role in the variable success of CPAP therapy on NCF, this is an important area to study further.

Acknowledgments We acknowledge the valuable input received from Dr. Berjinder Jay Sethi toward the completion of this chapter.

References

1. Douglas NJ, Polo O. Pathogenesis of obstructive sleep apnoea/hypopnoea syndrome. Lancet. 1994;344(8923):653–5. https://doi.org/10.1016/s0140-6736(94)92088-5. PMID: 7915351.
2. Dempsey JA, Veasey SC, Morgan BJ, O'Donnell CP. Pathophysiology of sleep apnea. Physiol Rev. 2010;90(1):47–112. https://doi.org/10.1152/physrev.00043.2008. Erratum in: Physiol Rev. 2010;90(2):797–8. PMID: 20086074; PMCID: PMC3970937.
3. Zhou J, Camacho M, Tang X, Kushida CA. A review of neurocognitive function and obstructive sleep apnea with or without daytime sleepiness. Sleep Med. 2016;23:99–108. https://doi.org/10.1016/j.sleep.2016.02.008. Epub 2016 Mar 2. PMID: 27288049.
4. Roth T, Hartse KM, Zorick F, Conway W. Multiple naps and the evaluation of daytime sleepiness in patients with upper airway sleep apnea. Sleep. 1980;3(3–4):425–39. PMID: 6111835.
5. Greenberg GD, Watson RK, Deptula D. Neuropsychological dysfunction in sleep apnea. Sleep. 1987;10(3):254–62. https://doi.org/10.1093/sleep/10.3.254. PMID: 3629088.
6. Naismith S, Winter V, Gotsopoulos H, Hickie I, Cistulli P. Neurobehavioral functioning in obstructive sleep apnea: differential effects of sleep quality, hypoxemia and subjective sleepiness. J Clin Exp Neuropsychol. 2004;26(1):43–54. https://doi.org/10.1076/jcen.26.1.43.23929. PMID: 14972693.
7. Johns MW. A new method for measuring daytime sleepiness: the Epworth sleepiness scale. Sleep. 1991;14(6):540–5. https://doi.org/10.1093/sleep/14.6.540. PMID: 1798888.
8. Hoddes E, Dement W, Zarcone V. The development and use of the Stanford sleepiness scale (SSS). Psychophysiology. 1972;9:150.
9. Espana R, Scammell T. Sleep neurobiology for the clinician. Sleep. 2004;27:811–20.

10. Chaytor N, Schmitter-Edgecombe M. The ecological validity of neuropsychological tests: a review of the literature on everyday cognitive skills. Neuropsychol Rev. 2003;13:181–97.

11. Stenfors CU, Marklund P, Magnusson Hanson LL, Theorell T, Nilsson LG. Subjective cognitive complaints and the role of executive cognitive functioning in the working population: a case-control study. PLoS One. 2013;8:e83351.

12. Waldorff FB, Siersma V, Waldemar G. Association between subjective memory complaints and health care utilisation: a three-follow up. BMC Geriatr. 2009;9:43.

13. Vaessen TJ, Overeem S, Sitskoorn MM. Cognitive complaints in obstructive sleep apnea. Sleep Med Rev. 2015;19:51–8. https://doi.org/10.1016/j.smrv.2014.03.008. Epub 2014 Apr 2. PMID: 24846772.

14. Ferini-Strambi L, Lombardi GE, Marelli S, Galbiati A. Neurological deficits in obstructive sleep apnea. Curr Treat Options Neurol. 2017;19(4):16. https://doi.org/10.1007/s11940-017-0451-8. PMID: 28374233.

15. Garbarino S, Durando P, Guglielmi O, Dini G, Bersi F, Fornarino S, Toletone A, Chiorri C, Magnavita N. Sleep apnea, sleep debt and daytime sleepiness are independently associated with road accidents. A cross-sectional study on truck drivers. PLoS One. 2016;11(11):e0166262. https://doi.org/10.1371/journal.pone.0166262. PMID: 27902703; PMCID: PMC5130193.

16. Bucks RS, Olaithe M, Eastwood P. Neurocognitive function in obstructive sleep apnoea: a meta-review. Respirology. 2013;18:61–70.

17. Jackson ML, McEvoy RD, Banks S, Barnes M. Neurobehavioral impairment and CPAP treatment response in mild-moderate obstructive sleep apneas. J Clin Sleep Med. 2018;14(1):47–56. https://doi.org/10.5664/jcsm.6878. PMID: 29198304; PMCID: PMC5734962.

18. Verstraeten E. Neurocognitive effects of obstructive sleep apnea syndrome. Curr Neurol Neurosci Rep. 2007;7:161–6.

19. Beebe DW, Gozal D. Obstructive sleep apnea and the prefrontal cortex: towards a comprehensive model linking nocturnal upper airway obstruction to daytime cognitive and behavioral deficits. J Sleep Res. 2002;11(1):1–16. https://doi.org/10.1046/j.1365-2869.2002.00289.x. PMID: 11869421.

20. Wang G, Goebel JR, Li C, Hallman HG, Gilford TM, Li W. Therapeutic effects of CPAP on cognitive impairments associated with OSA. J Neurol. 2020;267(10):2823–8. https://doi.org/10.1007/s00415-019-09381-2. Epub 2019 May 20. PMID: 31111204.

21. Koch H, Schneider LD, Finn LA, et al. Breathing disturbances without hypoxia are associated with objective sleepiness in sleep apnea. Sleep. 2017;40(11):zsx152.

22. Koehler U, Apelt S, Augsten M, et al. Daytime sleepiness in patients with obstructive sleep apnoea (OSA) – pathogenetic factors. Pneumologie. 2011;65:137–42.

23. Fong SY, Ho CK, Wing YK. Comparing MSLT and ESS in the measurement of excessive daytime sleepiness in obstructive sleep apnoea syndrome. J Psychosom Res. 2005;58(1):55–60. https://doi.org/10.1016/j.jpsychores.2004.05.004. PMID: 15771871.

24. Sharkey KM, Orff HJ, Tosi C, et al. Subjective sleepiness and daytime functioning in bariatric patients with obstructive sleep apnea. Sleep Breath. 2013;17:267–74.

25. Guilleminault C, Partinen M, Quera-Salva MA, et al. Determinants of daytime sleepiness in obstructive sleep apnea. Chest. 1988;94:32–7.

26. Kainulainen S, Töyräs J, Oksenberg A, Korkalainen H, Sefa S, Kulkas A, Leppänen T. Severity of desaturations reflects OSA-related daytime sleepiness better than AHI. J Clin Sleep Med. 2019;15(8):1135–42. https://doi.org/10.5664/jcsm.7806. PMID: 31482835; PMCID: PMC6707054.

27. Boland LL, Shahar E, Iber C, et al. Measures of cognitive function in persons with varying degrees of sleep-disordered breathing: the Sleep Heart Health Study. J Sleep Res. 2002;11:265–72.

28. Naegele B, Thouvard V, Pepin JL, et al. Deficits of cognitive executive functions in patients with sleep apnea syndrome. Sleep. 1995;18:43–52.

29. Sharma H, Sharma SK, Kadhiravan T, et al. Pattern & correlates of neurocognitive dysfunction in Asian Indian adults with severe obstructive sleep apnoea. Indian J Med Res. 2010;132:409–14.

30. Twigg GL, Papaioannou I, Jackson M, et al. Obstructive sleep apnea syndrome is associated with deficits in verbal but not visual memory. Am J Respir Crit Care Med. 2010;182:98–103.

31. Quan SF, Chan CS, Dement WC, et al. The association between obstructive sleep apnea and neurocognitive performance – the Apnea Positive Pressure Long-term Efficacy Study (APPLES). Sleep. 2011;34:303–14B.

32. Redline S, Strauss ME, Adams N, Winters M, Roebuck T, Spry K, Rosenberg C, Adams K. Neuropsychological function in mild sleep-disordered breathing. Sleep. 1997;20(2):160–7. https://doi.org/10.1093/sleep/20.2.160. PMID: 9143077.

33. Aloia MS, Arndt JT, Davis JD, Riggs RL, Byrd D. Neuropsychological sequelae of obstructive sleep apnea-hypopnea syndrome: a critical review. J Int Neuropsychol Soc. 2004;10(5):772–85. https://doi.org/10.1017/S1355617704105134. PMID: 15327723.

34. Lis S, Krieger S, Hennig D, Röder C, Kirsch P, Seeger W, Gallhofer B, Schulz R. Executive functions and cognitive subprocesses in patients with obstructive sleep apnea. J Sleep Res. 2008;17(3):271–80. https://doi.org/10.1111/j.1365-2869.2008.00660.x. Epub 2008 May 15. PMID: 18484964.

35. Ju Y-ES, Zangrilli MA, Finn MB, Fagan AM, Holtzman DM. Obstructive sleep apnea treatment, slow wave activity, and amyloid-β. Ann Neurol. 2019;85(2):291–5.

36. Bubu OM, Andrade AG, Umasabor-Bubu OQ, Hogan MM, Turner AD, de Leon MJ, et al. Obstructive sleep apnea, cognition and Alzheimer's disease: a systematic review integrating three decades of multidisciplinary research. Sleep Med Rev. 2020;50:101250.

37. Kolarova M, García-Sierra F, Bartos A, Ricny J, Ripova D. Structure and pathology of tau protein in Alzheimer disease [Internet]. Int J Alzheimers Dis. 2012;2012:1–13. Available from: https://doi.org/10.1155/2012/731526

38. Richards KC, Gooneratne N, Dicicco B, Hanlon A, Moelter S, Onen F, et al. CPAP adherence may slow 1-year cognitive decline in older adults with mild cognitive impairment and apnea. J Am Geriatr Soc. 2019;67(3):558–64.

39. Au CT, Zhang J, Cheung JYF, Chan KCC, Wing YK, Li AM. Familial aggregation and heritability of obstructive sleep apnea using children probands. J Clin Sleep Med. 2019;15(11):1561–70.

40. Mukherjee S, Saxena R, Palmer LJ. The genetics of obstructive sleep apnoea. Respirology. 2018;23(1):18–27.

41. Bekris LM, Yu C-E, Bird TD, Tsuang DW. Review article: Genetics of Alzheimer disease [Internet]. J Geriatr Psychiatry Neurol. 2010;23:213–27. Available from: https://doi.org/10.1177/0891988710383571

42. Kadotani H, Kadotani T, Young T, Peppard PE, Finn L, Colrain IM, et al. Association between apolipoprotein E epsilon4 and sleep-disordered breathing in adults. JAMA. 2001;285(22):2888–90.

43. Jackson ML, Howard ME, Barnes M. Cognition and daytime functioning in sleep-related breathing disorders. Prog Brain Res. 2011;190:53–68.

44. Lim DC, Veasey SC. Neural injury in sleep apnea. Curr Neurol Neurosci Rep. 2010;10:47–52.

45. Ayalon L, Ancoli-Israel S, Aka AA, et al. Relationship between obstructive sleep apnea severity and brain activation during a sustained attention task. Sleep. 2009;32:373–81.

46. Thomas RJ, Rosen BR, Stern CE, et al. Functional imaging of working memory in obstructive sleep-disordered breathing. J Appl Physiol. 2005;98:2226–34.

47. Khazaie H, Veronese M, Noori K, Emamian F, Zarei M, Ashkan K, Leschziner GD, Eickhoff CR, Eickhoff SB, Morrell MJ, Osorio RS, Spiegelhalder K, Tahmasian M, Rosenzweig I. Functional reorganization in obstructive sleep apnoea and insomnia: a systematic review of the resting-state fMRI. Neurosci Biobehav Rev. 2017;77:219–31. https://doi.org/10.1016/j.neubiorev.2017.03.013. Epub 2017 Mar 23. PMID: 28344075; PMCID: PMC6167921.

48. Sullivan CE, Issa FG, Berthon-Jones M, Eves L. Reversal of obstructive sleep apnoea by continuous positive airway pressure applied through the nares. Lancet. 1981;317(8225):862–5, ISSN 0140-6736. https://doi.org/10.1016/S0140-6736(81)92140-1.

49. Loredo JS, Ancoli-Israel S, Dimsdale JE. Effect of continuous positive airway pressure vs placebo continuous positive airway pressure on sleep quality in obstructive sleep apnea. Chest. 1999;116:1545–9.

50. Sin DD, Logan AG, Fitzgerald FS, et al. Effects of continuous positive airway pressure on cardiovascular outcomes in heart failure patients with and without Cheyne-Stokes respiration. Circulation. 2000;102:61–6.

51. Sanchez AI, Martinez P, Miro E, et al. CPAP and behavioral therapies in patients with obstructive sleep apnea: effects on daytime sleepiness, mood, and cognitive function. Sleep Med Rev. 2009;13:223–33.

52. Naegele B, Pepin JL, Levy P, et al. Cognitive executive dysfunction in patients with obstructive sleep apnea syndrome (OSAS) after CPAP treatment. Sleep. 1998;21:392–7.

53. Daurat A, Sarhane M, Tiberge M. Syndrome d'apnées obstructives du sommeil et cognition: une revue [Internet]. Neurophysiol Clin/ Clin Neurophysiol. 2016;46:201–15. Available from: https://doi.org/10.1016/j.neucli.2016.04.002

54. Matthews EE, Aloia MS. Cognitive recovery following positive airway pressure (PAP) in sleep apnea. Prog Brain Res. 2011;190:71–88.

55. Hendrick AM, Gibson MV, Kulshreshtha A. Diabetic retinopathy [Internet]. Prim Care. 2015;42:451–64. Available from: https://doi.org/10.1016/j.pop.2015.05.005

56. Antic NA, Catcheside P, Buchan C, Hensley M, Naughton MT, Rowland S, Williamson B, Windler S, McEvoy RD. The effect of CPAP in normalizing daytime sleepiness, quality of life, and neurocognitive function in patients with moderate to severe OSA. Sleep. 2011;34(1):111–9. https://doi.org/10.1093/sleep/34.1.111. PMID: 21203366; PMCID: PMC3001789.

57. Pan YY, Deng Y, Xu X, Liu YP, Liu HG. Effects of continuous positive airway pressure on cognitive deficits in middle-aged patients with obstructive sleep apnea syndrome: a meta-analysis of randomized controlled trials. Chin Med J. 2015;128(17):2365–73. https://doi.org/10.4103/0366-6999.163385.

58. Kushida CA, Nichols DA, Holmes TH, Quan SF, Walsh JK, Gottlieb DJ, Simon RD Jr, Guilleminault C, White DP, Goodwin JL, Schweitzer PK, Leary EB, Hyde PR, Hirshkowitz M, Green S, McEvoy LK, Chan C, Gevins A, Kay GG, Bloch DA, Crabtree T, Dement WC. Effects of continuous positive airway pressure on neurocognitive function in obstructive sleep apnea patients: the Apnea Positive Pressure Long-term Efficacy Study (APPLES). Sleep. 2012;35(12):1593–602. https://doi.org/10.5665/sleep.2226. Erratum in: Sleep. 2016;39(7):1483. PMID: 23204602; PMCID: PMC3490352.

59. Kribbs NB, Pack AI, Kline LR, Smith PL, Schwartz AR, Schubert NM, Redline S, Henry JN, Getsy JE, Dinges DF. Objective measurement of patterns of nasal CPAP use by patients with obstructive sleep apnea. Am Rev Respir Dis. 1993;147(4):887–95. https://doi.org/10.1164/ajrccm/147.4.887. PMID: 8466125.

60. Alchanatis M, Zias N, Deligiorgis N, Amfilochiou A, Dionellis G, Orphanidou D. Sleep apnea-related cognitive deficits and intelligence: an implication of cognitive reserve theory. J Sleep Res. 2005;14(1):69–75. https://doi.org/10.1111/j.1365-2869.2004.00436.x. PMID: 15743336.

61. Batool-Anwar S, Goodwin JL, Kushida CA, Walsh JA, Simon RD, Nichols DA, Quan SF. Impact of continuous positive airway pressure (CPAP) on quality of life in patients with obstructive sleep apnea (OSA). J Sleep Res. 2016;25(6):731–8. https://doi.org/10.1111/jsr.12430. Epub 2016 May 30. PMID: 27242272; PMCID: PMC5436801.

62. Rezaie L, Phillips D, Khazaie H. Barriers to acceptance and adherence to continuous positive airway pressure therapy in patients with obstructive sleep apnea: a report from Kermanshah province, western Iran. Patient Prefer Adherence. 2018;12:1299–304. https://doi.org/10.2147/PPA.S165905.

63. Kubicki S, Herrmann WM, Fichte K, Freund G. Reflections on the topics: EEG frequency bands and regulation of vigilance [Internet]. Pharmacopsychiatry. 1979;12:237–45. Available from: https://doi.org/10.1055/s-0028-1094615

64. Toth M, Kondakor I, Faludi B. Differences of brain electrical activity between moderate and severe obstructive sleep apneic patients: a LORETA study. J Sleep Res. 2016;25(5):596–604.

65. Kim JS, Seo JH, Kang MR, Seong MJ, Lee WG, Joo EY, Hong SB. Effect of continuous positive airway pressure on regional cerebral blood flow in patients with severe obstructive sleep apnea syndrome. Sleep Med. 2017;32:122–8. https://doi.org/10.1016/j.sleep.2016.03.010. Epub 2016 May 12. PMID: 28366323.

66. Shiota S, Inoue Y, Takekawa H, Kotajima M, Nakajyo M, Usui C, Yoshioka Y, Koga T, Takahashi K. Effect of continuous positive airway pressure on regional cerebral blood flow during wakefulness in obstructive sleep apnea. Sleep Breath. 2014;18(2):289–95. https://doi.org/10.1007/s11325-013-0881-9. Epub 2013 Sept 13. PMID: 24026964.

67. Piraino A, Sette G, D'Ascanio M, La Starza S, Aquilini M, Ricci A. Effect of OSAS on cerebral vasoreactivity and cIMT before and after CPAP treatment. Clin Respir J. 2019;13(9):555–9. https://doi.org/10.1111/crj.13057. Epub 2019 Jul 24. PMID: 31301263.

68. Canessa N, Castronovo V, Cappa SF, Aloia MS, Marelli S, Falini A, Alemanno F, Ferini-Strambi L. Obstructive sleep apnea: brain structural changes and neurocognitive function before and after treatment. Am J Respir Crit Care Med. 2011;183(10):1419–26. https://doi.org/10.1164/rccm.201005-0693OC. Epub 2010 Oct 29. PMID: 21037021.

69. Dalmases M, Solé-Padullés C, Torres M, Embid C, Nuñez MD, Martínez-Garcia MÁ, Farré R, Bargalló N, Bartrés-Faz D, Montserrat JM. Effect of CPAP on cognition, brain function, and structure among elderly patients with OSA: a randomized pilot study. Chest. 2015;148:1214–23.

70. Crawford-Achour E, Dauphinot V, Saint Martin M, Tardy M, Gonthier R, Barthelemy JC, Roche F. Protective effect of long-term CPAP therapy on cognitive performance in elderly patients with severe OSA: the PROOF study. J Clin Sleep Med. 2015;11(5):519–24.

71. Feng J, Wu Q, Zhang D, Chen BY. Hippocampal impairments are associated with intermittent hypoxia of obstructive sleep apnea. Chin Med J. 2012;125(4):696–701. PMID: 22490498.

72. Eriksson PS, Perfilieva E, Björk-Eriksson T, Alborn AM, Nordborg C, Peterson DA, Gage FH. Neurogenesis in the adult human hippocampus. Nat Med. 1998;4:1313–7.

73. Fotuhi M, Do D, Jack C. Modifiable factors that alter the size of the hippocampus with ageing. Nat Rev Neurol. 2012;8:189–202.

74. Aaronson JA, Hofman WF, van Bennekom CA, van Bezeij T, van den Aardweg JG, Groet E, Kylstra WA, Schmand B. Effects of continuous positive airway pressure on cognitive and functional outcome of stroke patients with obstructive sleep apnea: a randomized

controlled trial. J Clin Sleep Med. 2016;12(4):533–41. https://doi.org/10.5664/jcsm.5684. PMID: 26888587; PMCID: PMC4795280.

75. Kim H, Im S, Park JI, Kim Y, Sohn MK, Jee S. Improvement of cognitive function after continuous positive airway pressure treatment for subacute stroke patients with obstructive sleep apnea: a randomized controlled trial. Brain Sci. 2019;9(10):252. https://doi.org/10.3390/brainsci9100252. PMID: 31557935; PMCID: PMC6826775.

76. Brill AK, Horvath T, Seiler A, Camilo M, Haynes AG, Ott SR, Egger M, Bassetti CL. CPAP as treatment of sleep apnea after stroke: a meta-analysis of randomized trials. Neurology. 2018;90(14):e1222–30. https://doi.org/10.1212/WNL.0000000000005262. Epub 2018 Mar 9. PMID: 29523641.

77. Haba-Rubio J, Vujica J, Franc Y, Michel P, Heinzer R. Effect of CPAP treatment of sleep apnea on clinical prognosis after ischemic stroke: an observational study. J Clin Sleep Med. 2019;15(6):839–47. https://doi.org/10.5664/jcsm.7832. PMID: 31138378; PMCID: PMC6557650.

78. Richards KC, Gooneratne N, Dicicco B, Hanlon A, Moelter S, Onen FY, Sawyer A, Weaver T, Lozano A, Carter P, Johnson J. CPAP adherence may slow 1-year cognitive decline in older adults with mild cognitive impairment and apnea. J Am Geriatr Soc. 2019;67(3):558–64. https://doi.org/10.1111/jgs.15758. Epub 2019 Feb 6. PMID: 30724333; PMCID: PMC6402995.

79. Wang Y, Cheng C, Moelter S, Fuentecilla JL, Kincheloe K, Lozano AJ, Carter P, Gooneratne N, Richards KC. One year of continuous positive airway pressure adherence improves cognition in older adults with mild apnea and mild cognitive impairment. Nurs Res. 2020;69(2):157–64. https://doi.org/10.1097/NNR.0000000000000420. PMID: 32108738; PMCID: PMC7212768.

80. Lin CH, Lurie RC, Lyons OD. Sleep apnea and chronic kidney disease: a state-of-the-art review. Chest. 2020;157(3):673–85. https://doi.org/10.1016/j.chest.2019.09.004. Epub 2019 Sept 19. PMID: 31542452.

81. Drew DA, Weiner DE, Sarnak MJ. Cognitive impairment in CKD: pathophysiology, management, and prevention. Am J Kidney Dis. 2019;74(6):782–90. https://doi.org/10.1053/j.ajkd.2019.05.017. Epub 2019 Aug 1. PMID: 31378643; PMCID: PMC7038648.

82. Yaffe K, Ackerson L, Kurella Tamura M, Le Blanc P, Kusek JW, Sehgal AR, Cohen D, Anderson C, Appel L, Desalvo K, Ojo A, Seliger S, Robinson N, Makos G, Go AS, Chronic Renal Insufficiency Cohort Investigators. Chronic kidney disease and cognitive function in older adults: findings from the chronic renal insufficiency cohort cognitive study. J Am Geriatr Soc. 2010;58(2):338–45. https://doi.org/10.1111/j.1532-5415.2009.02670.x. Epub 2010 Jan 26. PMID: 20374407; PMCID: PMC2852884.

83. Sarnak MJ, Tighiouart H, Scott TM, Lou KV, Sorensen EP, Giang LM, Drew DA, Shaffi K, Strom JA, Singh AK, Weiner DE. Frequency of and risk factors for poor cognitive performance in hemodialysis patients. Neurology. 2013;80(5):471–80. https://doi.org/10.1212/WNL.0b013e31827f0f7f. Epub 2013 Jan 9. PMID: 23303848; PMCID: PMC3590049.

84. Park KS, Chang JH, Kang EW. Effects of 12 months of continuous positive airway pressure therapy on cognitive function, sleep, mood, and health-related quality of life in a peritoneal dialysis patient with obstructive sleep apnea. Kidney Res Clin Pract. 2018;37(1):89–93. https://doi.org/10.23876/j.krcp.2018.37.1.89. Epub 2018 Mar 31. PMID: 29629282; PMCID: PMC5875581.

85. Kerner NA, Roose SP. Obstructive sleep apnea is linked to depression and cognitive impairment: evidence and potential mechanisms. Am J Geriatr Psychiatry. 2016;24(6):496–508.

86. Harris M, Glozier N, Ratnavadivel R, Grunstein RR. Obstructive sleep apnea and depression [Internet]. Sleep Med Rev. 2009;13:437–44. Available from: https://doi.org/10.1016/j.smrv.2009.04.001

87. Labarca G, Saavedra D, Dreyse J, Jorquera J, Barbe F. Efficacy of CPAP for improvements in sleepiness, cognition, mood, and quality of life in elderly patients with OSA: systematic review and meta-analysis of randomized controlled trials. Chest. 2020;158(2):751–64. https://doi.org/10.1016/j.chest.2020.03.049. Epub 2020 Apr 11. PMID: 32289311.

88. Byrne P, Cullinan J, Gillespie P, Perera R, Smith SM. Statins for primary prevention of cardiovascular disease: modelling guidelines and patient preferences based on an Irish cohort. Br J Gen Pract. 2019;69(683):e373–80.

89. Rosenzweig I, Glasser M, Polsek D, Leschziner GD, Williams SCR, Morrell MJ. Sleep apnoea and the brain: a complex relationship [Internet]. Lancet Respir Med. 2015;3:404–14. Available from: https://doi.org/10.1016/s2213-2600(15)00090-9

90. Olaithe M, Bucks RS, Hillman DR, Eastwood PR. Cognitive deficits in obstructive sleep apnea: insights from a meta-review and comparison with deficits observed in COPD, insomnia, and sleep deprivation. Sleep Med Rev. 2018;38:39–49.

91. Neumannova K, Hobzova M, Sova M, Prasko J. Pulmonary rehabilitation and oropharyngeal exercises as an adjunct therapy in obstructive sleep apnea: a randomized controlled trial. Sleep Med. 2018;52:92–7.

92. Lorenzi-Filho G, Almeida FR, Strollo PJ. Treating OSA: current and emerging therapies beyond CPAP. Respirology. 2017;22(8):1500–7.

93. Chapman JL, Vakulin A, Hedner J, Yee BJ, Marshall NS. Modafinil/armodafinil in obstructive sleep apnoea: a systematic review and meta-analysis. Eur Respir J. 2016;47(5):1420–8.

94. Brownlow JA, Miller KE, Gehrman PR. Insomnia and cognitive performance [Internet]. Sleep Med Clin. 2020;15:71–6. Available from: https://doi.org/10.1016/j.jsmc.2019.10.002

95. Eckert DJ, White DP, Jordan AS, Malhotra A, Wellman A. Defining phenotypic causes of obstructive sleep apnea. Identification of novel therapeutic targets. Am J Respir Crit Care Med. 2013;188(8):996–1004.

Sleep Apnea and Cardiovascular Disease: The Role of CPAP and CPAP Adherence

Lee A. Surkin, Asmaa M. Abumuamar, and Kathryn Hansen

16.1 Introduction

Obstructive sleep apnea is a common sleep disorder with significant healthcare burden [1] and cardiovascular consequences [2]. Understanding the physiology of sleep, respiratory function, and autonomic control of nocturnal heart rate and rhythm is crucial for understanding the pathophysiological changes of OSA and their effect on the cardiovascular system.

During sleep, there is an increase in upper airway resistance, which is controlled by pharyngeal muscles, due to decreased tonic excitatory drive to upper airway muscles [3]. In individuals with structural narrowing of upper airways, these physiological changes may precipitate airflow limitation, hypoventilation, and obstructive apneas.

Obstructive sleep apnea is characterized by recurrent obstructive events which result in reduced airflow, hypoxemia, and hypercapnia. During obstruction, individuals maintain continuous, ineffective inspiratory effort resulting in arousal from sleep and sympathetic overstimulation. Respiration is regulated by central and peripheral chemoreceptors [4], which respond to hypoxemia, hypercapnia, systemic blood pressure changes, and acid-base imbalance [3].

In response to hypoxemia and hypercapnia, central chemoreceptors are activated and result in an increased rate and depth of breathing. This also stimulates sympathetic activity affecting the cardiovascular system, which increases blood pressure. It is known that the chemoreceptor reflex is impaired in OSA, resulting in parasympathetic stimulation of the heart causing bradycardia and coronary vasodilation and increases sympathetic outflow to the vascular system resulting in vasoconstriction. Consequently, the associated cerebral ischemia activates the central chemoreceptors leading to a concurrent activation of sympathetic and vagal nerves to the cardiovascular system. The net result is autonomic instability characterized by variability of heart rate, blood pressure, and vascular tone [5].

In addition, REM sleep is characterized by low-frequency variability of the heart rate which reflects the dominance of sympathetic stimulation during this stage. REM sleep is also characterized by a suppressed ventilatory response to hypoxia and hypercapnia and variable respiratory rate and muscle activity [3, 6]. Autonomic instability during sleep in patients with OSA creates a favorable milieu for the development of cardiac disorders.

16.2 OSA and Cardiovascular Complications: Association and Mechanism

The mechanism of cardiovascular disorders associated with OSA is complicated and not fully understood. The main pathophysiological changes of OSA include hypoxia and oxidative stress [7], intrathoracic pressure swings [8], autonomic instability [9], and inflammation. These changes induce electrical and structural remodeling of the cardiovascular (CV) system [8] resulting in an increased risk for resistant hypertension, arrhythmia, CAD, HF, stroke, post-cardiac surgery complications, and CV mortality [10, 11]. Therefore, screening and detection of OSA in patients with CV risk factors and/or patients with cardiovascular disorders is clinically important [12, 13].

Due to obstructive apneas, hypoxia induces reflex bradycardia and increases blood pressure [7]. The effects of hypoxia and hypercapnia include prolonged atrial refractory

L. A. Surkin (✉)
Empire Sleep Medicine, New York, NY, USA

CardioSleep Diagnostics, Greenville, NC, USA

American Academy of Cardiovascular Sleep Medicine, Greenville, NC, USA

A. M. Abumuamar
Department of Medicine, University of Toronto, Toronto, ON, Canada

K. Hansen
American Academy of Cardiovascular Sleep Medicine, Greenville, NC, USA

Society of Behavioral Sleep Medicine, Lexington, KY, USA

C. M. Shapiro et al. (eds.), *CPAP Adherence*, https://doi.org/10.1007/978-3-030-93146-9_16

periods, slow and delayed conduction, and increased heterogeneity of conduction. As an example, nocturnal hypoxemia is an independent risk factor for new-onset atrial fibrillation (AF) [13]. The resultant oxidative stress in OSA may also cause myocardial injury, ischemia, and abnormal excitability [14, 15].

The role of inflammation in OSA has emerged as a contributing factor of cardiovascular consequences. OSA is associated with higher levels of C-reactive protein (CRP), which is a marker of vascular inflammation [16]. CRP level has been identified as an independent risk factor for coronary artery disease and recurrent AF after electrical cardioversion [17]. Moreover, CRP is associated with a higher risk of thromboembolism in patients with AF [18].

16.3 OSA and CPAP

The most common treatment of OSA has historically been continuous positive airway pressure therapy (CPAP). Early data suggested that CPAP treatment decreased cardiovascular (CV) morbidity and mortality [19]. Studies showed that effective CPAP treatment may reverse the adverse physiological sequelae of OSA including oxidative stress [20], sympathetic hyperstimulation [21, 22], and CV remodeling [23].

Moreover, several studies showed the effects of CPAP on markers of sympathetic activity. Kohler et al. found that CPAP reduced the level of 24-hour urinary catecholamines [21]. Similar studies reported a reduction in urinary norepinephrine levels [24].

In addition to the potential role of CPAP in mitigating the pathophysiological sequelae of OSA, the clinical benefits of CPAP in patients with hypertension (HTN), cardiac arrhythmia, CAD, HF, and stroke have been investigated. A summary of evidence is presented in the following sections.

16.4 Hypertension

OSA has been detected in 50% of patients with HTN [25] and up to 83% of patients with resistant HTN [26]. The seventh report of the Joint National Committee on Prevention, Detection, Evaluation and Treatment of High Blood Pressure (JNC7) defined OSA as a secondary cause of HTN [27]. Increasing severity of OSA is associated with higher incidence of HTN [28].

The following case study represents the importance of a clinical assessment to evaluate the relationship between OSA and HTN.

Several studies have shown that CPAP treatment decreases blood pressure in patients with resistant HTN [29, 30]. Most of the clinical studies have shown a modest reduction of sys-

Box 16.1 Clinical Vignette: A Patient with HTN

A 42-year-old male presented to his primary care physician for an annual physical exam. He reported symptoms of daily frontal and temporal headaches that he attributed to a high-stress job. In general, he reported feeling tired in the afternoons requiring him to drink a couple of caffeinated beverages to make it through the day. He admitted to snoring as reported by his wife who sleeps in another room. The patient brought a log of his ambulatory blood pressure readings over the past 2 months which revealed a consistent elevated blood pressure in the 150–160/90–110 range.

His exam was remarkable for a blood pressure of 158/98, heart rate of 86, and a BMI of 31, and he had an S4 gallop on his cardiac exam with a normal fundoscopic and neurologic exam. He has been compliant with his antihypertensive regimen which included a thiazide diuretic, an ACE inhibitor, and a calcium channel blocker, all of which at maximal therapeutic dosing.

He was referred for a polysomnogram which revealed severe obstructive sleep apnea with an apnea hypopnea index of 38 and a nadir O2 saturation of 71%. He was started on an auto-titrating CPAP machine and was adherent and on optimal therapy based on objective data extracted from the machine.

A follow-up at 6 months into therapy revealed better control of his blood pressure with readings in the 135–145/85–90 range. Subjectively, the headaches, snoring, and afternoon tiredness had resolved.

tolic and diastolic blood pressure of 2–3 mmHg with the use of CPAP in patients with OSA [31]. These modest effects, however, significantly reduce CV and cerebrovascular risk and mortality [32].

For example, a randomized clinical trial (RCT) included 194 patients with resistant HTN and moderate-to-severe OSA. Patients were randomized to receive CPAP or no CPAP, in addition to optimal medical therapy. After 12 weeks, there was a greater reduction in 24-hour mean and diastolic blood pressure and improvement in nocturnal blood pressure pattern in CPAP-treated patients compared with untreated patients. Also, there was a significant positive correlation between hours of CPAP use and a decrease in 24-hour mean blood pressure (MBP) [33]. Another RCT showed similar results among patients with ambulatory blood pressure monitoring-confirmed resistant HTN who used CPAP more than 5.8 hours/night for 3 months [34].

A 2007 meta-analysis reviewed the effect of CPAP treatment on 24-hour ambulatory MBP in a total of 572 patients with OSA and HTN from 12 RCTs. The results indicated a total reduction of 1.60 mmHg. The findings also showed a greater reduction in ambulatory MBP in patients with more severe OSA and with increased adherence to nightly use of CPAP treatment [35].

In 2014, a patient-level meta-analysis included 968 individuals with OSA from 8 RCTs. CPAP treatment resulted in a 2.27 reduction in systolic blood pressure (SBP) and 1.78 reduction in diastolic blood pressure (DBP). After adjusting for the severity of OSA, age, BMI, BP medications, and adherence to CPAP therapy, patients with uncontrolled HTN had a substantial reduction of SBP by 7.1 mmHg and DBP by 4.3 mmHg [36]. Therefore, patients with uncontrolled HTN and OSA are likely to have greater benefits with use of CPAP.

In a 2017 metanalysis of six controlled trials, CPAP treatment resulted in a significant reduction in mean and diastolic blood pressure in patients with resistant hypertension and OSA [37]. Therefore, it is crucial to detect undiagnosed OSA in patients with resistant hypertension. CPAP therapy has proven benefits on blood pressure control in these patients.

16.5   Cardiac Arrhythmia

In patients with cardiac arrhythmia, most studies involve patients with atrial fibrillation (AF), which is the most common form of arrhythmia and is highly prevalent in patients with OSA [38]. Several studies showed that CPAP therapy decreases the recurrence and severity of AF [38–41]. The main duration of follow-up in these studies ranged between 4 weeks [41] and up to 24 months [40].

The following case study correlates the importance of a diagnostic testing to diagnose OSA for effective management of AF.

Box 16.2 Clinical Vignette: A Patient with AF

A 63-year-old female with a history of HTN, paroxysmal AF, and obesity presented to her cardiologist for a requested follow-up due to frequent palpitations associated with reduced exercise capacity. She has had a history of paroxysmal AF for less than 1 year which has been more symptomatic in the past month. She underwent a successful cardioversion 6 months prior to the current visit. Her ECG in the office revealed recurrent AF with a heart rate of 105. On ambulation, her pulse rapidly increased to 140 with symptoms.

On further questioning, she reported snoring and waking feeling unrefreshed with excessive daytime sleepiness.

The cardiologist increased her medical regimen for rate control and referred her for a formal sleep medicine consultation.

The patient underwent a home sleep apnea test which revealed moderate OSA with an (apnea hypopnea index) AHI of 22 and a nadir O2 saturation of 78%. She was started on an auto-titrating CPAP machine. At her 1 month follow-up with the sleep physician, her vital signs revealed a heart rate of 86 and irregular with an otherwise normal exam. Her prior sleep apnea symptoms had significantly improved, and she was adherent and on optimal therapy.

One month later, she was seen by her cardiologist and was still in AF with a controlled heart rate. Options of a repeat cardioversion or a referral for an ablation were discussed, and she opted for an electrophysiology referral and underwent a successful ablation. She has remained in sinus rhythm at subsequent follow-up visits and continues on PAP therapy.

A randomized controlled trial [42] included two groups of patients with OSA matched for age, BMI, the severity of OSA, and cardiovascular risk factors. After 4 weeks of follow-up, there was significantly better control of the average heart rate among the group treated with effective CPAP compared to those in the sub-therapeutic CPAP group [42]. The effects of CPAP on the burden of atrial fibrillation were linked to achieving better control of heart rate [39]. Since heart rate control is an important aspect in the management of AF, CPAP treatment has been shown to be beneficial.

Several observational studies have shown a significant reduction in the recurrence of AF [43], improved AF-free survival [44], and increased success rate of AF ablation procedures [45]. A meta-analysis of studies including patients undergoing surgical ablation of AF showed a higher AF recurrence among patients with untreated OSA compared to patients with CPAP-treated OSA. In addition, there was a similar efficacy of the procedure among CPAP-treated patients compared to patients without OSA [46].

Further, Abumuamar et al. found that CPAP treatment resulted in a significant reduction in atrial and ventricular ectopy count/24 hours in patients with AF and OSA at 3 and 6 months of CPAP treatment compared to baseline [13, 47]. The reduction of average atrial ectopy count in patients with paroxysmal AF may decrease occurrence and/or recurrence of AF.

The effects of CPAP therapy on other cardiac arrhythmias have been also investigated. Observational studies showed that CPAP treatment decreased the recurrence of nocturnal bradycardia, sinus pauses, and heart block [48]. However, a randomized controlled trial did not show a significant decrease of bradyarrhythmia, but there was a positive trend toward the reduction of nocturnal sinus bradycardias/pauses among patients treated with CPAP [42].

In patients with OSA and CHF, a RCT showed a significant reduction in the frequency of nocturnal ventricular premature beats (VPBs) among CPAP-treated patients [11]. Furthermore, CPAP treatment reversed ventricular repolarization measures, which may decrease the risk of ventricular arrhythmia [49]. Withdrawal of CPAP treatment was found to prolong cardiac repolarization measures, which increase the risk of ventricular arrhythmias [50]. Craig et al. showed that CPAP treatment was associated with a positive trend toward a reduction of daytime ventricular tachycardia [42].

The number of RCTs in patients with OSA and cardiac arrhythmia is still limited. CPAP treatment's ability to reverse cardiac remodeling induced by OSA and the degree of CPAP's impact on hypertension and arrhythmia may be affected by several factors. These factors include the severity and duration of OSA, baseline cardiovascular structure and function, treatment and optimization of comorbid conditions, and adherence to and duration of CPAP treatment. These factors in addition to the heterogeneity of data as well as the lack of well-designed trials have resulted in inconsistent results. However, the evidence points toward positive effects of CPAP treatment on cardiovascular structure and function [10]. Longer duration and more severe OSA may result in irreversible cardiac remodeling; therefore, early detection and treatment of OSA are imperative especially when considering cardiac arrhythmias.

16.6 Coronary Artery Disease

The strong association between OSA and CAD has been widely accepted for many decades. A study by Hung in 1990 studied 101 male survivors of myocardial infarction (MI) compared to 53 males without known heart disease, performed sleep testing and adjusted the data for age, BMI, HTN, smoking, and cholesterol, and determined that the relative risk for MI was 23.3 in the OSA population. The next closest was smoking with an odds ratio of 11.1 [51].

Box 16.3 Clinical Vignette: A Patient with CAD

A 64-year-old male with a past medical history significant for hypertension, hypercholesterolemia, and obesity was in his usual state of health when he awakened at 4 AM with substernal chest pain, shortness of breath, and diaphoresis. 911 was called, and the patient was having an acute myocardial infarction. He was taken directly to the Cath Lab for primary intervention and underwent successful percutaneous coronary intervention with a drug-eluting stent to the mid LAD. He had preserved left ventricular function.

While recovering in the hospital, witnessed apneas were noted associated with significant desaturations. Prior to discharge he underwent a polysomnogram which revealed moderate obstructive sleep apnea with an apnea-hypopnea index of 22 and a nadir oxygen saturation of 74%. An auto-titrating CPAP machine was ordered.

The following case study underscores the importance of a clinical assessment to evaluate the relationship between OSA and CAD.

Kasai reported on the marked stress imposed on both ventricles and pulmonary arteries due to airway obstruction yielding even more compelling pathophysiologic evidence to the strong association [52]. He also described the CV autonomic effects of OSA concluding that there were direct effects from hypoxia, hypercarbia, arousals, transient hypotension, and transient decrease in stroke volume that all lead to increases in sympathetic nerve activity ultimately increasing the risk of CV-related mortality [52].

To correlate this on a more cellular level, as stated earlier, there is evidence showing that individuals with OSA have significantly increased markers of inflammation based on elevated CRP levels that have been directly implicated in coronary artery disease risk [53]. As inflammation takes hold in the arterial wall, plaque forms and the cascade of CAD is established. Research on factors that increase the risk of plaque rupture and subsequent acute MI identifies certain plaques as being "vulnerable" to rupture and infarction. In a study, coronary CT scans, which can identify vulnerable plaques, were obtained on patients presenting with atypical chest pain or prior equivocal physiological testing for CAD. The subjects then underwent sleep testing. The results indicated that 55% of patients with OSA had vulnerable plaques compared to 28% of non-OSA patients [54].

A seminal study investigated timing of MI in patients with and without OSA. The study prospectively followed 92 patients with MI and identified the time of chest pain onset. The group with OSA experienced a MI between midnight and 6 am compared to those without OSA. There was a six times greater likelihood for the event between midnight and 6 am than during the rest of the 24-hour period. In addition, 91% of the patients who experienced a MI had OSA [55].

The early data presented very compelling claims of a strong association between OSA and CAD. What remained unanswered during this period was whether there is a favorable impact of treatment with CPAP.

Evidence also demonstrated that major adverse cardiac events (MACE) defined as death, acute coronary syndrome, CHF, hospitalization, or the need for revascularization was significantly reduced in moderate or severe OSA patients treated with CPAP or ENT surgery. Specifically, OSA treated patients had a 33% reduced risk of MACE compared to untreated patients [56].

In the early 1990s, a group of researchers collaborated on the launch of the Sleep Heart Health Study (SHHS), a multicenter prospective study of CV outcomes associated with OSA, enrolling 4422 people, 1927 males and 2495 females, who were studied for approximately 9 years. The findings demonstrated a significant association between CV events with AHI in male subjects, but not in the female subjects controlling for age, race, prior MI, and smoking. The association in male participants, however, was not significant when controlling for diabetes. In male participants less than or equal to 70 years of age, the association with the AHI was stronger. When combining males and females in a single model adjusting for all covariates, the interaction between sex and AHI was of borderline significance. Of additional interest was that all-cause mortality was greater as OSA worsened with the greatest effect in men less than 70 years of age [57].

An observational study by Marin of 1651 patients followed for 10 years compared healthy male controls with those with untreated mild-to-moderate OSA, untreated severe OSA, and CPAP-treated OSA. The study showed that severe OSA was associated with significantly increased risk of fatal and non-fatal CV events and was reduced with CPAP use [58].

The findings were confirmed by another observational cohort study by Campos-Rodriguez on 1116 females. In the study, control subjects with an AHI of less than 10 events/hour were compared to subjects who had mild-to-moderate and severe OSA. It documented the impact of CPAP adherence at greater than or equal to 4 hours/day, as well as non-adherence for an 11-year follow-up. The study revealed that, compared to the control group, the adjusted hazard ratios for CV mortality were 3.54 for untreated severe OSA, 0.55 for treated severe OSA, 1.6 for untreated mild-to-moderate OSA, and 0.19 for treated mild-to-moderate OSA [59].

Therefore, a number of observational studies conducted over variable periods suggested the possibility that treating moderate-to-severe OSA may result in a beneficial long-term effect with regard to CAD. More definitive data through randomized control trials was required to confirm the findings of the observational studies.

A randomized controlled trial looked at the effects of CPAP on HTN and CV events and non-sleepy patients with OSA. 725 consecutive patients were studied with an AHI of greater than or equal to 20 and an Epworth sleepiness scale of less than or equal to 10 with no prior cardiac history. After a 3-to-5-year follow-up, the study concluded that there was no difference in new HTN or CV events in non-sleepy moderate-to-severe OSA patients. Of significant interest was that a post hoc analysis revealed that in CPAP-adherent subjects (>4 hours/day), the primary outcome odds ratio was 0.72. In CPAP-non-adherent subjects (<4 hours/day), the primary outcome odds ratio was 1.13. The analysis also reviewed the effect of CPAP adherence coupled with the impact of time spent with abnormal oxygen saturation controlling for AHI and divided the groups based on a >6.8% time with an oxygen saturation <90%. This analysis revealed that adherent use of CPAP had improved cardiac outcomes with an odds ratio of 0.71 compared to the non-adherent group with an odds ratio of 1.89 [60].

The largest randomized controlled trial to date called Sleep Apnea Cardiovascular Endpoints Trial (SAVE) enrolled 2717 non-sleepy adults aged 45–75 with moderate-to-severe OSA and CAD or CV disease with a mean follow-up of 3.7 years. The study compared CPAP plus usual care versus usual care alone with primary endpoints of CV death, MI, stroke, hospitalization for unstable angina, heart failure, or TIA. Secondary endpoints investigated were other CV outcomes, quality of life, snoring symptoms, daytime sleepiness, and mood. The average duration of CPAP use was 3.3 hours/day. The average AHI declined from 29 to 3.7 in treated patients. The study revealed that the hazard ratio on CPAP was equal to 1.10 compared to usual care demonstrating no significant effect on any individual or composite endpoint. The conclusion was that CPAP in addition to usual care was not superior to usual care alone for secondary prevention of CV events in patients with established CAD and CV disease and moderate-to-severe OSA. CPAP use decreased snoring and daytime sleepiness and improved quality of life and mood. On an adjusted propensity analysis, it appeared that there may be a benefit in patients using at least 4 hours of CPAP every night on average [61].

Another RCT titled Randomized Intervention with CPAP and Coronary Artery Disease and Sleep Apnea (RICCADSA) studied 244 individuals with a history of CAD and/or CV disease with a history of revascularization within the prior 6 months and compared participants without sleep apnea to those with moderate-to-severe, non-sleepy sleep apnea treated with CPAP. The median follow-up was 57 months. The endpoints were repeat revascularization, MI, stroke, and CV mortality. There were 49 patients who reached the endpoint. Of those, 22 were in the CPAP arm, and 27 were in the untreated arm revealing no statistical significance. Data in the group who used CPAP with a 3-hour cutoff revealed no significant difference, but a significant difference was discovered in the group who used CPAP greater than 4 hours (6 events) versus no CPAP (43 events). Adjusting for variables, the incidence of the composite endpoint was 2.31 per 100 patient years for CPAP use greater than 4 hours and 5.32 per 100 patient years for CPAP use less than 4 hours or no usage.

The conclusion in this group was that there was a significant reduction in endpoints after adjustment for baseline comorbidities and adherence with CPAP [62].

In summary, the association between OSA and CV disease is widely accepted. Early observational studies revealed mixed results regarding the effect of CPAP treatment as a long-term benefit for cardiovascular disease. Randomized controlled trials have failed to demonstrate treatment efficacy.

A recent review proposed alterations in the design of future randomized controlled trials to more accurately and reliably assess if CPAP provides a statistically significant benefit in mitigating coronary artery disease [63]. The review suggests that future study designs should enroll patients from sleep clinics since they reflect a real-world representation of the sleep apnea patient, namely, those who manifest excessive daytime sleepiness. This population would be anticipated to experience subjective benefit from CPAP therapy and therefore improved adherence. He also proposed that those with severe sleepiness may need to be excluded due to randomization concerns. In addition, it was suggested that the focus should be on those individuals with more severe OSA at least initially based on population studies that have shown a higher degree of CV mortality as well as those patients with a greater degree of hypoxia. The final suggestion raised was to include patients who are younger to allow for long-term follow-up data.

The next generations of clinical trials are being planned or are underway. Given the clear associations between OSA and CAD, it is anticipated that results of these future trials will reveal efficacious treatments which will then lead clinicians to screen patients for OSA to the same degree as other established CV risk factors such as HTN, hyperlipidemia, and diabetes.

16.7 Heart Failure

CHF is one of the most common diagnoses resulting in hospital admission in the USA and is more prevalent in the geriatric population. Data from the Atherosclerosis Risk in Communities study have shown that approximately 915,000 new cases of HF occur each year in the USA [64]. Healthcare costs are greater than $30 billion per year and are anticipated to exceed $70 billion by 2030 [65].

The association between HF and both central sleep apnea (CSA) and OSA is well documented and accepted. One of the first studies to utilize formal in-lab sleep testing was conducted by Javaheri et al. and prospectively studied 81 male patients with left ventricular ejection fraction (LVEF) less than 45% and HF. The results indicated that 51% of the patients with stable heart failure had evidence of sleep-related breathing disorders: 40% had CSA and 11% had OSA [66].

A common breathing abnormality in HF characterized by periods of central apneas followed by a crescendo-decrescendo breathing pattern is usually referred to as Cheyne-Stokes breathing or Cheyne-Stokes respiration. It was initially described by John Hunter in 1781 followed by John Cheyne in 1818 and then William Stokes in 1854. The historically accurate name should be Hunter-Cheyne-Stokes breathing.

HF is further described based on the status of the LVEF. HF with preserved ejection fraction (HFpEF) has a normal ejection fraction, which, by convention, is greater than or equal to 50%. HF with reduced ejection fraction (HFrEF) is associated with an ejection fraction of less than 50%. This is significant because sleep apnea is associated with both forms of HF (HFpEF and HFrEF), and the presentation and treatment can vary. An intriguing and not entirely clear fact is that HF patients typically do not experience the excessive daytime sleepiness that is commonly associated with sleep apnea. This is thought to be secondary to enhanced sympathetic tone [67].

The following case study correlates the association between sleep apnea, CPAP, and HF.

The aforementioned Sleep Heart Health Study revealed a 2.38 times increased risk in the likelihood of having HF in individuals with OSA. This was independent of other known risk factors [67]. Bradley et al. concluded in a two-part review that OSA may play a role in the cause and progression of HF and called for more research [68]. Another review concluded that those with HF and moderate-to-severe

---

Box 16.4 Clinical Vignette: A Patient with OSA and Decompensated Congestive Heart Failure

A 69-year-old female was admitted to the cardiac intensive care unit with decompensated congestive heart failure (CHF). She noted progressive weight gain, lower extremity edema, orthopnea, frequent nocturia, and paroxysmal nocturnal dyspnea for 2 weeks prior to admission. She denied any known history of sleep disordered breathing or associated symptoms such as snoring, awakening feeling unrefreshed, excessive daytime sleepiness, or witnessed apneas.

Her hospital course was remarkable for symptomatic improvement with diuresis. There were witnessed apneas both in the ICU and stepdown units associated with desaturations. In-hospital cardiac testing revealed a LVEF of 34%, no evidence of CAD, and no significant coronary artery disease.

Approximately 2 weeks after discharge, the patient underwent a polysomnography, which revealed moderate CSA with Hunter-Cheyne-Stokes breathing. She was referred for a sleep medicine consultation to discuss treatment options.

The patient underwent a CPAP titration study which revealed that both OSA and CSA were effectively eliminated with the use of bilevel PAP at a setting of 15/11 cm H$_2$O. The patient was started on therapy and remained clinically stable from a CHF standpoint. She underwent a repeat assessment of her left ventricular function by echocardiography 6 months later which revealed an improvement in her LVEF from 34% to 48%.

untreated OSA had a higher mortality [69]. In general, the prevalence of sleep apnea in HF ranges from 50% to 70% with approximately two-thirds being CSA.

Several randomized controlled studies evaluated different types of positive airway pressure modalities in treating CSA in the HFrEF patient populations. The CANPAP study (Canadian Continuous Positive Airway Pressure for Patients with Central Sleep Apnea and Heart Failure) randomized 258 patients to receive either standard therapy for HF or standard therapy for HF with CPAP. This study showed that CPAP decreased central apneic events, improved overnight oxygen levels, increased the LVEF, and increased the distance walked in 6 minutes, yet did not improve mortality [70]. Of interest is that a post hoc analysis showed a mortality benefit in those patients who had more effective suppression of apneic events (AHI < 15) [71, 72].

Technological advancements in the treatment of sleep disordered breathing have resulted in a modality called adaptive servo-ventilation (ASV). This is a noninvasive ventilator that detects variations in airflow in patients with obstructive, central, and Hunter-Cheyne-Stokes breathing and normalizes it through a complex algorithm.

In 2015, a seminal trial titled Treatment of Sleep Disordered Breathing with Predominant Central Sleep Apnea by Adaptive Servo Ventilation in Patients with Heart Failure or SERVE-HF was stopped prematurely due to an increase in mortality. This study randomized 1300 patients with chronic HF and a LVEF of less than or equal to 45%. Subjects had New York Heart Association Class III or IV heart failure or Class II heart failure with greater than one hospitalization for HF in the previous 24 months. Enrolled patients had predominantly CSA defined as an AHI of greater than or equal to 15 with greater than or equal to 50% central events and a central index of greater than 10/hour. Subjects were randomized to usual care or ASV treatment.

As noted, the study was stopped prematurely when it was discovered that all-cause and CV mortality were significantly higher in the ASV group compared to control with a hazard ratio for death from any cause of 1.28 and 1.34 for CV death. There was no statistically significant difference between patients randomized to ASV therapy and those in the control group in the primary endpoint of time to all-cause mortality or unplanned hospitalization for worsening HF. The results revealed an increase in CV mortality by 2.5% in the treated group of patients with symptomatic CHF (10% versus 7.5%) [73].

As a result of this trial, it was recommended that physicians stop prescribing ASV for patients with a LVEF of less than or equal to 45% HF symptoms and CSA. It was also recommended that a cardiac assessment for HF and LVEF is obtained prior to prescribing ASV, and all patients previously treated were advised to follow up with their prescribing provider.

Many experts have questioned the results of SERVE-HF based on the study design and the actual ASV algorithm used, which may have led to possible reduced cardiac output secondary to higher PAP pressures and hyperventilation [74].

An ongoing study called Effect of Adaptive Servo Ventilation on Survival and Hospital Admissions in Heart Failure or ADVENT-HF is studying HF in patients with CSA or non-sleepy OSA treated with ASV. This study is ongoing as of the time of this publication and has not been halted prematurely.

An innovative technology to treat CSA is phrenic nerve pacing, which has been shown to effectively suppress central apnea and has been studied in a multicenter trial in the USA and Europe in male patients with CSA in which two-thirds had HF. The study revealed that there was at least a 50% reduction in the AHI [75]. Data from a subsequent randomized controlled trial revealed an 81% reduction in the central apnea index, a 44% reduction in the oxygen desaturation index, and a 44% reduction in the mean arousal index with an associated 17% increase in REM sleep [76]. This treatment is now approved for moderate-to-severe CSA.

Research into effective treatments is now focusing on several different phenotypes of OSA including increased loop gain and chemosensitivity, reduced pharyngeal dilator muscle tone, anatomically narrow airway, and low respiratory arousal threshold. There are different targeted treatments under evaluation which will hopefully provide more specific and efficacious treatment options in the future.

16.8 Stroke

Sleep-disordered breathing (SDB) is an established risk factor after a stroke and if left untreated is associated with a poor prognosis secondary to a worsening of the neurological state. This is assumed to be exacerbated by apnea-induced hypercapnia and cerebral vasodilatation in the area of the ischemia [77].

The estimated prevalence of OSA after stroke or TIA is over 70% [78]. The reasons for these increased rates are not clear, yet may be partly related to positional sleep apnea, stroke-related upper airway tone changes, or untreated OSA preceding the stroke. Multiple studies suggest that OSA is more often a preexisting condition before a stroke rather than the consequence of brain injury. The findings from a prospective study of sleep apnea evaluations both before and after a stroke and TIA show a similar frequency of OSA, suggesting it is a common predisposing condition [79].

The feasibility for use of CPAP as a treatment with acute stroke may be beneficial; however, studies on the efficacy of CPAP therapy after stroke are limited.

One randomized open-label, parallel-group feasibility study to evaluate the efficacy of CPAP treatment following the ischemic event assigned 50 patients to receive intervention with standard stroke care or assigned to a control group plus standard care [77]. The patients in the treatment group received noninvasive auto-adjusting positive airway pressure (APAP) for three nights starting the first night post stroke. Both groups of patients were studied in a sleep lab the fourth night post stroke. Patients receiving APAP with an AHI greater than 10/hour remained on therapy plus standard care.

The endpoint of feasibility was defined as a reduction in AHI with APAP within the first three nights and used for greater than 4 hours/night. Compared to the control group, the patients receiving therapy experienced a significant reduction of AHI when compared to the AHI on night four. Additionally, all patients were assessed using the National Institutes of Health Stroke Scale (NIHSS) scores, and improvement was recorded on day 8 post stroke in the group receiving therapy when compared to the control group [64].

These findings confirm that CPAP therapy contributed to reduction in AHI and might improve the clinical outcome after stroke. Yet, there is limited research data available about the impact of OSA and recurrent stroke, especially adjusting for diverse populations, larger samples, age, or population-based data.

The role of sleep disorders in stroke outcome and recurrence has become a challenging question. Despite studies that estimate a greater than 70% prevalence of sleep disorders after stroke, only about 6% of stroke survivors are offered formal sleep testing, and an estimated 2% complete such testing in the 3-month post-stroke period [65]. The reasons for the low rate of screening are at least partly related to the lack of awareness about sleep disorders among stroke patients [79].

16.9 Conclusion

The prevalence of obstructive sleep apnea is increasing worldwide and represents an epidemic healthcare crisis. There are clear associations with cardiovascular disorders such as hypertension, coronary artery disease, heart failure, arrhythmia, and stroke. Yet, despite the clear associations between obstructive sleep apnea and cardiovascular disease, randomized controlled trials to date have not demonstrated a statistically significant reduction in major adverse cardiac events in those individuals with cardiovascular disease.

Evidence supports CPAP therapy-related improvement in individuals with obstructive sleep apnea and hypertension. In addition, the research presented supports screening and CPAP therapy in patients with cardiac arrhythmias, the most common of which is atrial fibrillation.

While CPAP is the most common and long-standing treatment option for obstructive sleep apnea, it is not the only treatment. There are multiple other treatment options including oral appliance therapy, ENT head and neck surgery, maxillomandibular advancement surgery, medical and surgical weight loss techniques, hypoglossal nerve stimulation, phrenic nerve pacing for central sleep apnea, and even supplemental nocturnal oxygen in appropriate patients. There are also other new and innovative treatments being actively researched.

Despite the lack of data that would support improved cardiovascular outcomes as a result of treating sleep apnea with CPAP, the high prevalence of both disorders and clear associations highlight the importance of routine screening for obstructive sleep apnea in patients with established cardiovascular disease.

The importance of designing more sophisticated randomized controlled trials is paramount so that standard practice guidelines can be enhanced and refined. We are entering a new paradigm of clinical research involving phenotyping given the variable pathogenesis of obstructive sleep apnea. This involves an individualized or personal approach to therapy based on a clear understanding of the mechanism of the underlying disease. This may also involve combination therapy for more complicated cases.

An interdisciplinary and collaborative approach is critical for the future since approximately 80–85% of individuals with sleep apnea remain undiagnosed. As our population ages with an increasing prevalence of obesity, both obstructive sleep apnea and cardiovascular disease will continue to be at the forefront of morbidity and mortality.

Sleep disorders need to be a focus of individualized screening by primary care providers, physician extenders, specialists, and other healthcare providers including dentists. This collaboration will result in enhanced diagnostic capability which, along with more sophisticated clinical research guiding efficacious treatments, will enable patients with sleep apnea and cardiovascular disease enjoy improved quality of life and extended life expectancy.

References

1. Virani SS, Alonso A, Benjamin EJ, Bittencourt MS, Callaway CW, Carson AP, et al. Heart disease and stroke statistics – 2020 update: a report from the American Heart Association. Circulation. 2020;141:e139–596.
2. Floras JS. Sleep apnea and cardiovascular disease. Circulation Research 2018;122(12):1741–64. https://doi.org/10.1161/CIRCRESAHA.118.310783.
3. Horner RL. Chapter 21: Respiratory physiology: central neural control of respiratory neurons and motoneurons during sleep. In: Kryger MH, Roth T, Dement WC, editors. Principles and practice of sleep medicine [Internet]. 5th ed. Philadelphia: W.B. Saunders; 2011. p. 237–49. Available from: http://www.sciencedirect.com/science/article/pii/B9781416066453000219.
4. Duffin J. Functional organization of respiratory neurones: a brief review of current questions and speculations. Exp Physiol. 2004;89(5):517–29.
5. Snyder F, Hobson JA, Morrison DF, Goldfrank F. Changes in respiration, heart rate, and systolic blood pressure in human sleep. J Appl Physiol. 1964;19:417–22.
6. Horner RL. Neuromodulation of hypoglossal motoneurons during sleep. Respir Physiol Neurobiol. 2008;164(1–2):179–96.
7. McNicholas WT, Bonsigore MR, Bonsignore MR, Management Committee of EU COST ACTION B26. Sleep apnoea as an independent risk factor for cardiovascular disease: current evidence, basic mechanisms and research priorities. Eur Respir J. 2007;29(1):156–78.
8. Chan KH, Wilcox I. Obstructive sleep apnea: novel trigger and potential therapeutic target for cardiac arrhythmias. Expert Rev Cardiovasc Ther. 2010;8(7):981–94.
9. Vanninen E, Tuunainen A, Kansanen M, et al. Cardiac sympathovagal balance during sleep apnea episodes. Clin Physiol Oxf Engl. 1996;16(3):209–16.
10. Asmaa M, Abumuamar Tatyana, Mollayeva Paul, Sandor David, Newman Kumaraswamy, Nanthakumar Colin M, Shapiro (2017) Efficacy of Continuous Positive Airway Pressure Treatment in Patients with Cardiac Arrhythmia and Obstructive Sleep Apnea: What is the Evidence?. Clinical Medicine Insights: Therapeutics 91179559X1773422-10.1177/1179559X17734227.
11. Ryan CM. Effect of continuous positive airway pressure on ventricular ectopy in heart failure patients with obstructive sleep apnoea. Thorax 2005;60(9):781–85. https://doi.org/10.1136/thx.2005.040972.
12. Abumuamar AM, Sandor P, Dorian P, Newman D, Shapiro C. Obstructive sleep apnea is highly undetected in non-obese patients with atrial fibrillation. Sleep Med. 2017;40:e4.
13. Abumuamar AM, Newman D, Dorian P, Shapiro CM. Cardiac effects of CPAP treatment in patients with obstructive sleep apnea and atrial fibrillation. J Interv Card Electrophysiol. 2019;54(3):289–97.
14. Peng Y, Yuan G, Overholt JL, Kumar GK, Prabhakar NR. Systemic and cellular responses to intermittent hypoxia: evidence for oxidative stress and mitochondrial dysfunction. Adv Exp Med Biol. 2003;536:559–64.
15. Jeong E-M, Liu M, Sturdy M, Gao G, Varghese ST, Sovari AA, et al. Metabolic stress, reactive oxygen species, and arrhythmia. J Mol Cell Cardiol. 2012;52(2):454–63.
16. Li K, Wei P, Qin Y, Wei Y. Is C-reactive protein a marker of obstructive sleep apnea?: a meta-analysis. Medicine (Baltimore). 2017;96(19):e6850.
17. Schotten U, Verheule S, Kirchhof P, Goette A. Pathophysiological mechanisms of atrial fibrillation: a translational appraisal. Physiol Rev. 2011;91(1):265–325.
18. Chang S-N, Lai L-P, Chiang F-T, Lin J-L, Hwang J-J, Tsai C-T. The C-reactive protein gene polymorphism predicts the risk of thrombo-embolic stroke in atrial fibrillation: a more than 10-year prospective follow-up study. J Thromb Haemost. 2017;15(8):1541–6.
19. Marin JM, Carrizo SJ, Vicente E, Agusti AGN. Long-term cardiovascular outcomes in men with obstructive sleep apnoea-hypopnoea with or without treatment with continuous positive airway pressure: an observational study. Lancet. 2005;365(9464):1046–53.
20. Alonso-Fernández A, García-Río F, Arias MA, Hernanz A, de la Peña M, Piérola J, et al. Effects of CPAP on oxidative stress and nitrate efficiency in sleep apnoea: a randomised trial. Thorax. 2009;64(7):581–6.
21. Kohler M, Pepperell JCT, Casadei B, Craig S, Crosthwaite N, Stradling JR, et al. CPAP and measures of cardiovascular risk in males with OSAS. Eur Respir J. 2008;32(6):1488–96.
22. Kohler M, Stoewhas A-C, Ayers L, Senn O, Bloch KE, Russi EW, et al. Effects of continuous positive airway pressure therapy withdrawal in patients with obstructive sleep apnea: a randomized controlled trial. Am J Respir Crit Care Med. 2011;184(10):1192–9.
23. Baranchuk A, Pang H, Seaborn GEJ, Yazdan-Ashoori P, Redfearn DP, Simpson CS, et al. Reverse atrial electrical remodelling induced by continuous positive airway pressure in patients with severe obstructive sleep apnoea. J Interv Card Electrophysiol. 2013;36(3):247–53.
24. Phillips CL, Yee BJ, Marshall NS, Liu PY, Sullivan DR, Grunstein RR. Continuous positive airway pressure reduces postprandial lipidemia in obstructive sleep apnea: a randomized, placebo-controlled crossover trial. Am J Respir Crit Care Med. 2011;184(3):355–61.
25. Masood, Ahmad Devan, Makati Sana, Akbar (2017) Review of and Updates on Hypertension in Obstructive Sleep Apnea. International Journal of Hypertension 2017;1–13. https://doi.org/10.1155/2017/1848375.
26. Alexander G., Logan Sandra M., Perlikowski Andrew, Mente Andras, Tisler Ruzena, Tkacova Mitra, Niroumand Richard S. T., Leung T. Douglas, Bradley High prevalence of unrecognized sleep apnoea in drug-resistant hypertension. Journal of Hypertension 2001;19(12):2271–77. https://doi.org/10.1097/00004872-200112000-00022.
27. Aram V, Chobanian George L, Bakris Henry R, Black William C, Cushman Lee A, Green Joseph L, Izzo Daniel W, Jones Barry J, Materson Suzanne, Oparil Jackson T., Wright Edward J., Roccella. Seventh Report of the Joint National Committee on Prevention Detection Evaluation and Treatment of High Blood Pressure. Hypertension 2003;42(6):1206–52. https://doi.org/10.1161/01.HYP.0000107251.49515.c2.
28. Khin Mae, Hla Terry, Young Laurel, Finn Paul E., Peppard Mariana, Szklo-Coxe Maryan, Stubbs. Longitudinal Association of Sleep-Disordered Breathing and Nondipping of Nocturnal Blood Pressure in the Wisconsin Sleep Cohort Study. Sleep 2008;31(6):795–800 https://doi.org/10.1093/sleep/31.6.795.
29. Liu L, Cao Q, Guo Z, Dai Q. Continuous positive airway pressure in patients with obstructive sleep apnea and resistant hypertension: a meta-analysis of randomized controlled trials. J Clin Hypertens (Greenwich). 2016;18(2):153–8.
30. Dhillon S, Chung SA, Fargher T, Huterer N, Shapiro CM. Sleep apnea, hypertension, and the effects of continuous positive airway pressure. Am J Hypertens. 2005;18(5 Pt 1):594–600.
31. Sydney B, Montesi Bradley A, Edwards Atul, Malhotra Jessie P, Bakker. The Effect of Continuous Positive Airway Pressure Treatment on Blood Pressure: A Systematic Review and Meta-Analysis of Randomized Controlled Trials. Journal of Clinical Sleep Medicine 2012;08(05):587–96 https://doi.org/10.5664/jcsm.2170.
32. Joaquín, Durán-Cantolla Felipe, Aizpuru Cristina, Martínez-Null Ferrán, Barbé-Illa. Obstructive sleep apnea/hypopnea and systemic hypertension. Sleep Medicine Reviews 2009;13(5):323–31 10.1016/j.smrv.2008.11.001.

33. Martínez-García M-A, Capote F, Campos-Rodríguez F, Lloberes P, Díaz de Atauri MJ, Somoza M, et al. Effect of CPAP on blood pressure in patients with obstructive sleep apnea and resistant hypertension: the HIPARCO randomized clinical trial. JAMA. 2013;310(22):2407–15.

34. Lozano L, Tovar JL, Sampol G, Romero O, Jurado MJ, Segarra A, et al. Continuous positive airway pressure treatment in sleep apnea patients with resistant hypertension: a randomized, controlled trial. J Hypertens. 2010;28(10):2161–8.

35. Haentjens P. The Impact of Continuous Positive Airway Pressure on Blood Pressure in Patients With Obstructive Sleep Apnea Syndrome. Archives of Internal Medicine 2007;167(8):757-10.1001/archinte.167.8.757.

36. Jessie P, Bakker Bradley A, Edwards Shiva P, Gautam Sydney B, Montesi Joaquín, Durán-Cantolla Felipe Aizpuru, Barandiarán Ferran, Barbé Manuel, Sánchez-de-la-Torre Atul, Malhotra. Blood Pressure Improvement with Continuous Positive Airway Pressure is Independent of Obstructive Sleep Apnea Severity. Journal of Clinical Sleep Medicine 2014;10(04):365–69 https://doi.org/10.5664/jcsm.3604.

37. Lei Q, Lv Y, Li K, Ma L, Du G, Xiang Y, et al. Effects of continuous positive airway pressure on blood pressure in patients with resistant hypertension and obstructive sleep apnea: a systematic review and meta-analysis of six randomized controlled trials. J Bras Pneumol. 2017;43(5):373–9.

38. Abumuamar AM, Dorian P, Newman D, Shapiro CM. The prevalence of obstructive sleep apnea in patients with atrial fibrillation. Clin Cardiol. 2018;41(5):601–7.

39. Dediu GN, Dumitrache-Rujinski S, Lungu R, Frunză S, Diaconu C, Bartoş D, et al. Positive pressure therapy in patients with cardiac arrhythmias and obstructive sleep apnea. Pneumologia. 2015;64(1):18–22.

40. Holmqvist F, Guan N, Zhu Z, Kowey PR, Allen LA, Fonarow GC, et al. Impact of obstructive sleep apnea and continuous positive airway pressure therapy on outcomes in patients with atrial fibrillation-results from the Outcomes Registry for Better Informed Treatment of Atrial Fibrillation (ORBIT-AF). Am Heart J. 2015;169(5):647–654.e2.

41. Abe H, Takahashi M, Yaegashi H, Eda S, Tsunemoto H, Kamikozawa M, et al. Efficacy of continuous positive airway pressure on arrhythmias in obstructive sleep apnea patients. Heart Vessel. 2010;25(1):63–9.

42. Craig S, Pepperell JCT, Kohler M, Crosthwaite N, Davies RJO, Stradling JR. Continuous positive airway pressure treatment for obstructive sleep apnoea reduces resting heart rate but does not affect dysrhythmias: a randomised controlled trial. Journal of Sleep Research 2009;18(3):329–36. https://doi.org/10.1111/j.1365-2869.2008.00726.x.

43. Naruse Y, Tada H, Satoh M, Yanagihara M, Tsuneoka H, Hirata Y, Ito Y, Kuroki K, Machino T, Yamasaki H, Igarashi M, Sekiguchi Y, Sato A, Aonuma K. Concomitant obstructive sleep apnea increases the recurrence of atrial fibrillation following radiofrequency catheter ablation of atrial fibrillation: Clinical impact of continuous positive airway pressure therapy. Heart Rhythm 2013;10(3):331–37. https://doi.org/10.1016/j.hrthm.2012.11.015.

44. Fein AS, Shvilkin A, Shah D, Haffajee CI, Das S, Kumar K, Kramer DB, Zimetbaum PJ, Buxton AE, Josephson ME, Anter E. Treatment of Obstructive Sleep Apnea Reduces the Risk of Atrial Fibrillation Recurrence After Catheter Ablation. Journal of the American College of Cardiology 2013;62(4):300–05. https://doi.org/10.1016/j.jacc.2013.03.052.

45. Matiello M, Nadal M, Tamborero D, Berruezo A, Montserrat J, Embid C, Rios, J Villacastín J, Brugada J, Mont L. Low efficacy of atrial fibrillation ablation in severe obstructive sleep apnoea patients. Europace 2010;12(8):1084–89. https://doi.org/10.1093/europace/euq128.

46. Li L, Wang Z-w, Li J, Ge X, Guo L-z, Wang Y, Guo W-h, Jiang C-x, Ma C-s. Efficacy of catheter ablation of atrial fibrillation in patients with obstructive sleep apnoea with and without continuous positive airway pressure treatment: a meta-analysis of observational studies. Europace 2014;16(9):1309–14. https://doi.org/10.1093/europace/euu066.

47. Yaranov DM, Smyrlis A, Usatii N, Butler A, Petrini JR, Mendez J, et al. Effect of obstructive sleep apnea on frequency of stroke in patients with atrial fibrillation. Am J Cardiol. 2015;115(4):461–5.

48. Wu X, Liu Z, Chang SC, Cuiping Fu SC, Li, W Jiang H, Jiang L, Li S. Screening and managing obstructive sleep apnoea in nocturnal heart block patients: an observational study. Respiratory Research 2016;17(1). https://doi.org/10.1186/s12931-016-0333-8.

49. Roche F, Barthélémy J-C, Garet M, Duverney D, Pichot V, Sforza E. Continuous Positive Airway Pressure Treatment Improves the QT Rate Dependence Adaptation of Obstructive Sleep Apnea Patients. Pacing and Clinical Electrophysiology 2005;28(8):819–25 https://doi.org/10.1111/j.1540-8159.2005.00188.x.

50. Rossi VA, Stoewhas A-C, Camen G, Steffel J, Bloch KE, Stradling JR, Kohler M. The effects of continuous positive airway pressure therapy withdrawal on cardiac repolarization: data from a randomized controlled trial. European Heart Journal 2012;33(17):2206–12. https://doi.org/10.1093/eurheartj/ehs073.

51. Hung J, Whitford EG, Parsons RW, et al. Association of sleep apnoea with myocardial infarction in men. Lancet. 1990;336(8710):261–4. https://doi.org/10.1016/0140-6736(90)91799-g.

52. Kasai T, Bradley TD. Obstructive sleep apnea and heart failure: pathophysiologic and therapeutic implications. J Am Coll Cardiol. 2011;57(2):119–27.

53. Shamsuzzaman ASM, Winnicki M, Lamfranchi P, et al. Elevated C-reactive protein in patients with obstructive sleep apnea. Circulation. 2002;105:2462–4.

54. Sharma S, Schoepf JU, Armstrong AM, Parker AT, Abro JA. Independent association between obstructive sleep apnea and vulnerable plaque demonstrated by non-invasive coronary CT angiography. Chest. 2009;136(4_MeetingAbstracts):67S-f-68S.

55. Sert Kuniyoshi FH, Garcia-Touchard A, Gami A, et al. Day-night variation of acute myocardial infarction in obstructive sleep apnea. J Am Coll Cardiol. 2008;52:343–6.

56. Milleron O, Pillière R, Foucher A, et al. Benefits of obstructive sleep apnoea treatment in coronary artery disease: a long-term follow-up study. Eur Heart J. 2004;25:728–34.

57. Gottlieb DJ, Yenokyan G, Newman AB, et al. Prospective study of obstructive sleep apnea and incident coronary heart disease and heart failure: the Sleep Heart Health Study. Circulation. 2010;122:352–60.

58. Marin JM, Carrizo SJ, Vincente E, et al. Long-term cardiovascular outcomes in men with obstructive sleep apnoea-hypopnoea with or without treatment with continuous positive airway pressure: an observational study. Lancet. 2005;365:1046–53.

59. Campos-Rodriguez F, Martinez-Garcia MA, de la Cruz-Moron I, et al. Cardiovascular mortality in women with obstructive sleep apnea. Ann Intern Med. 2020;156(2):115–22.

60. Barbe F, Cantolla JD, Sanchez-de-la-Torre M, et al. Effect of continuous positive airway pressure on the incidence of hypertension and cardiovascular events in nonsleepy patients with obstructive sleep apnea: a randomized controlled trial. JAMA. 2012;307:2161–8.

61. McEvoy N, Antic NA, et al. CPAP for prevention of cardiovascular events in obstructive sleep apnea. N Engl J Med. 2016;375:919–31.

62. Peker Y, Glantz H, Eulenburg C, et al. Effect of positive airway pressure on cardiovascular outcomes in coronary artery disease patients with nonsleepy obstructive sleep apnea. The RICCADSA randomized controlled trial. Am J Respir Crit Care Med. 2016;194:613–20.

63. Javaheri S, Martinez-Garcia MA, Campos-Todriguez F, et al. CPAP treatment and cardiovascular prevention. Chest. 2019;156(3):431–7.

64. Mozaffarian D, Benjamin EJ, Go AS, et al. Heart disease and stroke statistics – 2016 update: a report from the American Heart Association. Circulation. 2016;133(4):e38–360.

65. Heidenreich PA, Albert NM, Allen LA, Bluemke DA, Butler J, Fonarow GC, Ikonomidis JS, Khavjou O, Konstam MA, Maddox TM, Nichol G, Pham M, Piña IL, Trogdon JG. Forecasting the Impact of Heart Failure in the United States. Circulation: Heart Failure 2013;6(3):606–19. https://doi.org/10.1161/HHF.0b013e318291329a.

66. Javaheri S, Teramoto S, Ouchi Y, et al. Clinical significance of arterial blood gas analysis for detection and/or treatment of central sleep apnea in patients with heart failure. Circulation. 1998;97:2154–9.

67. Shahar E, Whitney CW, Redline S, et al. Sleep-disordered breathing and cardiovascular disease: cross-sectional results of the Sleep Heart Health Study. Am J Respir Crit Care Med. 2001;163:19–25.

68. Bradley TD, Floras JS. Sleep apnea and heart failure. Circulation. 2003;107:1671–8.

69. Kasai T, Arcand J, Allard JPO, et al. Sleep apnea and cardiovascular disease. J Am Coll Cardiol. 2011;57:119–27.

70. Bradley TD, Kimoff RJ, et al. Continuous positive airway pressure for central sleep apnea. N Engl J Med. 2005;353:2025–33.

71. Kasai T, et al. Sleep apnea and cardiovascular disease: a bidirectional relationship. Circulation. 2012;124:1495–510.

72. Arzt M, Flores JS, Logan AG, et al. Sleep disordered breathing and cardiovascular disease. Circulation. 2007;115:3173–80.

73. Cowie MR, Woehrle H, Wegscheider K, et al. Adaptive servo-ventilation for central sleep apnea in systolic heart failure. N Engl J Med. 2015;373:1095–105.

74. Javaheri S, Brown LK, Randerath W, et al. SERVE-HF: more questions. Chest. 2016;149:900–4.

75. Abraham WT, Jagielski D, Oldenburg D, et al. Phrenic nerve stimulation for central sleep apnea. JACC Heart Fail. 2015;3(5):360–9.

76. Costanzo M, Ponikowski P, Jacaheri S, et al. Transvenous neurostimulation for central sleep apnoea: a randomized controlled trial. Lancet. 2016;388:974–82; Am J Cardiol. 2018;121:1400–8.

77. Minnerup J, Ritter AR, et al. Continuous positive airway pressure ventilation for acute ischemic stroke: a randomized feasibility study. Stroke. 2012;43(4):1137–9. http://stroke.ahajournals.org/lookup/suppl/doi:10.1161/STRROKEAHA.111.637611/-/DC1.

78. Khot SP, Morgenstern LB. Sleep and stoke. Stroke. 2019;50:1612–7.

79. Brown DL, Jiang X, Li C, Case E, Sozener CB, Chervin RD, et al. Sleep apnea screening is uncommon after stroke. Sleep Med. 2019;59:90–3.

Cognitive Behavioral Therapy for Insomnia in Patients with Comorbid Insomnia and Obstructive Sleep Apnea

Jean-Philippe Gouin

Obstructive sleep apnea (OSA) is typically conceptualized as a disorder of excessive sleepiness. In contrast, insomnia is often presented as a disorder of hyperarousal. Given that some of the nighttime and daytime complaints associated with insomnia and OSA are similar, the presence of insomnia symptoms among OSA patients can be easily overlooked [1]. Nonetheless, a substantial proportion of individuals with OSA present with clinically significant insomnia symptoms. A meta-analysis suggests that about 38% of OSA patients meet criteria for an insomnia disorder [2]. These insomnia symptoms have important consequences for the patient's functioning, quality of life, and adherence to positive airway pressure (PAP) treatment.

One of the challenges in diagnosing insomnia disorder among OSA patients is related to the shared symptoms that are present in both disorders [3]. Insomnia disorder and OSA include both nighttime and daytime symptoms. The nighttime insomnia symptoms include difficulty falling asleep, staying asleep, and early morning awakenings. In OSA, frequent post-apneic nocturnal awakenings may mimic sleep maintenance difficulties. Nonrestorative sleep is reported by both OSA and insomnia patients. Furthermore, many of daytime symptoms of insomnia, such as mood disturbances, fatigue, complaints of impaired attention, concentration, and memory, can also be signs and symptoms of OSA. Insomnia symptoms can therefore be easily confounded by OSA symptoms [1].

The management of insomnia symptoms is important in OSA patients. First, individuals with insomnia comorbid with OSA present more sleep disturbances than patients with OSA alone. This includes shorter total sleep time, less N2 sleep, and more wake after sleep onset during polysomnography [4]. They also present with more depressive symptoms, more psychiatric comorbidities, more daytime impairment, and lower quality of life than patients with OSA

alone [5–9]. Furthermore, the presence of insomnia symptoms has been associated with poorer adherence to PAP treatment [10–12].

Although insomnia symptoms were previously considered "secondary" to OSA, in many cases, they are actually symptoms of a distinct disorder rather than an epiphenomenon of OSA. In different observational cohort studies, patients with OSA using PAP regularly experienced a decrease in sleep maintenance insomnia symptoms over time, with greater hours of PAP use per week being associated with larger decrease in insomnia symptoms severity [10]. However, difficulty with sleep initiation and early morning awakenings persisted despite PAP use [13, 14]. Notably, a substantial proportion of OSA patients display residual insomnia symptoms above the clinical cutoff for an insomnia disorder despite PAP use. Insomnia thus appears to be a distinct, self-sustaining disorder that requires its own specific treatment.

Cognitive behavioral therapy for insomnia (CBTi) is currently the recommended first-line treatment for an insomnia disorder [15]. Cohort studies indicate that OSA severity is not associated with the effectiveness of CBTi [3, 16, 17]. The efficacy of CBTi in patients with OSA has been confirmed in randomized controlled trials. Sweetman and colleagues [18] showed that a four-session CBTi administered before starting PAP treatment was associated with a larger reduction in insomnia severity, compared to treatment as usual. Similarly, Ong et al. [19] observed that CBTi administered before or concurrent to PAP treatment was associated with greater decreases in insomnia severity, compared to PAP treatment alone. In contrast, Bjorvatn and colleagues [20] reported that a CBTi self-help book was not associated with greater reduction in insomnia among OSA patients, compared to sleep hygiene education. These results suggest that therapist-assisted CBTi is an effective treatment for insomnia disorder comorbid to OSA.

There are mixed findings regarding whether CBTi is associated with improved acceptance and adherence to PAP. Sweetman et al. [18] reported that CBTi prior to PAP

J.-P. Gouin (✉)
Department of Psychology, Concordia University, Montreal, QC, Canada
e-mail: JP.Gouin@concordia.ca

initiation was associated with greater PAP acceptance and adherence 6 months later. In contrast, Ong et al. [19] did not observe differences in PAP adherence among groups who received either CBTi prior to PAP initiation, CBTi concomitant to PAP treatment, or PAP alone. In these two randomized trials, a standard CBTi protocol focusing only on insomnia symptoms was used. Interventionists were explicitly told not to address PAP use issues in order to isolate the effect of CBTi on PAP adherence. In contrast, Alessi and colleagues [21] trained non-clinician sleep coaches, supervised by sleep specialists, to deliver a 5-week CBTi intervention that also included behavioral strategies to increase PAP adherence. The sleep coach intervention was associated with larger improvement in self-reported sleep quality as well as greater PAP use over the 6-month follow-up assessment, compared to a sleep education control condition. Although replication of these results is paramount, these findings suggest that a CBTi intervention combined with behavioral strategies to enhance PAP compliance may be most appropriate to address both insomnia symptoms and PAP compliance issues among patients with OSA.

The Spielman 3-P model of insomnia [22] is a helpful conceptual framework to understand the development and maintenance of insomnia over time, including among OSA patients. This model considers predisposing, precipitating, and perpetuating factors impacting the evolution of insomnia symptoms. The model postulates that predisposing conditions, such as high anxiousness, may make some individuals at greater risk for insomnia. Precipitating circumstances are events that trigger the onset of an insomnia episode. These can be stressful life events, schedule changes causing sleep disruptions, or, in the context of OSA, repeated nocturnal awakenings following apneic events, nocturia, or apnea and PAP-related anxiety and frustration at night. Perpetuating factors are maladaptive cognitive and behavioral strategies that the person adopts to cope with these initial insomnia symptoms, such as taking prolonged naps during the day, staying in bed for several hours to compensate for lack of sleep, or consuming large amount of caffeine to cope with daytime fatigue and sleepiness. These maladaptive strategies, while helpful at relieving some of the negative consequences of insomnia in the short-term, tend to maintain the insomnia symptoms in the long term. CBTi targets these perpetuating factors maintaining insomnia disorder over time.

CBTi is a multicomponent intervention that typically includes education about sleep, stimulus control strategies, sleep restriction strategies, and cognitive therapy, administered during 4–8 weekly sessions [23]. Relaxation strategies, such diaphragmatic breathing, progressive muscle relaxation, or guided imagery, are also sometimes included in the treatment protocol. Dismantling studies suggest that stimulus control, sleep restriction strategies, and cognitive therapy are the most effective components of the intervention [24–

26]. Brief behavioral therapy for insomnia focusing on stimulus control and sleep restriction strategies administered in 1–4 sessions are also effective at reducing insomnia severity [23]. However, multicomponent interventions appear to be more effective than single-component interventions [23].

A CBTi protocol typically starts with education about sleep. Borbély et al.'s two-process model of sleep regulation [27] is presented in layman terms to provide a rationale for the treatment strategies. Patients are instructed that their likelihood of being able to fall and remain asleep on a given night is dependent on two main factors, the homeostatic sleep pressure and the circadian drive regulated by the internal clock. The behavioral strategies will thus target these two processes. Classical conditioning principles are briefly presented to explain the concept of conditioned arousal and provide a rationale for the stimulus control strategies. Given that, relative to their total sleep time, the patients spend a long time in bed awake and anxious or frustrated about not being able to sleep, and their sleep environment becomes implicitly associated with wakefulness rather than sleep. The clinician highlights that the body will create new associations with the sleep environment after the bed has been *repeatedly* associated with sleep rather than wakefulness. This sets the stage for requiring the patient to maintain these behavioral strategies over several consecutive days.

Stimulus control strategies aim at reducing the conditioned or learned associations between the sleep environment, i.e., the bed, and arousal. The main goal of this set of strategies is to reduce the time spent in bed while not asleep. This will help strengthen the association between the bed environment and sleep as well as reducing the association between the sleep environment and arousing activities that interfere with sleep onset and maintenance. Six strategies are used to implement the stimulus control intervention.

1. Lie down in bed to go to sleep only when you are feeling sleepy. Here it is helpful to discuss the difference between fatigue, a state of low energy level, from sleepiness, a state when it becomes difficult to stay awake.
2. If you are unable to fall asleep within 10–15 minutes, get out of bed. Return to bed only when you are sleepy again.
3. If you wake up in the middle of the night and are unable to fall back asleep, get out of bed. Return to bed only when you are sleepy again.
4. Get up at up the same time everyday regardless of the amount of sleep that you had during the night. This will help anchor your circadian rhythm. Most patients will have to set up an alarm clock to follow this recommendation. This strategy should be applied both during weekdays and weekends.
5. Avoid napping during the day. Some patients with OSA may want to nap in order to reduce the excessive sleepiness during the day. If they decide to nap, they should

plan to sleep for only 15–20 minutes about 7–9 hours before the desired bedtime. This requires setting an alarm clock to avoid oversleeping during the day.

6. Do not use the bed for activities other than sleep and sex. Avoid eating, reading, watching television, browsing on your phone and tablet, or worrying in bed.

In order to change the learned, conditioned associations between the sleep environment and conditioned arousal, the stimulus control strategies must be applied for several consecutive nights. It is thus important to tell the patient that they should not expect to see an immediate improvement in insomnia symptoms. Rather, it is crucial that they maintain these strategies for at least 2 weeks in order to evaluate their efficacy.

The sleep restriction strategies, often presented as sleep consolidation strategies to the patient, aim at increasing the homeostatic sleep drive by setting a time in bed window that is close to the time actually spent asleep. This strategy will lead to an initial sleep deprivation that will eventually lead to deeper sleep during the sleep window, reduce compensatory sleep behaviors, and enhance the regularity of sleep-wake cycles. To determine the prescribed time in bed window, the patient is asked to fill out a sleep diary during at least 7 consecutive days. The patient is asked to record the time they went to bed, sleep onset latency, number of nocturnal awakenings, total wake time after sleep onset, final awakening, as well as the time that they got out of bed. The sleep diary data allows the clinician to estimate the average sleep time per night as well as the patient's sleep efficiency. Sleep efficiency refers to the ratio of total sleep time over the total time in bed.

The following instructions are given to determine the maximum amount of time in bed allocated:

1. Looking at your sleep diary, calculate the average total sleep time (TST) as well as total time in bed (TIB) per night for the past week. The initial length of your sleep window is determined using the formula: TIB = average TST + 30 minutes. Adding 30 minutes to the average sleep time allows for normal sleep onset latency and brief nocturnal awakenings. Your sleep window should not be less than 5.5 hours per night.

2. Choose a consistent wake-up time. You will be asked to get out of bed no later than 15 minutes after your wake-up time, every day of the week including weekends. Using the TIB calculated above, count backward from your desired wake-up time. This will be your earliest bedtime. We will ask you to strictly adherence to these prescribed times in and out of bed for at least 1 week in order to experience the sleep consolidation effect.

3. Each week, your sleep window can be adjusted as a function of your sleep efficiency. Sleep efficiency is calculated by dividing the average time that you actually slept by that average time that you spent in bed per night. If your sleep efficiency is greater than 85% and you feel you are not getting enough sleep for optimal daytime functioning, increase your allowed time in bed by 15 minutes at either end of the sleep window. If your sleep efficiency is lower than 85%, you decrease your time in bed by 15 minutes at either end of the sleep window. You should maintain your new sleep window for at least 7 nights before making new changes.

The length of the sleep window should be largely based on sleep diary data. However, the timing of the sleep window should be based on patient's circadian preferences and social and occupational responsibilities. Some patients will prefer staying up late and others getting up early. The timing of the initial sleep window can then be adjusted accordingly.

Although very effective in reducing insomnia symptoms, sleep restriction is not tolerated by all patients. Furthermore, it is not recommended for individuals with bipolar or seizure disorder or among heavy equipment operators because it could increase risk for relapse or occupational accidents. With these patients, sleep compression strategies can be used. Instead of starting by reducing the sleep window and gradually expanding it, the sleep compression strategy aims at gradually reducing the total time in bed every week in order to achieve a sleep efficiency of 85%. For most patients, it helps to set a fixed waking up time and then gradually delay their earliest bedtime based on the change in sleep efficiency each week. However, for patients who initially wake up late into the day, a gradual change of both bedtime and rising time may be most appropriate.

For both stimulus control and sleep restriction, it is expected that these strategies will lead to some degree of sleep deprivation after the initiation of these strategies. However, over time, the increased sleep pressure will reduce sleep onset latency as well as wake after sleep onset. It is thus important to tell the patients to maintain these strategies for at least 2 weeks in order to evaluate their efficacy. If the patient questions whether these strategies will be helpful for them, the clinician can encourage the patient to treat these strategies as an experiment and to collect data to learn what the key factors are that influence their sleep. Furthermore, to promote adherence to these recommendations, it is helpful to identify barriers to the implementation of these strategies and engage in problem-solving with the patient to determine how to deal with these barriers. Notably, it is helpful to identify ahead of time some calm, non-arousing activities that the patient can do when they get out of bed in the middle of the night or what they will do now that they are spending much less time in bed trying to sleep.

The cognitive therapy strategies aim at identifying and changing dysfunctional beliefs about sleep held by patients.

Individuals with insomnia may hold catastrophic beliefs about the consequences of poor sleep. For example, patients may think that if they don't sleep 8 hours per night, they won't be able to function the next day. These beliefs, in turn, make them experience increased sleep-related worry and anxiety that can interfere with sleep onset and maintenance. These beliefs may also lead them to engage in different compensatory behaviors to deal with sleep loss. For example, a patient may regularly cancel social and occupational commitments after a poor night of sleep. These compensatory behaviors, while aimed at minimizing the consequences of insomnia in the short term, may paradoxically increase sleep-related anxiety and interfere with sleep in the long term.

In cognitive therapy, Socratic questioning can be used to help patients reduce black-and-white thinking with regard to insomnia. For example, the clinician may ask the patient to identify times when they were able to function well after a night of severe insomnia. The clinician can also ask the patient to engage in a series of behavioral experiments to test their beliefs about sleep. For example, with a patient who is concerned about the consequences of sleep loss, the clinician could ask them to identify how they think they will function if they don't sleep enough. Then, the patient is asked to force themselves to sleep no more than 6 hours on one night to evaluate how they actually function the next day. After this behavioral experiment, the patient evaluates to what extent the feared consequences actually happened. Although the patient may not be functioning optimally, the patient often realizes that they can still function fairly well despite some sleep deprivation. These experiments can help reduce nighttime catastrophic thinking and anxiety regarding sleep loss.

Patients with an insomnia disorder comorbid to OSA may be concerned that wearing a PAP mask may interfere with their ability to fall and remain asleep. It is important to have an explicit discussion about how PAP use may interfere with the application of some of the CBTi strategies (e.g., remove and replacing the PAP mask when getting out of bed in the middle of the night) and to engage in collaborative problem-solving with the patient to create specific plans on how to deal with the patient-reported barriers to CBTi associated with PAP use. For patients who are refusing PAP treatment or demonstrate issues with PAP compliance, motivation enhancement and problem-solving strategies can be helpful (see Chap. 6). Some patients may be resistant to PAP use because of anxiety, claustrophobia, and physical discomfort when using PAP device. In these situations, exposure therapy may help address these issues (see Chap. 6).

In summary, more than a third of OSA patients present with a comorbid insomnia disorder. These insomnia symptoms are associated with poorer sleep, worse daytime functioning, and poorer adherence to PAP treatment. Rather than being secondary to OSA, insomnia is often a distinct, self-perpetuating disorder that requires its own specific treatment. CBTi is an effective non-pharmacological treatment of insomnia disorder among patients with OSA.

Acknowledgments Preparation of this chapter was supported by a project grant from the Canadian Institutes for Health Research awarded to JPG. The author would like to thank Dr. Thien Thanh Dang Vu for comments on an earlier version of the chapter.

References

1. Luyster FS, Buysse DJ, Strollo PJ. Comorbid insomnia and obstructive sleep apnea: challenges for clinical practice and research. J Clin Sleep Med. 2010;6(2):196–204.
2. Zhang Y, Ren R, Lei F, Zhou J, Zhang J, Wing YK, Sanford LD, Tang X. Worldwide and regional prevalence rates of co-occurrence of insomnia and insomnia symptoms with obstructive sleep apnea: a systematic review and meta-analysis. Sleep Med Rev. 2019;45:1–17. https://doi.org/10.1016/j.smrv.2019.01.004.
3. Sweetman A, Lack LC, Catcheside PG, Antic NA, Chai-Coetzer CL, Smith SS, Douglas JA, McEvoy RD. Developing a successful treatment for co-morbid insomnia and sleep apnoea. Sleep Med Rev. 2017;33:28–38. https://doi.org/10.1016/j.smrv.2016.04.004.
4. Bianchi MT, Williams KL, McKinney S, Ellenbogen JM. The subjective-objective mismatch in sleep perception among those with insomnia and sleep apnea. J Sleep Res. 2013;22(5):557–68. https://doi.org/10.1111/jsr.12046.
5. Cho YW, Kim KT, Moon HJ, Korostyshevskiy VR, Motamedi GK, Yang KI. Comorbid insomnia with obstructive sleep apnea: clinical characteristics and risk factors. J Clin Sleep Med. 2018;14(3):409–17. https://doi.org/10.5664/jcsm.6988.
6. Krakow B, Melendrez D, Ferreira E, Clark J, Warner TD, Sisley B, Sklar D. Prevalence of insomnia symptoms in patients with sleep-disordered breathing. Chest. 2001;120(6):1923–9. https://doi.org/10.1378/chest.120.6.1923.
7. Philip R, Catcheside P, Stevens D, Lovato N, McEvoy D, Vakulin A. Comorbid insomnia and sleep apnoea is associated with greater neurocognitive impairment compared with OSA alone. J Sleep Res. 2017;40:e260.
8. Sivertsen B, Björnsdóttir E, Øverland S, Bjorvatn B, Salo P. The joint contribution of insomnia and obstructive sleep apnoea on sickness absence. J Sleep Res. 2013;22(2):223–30. https://doi.org/10.1111/j.1365-2869.2012.01055.x.
9. Tasbakan MS, Gunduz C, Pirildar S, Basoglu OK. Quality of life in obstructive sleep apnea is related to female gender and comorbid insomnia. Sleep Breath. 2018;22(4):1013–20. https://doi.org/10.1007/s11325-018-1621-y.
10. Björnsdóttir E, Janson C, Sigurdsson JF, Gehrman P, Perlis M, Juliusson S, Arnardottir ES, Kuna ST, Pack AI, Gislason T, Benediktsdóttir B. Symptoms of insomnia among patients with obstructive sleep apnea before and after two years of positive airway pressure treatment. Sleep. 2013;36(12):1901–9. https://doi.org/10.5665/sleep.3226.
11. Wallace DM, Sawyer AM, Shafazand S. Comorbid insomnia symptoms predict lower 6-month adherence to CPAP in US veterans with obstructive sleep apnea. Sleep Breath. 2018;22(1):5–15. https://doi.org/10.1007/s11325-017-1605-3.
12. Wickwire EM, Smith MT, Birnbaum S, Collop NA. Sleep maintenance insomnia complaints predict poor CPAP adherence: a clinical case series. Sleep Med. 2010;11(8):772–6. https://doi.org/10.1016/j.sleep.2010.03.012.

13. Glidewell RN, Renn BN, Roby E, Orr WC. Predictors and patterns of insomnia symptoms in OSA before and after PAP therapy. Sleep Med. 2014;15(8):899–905. https://doi.org/10.1016/j.sleep.2014.05.001.

14. Krakow BJ, McIver ND, Obando JJ, Ulibarri VA. Changes in insomnia severity with advanced PAP therapy in patients with post-traumatic stress symptoms and comorbid sleep apnea: a retrospective, nonrandomized controlled study. Mil Med Res. 2019;6(1):15. https://doi.org/10.1186/s40779-019-0204-y.

15. Schutte-Rodin S, Broch L, Buysse D, Dorsey C, Sateia M. Clinical guideline for the evaluation and management of chronic insomnia in adults. J Clin Sleep Med. 2008;4(5):487–504. https://doi.org/10.5664/jcsm.27286.

16. Krakow B, Melendrez D, Lee SA, Warner TD, Clark JO, Sklar D. Refractory insomnia and sleep-disordered breathing: a pilot study. Sleep Breath. 2004;8(1):15–29. https://doi.org/10.1007/s11325-004-0015-5.

17. Fung CH, Martin JL, Josephson K, Fiorentino L, Dzierzewski JM, Jouldjian S, Tapia JC, Mitchell MN, Alessi C. Efficacy of cognitive behavioral therapy for insomnia in older adults with occult sleep-disordered breathing. Psychosom Med. 2016;78(5):629–39. https://doi.org/10.1097/PSY.0000000000000314.

18. Sweetman A, Lack L, Catcheside PG, Antic NA, Smith S, Chai-Coetzer CL, Douglas J, O'grady A, Dunn N, Robinson J, Paul D, Williamson P, McEvoy RD. Cognitive and behavioral therapy for insomnia increases the use of continuous positive airway pressure therapy in obstructive sleep apnea participants with comorbid insomnia: a randomized clinical trial. Sleep. 2019;42(12):zsz178. https://doi.org/10.1093/sleep/zsz178.

19. Ong JC, Crawford MR, Dawson SC, Fogg LF, Turner AD, Wyatt JK, Crisostomo MI, Chhangani BS, Kushida CA, Edinger JD, Abbott SM, Malkani RG, Attarian HP, Zee PC. A randomized controlled trial of CBT-I and PAP for obstructive sleep apnea and comorbid insomnia: Main outcomes from the MATRICS study. Sleep. 2020;43(9):zsaa041. https://doi.org/10.1093/sleep/zsaa041.

20. Bjorvatn B, Berge T, Lehmann S, Pallesen S, Saxvig IW. No effect of a self-help book for insomnia in patients with obstructive sleep apnea and comorbid chronic insomnia - a randomized controlled trial. Front Psychol. 2018;9:2413. https://doi.org/10.3389/fpsyg.2018.02413.

21. Alessi CA, Fung CH, Dzierzewski JM, Fiorentino L, Stepnowsky C, Rodriguez Tapia JC, Song Y, Zeidler MR, Josephson K, Mitchell MN, Jouldjian S, Martin JL. Randomized controlled trial of an integrated approach to treating insomnia and improving use of positive airway pressure therapy in veterans with comorbid insomnia disorder and obstructive sleep apnea. Sleep. 2020:zsaa235. https://doi.org/10.1093/sleep/zsaa235.

22. Spielman A. Assessment of insomnia. Clin Psychol Rev. 1986;6(1):11–25. https://doi.org/10.1016/0272-7358(86)90015-2.

23. Edinger JD, Arnedt JT, Bertisch SM, et al. Behavioral and psychological treatments for chronic insomnia disorder in adults: an American Academy of Sleep Medicine systematic review, meta-analysis, and GRADE assessment. J Clin Sleep Med. 2021;17(2):263–98. https://doi.org/10.5664/jcsm.8988.

24. Epstein DR, Sidani S, Bootzin RR, Belyea MJ. Dismantling multicomponent behavioral treatment for insomnia in older adults: a randomized controlled trial. Sleep. 2012;35(6):797–805. https://doi.org/10.5665/sleep.1878.

25. Harvey AG, Bélanger L, Talbot L, Eidelman P, Beaulieu-Bonneau S, Fortier-Brochu É, Ivers H, Lamy M, Hein K, Soehner AM, Mérette C, Morin CM. Comparative efficacy of behavior therapy, cognitive therapy, and cognitive behavior therapy for chronic insomnia: a randomized controlled trial. J Consult Clin Psychol. 2014;82(4):670–83. https://doi.org/10.1037/a0036606.

26. Sunnhed R, Hesser H, Andersson G, Carlbring P, Morin CM, Harvey AG, Jansson-Fröjmark M. Comparing internet-delivered cognitive therapy and behavior therapy with telephone support for insomnia disorder: a randomized controlled trial. Sleep. 2020;43(2):zsz245. https://doi.org/10.1093/sleep/zsz245.

27. Borbély AA, Daan S, Wirz-Justice A, Deboer T. The two-process model of sleep regulation: a reappraisal. J Sleep Res. 2016;25:131–43. https://doi.org/10.1111/jsr.12371.

Overview of Medication Treatment for Co-Morbid Insomnia and Sleep Apnea (COMISA)

Alan D. Lowe and Megan S. Lowe

18.1 Co-Morbid Insomnia and Sleep Apnea (COMISA)

Despite the frequent presentation of both sleep apnea and insomnia in the same patient, it was not immediately recognized that their combined presence could exacerbate and intensify the symptoms of each. COMISA was first identified by Guilleminault, Eldridge, and Dement [1, 2]. The article alerted clinicians to the possibility that patients with insomnia might be unaware of their sleep apnea symptoms and thus of the consequent risk of misdiagnosing the condition as a case of uncomplicated insomnia. The article had a very limited impact over the next 30 years until the publication of findings in 1999 and 2001 showing that insomnia and obstructive sleep apnea (OSA) have 30% to 50% comorbidity rates [3–6]. Since 1999 a substantial number of studies have further documented the considerable overlap and bidirectional relationship of comorbid insomnia and OSA [6].

COMISA has remained a persistent challenge to treat well. This observation emphasizes the importance of screening for insomnia in a "sleep apnea clinic," most expeditiously by providing the patient with a screening questionnaire prior to the interview. When compared to patients with OSA who do not have insomnia, COMISA patients frequently show poor adherence with using continuous positive airway pressure (CPAP) therapy [6–13]. A major part of the challenge of dealing with this patient group thus relates to how to increase the initial acceptance of and subsequent use of CPAP therapy. This has led to advocacy of the importance of treating insomnia disorder prior to or concurrently with initiating CPAP treatment [6–13].

First-line treatment of chronic insomnia is cognitive behavioral therapy for insomnia (CBT-I). Chapter 17

Part 3 in this book describe the use and efficacy of CBT-I in COMISA patients. When CBT-I is not available, hypnotic agents may need to be considered.

18.2 Sedative/Hypnotic Agents in Patients with OSA

18.2.1 Overall Effects

A literature review of studies by Mason et al. contained in the Cochrane Airways Group Specialized Register of Trials found that a wide range of medications, including remifentanil 0.75 mcg/kg/hr (infused opioid), eszopiclone 3 mg, zolpidem 10 and 20 mg, brotizolam 0.25 mg, flurazepam 30 mg, nitrazepam 10 mg to 15 mg, temazepam 10 mg, triazolam 0.25 mg, ramelteon 8 mg and 16 mg, and sodium oxybate 4.5 g and 9 g, did not produce a deleterious effect on OSA severity as measured by change in apnea-hypopnea index (AHI) or oxygen desaturation index (ODI) [14–23]. Zolpidem at 20 mg, flurazepam 30 mg, remifentanil infusion, and triazolam 0.25 mg, however, did result in significant oxygen desaturations statistically and clinically suggesting caution with these agents at these doses. In two clinical trials, eszopiclone 3 mg and sodium oxybate 4.5 g decreased AHI (compared to placebo) [14]. The reviewers concluded that no evidence existed that these pharmacological compounds produced significant adverse changes in the AHI or ODI and thus did not severely effect OSA severity [14]. Caution was still suggested because the studies reviewed were small and short duration, and there are instances where oxygen desaturation could occur with particular agents at certain doses, such as zolpidem at higher than therapeutically recommended doses, which should not be used. The authors suggested that further investigation of agents which decreased AHI as a therapeutic option may be worthwhile for a subgroup of OSA patients [14].

A. D. Lowe (✉)
University of Toronto, Toronto, ON, Canada
e-mail: alan.lowe@nygh.on.ca

M. S. Lowe
McMaster University, Hamilton, ON, Canada

© The Author(s), under exclusive license to Springer Nature Switzerland AG 2022
C. M. Shapiro et al. (eds.), *CPAP Adherence*, https://doi.org/10.1007/978-3-030-93146-9_18

18.2.2 Benzodiazepines (BZDs)

Efforts to treat insomnia in the context of obstructive sleep apnea used to be focused on benzodiazepines (BZDs) before the advent of non-benzodiazepine hypnotics. There are many concerns with BZD's treatment for insomnia in general which include abuse, dependence, addiction, withdrawal, rebound insomnia, falls, cognitive impairment, and adverse changes in sleep architecture such as promoting light sleep while reducing deep and REM sleep [24, 25]. In addition to the overall adverse central nervous system (CNS) depressant effect of these agents, concerns for COMISA patients also include the decreased ventilatory response to hypoxia and reduced upper airway muscle tone as well as any other mechanisms exacerbating sleep disordered breathing [26–30].

Some studies have found adverse changes with some BZDs such as flurazepam and triazolam while others not, such as with temazepam in mild OSA and nitrazepam in mild to mod OSA patients [16–19]. A study by Berry et al. focused on the effects of triazolam (0.25 mg) in 12 patients with severe sleep apnea in a randomized crossover study [19]. Measurements of sleep were determined by polysomnography. Triazolam was found to increase the arousal threshold to airway occlusion, and this produced only a modest prolongation in the duration of events in this patient group.

There is a body of evidence against the use of BZDs in COMISA patients. For example, a recent study by Wang et al. performed a retrospective case review using the Taiwan National Health Insurance Database from 1996 to 2013 with the purpose of quantifying the extent of acute respiratory events among COMISA patients who were users of hypnotics [31]. The case group included 216 hypnotic users who were diagnosed as having experienced acute respiratory events, including pneumonia and respiratory failure. The hypnotics used included both benzodiazepines (BZDs) and non-benzodiazepines (non-BZDs). Following an adjusted multivariate analysis, the authors concluded that long-term BZD use may increase the risk of acute respiratory failure in OSA patients.

Although the effects of BZDs on OSA may be modest, BZDs are not ideally recommended for the treatment of insomnia in general or to patients with COMISA. There may however be instances when they may need to be prescribed like when there are severe comorbid refractory disorders of anxiety or PTSD with COMISA, although further studies are needed.

18.2.3 Non-benzodiazepines (Non-BZDs)

Non-benzodiazepines are a better treatment choice than BZDs for treatment of insomnia in general and in particular for COMISA patients.

Various studies have shown that non-benzodiazepines compared to BZDs can increase total sleep time, improve sleep continuity along with sleep architecture, and have fewer adverse effects and fewer interactions [32–39].

Given the limitations of BZDs, various studies have been carried out concerning the safety and efficacy of non-BZDs for insomnia in the context of sleep disordered breathing or obstructive sleep apnea. GABAergic non-benzodiazepine agents, zolpidem, zaleplon, and eszopiclone, have been investigated in OSA patients. There is evidence that non-BZDs are a better alternative to BZDs and may improve sleep without causing respiratory depression. The advantage of these agents are that they may have only limited muscle relaxant effects, which is a benefit to treating the core breathing problems of OSA.

Further, there is some evidence that these agents may not worsen sleep apnea and may alternatively decrease AHI in certain populations with potential to improve tolerance and adherence to CPAP therapy [40–53].

A meta-analysis by Nigram et al. of published studies over the 30-year period between 1988 and 2017 evaluated the efficacy and safety of non-benzodiazepine sedative hypnotics (NBSHs), included agents such as zolpidem, zaleplon, and eszopiclone [54]. The meta-analysis, comprising data from a total of 2099 patients, found that the NBSH drugs did not increase AHI, regardless of the baseline AHI values (mild, moderate, severe, or no OSA). The AHI was found to improve minimally with use of NBSH drugs, but eszopiclone showed the greatest difference, having an MD of −5.73 events/h.

Another literature review identified eight controlled clinical trials (with 448 patients) on the effect of non-BZDs on sleep quality and severity of OSA symptoms, including the AHI index and the nadir of arterial oxygen saturation (SaO2) [55]. The review by Zhang et al. supported the conclusion that non-BZDs in typically recommended doses improved sleep quality without worsening sleep apnea in OSA patients.

18.2.4 Non-benzodiazepines for OSA Without CPAP

A small pilot study ($n = 22$) by Rosenberg et al. was conducted prior to larger OSA/COMISA studies for eszopiclone [56]. The objective of the study was to evaluate the effect of eszopiclone 3 mg on respiration, sleep, and safety in mild-moderate OSA patients who were withdrawn from CPAP. The study was a double-blind, randomized crossover design with patients (35–64 years) receiving eszopiclone 3 mg or placebo on two consecutive nights in the sleep laboratory. There was a 5–7 day washout between the two treatments. Eszopiclone administration without CPAP did not worsen AHI and was found to improve sleep maintenance and efficiency.

An open label trial investigated the effect of zolpidem 10 mg over a period of 9 weeks on 20 patients who were suffering from idiopathic central sleep apnea [57]. Although three patients experienced significant increases in obstructive events, the majority of patients showed decreases in central apnea/hypopneas and associated symptoms with zolpidem. They also had improved sleep continuity and decreased subjective daytime sleepiness.

18.2.5 Non-benzodiazepines for OSA Treated with CPAP

The first large (*n* = 226), randomized, double-blind, placebo-controlled study of eszopiclone in OSA patients receiving diagnostic polysomnography (PSG) or CPAP titration investigated the effects of eszopiclone 3 mg on various parameters of sleep quality among the 226 patients to evaluate whether such treatment would improve the quality of diagnostic PSG and CPAP titration studies [58]. Either eszopiclone or placebo was administered once on the night of testing, just before polysomnography. Compared to placebo, pretreatment with eszopiclone improved CPAP titrations and produced fewer residual events/h (5.7 vs. 11.9) and fewer incomplete titrations (31.1% vs. 48.0%). There was also a trend for more non-usable studies with placebo than with eszopiclone (7.1% vs. 2.7%) with the authors concluding routine use of non-benzodiazepines as premedication for PSG should be considered.

In another placebo-controlled study, the 16 participants with severe OSA and on CPAP therapy for at least 6 months received zolpidem 10 mg [59]. All patients were tested during one night of CPAP use. Sleep architecture, AHI, and arterial oxygen saturation showed no differences between zolpidem and placebo.

18.3   Hypnotic Agents and CPAP Adherence

18.3.1 Hypnotic Medications (Type Not Specified)

In a retrospective chart review of short-term CPAP therapy among 400 consecutive patients, only age and one-time sedative/hypnotic use during titration polysomnography were found to correlate with short-term compliance [48].

18.3.2 Non-benzodiazepines

Bradshaw et al. in 2006 investigated the effects of zolpidem, placebo, or standard care on compliance with CPAP therapy among 72 male patients who had been referred for CPAP treatment [47]. The duration of the study period was 14 days. Among this group of new CPAP users, those who had been given zolpidem did not show increased compliance to CPAP

therapy when compared to the placebo or standard care group. Similarly, Park et al. studied 134 patients undergoing their first night of CPAP therapy [60]. The investigators sought to determine the effects on CPAP compliance of a single dose of zaleplon 10 mg among 73 patients. It was found that, at 1 month, zaleplon improved sleep latency and had beneficial effects on sleep quality on self-report inventories, when compared to placebo, but did not improve adherence to CPAP therapy.

However, Lettieri et al. (2009), in a second double-blind, randomized, placebo-controlled trial of eszopiclone, compared the effect of eszopiclone 3 mg with a matching placebo in 117 participants (of whom 98 completed the study) prior to CPAP titration polysomnography with respect to short-term CPAP compliance [49]. Compared to placebo, eszopiclone 3 mg improved residual obstructive events at the final CPAP pressure (eszopiclone, 6.4 events/ h vs. placebo, 12.8 events/ h) and improved short-term CPAP compliance during the first 4 to 6 weeks of therapy. Eszopiclone was found to improve mean sleep efficiency to a greater extent over placebo (87.8% vs. 80.1%).

An additional double-blind, randomized, placebo-controlled trial by Lettieri et al. was conducted to determine if a short course of eszopiclone 3 mg during the first 2 weeks of CPAP therapy, compared to placebo, would improve long-term adherence to CPAP in 160 adults who had severe OSA (mean AHI, 36.9 events/h) [50]. Adherence to CPAP in the eszopiclone group was found to be superior to the placebo group, in which patients used CPAP for 20.8% more nights. Further, eszopiclone patients used CPAP for 1.1 hours more than the placebo group over the course of 6 months.

These findings suggest that although there may be differences among the non-benzodiazepines in terms of effect and compliance in COMISA patients, eszopiclone therapy may potentially improve more consistently response, short- and longer-term compliance with CPAP therapy [47–53].

18.3.3 New Dual Orexin Receptor Antagonists (DORAs, Suvorexant, Lemborexant)

Orexin receptor antagonists appear to facilitate sleep by acting selectively on and blocking the wake system of the brain, which is mediated by orexin receptors. These receptors originate in the lateral hypothalamus and project throughout the brain, including to respiratory centers in the brainstem. It has thus been hypothesized that orexin receptors are involved in the cardiorespiratory response to acute stressors [61].

One study showed that single-use suvorexant was a safe and effective hypnotic for 84 patients with suspected OSA and who experienced insomnia during overnight PSG by Matsumura et al. [62, 63]. Patients who had difficulty falling asleep were permitted to take suvorexant and if they continued to experience insomnia (greater than one hour to fall asleep) were optionally permitted to take zolpidem. The resultant groupings were 44 achieved sufficient sleep with single-use suvorexant alone and 40 who needed suvorexant plus zolpidem. PSG results of 144 patients with AHI >= 5 events/h, revealed 63.1% in the insomnia group had severe OSA versus 70.8% in the non-insomnia comparison group. When the insomnia and non-insomnia groups were compared, there were no differences found in terms of subjectively assessed sleep time or morning mood. The results were interpreted to support the conclusion that single-use suvorexant is a safe and effective hypnotic for laboratory PSG in suspected OSA patients who suffer from insomnia.

Cheng et al. carried out a randomized, double-blind, placebo-controlled, two-period crossover study to examine respiratory safety parameters of lemborexant 10 mg (a DORA with more OX2 orexin receptor blocking affinity than OX1) in 39 individuals who had mild OSA [64]. The subjects were assigned to one of two treatment conditions to receive either lemborexant or placebo and continued on this for 8 days. This was followed by a washout period of 14 days, after which the subjects crossed over to receive the comparison agent. Lemborexant was not found to worsen mean AHI index nor reduce mean oxygen saturation following single or multiple doses when compared to placebo. These findings supported the conclusion that lemborexant at the 10 mg dose demonstrated respiratory safety in this adult and elderly mild OSA study population.

Recently, Moline et al. conducted a multi-centre, randomized, double-blind, placebo-controlled, two-period crossover study on the effects of lemborexant in 33 subjects with untreated moderate to severe OSA; data from the cohort of patients showed no increase in AHI or decrease in peripheral capillary oxygen saturation following single dose or 8 nights of treatment [65]. Given these safety findings and that lemborexant has been shown to significantly increase REM sleep compared to placebo in early trials, there is a suggestion it could play a significant role improving CPAP compliance by alleviating middle and late insomnia in particular, lessening REM-related obstructive sleep apnea through better compliance, possibly helping decrease REM-related OSA's cardiovascular risk and complications in those predisposed, although more studies are needed [66, 67]. Positive long term 12 month sleep data for initial, middle and late insomnia along with positive early phase multiple PSG data (7 PSGs in Sunrise 1) with lemborexant suggests a potential long-term CPAP compliance study would be feasible and informative [68–71].

18.3.4 Antidepressants and OSA (Trazodone and Mirtazapine)

In various studies of both clinical and community-based populations, high rates of depression have been found in individuals diagnosed with OSA [72, 73]. While hypotheses for the linkage between the two conditions have been advanced, the exact mechanisms underlying the association have not been established [72, 73]. Additionally, the effect of antidepressants on OSA has only been minimally studied, possibly due to conceptual concerns that sedatives might worsen OSA in some patients. Nevertheless, some preliminary efforts have examined how trazodone might alter the arousal threshold and OSA severity in patients with OSA. Trazodone is a widely prescribed antidepressant which possesses hypnotic properties with associated increases in the arousal threshold.

Limited work in animal models and small-sample size clinical studies suggested to Smales et al. that these effects would not alter upper airway muscular activity and thus that the agent would have potential for reducing symptoms of OSA [74]. The investigators thus studied the effect of 1 week of trazodone or placebo administration in 15 OSA patients in a randomized crossover design study. Compared to placebo, trazodone was found to reduce the AHI index without worsening oxygen saturation or respiratory event duration. Eckert et al. studied the effects of trazodone in seven patients with OSA who had a low arousal threshold using a within subjects crossover design [75]. Trazodone was found to increase the respiratory threshold, but did not alter the AHI index, nor did it affect dilator muscle activity. This improvement in arousal threshold was not sufficient however to overcome the restrictive upper airway anatomy of these patients.

Similar to trazodone, mirtazapine has been the focus of relatively few studies regarding its efficacy for the treatment of sleep disordered breathing or OSA. Carley et al. studied the effect of mirtazapine on OSA symptoms in 12 newly diagnosed OSA patients [76]. The patients self-administered mirtazapine, either 4.5 mg or 15 mg, or placebo each night for three consecutive 7-day treatment periods. The order of treatments was randomized for all patients. While both dosages of mirtazapine were found to be superior to placebo, the 15 mg dosage was better than 4.5 mg for reducing the AHI, while only the 15 mg dosage reduced the degree of sleep fragmentation. The investigators concluded that in spite of these improvements, they could not offer an unqualified endorsement of mirtazapine in view of side effects of sedation and weight gain. In a follow-up study, Marshall et al. extended the basic experimental design of the Carley et al. (2007) investigation but increased the number of dosage regimens [77]. In the first component of the study, a three-way crossover design was applied: 20 OSA patients were asked to self-administer 7.5, 15, 30, and/or 45 mg or placebo before going to bed for 2 weeks at each dose. In a second parallel study, 65 OSA patients were asked to self-administer mirtazapine 15 mg or mirtazapine 15 mg plus compound CD0012 or placebo for 4 weeks. The investigators were unable to find any improvement in measures of sleep apnea following any of the dosage courses of mirtazapine and thus were not able to recommend the drug for treating OSA symptoms.

In a randomized, double blind crossover study on venlafaxine by Schmickl et al., it was found that AHI improved by 19% in patients with high arousal threshold (-10.9 events/h) but tended to increase in patients with a low arousal threshold ($+7$ events/ h) with other predictors including elevated AHI and less collapsible upper airway at baseline, concluding that venlafaxine simultaneously worsened and improved various pathophysiological traits, resulting in a zero net effect, and that careful patient selection based on pathophysiologic traits or combination therapy with drugs countering its alerting effects may produce a more robust response [78].

18.4 Medications for COMISA Conclusion

COMISA is a complex but common sleep disorder, which can result in increased morbidity and mortality more so than if either insomnia or obstructive sleep apnea were present alone. The presence of both disorders can make clinical diagnosis and treatment of each more difficult. Given the bidirectional nature of the disorder, optimal treatment of COMISA is multidisciplinary. CBT-I is not only first line for treatment of insomnia but also for insomnia of COMISA with the addition of CPAP contemporaneously or after, which may also improve CPAP compliance.

However, given the complexity, severity, chronicity, and refractoriness of the disorder along with comorbidities and the practical issues of CBT-I availability, sedative/hypnotics may be needed. The role of non-benzodiazepines for treatment of insomnia may need to be considered, and preliminary evidence suggests certain ones such as eszopiclone and zolpidem may be safe and effective at proper therapeutic doses and duration, in untreated and treated patients on CPAP, with eszopiclone possibly improving CPAP compliance and lowering AHI more in untreated patients. This may give relief to initial prescribers when insomnia severity warrants it and sleep apnea is not completely known waiting for a PSG, although caution is always exercised when starting any sedative/hypnotic agent.

DORAs look promising for treating COMISA, as studies for lemborexant 10 mg single use and up to 8 nights did not worsen AHI or lower mean oxygen saturation in adult or elderly untreated patients with mild, moderate or severe sleep apnea. Even suvorexant in combination with zolpidem was found to be safe and effective in a single use PSG laboratory context.

Given the many neurotransmitter systems involved in the sleep-wake cycle and sedative/hypnotics with different mechanisms of action, more research is certainly needed in this complex area such as which agent, class, or combination is optimal, the dosing, timing, and duration of treatment in relation to patient insomnia type, severity, complexity, and duration, along with whether CPAP or other therapy is present or not. Effects on compliance and overall treatment response will also need to be examined with the various treatment agents, comparing different classes and particular agents.

References

1. Guilleminault C, Eldridge FL, Dement WC. Insomnia with sleep apnea: a new syndrome. Science. 1973;181(4102):856–8. https://doi.org/10.1126/science.181.4102.856. PMID: 4353301.
2. Guilleminault C, Davis K, Huynh NT. Prospective randomized study of patients with insomnia and mild sleep disordered breathing. Sleep. 2008;31(11):1527–33. https://doi.org/10.1093/sleep/31.11.1527. PMID: 19014072.
3. Lichstein KL, Riedel BW, Lester KW, et al. Occult sleep apnea in a recruited sample of older adults with insomnia. J Consult Clin Psychol. 1999;67(3):405–10. PubMed:10369061.
4. Krakow B, Melendez D, Ferreira E, et al. Prevalence of insomnia symptoms in patients with sleep-disordered breathing. Chest. 2001;120(6):1923–9. PubMed: 11742923.
5. Krakow B, Melendrez D, Lee SA, Warner TD, Clark JO, Sklar D. (2004). Refractory insomnia and sleep-disordered breathing: a pilot study. Sleep Breath. 2004;8(1):15–29. https://doi.org/10.1007/s11325-004-0015-5. PMID: 150269350.
6. Ong JC, Crawford MR. Insomnia and obstructive sleep apnea. Sleep Med Clin. 2013;8(3):389–98. https://doi.org/10.1016/j.jsmc.2013.04.004.
7. Sweetman A, Lack L, Bastien C. Co-Morbid Insomnia and Sleep Apnea (COMISA): prevalence, consequences, methodological considerations, and recent randomized controlled trials. Brain Sci. 2019;9(12):371. https://doi.org/10.3390/brainsci9120371. PMID: 31842520.
8. Sweetman A, Lack L, Catcheside PG, Antic NA, Smith S, Chai-Coetzer CL, Douglas J, O'grady A, Dunn N, Robinson J, Paul D, Williamson P, McEvoy RD. Cognitive and behavioral therapy for insomnia increases the use of continuous positive airway pressure therapy in obstructive sleep apnea participants with comorbid insomnia: a randomized clinical trial. Sleep. 2019;42(12):zsz178. https://doi.org/10.1093/sleep/zsz178. PMID: 31403168.
9. Sweetman A, Lack L, Lambert S, Gradisar M, Harris J. Does comorbid obstructive sleep apnea impair the effectiveness of cognitive and behavioral therapy for insomnia? Sleep Med. 2017;39:38–46. https://doi.org/10.1016/j.sleep.2017.09.003. Epub 2017 Sep 22. PMID: 29157586.
10. Sweetman A, Lack L, McEvoy RD, Antic NA, Smith S, Chai-Coetzer CL, Douglas J, O'Grady A, Dunn N, Robinson J, Paul D, Eckert D, Catcheside PG. Cognitive behavioural therapy for insomnia reduces sleep apnoea severity: a randomised controlled trial. ERJ Open Res. 2020;6(2):00161–2020. https://doi.org/10.1183/23120541.00161-2020. eCollection 2020 Apr. PMID: 32440518.
11. Sweetman AM, Lack LC, Catcheside PG, Antic NA, Chai-Coetzer CL, Smith SS, Douglas JA, McEvoy RD. Developing a successful treatment for co-morbid insomnia and sleep apnoea. Sleep Med Rev. 2017;33:28–38. https://doi.org/10.1016/j.smrv.2016.04.004. Epub 2016 May 6. PMID: 27401786.
12. Bahr K, Carmara RJ, Gouveris H, Tuin I. Current treatment of comorbid insomnia and obstructive sleep apnea with CBTI and PAP-therapy: a systematic review. Front Neurol. 2018;9:804. https://doi.org/10.3389/fneur.2018.00804. PMID: 30420826.
13. Crawford MR, Turner AD, Wyatt JK, Fogg LF, Ong JC. Evaluating the treatment of obstructive sleep apnea comorbid with insomnia disorder using an incomplete factorial design. Contemp Clin Trials.

2016;47:146–52. https://doi.org/10.1016/j.cct.2015.12.017. Epub 2015 Dec 28. PMID: 26733360.

14. Mason M, Cates CJ, Smith I. Effects of opioid, hypnotic and sedating medications on sleep-disordered breathing in adults with obstructive sleep apnoea. Cochrane Database Syst Rev. 2015;(7):CD011090. https://doi.org/10.1002/14651858. CD011090.pub2. PMID: 26171909.

15. Cirignotta F, Mondini S, Gerardi R, Zucconi M. Effect of brotizolam on sleep-disordered breathing in heavy snorers with obstructive apnea. Curr Therap Res Clin Exp. 1992;51(3):360–6.

16. Dolly FR, Block AJ. Effects of flurazepam on sleep-disordered breathing and nocturnal oxygen desaturation in asymptomatic subjects. Am J Med. 1982;73:239–43.

17. Höijer U, Hedner J, Ejnell H, Grunstein R, Odelberg E, Elam M. Nitrazepam in patients with sleep apnoea: a double-blind placebo-controlled study. Eur Respir J. 1994;7(11):2011–5.

18. Camacho ME, Morin CM. The effect of Temazepam on respiration in elderly insomniacs with mild sleep apnea. Sleep. 1995;18:644–5. https://doi.org/10.1093/sleep/18.8.644.

19. Berry RB, Kouchi K, Bower J, Prosise G, Light RW. Triazolam in patients with obstructive sleep apnea. Am J Respir Crit Care Med. 1995;151(2 Pt 1):450–4. https://doi.org/10.1164/ajrccm.151.2.7842205. PMID: 7842205.

20. Kryger M, Wang-Weigand S, Roth T. Safety of ramelteon in individuals with mild to moderate obstructive sleep apnea. Sleep Breath. 2007;11:159–64.

21. Gooneratne NS, Gehrman P, Gurubhagavatula I, Al-Shehabi E, Marie E, Schwab R. Effectiveness of ramelteon for insomnia symptoms in older adults with obstructive sleep apnea: a randomized placebo-controlled pilot study. J Clin Sleep Med. 2010;6(6):572–80.

22. George CFB, Feldman N, Zheng Y, Steininger TL, Grzeschik SM, Lai C, Inhaber N. A 2-week, polysomnographic, safety study of sodium oxybate in obstructive sleep apnea syndrome. Published online: 18 January 2010. This article is published with open access at Springerlink.com.

23. George CFP, Feldman N, Inhaber N, Steininger TL, Grzeschik SM, Lai C, Zheng Y. A safety trial of sodium oxybate in patients with obstructive sleep apnea: acute effects on sleep-disordered breathing. Sleep Med. 2010;11(1):38–42. https://doi.org/10.1016/j.sleep.2009.06.006. Epub 2009 Nov 7.

24. Janhsen K, Roser P, Hoffmann K. The problems of long-term treatment with benzodiazepines and related substances. Dtsch Arztebl Int. 2015;112(1–2):1–7. https://doi.org/10.3238/arztebl.2015.0001. PMID: 25613443.

25. Riemann D, Perlis ML. The treatments of chronic insomnia: a review of benzodiazepine receptor agonists and psychological and behavior therapies. Sleep Med Rev. 2009;13(3):205–14. https://doi.org/10.1016/j.smrv.2008.06.001.

26. Bonora M, St John WM, Bledsoe TA. Differential elevation by protriptyline and depression by diazepam of upper airway respiratory motor activity. Am Rev Respir Dis. 1985;131:41–5.

27. Leiter JC, Knuth SL, Krol RC, Bartlett D Jr. The effect of diazepam on genioglossal muscle activity in normal human subjects. Am Rev Respir Dis. 1985;132:216–9.

28. Hanly P, Powles P. Hypnotics should never be used in patients with sleep apnea. J Psychosom Res. 1993;37:59–65.

29. Lu B, Budhiraja R, Parthasarathy S. Sedating medications and undiagnosed obstructive sleep apnea: physician determinants and patient consequences. J Clin Sleep Med. 2005;1:367–71.

30. Luyster FS, Buysse DJ, Strollo PJ Jr. Comorbid insomnia and obstructive sleep apnea: challenges for clinical practice and research. J Clin Sleep Med. 2010;6(2):196–204. PMID: 20411700.

31. Wang SH, Chen WS, Tang SE, Lin HC, Peng CK, Chu HT, Kao CH. Benzodiazepines associated with acute respiratory failure in patients with obstructive sleep apnea. Front Pharmacol. 2019;9:1513. https://doi.org/10.3389/fphar.2018.01513. eCollection 2018. PMID: 30666205.

32. Nutt DJ, Stahl SM. Searching for perfect sleep: the continuing evolution of GABAa receptor modulators as hypnotics. J Psychopharmacol. 24(11):1601–12. https://doi.org/10.1177/0269881109106927.

33. Qaseem A, Kansagara D, Forciea MA, Cooke M, Denberg TD, Clinical Guidelines Committee of the American College of Physicians. Management of chronic insomnia disorder in adults: a clinical practice guideline from the American College of Physicians. Ann Intern Med. 2016;165(2):125–33. https://doi.org/10.7326/M15-2175. Epub 2016 May 3. PMID: 27136449.

34. Sateia MJ, Buysse DJ, Krystal AD, Neubauer DN, Heald JL. Clinical practice guideline for the pharmacologic treatment of chronic insomnia in adults: an American Academy of Sleep Medicine Clinical Practice Guideline. J Clin Sleep Med. 2017;13(2):307–49. https://doi.org/10.5664/jcsm.6470. PMID: 27998379.

35. MacFarlane J. Taking control of acute insomnia- restoring healthy sleep patterns. The Canadian Sleep Society, Insomnia Rounds. 2012;1(2).

36. MacFarlane J. The effects of psychotropic and neurotropic medications on sleep. Sleepreviewmag.com. 2019, Aug/Sep, 22–24.

37. NIH State of the Science Conference Statement on manifestations and management of chronic insomnia in adults statement. J Sleep Med. 2005; 1(4):412–421. PMID 17308547 https://consensus.nih.gov/2005/insomniastatement.htm.

38. Pagel JF, Pandi-Perumal SR, Monti JM. Review: treating insomnia with medications. Sleep Sci Pract. 2018;2:5.BMC. https://doi.org/10.1186/s41606-018-0025-z.

39. Janseen HCJP, Venekamp LN, Peeters GAM, Pijpers A, Pevernagie AA. Management of insomnia in sleep disordered breathing. Eur Respir Rev. 2019;28:190080. https://doi.org/10.1183/16000617.0080-2019.

40. Eckert DJ, Owens RL, Kehlmann GB, Wellman A, Rahangdale S, Yim-Yeh S, White DP, Malhotra A. Eszopiclone increases the respiratory arousal threshold and lowers the apnoea/hypopnoea index in obstructive sleep apnoea patients with a low arousal threshold. Clin Sci (Lond). 2011;120(12):505–14. https://doi.org/10.1042/CS20100588.

41. Smith PR, Sheikh KL, Costan-Toth C, Forsthoefel D, Bridges E, Andrada TF, Holley AB. Eszopiclone and zolpidem do not affect the prevalence of the low arousal threshold phenotype. J Clin Sleep Med. 13(1):115–9. https://doi.org/10.5664/jcsm.6402.

42. Eckert DJ, Malhotra A. Pathophysiology of adult obstructive sleep apnea. Proc Am Thorac Soc. 2008;5:144–53.

43. Eckert DJ, Sweetman A. Impaired central control of sleep depth propensity as a common mechanism for excessive overnight wake time: implications for sleep apnea, insomnia and beyond. J Clin Sleep Med. 2020;16(3):341–3. https://doi.org/10.5664/jcsm.8268. Epub 2020 Jan 14. PMID: 32003739.

44. Hagen C, Patel A, McCall WV. Prevalence of insomnia symptoms in sleep laboratory patients with and without sleep apnea. Psychiatry Res. 2009;170(2–3):276–7. https://doi.org/10.1016/j.psychres.2009.02.001. Epub 2009 Nov 6. PMID: 19896722.

45. Lofaso F, Goldenberg F, Thebault C, Janus C, Harf A. Effect of zopiclone on sleep, night-time ventilation, and daytime vigilance in upper airway resistance syndrome. Eur Respir J. 1997;10:2573–7.

46. Cirignotta F, Mondini S, Zucconi M, Gerardi R, Farolfi A, Lugaresi E. Zolpidem-polysomnographic study of the effect of a new hypnotic drug in sleep apnea syndrome. Pharmacol Biochem Behav. 1988;29(4):807–9. https://doi.org/10.1016/0091-3057(88)90212-2. PMID: 3413202.

47. Bradshaw DA, Ruff GA, Murphy DP. An oral hypnotic medication does not improve continuous positive airway pressure compliance in men with obstructive sleep apnea. Chest. 2006;130(5):1369–76. https://doi.org/10.1378/chest.130.5.1369. PMID: 17099012.

48. Collen J, Lettieri C, Kelly W, Roop S. Clinical and polysomnographic predictors of short-term continuous positive airway pressure compliance. Chest. 2009;135(3):704–9. https://doi.org/10.1378/chest.08-2182. Epub 2008 Nov 18. PMID: 19017888.

49. Lettieri CJ, Collen JF, Eliasson AH, Quast TM. Sedative use during continuous positive airway pressure titration improves subsequent compliance: a randomized, double-blind, placebo-controlled trial. Chest. 2009;136(5):1263–8. https://doi.org/10.1378/chest.09-0811. Epub 2009 Jun 30. PMID: 19567493.

50. Lettieri CJ, Shah AA, Holley AB, Kelly WF, Chang AS, Roop SA. Effects of a short course of eszopiclone on continuous positive airway pressure adherence: a randomized tria. Ann Intern Med. 2009;151(10):696–702. https://doi.org/10.7326/0003-4819-151-10-200911170-00006. PMID: 19920270.

51. Nguyên XL, Chaskalovic J, Rakotonanahary D, Fleury B. Insomnia symptoms and CPAP compliance in OSAS patients: a descriptive study using data mining methods. Sleep Med. 2010;11(8):777–84. https://doi.org/10.1016/j.sleep.2010.04.008. Epub 2010 Jul 6. PMID: 20599419.

52. Pieh C, Bach M, Popp R, Jara C, Crönlein T, Hajak G, Geisler P. Insomnia symptoms influence CPAP compliance. Sleep Breath. 2013;17(1):99–104. https://doi.org/10.1007/s11325-012-0655-9. Epub 2012 Feb 4. PMID: 22311553.

53. Wallace DM, Vargas SS, Schwartz SJ, Aloia MS, Shafazand S. Determinants of continuous positive airway pressure adherence in a sleep clinic cohort of South Florida Hispanic veterans. Sleep Breath. 2013;17(1):351–63. https://doi.org/10.1007/s11325-012-0702-6. Epub 2012 Apr 17. PMID: 22528953.

54. Nigam G, Camacho M, Riaz M. The effect of nonbenzodiazepines sedative hypnotics on apnea-hypopnea index: a meta-analysis. Ann Thorac Med. 2019;14(1):49–55. https://doi.org/10.4103/atm.ATM_198_18. PMID: 30745935.

55. Zhang XJ, Li QY, Wang Y, Xu HJ, Lin YN. The effect of non-benzodiazepine hypnotics on sleep quality and severity in patients with OSA: a meta-analysis. Sleep Breath. 2014;18(4):781–9. https://doi.org/10.1007/s11325-014-0943-7. Epub 2014 Jan 29. PMID: 24474447.

56. Rosenberg R, Roach JM, Scharf M, Amato DA. A pilot study evaluating acute use of eszopiclone in patients with mild to moderate obstructive sleep apnea syndrome. Sleep Med. 2007;8(5):464–70. https://doi.org/10.1016/j.sleep.2006.10.007. Epub 2007 May 18. PMID: 17512799.

57. Quadri S, Drake C, Hudgel DW. Improvement of idiopathic central sleep apnea with zolpidem. J Clin Sleep Med. 2009;5(2):122–9. PMID: 19968044.

58. Lettieri CJ, Quast TN, Eliasson AH, Andrada T. Eszopiclone improves overnight polysomnography and continuous positive airway pressure titration: a prospective, randomized, placebo-controlled trial. Sleep. 2008;31(9):1310–6. PMID: 18788656.

59. Berry RB, Patel PB. Effect of zolpidem on the efficacy of continuous positive airway pressure as treatment for obstructive sleep apnea. Sleep. 2006;29(8):1052–6. https://doi.org/10.1093/sleep/29.8.1052. PMID: 16944674.

60. Park JG, Olson EJ, Morgenthaler TI. Impact of Zaleplon on continuous positive airway pressure therapy compliance. J Clin Sleep Med. 2013;9(5):439–44. https://doi.org/10.5664/jcsm.2660. PMID: 23674934.

61. Carrive P, Kuwaki T. Orexin and Central Modulation of Cardiovascular and Respiratory Function. Curr Top Behav Neurosci. 2017;33:157–196. https://doi.org/10.1007/7854_2016_46.

62. Matsumura T, Terada J, Yoshimura C, Koshikawa K, Kinoshita T, Yahaba M, Nagashima K, Sakao S, Tatsumi K. Single-use suvorexant for treating insomnia during overnight polysomnography in patients with suspected obstructive sleep apnea: a single-center experience. Drug Des Devel Ther. 2019;13:809–16. https://doi.org/10.2147/DDDT.S197237. eCollection 2019. PMID: 30880914.

63. Sun H, Palcza J, Card D, Gipson A, Rosenberg R, Kryger M, Lines C, Wagner JA, Troyer MD. Effects of suvorexant, an orexin receptor antagonist, on respiration during sleep in patients with obstructive sleep apnea. J Clin Sleep Med. 2016;12(1):9–17.

64. Cheng JY, Filippov G, Moline M, Zammit GZ, Bsharat M, Hall N. Respiratory safety of lemborexant in healthy adult and elderly

subjects with mild obstructive sleep apnea: a randomized, double blind, placebo-controlled, crossover study. J Sleep Res. 2020;29(4):e13021. https://doi.org/10.1111/jsr.13021.

65. Moline M, Cheng JY, Lorch D, Hall N, Shah D. Respiratory Safety of Lemborexant in Adult and Elderly Subjects with Moderate to Severe Obstructive Sleep Apnea. Poster presented at: American College of Neuropsychopharmacology Congress; Dec 5–8, 2021; San Juan, Puerto Rico.

66. Murphy PJ, Moline M, Pinner K, Hong Q, Yardley J, Zammit G, Satlin A. Effects of Lemborexant on sleep architecture in subjects with insomnia disorder. Poster session presented at: SLEEP 2016; Jun 11–15; Denver, CO, USA.

67. Murphy P, Kumar D, Zammit G, Rosenberg R, Moline M. Safety of lemborexant versus placebo and zolpidem: effects on auditory awakening threshold, postural stability, and cognitive performance in healthy older participants in the middle of the night and upon morning awakening. J Clin Sleep Med. 2020;16(5):765–73.

68. Murphy P, Moline M, Mayleben D, et al. Lemborexant, a dual orexin receptor antagonist (DORA) for treatment for insomnia disorder: results from a Bayesian, adaptive, randomized, double-blind, placebo-controlled study. J Clin Sleep Med. 2017;13(11):1289–99. https://doi.org/10.5564/jcsm.6800. PMID: 29065953.

69. Yardley J, Mikko K, Inoue Y, Pinner K, Perdomo C, Ishikawa K, Filippov N, Moline M. Long-term effectiveness and safety of lemborexant in adults with insomnia disorder: results from a phase 3 randomized clinical trial. Sleep Med. 2021;80:333–42. https://doi.org/10.1016/j.sleep.2021.01.048.

70. Rosenberg R, Murphy P, Zammit G, et al. Comparison of lemborexant with placebo and zolpidem tartrate extended release for the treatment of older adults with insomnia disorder: a phase 3 randomized clinical trial. JAMA Netw Open. 2019;2:e1918254. https://doi.org/10.1001/jamanetworkopen.2019.18254.

71. Karppa M, Yardley J, Pinner K, et al. Long-term efficacy and tolerability of lemborexant compared with placebo in adults with insomnia disorder: results from the phase 3 randomized clinical trial SUNRISE-2. Sleep. 2020; https://doi.org/10.1093/sleep/zsaa123.

72. Harris M, Glozier N, Ratnavadivel R, Grunstein RR. Obstructive sleep apnea and depression. Sleep Med Rev. 2009;13(6):437–44. https://doi.org/10.1016/j.smrv.2009.04.001. Epub 2009 Jul 10. PMID: 19596599.

73. Ong JC, Gress JL, San Pedro-Salcedo MG, Manber R. Frequency and predictors of obstructive sleep apnea among individuals with major depressive disorder and insomnia. J Psychosom Res. 2009;67(2):135–41. https://doi.org/10.1016/j.jpsychores.2009.03.011. Epub 2009 Apr 25. PMID: 19616140.

74. Smales ET, Edwards BA, Deyoung PN, McSharry DG, Wellman A, Velasquez A, Owens R, Orr JE, Malhotra A. Trazodone effects on obstructive sleep apnea and non-REM arousal threshold. Ann Am Thorac Soc. 2015;12(5):758–64.

75. Eckert DJ, Malhotra A, Wellman A, White DP. Trazodone increases the respiratory arousal threshold in patients with obstructive sleep apnea and a low arousal threshold. Sleep. 2014;37(4):811–9. https://doi.org/10.5665/sleep.3596.

76. Carley DW, Olopade C, Ruigt GS, Radulovacki M. Efficacy of mirtazapine in obstructive sleep apnea syndrome. Sleep. 2007;30(1):35–41. https://doi.org/10.1093/sleep/30.1.35.

77. Marshall NS, Yee BJ, Desai AV, Buchanan PR, Wong KKH, Crompton R, et al. Two randomized placebo-controlled trials to evaluate the efficacy and tolerability of mirtazapine for the treatment obstructive sleep apnea. Sleep. 2008;31(6):824–31. https://doi.org/10.1093/sleep/31.6.824.

78. Schmickl CN, Yanru L, Orr JE, Jen R, Sands SA, Bradley EA, DeYoung P, Owens RL, Malhotra A. Effects of venlafaxine on apnea-hypopnea index in patients with sleep apnea: a randomized. Double-Blind Crossover Study Chest. 2020;158(2):765–75. https://doi.org/10.1016/j.chest.2020.02.074.Epub. 2020 Apr 9.

CPAP Adherence in Patients with Obstructive Sleep Apnea and Depression

19

Danielle Penney and Joseph Barbera

Key Terms

OSA	*Obstructive sleep apnea:* A chronic sleep disorder involving repeated episodes of airway obstruction and hypoxia.
EDS	*Excessive daytime sleepiness*: One of the key symptoms associated with OSA.
REM sleep	*Rapid eye movement sleep*: A stage of sleep characterized by random rapid eye movements accompanied by low muscle tone in the body.
CPAP	*Continuous positive airway pressure*: a machine used in the treatment of sleep apnea that applies mild positive pressure to keep the airways open during sleep.
SWS	*Slow wave sleep:* a stage of the sleep cycle commonly referred to as 'deep sleep', and characterized by delta brain waves on electroencephalography.

19.1 Introduction

For over hundreds of years, humans have appreciated some kind of relationship between sleep and mental health. Over the past century, this association has been studied more systematically, and the reciprocal association between sleep and mental health has been confirmed. For example, many studies of people experiencing depression and anxiety have consistently shown significant sleep pattern disruption, and multiple studies have reliably found that individuals experiencing insomnia often also have difficulties with depression and anxiety and that insomnia can lead to depression [1].

Reports of sleep disorders involving apneic events during sleep have been described for over 150 years—in the late 1800s, the term "Pickwickian syndrome" was used to describe apneic symptoms in obese patients. In 1965, the first polysomnograph recorded apneas during sleep, leading to the recognition of what we now know as obstructive sleep apnea [2]. The discovery of sleep apnea in 1965 is now regarded as one of the most important advances in the history of sleep medicine.

Obstructive sleep apnea (OSA) is a chronic sleep disorder characterized by repeated episodes of upper airway obstruction, resulting in the reduction (hypopnea) or cessation (apnea) of breathing during sleep. The sequelae of OSA consist of an interconnected myriad of both medical and psychological factors. Well-recognized medical consequences and of OSA include obesity, cardiac arrhythmias, and hypertension. It is almost a sin quo non in some conditions, such as in retinal vein thrombosis. However, OSA also consists of cognitive and psychological features related to waking behavior: such as excessive daytime sleepiness (EDS), mood changes, depression and anxiety, and decreased productivity (Fig. 19.1). OSA is regarded as a highly prevalent disorder throughout the general population, as it is currently estimated to affect 34% of men and 17% of women [3]. This figure also increases with age, as the rate of OSA in elderly populations is estimated to be between 30 and 40%. In patients with cardiovascular disease specifically, the prevalence of OSA is as high as 40% to 60% [4]. Furthermore, the general prevalence of OSA is increasing, likely owing to the global obesity epidemic coupled with an aging population. Over the past two decades, OSA prevalence rates have experienced relative increases between 14% and 55%, depending on subgroup [2].

Aside from being one of the most common sleep disorders, sleep apnea has a significant negative impact on both the individual and from a public health perspective. From the perspective of the individual, there are numerous short-term and long-term health consequences associated with sleep apnea. Studies have shown that individuals with OSA have an increased mortality and morbidity risk [5]. There are multiple interrelated mechanisms to explain the symptoms of OSA, but a significant number of these symptoms and risks stem from intermittent hypoxia due to repeated apneas, coupled with sleep fragmentation from microarousals (Fig. 19.2).

D. Penney (✉)
McMaster University, Youthdale Child & Adolescent Sleep Centre, Toronto, ON, Canada
e-mail: danielle.penney@medportal.ca

J. Barbera
Department of Psychiatry, University of Toronto, Toronto, ON, Canada

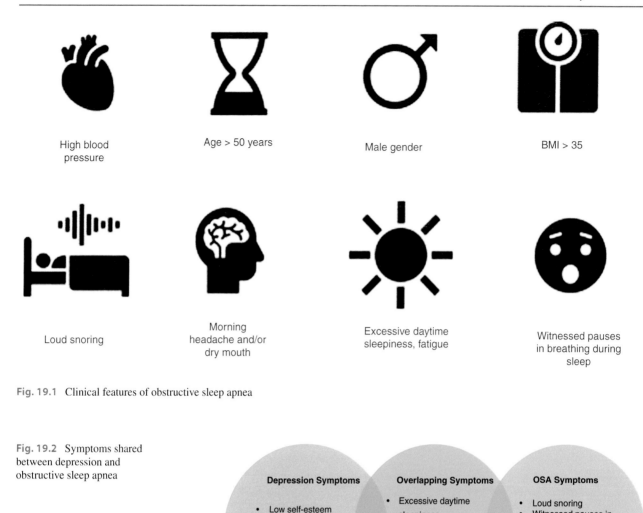

Fig. 19.1 Clinical features of obstructive sleep apnea

Fig. 19.2 Symptoms shared between depression and obstructive sleep apnea

These episodes of nocturnal hypoxemia can lead to spikes in sympathetic activity, which can increase heart rate and blood pressure.

Taken as a whole, these changes seen in OSA can lead to loss of the "restorative" function of sleep [6]. Clinically, this results in one of the cardinal symptoms of OSA: excessive daytime sleepiness. EDS has a number of far reaching effects, which can include disturbed mood, difficulty focusing, absence from work, or decreased work productivity. OSA has been associated with a poor quality of life, cognitive impairment [7], an increased risk of numerous cardiovascular diseases, and an increased risk of developing a number of chronic conditions [8].

From a public health perspective, individuals with OSA are predisposed to cause motor vehicle accidents as a result of their daytime sleepiness. A 2004 study by Sassani et al. reported that sleep apnea may cost 1400 lives annually due to car accidents in the United States (US) alone [9]. OSA has both direct and indirect economic impacts, such as decreased work productivity, increased motor vehicle and workplace accidents, increased healthcare utilization and medical costs, and traffic accidents [10].

19.2   Sleep and Depression

One of the most challenging aspects when examining sleep difficulties, from both a clinical and research perspective, is the identification of etiological factors. In reality, the root cause of a patient's sleep issues are often multifactorial and comprise of several medical, environmental, and psychological factors.

A number of studies have demonstrated an increased risk of depression with a number of sleep disorders including insomnia, restless leg syndrome, and delayed sleep phase syndrome [1]. Since its infancy, the scientific literature produced by the field of sleep apnea research has been primarily focused on the relationship between OSA and other medical conditions—such as hypertension and diabetes—as opposed to psychological factors. Over the last few decades, however, the body of knowledge concerning the relationship between OSA and psychological factors such as psychiatric symptoms has grown significantly. Multiple studies of patients with OSA have found the rates of psychiatric disorders to be as high as 60%, with depression being one of the most common [11].

Sleep disorders have traditionally been thought to be a consequence of mood disorders. In the 5th edition of the *Diagnostic and Statistical Manual of Mental Disorders* (DSM-5), sleep disturbances are listed as symptoms of multiple mood disorders. Numerous studies have asserted that sleep disturbances themselves, such as insomnia or sleep apnea, have been shown to be risk factors for the onset of mood disorders [12]. If sleep disorders were in fact a consequence of mood disorders, then it logically follows that successful treatment of the mood disorder should significantly improve, if not totally ameliorate, a patient's sleep difficulties. However, this is quite often not the reality. Studies have shown that in many cases, treating a patient's mood disorder does not resolve their sleep issues [13]. However, advancements in the scientific literature over the last two decades have led to a shift in understanding, towards viewing sleep disorders as comorbid conditions—not merely symptoms—of mood disorders. Furthermore, there is also evidence to suggest that in many cases, the sleep disorder may in fact be the underlying cause of the mood disorder.

Sleep disturbances and psychiatric disorders are closely related. Various forms of sleep disturbances are present in a number of psychiatric conditions, from mood disorders and post-traumatic stress disorders to substance abuse disorder and schizophrenia. Furthermore, hallmark polysomnographic changes during sleep have been noted in individuals who have specific psychiatric conditions. For example, several studies have shown an association between shortened rapid eye movement (REM) latencies in patients suffering a variety of psychiatric disorders, such as schizophrenia, panic disorder, and depression [14–16]. Depressed patients have been found to have reduced amounts of slow wave sleep (SWS) and increased REM sleep [24, 34]. Hatzinger and colleagues found that depressed patients with reduced SWS and increased REM sleep experienced a higher recurrence rate of their depression.

19.3 Depression and OSA

Both OSA and depressive disorders are common among adults throughout the general population. OSA patients exhibit a high incidence of depression, with reports suggesting that up to half of patients experience elevated depressive symptoms [17]. Major depressive disorder is characterized by a persistent sad mood or loss of interest in previously pleasurable activities, in addition to affective, cognitive, and neurovegetative changes that impact daily functioning. In studies examining depression in patients with OSA, depression has been assessed a number of ways, including clinical questionnaires for mood disorders, clinician assessments, or patients' self-reported symptoms. Studies that have assessed depression in OSA patients have had a range of results. However, this is most likely due to the fact that these studies varied significantly in terms of their methodologies. Since many symptoms asked about in general depression questionnaires could also be attributed to OSA in addition to depression, this represents a potential source of false positives. Questionnaires that have commonly been used in studies of OSA patient populations include the Center for Epidemiological Studies Depression (CES-D) Scale, the Hospital Anxiety and Depression Scale (HADS), and the Patient Health Questionnaire (PHQ-9).

Although there exists some variation in the results, the vast majority of studies—including a number of large, multicenter studies that have been published within the last decade—have concluded a positive correlation between OSA and depressive symptoms [7, 18, 19]. This also appears to be the generally accepted view among clinicians in the field of sleep medicine.

In a European study of over 18,000 adults, the prevalence of major depressive disorder in individuals with a diagnosis of OSA or other breathing-related sleep disorders was 17.6% [20]. This study also further stated that 18% of individuals with a diagnosis of major depressive disorder met the criteria for breathing-related sleep disorders [20]. Furthermore, this relationship persisted even after controlling for obesity and hypertension. A large retrospective study of patients diagnosed with OSA found that 21.8% also had physician-diagnosed depressive disorder—nearly three times the prevalence for patients without OSA [21]. In the setting of a sleep clinic, these numbers are even higher; a study of 167 Dutch sleep clinic referrals found that 47% of male and 55% of female OSA patients had a Beck Depression Inventory (BDI) score of ≥10, which is indicative of probable depression [22]. In a study of over 400 OSA patients at a US sleep clinic, 38% of the women and 26% of the men had self-reported depression [23].

The prevalence of OSA in males is twice as high when compared to females. Conversely, depression rates are higher in women than in men in the general population [24]. Women with OSA have been shown to be at higher risk of having comorbid depression compared to women without OSA [25]. To further complicate things, sleep apnea is more likely to be misdiagnosed as depression among women, likely due to the overlap in psychological symptoms [16].

All in all, the sum total of the evidence points towards there being higher rates of depression among OSA patients in both the community and sleep clinic settings than in the general population. Furthermore, some evidence also suggests an association/correlation between OSA severity (measured by apnea-hypopnea index) and depressive symptoms [26].

19.4 Potential Mechanisms

The relationship between OSA and depression is further complicated by the fact that these disorders have overlapping symptoms, especially when it comes to vegetative symptoms such as fatigue, poor concentration, loss of interest, insomnia, and decreased libido. Both depression and OSA share common comorbid medical conditions such as obesity, metabolic syndrome, and systemic inflammation (Fig. 19.3) [27]. While the exact mechanism of the association between OSA and depression is unknown, the reality is that the answer is likely interrelated and multifactorial, given the complexity of each disorder on its own, as well as their multiple overlapping symptoms. Currently, a number of possible mechanisms have been proposed.

It is well-known that sleep deprivation and fragmentation are linked to mood problems. One possible mechanism is that the frequent arousals and poor sleep quality during sleep that is seen in patients with OSA may affect mood. Specifically, the intermittent hypoxemia associated with OSA has been proposed to be a key factor in influencing mood changes. In a randomized controlled trial of OSA patients with comorbid depression, CPAP treatment and

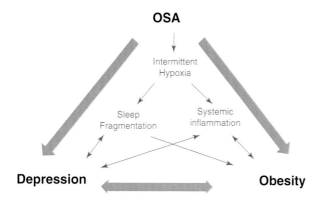

Fig. 19.3 Potential mechanisms behind the links between OSA, obesity, and depression

oxygen supplementation resulted in decreased psychological symptoms [23]. Since both of these treatments function to reduce hypoxia and subsequently increase blood oxygen saturation, this suggests that hypoxemia may play a role in the development of depression among OSA patients.

A 2008 study using fMRI technology showed differences in neural injury in the brains of OSA patients with and without depressive symptoms [28]. In the OSA patients with depressive characteristics, damage was evident in a number of neural structures, such as the hippocampus and caudate nuclei, thalamus, right internal capsule, as well as the medial pons and corpus callosum. This damage to several regions of white matter, such as the corpus callosum and the internal capsule, may reflect injury caused by the intermittent hypoxia associated with OSA [28].

The fact that there is significant overlap in the neurochemical pathways for both mood processes and sleep further adds legitimacy to this theory. In the brain, some inhibitory and excitatory neurotransmitters, such as serotonin, norepinephrine, and γ-aminobutyric acid (GABA), have been shown to be involved in both the sleep/wake cycle and mood regulation [28]. The locations of injury and aberrant function seen in OSA also happen to be parts of the brain that are affected in depression [28]. Thus, we are left with a variant of the classic "chicken or the egg" conundrum: it is possible that the depressive symptoms lead to the neural alterations seen in OSA, or conversely, it could also be that the neuropathology associated with OSA is what fosters depressive symptoms.

Aberrant function of the adrenal system also holds promise as a potential mechanism. Dysregulation of the hypothalamic-pituitary-adrenal (HPA) axis, a neuroendocrine system which plays a role in stress response, is a strong biological marker of depression. Hatzinger and colleagues found a significant association between dysregulated HPA system and sleep disturbances. It has previously been proposed that increased autonomic activity caused by the nocturnal awakenings and intermittent hypoxia of untreated OSA results in elevated cortisol levels and a disrupted HPA system, which could reasonably lead to a depressed mood [29]. Given this evidence, it is likely that for some patients with sleep disturbances and depression, the underlying neuroendocrine pathophysiology may be quite similar.

Systemic inflammation is also a possible link between the two conditions. OSA is associated with increased levels of pro-inflammatory cytokines such as IL-6 and tumor necrosis factor [30]. In individuals with depression, a similar immune profile has been noted, involving pro-inflammatory cytokines such as IL-1, IL-6, and interferons [31].

Since other comorbid chronic conditions have been recognized as both causes and consequences of obstructive sleep apnea—as is the case with hypertension—this could also be a factor involved in the correlation of OSA and depression, as depression has been shown to be prevalent among patients with chronic medical diseases.

While depression is common across patients with chronic conditions, obesity particularly holds considerable promise as a potential moderating variable between OSA and depression. Recent evidence confirms that obesity is a significant contributor to the development of OSA [32]. Not only is obesity a significant risk factor in the development of OSA, but evidence suggests that obesity level could influence sleep apnea severity [33]. A study evaluating the body mass index (BMI) of OSA patients found that overall, obese OSA patients had an apnea-hypopnea index double that of their non-obese counterparts. Aside from its relationship with OSA, there are significant suggestions in the research literature that an independent relationship between depression and obesity does exist [34–36]. For example, adolescents with depression have been shown to have an increased risk of becoming obese [37], and obese individuals have an increased risk of developing depression [38]. Since obesity appears to coexist with depression, it therefore follows that OSA might also covary with both conditions.

Evidence indicates that health-related difficulties mediate the relationship between OSAS and depression. For example, Akashiba et al. noted that in their study that scores on the SF-36 (a quality of life scale) were significantly lower in patients with OSAS when compared to age- and gender-matched controls [39].

Bardwell et al. (2003) used the CESD scale and found that one-third of the people they assessed with OSAS had significant levels of depression and that this level of depression predicted their fatigue [26]. Hence, while the exact mechanism of the relationship remains uncertain, it is clear that depression does play a role in the overall expression of OSAS. In reality, this link is likely complex and reciprocal.

19.5 Treatment of OSA

Although OSA is a prevalent and serious health problem, there fortunately exist a number of treatment options at present. The treatment options are widely varied and range from conservative measures such as weigh loss to invasive methods such as surgery (e.g., uvulopalatopharyngoplasty). Somewhere midway along this spectrum, other options include nightly use of a mandibular advancement appliance or an intranasal continuous positive airway pressure (CPAP) device. While there exists a number of possible treatments for OSA, nightly CPAP therapy remains the gold standard therapy in clinical practice, largely due to its high efficacy and low-risk profile [40]. CPAP therapy involves using a mask, or mask alternative, worn on the face and connected to an airflow source that supplies positive air pressure to keep the airway patent and prevent upper airway obstruction during sleep.

Current scientific literature overwhelmingly shows that CPAP therapy is necessary not only to reduce the harmful biological effects of OSA but also to improve mortality. In untreated OSA, mortality rates are around 20%, but this figure drastically falls to 3% in OSA patients on CPAP therapy [41]. Consistent CPAP use at the appropriate pressure level has been shown to reduce EDS, oxyhemoglobin desaturations, heart rate, and blood pressure while improving endothelial function [42], cognitive and sexual performance, and quality of life for the patient [7]. Furthermore, studies have shown that CPAP treatment also improves quality of life for the patient's bed partner [43] and decreases marital conflict [44]. Consistent CPAP therapy is associated with significant reductions in physician claims and hospital stays, as well as a reduction in motor vehicle accidents [45]. If all drivers with OSA in the United States were treated with CPAP, 980 lives and $11.1 billion in collision costs would be saved annually [9].

Numerous studies have examined the efficacy of CPAP treatment on symptoms such as EDS, hypertension, and heart rate. However, the impact of CPAP on depression has received comparatively less attention in the literature.

If a causal relationship exists between OSA and depression, it then logically follows that depression should be expected to improve with effective OSA therapy. The current evidence is in line with this assertion: most of the observational studies of depressive symptoms in OSA patients have shown that CPAP use has been associated with a reduction in depressive symptoms [46]. CPAP treatment has been shown to have a positive effect on depression levels in OSA patients, after as little time as one to 3 months [47].

A study of 41 OSA patients found that CPAP treatment significantly improved the psychological status of patient, seen as improved depression scores on the CES-D, and higher scores on the World Health Organization (WHO) quality of life scale, specifically in the domains of physical health, level of independence, and psychological health [7].

The exact mechanism by which this treatment benefit occurs is currently unknown. However, the improvement in depressive symptoms in OSA seems to involve the mitigation of the effects of obstructive hypoxia such as neural injury, sleepiness, fatigue, loss of libido, and impaired concentration [46, 48].

19.6 CPAP Therapy Adherence

It is clear that CPAP therapy effectively treats a number of symptoms associated with OSA and appears to especially improve adverse psychological features, such as depressive symptoms. However, all the aforementioned benefits of

CPAP therapy rely on consistent CPAP use. While there are undoubtedly numerous benefits of CPAP treatment, this is a moot point if patients do not adhere to this treatment.

Adherence with CPAP treatment is qualitatively defined as a regular, consistent CPAP use. Objectively, "ideal" usage is generally said to be around 6 to 8 hours per night. In some studies, researchers have defined CPAP adherence to be as little as 4 hours per night for 70% of nights [29].

Poor adherence with CPAP therapy is the biggest barrier to effective treatment of OSA, with patients typically discontinuing therapy during the first 4 weeks of treatment. It is estimated that only 50% of patients who are started on CPAP therapy will still be using it a year later, and even within that 50%, most will not be using their CPAP machine for the entire night [49]. Of this 50%, average compliance rates range from 4.7 to 6 hours per night, globally [50].

The most common reasons for non-compliance reported by patients include adverse side effects of treatment (e.g., discomfort, nasal dryness) and difficulty adapting to the pressure setting (i.e., difficulty exhaling or air swallowing) [40]. There are a vast number of factors that influence patient adherence. These factors can generally be divided into three categories: patient/sociodemographic, apnea-related (e.g., severity), and CPAP-related (e.g., pressure level).

19.7 Depression and CPAP Adherence

There are also a number of psychological variables related to CPAP adherence that have recently been identified. A patient having a greater internal locus of control, a higher health value, greater social support, and self-referred for OSA assessment (as opposed to a partner-initiated referral) has been associated with increased CPAP compliance [40]. Additionally, the occurrence of major life events beginning prior to CPAP therapy predicts poorer adherence [51]. Incidentally, these factors have also been shown to play a role in the depression; having a greater external locus of control and having a decreased amount of social support have been shown to be associated with depression [58]. Significant life events are also associated with first episodes of depression, as well as greater symptom severity [52]. Since the factors that contribute to OSA non-compliance also play a role in depression, this further adds to a potential link between the two.

Across a range of chronic conditions, depression is a known risk factor for medication non-compliance [53]. Since depression is a both a prevalent comorbidity in patients with OSA and a risk factor for non-compliance, the effect of depression on treatment compliance in sleep apnea warrants special attention. Studies using self-report depression scales have found that higher depression scores predicted significantly fewer hours of CPAP use (54s). This has been further supported by a 2014 study which found an independent association between depression and lower adherence during a home-based autoPAP titration [54]. A study of 28 male veterans reported that a number of variables, including depressive personality traits, explained 62% of the total variance of CPAP adherence [55].

Several mechanisms may be responsible for the association of depression and low adherence with CPAP treatment. As previously discussed, fatigue is a key symptom that is common to both depression and OSA. A number of studies have shown that the fatigue experienced by OSA patients is more closely related to the presence of depressive symptoms, rather than the severity of the OSA itself [26].

Reduction in sleepiness is the greatest known factor associated with increased adherence. While EDS and fatigue are distinct concepts, untreated depression-related fatigue may be confused with sleepiness from OSA by the general public, and fatigue due to depression may be interpreted as sleepiness from OSA. Thus, improvement of sleepiness symptoms on CPAP therapy may not be as noticeable for the patient if depression-related fatigue is still present. If the depression and its related fatigue are untreated, a patient may incorrectly conclude that the CPAP therapy was ineffective and abandon treatment. This is yet another of why depression screening in OSA patients is absolutely paramount.

It is well-known that the negative side effects of CPAP therapy are one of the most common reasons for patient non-compliance. Commonly experienced side effects include mask discomfort, claustrophobia, nasal congestion, and dry mouth. Research has shown that individuals with depression tend to report more symptoms regardless of the objective severity of the condition [56]. Thus, it is possible that OSA patients with depression are less tolerant of the negative side effects of CPAP therapy, causing them to terminate therapy prematurely compared to their non-depressed counterparts.

As previously discussed, since obesity is a common denominator between both OSA and depression, it is also possible that obesity could be having an effect on compliance levels.

Having a greater internal locus of control has been shown to be important in increasing CPAP adherence [57]. However, obesity has been found to be significantly associated with a greater external locus of control, as well as lower self-efficacy [58].

In summary, a patient's decision to use, or not use, CPAP is multifaceted, and the body of knowledge concerning the cognitive and psychological factors that influence CPAP adherence continues to expand.

19.8 Clinical Application

From a clinical perspective, it is important to understand how depression could potentially be a barrier to CPAP treatment, to aid in developing effective strategies to address and mitigate this non-compliance risk, to improve patient compliance and subsequently lower morbidity and mortality.

Many patients present with both OSA and major depression together. The most common symptoms of OSA and depression are fatigue and sleep disturbance. Both of these problems can disguise each other because of their similar symptoms, which presents a problem for the treating clinician. In higher-risk populations such as elderly patients, some clinicians have advocated for the ruling out of OSA *before* antidepressant treatment is initiated, since antidepressant medications do not help improve depressive symptoms due to OSA, coupled with the fact that OSA already has a high prevalence in older populations. Since CPAP has been shown to be an extremely effective treatment for OSA, the presentation of an OSA patient who does not seem to be improving on CPAP therapy should raise flags in the clinician's mind to initiate depression screening.

Since depression has been found to covary with OSA, it therefore follows that regular, proactive screening and treatment of depression prior to, or concurrent with, the initiation of CPAP therapy may hold potential as a promising method of increasing CPAP adherence. This is a small step that if taken by clinicians involved in the care of patients with sleep apnea could significantly improve patients' CPAP adherence, thus reducing their risk for the increased morbidity and mortality associated with untreated sleep apnea. However, further investigation is needed to determine if screening and treating depression improves outcomes in OSA patients.

Conversely, it should be emphasized to the patient with comorbid depression and OSA that the treatment of the OSA should be considered an essential part of their psychiatric treatment, along with any concurrent psychopharmacology or psychotherapy measures being undertaken. The effective treatment of sleep apnea should be seen as a necessary if not sufficient condition for the resolution of depressive symptoms. In addition to supportive psychotherapy measures, such patients may also benefit from an intensification of more specific psychological strategies designed to improve CPAP adherence such as motivation enhancement therapy [59] and cognitive behavioral therapy [60, 61].

19.9 Conclusion

Obstructive sleep apnea is associated with an increased prevalence of depression. The recognition of the coexistence of these conditions within a given patient is complicated by the overlapping nature of their respective symptom profiles. The recognition of depression in a patient with an OSA, and an appreciation of the interaction between these two conditions, is essential for the clinician in the management of such complex patients, including the addressing of barriers to CPAP adherence.

References

1. Ahmadi N, Saleh P, Shapiro CM. The association between sleep disorders and depression: implications for treatment. Sleep and mental illness. Cambridge, UK: Cambridge University Press; 2010. p. 154–64.
2. Jung R, Kuhlo W. Neurophysiological studies of abnormal night sleep and the Pickwickian syndrome. In: Akert K, Bally C, Schadé JP, editors. Progress in brain research [Internet]. Elsevier; 1965 [cited 2020 May 24]. p. 140–59. (Sleep Mechanisms; vol. 18). Available from: http://www.sciencedirect.com/science/article/pii/S0079612308635906.
3. Peppard PE, Young T, Barnet JH, Palta M, Hagen EW, Hla KM. Increased prevalence of sleep-disordered breathing in adults. Am J Epidemiol. 2013;177(9):1006–14.
4. Johnson KG, Johnson DC. Frequency of sleep apnea in stroke and TIA patients: a meta-analysis. J Clin Sleep Med. 2010;6(2):131–7.
5. Sleep apnea as an independent risk factor for all-cause mortality: the Busselton Health Study | Sleep | Oxford Academic [Internet]. [cited 2020 Sep 4]. Available from: https://academic.oup.com/sleep/article/31/8/1079/2454239.
6. Prevalence and correlates of nonrestorative sleep complaints | Sleep Medicine | JAMA Internal Medicine | JAMA Network [Internet]. [cited 2020 Sep 4]. Available from: https://jamanetwork.com/journals/jamainternalmedicine/article-abstract/486352.
7. Diamanti C, Manali E, Ginieri-Coccossis M, Vougas K, Cholidou K, Markozannes E, et al. Depression, physical activity, energy consumption, and quality of life in OSA patients before and after CPAP treatment. Sleep Breath. 2013;17(4):1159–68.
8. Tietjens JR, Claman D, Kezirian EJ, De Marco T, Mirzayan A, Sadroonri B, et al. Obstructive sleep apnea in cardiovascular disease: a review of the literature and proposed multidisciplinary clinical management strategy. J Am Heart Assoc [Internet]. 2018 [cited 2020 May 24];8(1). Available from: https://www.ncbi.nlm.nih.gov/pmc/articles/PMC6405725/.
9. Sassani A, Findley LJ, Kryger M, Goldlust E, George C, Davidson TM. Reducing motor-vehicle collisions, costs, and fatalities by treating obstructive sleep apnea syndrome. Sleep. 2004;27(3):453–8.
10. Scalzitti NJ, O'Connor PD, Nielsen SW, Aden JK, Brock MS, Taylor DM, et al. Obstructive sleep apnea is an independent risk factor for hospital readmission. J Clin Sleep Med. 2018;14(05):753–8.
11. Pillar G, Lavie P. Psychiatric symptoms in sleep apnea syndrome: effects of gender and respiratory disturbance index. Chest. 1998;114(3):697–703.
12. Möller PH-J. Outcomes in major depressive disorder: the evolving concept of remission and its implications for treatment. World J Biol Psychiatry. 2008;9(2):102–14.
13. Becker PM. Treatment of sleep dysfunction and psychiatric disorders. Curr Treat Options Neurol. 2006;8(5):367–75.
14. Zarcone VP, Benson KL, Berger PA. Abnormal rapid eye movement latencies in Schizophrenia. Arch Gen Psychiatry. 1987;44(1):45–8.
15. Berger M, Calker DV, Riemann D. Sleep and manipulations of the sleep–wake rhythm in depression. Acta Psychiatr Scand. 2003;108(s418):83–91.

16. Stefos G, Staner L, Kerkhofs M, Hubain P, Mendlewicz J, Linkowski P. Shortened REM latency as a psychobiological marker for psychotic depression? An age-, gender-, and polarity-controlled study. Biol Psychiatry. 1998;44(12):1314–20.

17. Harris M, Glozier N, Ratnavadivel R, Grunstein RR. Obstructive sleep apnea and depression. Sleep Med Rev. 2009;13(6):437–44.

18. Asghari A, Mohammadi F, Kamrava SK, Tavakoli S, Farhadi M. Severity of depression and anxiety in obstructive sleep apnea syndrome. Eur Arch Otorhinolaryngol. 2012;269(12):2549–53.

19. Jehan S, Auguste E, Pandi-Perumal SR, Kalinowski J, Myers AK, Zizi F, et al. Depression, obstructive sleep apnea and psychosocial health. Sleep Med Disord [Internet]. 2017 [cited 2020 May 24];1(3). Available from: https://www.ncbi.nlm.nih.gov/pmc/articles/PMC5836734/.

20. Ohayon MM. The effects of breathing-related sleep disorders on mood disturbances in the general population. J Clin Psychiatry. 2003;64(10):1195–200; quiz, 1274–6.

21. Sharafkhaneh A, Giray N, Richardson P, Young T, Hirshkowitz M. Association of psychiatric disorders and sleep apnea in a large cohort. Sleep. 2005;28(11):1405–11.

22. Vandeputte M, de Weerd A. Sleep disorders and depressive feelings: a global survey with the Beck depression scale. Sleep Med. 2003;4(4):343–5.

23. Wahner-Roedler DL, Olson EJ, Narayanan S, Sood R, Hanson AC, Loehrer LL, et al. Gender-specific differences in a patient population with obstructive sleep apnea-hypopnea syndrome. Gend Med. 2007;4(4):329–38.

24. Albert PR. Why is depression more prevalent in women? J Psychiatry Neurosci. 2015;40(4):219–21.

25. Maria B, Hung-Mo L, Slobodanka P, Alexios S, Bixler EO, Vgontzas AN. Lack of regular exercise, depression, and degree of apnea are predictors of excessive daytime sleepiness in patients with sleep apnea: sex differences. J Clin Sleep Med. 2008;04(01):19–25.

26. Bardwell WA, Moore P, Ancoli-Israel S, Dimsdale JE. Fatigue in obstructive sleep apnea: driven by depressive symptoms instead of apnea severity? Am J Psychiatry. 2003;160(2):350–5.

27. Andrews JG, Oei TP. The roles of depression and anxiety in the understanding and treatment of obstructive sleep apnea syndrome. Clin Psychol Rev. 2004;24(8):1031–49.

28. Cross RL, Kumar R, Macey PM, Doering LV, Alger JR, Yan-Go FL, et al. Neural alterations and depressive symptoms in obstructive sleep apnea patients. Sleep. 2008;31(8):1103–9.

29. Hatzinger M, Hemmeter UM, Brand S, Ising M, Holsboer-Trachsler E. Electroencephalographic sleep profiles in treatment course and long-term outcome of major depression: association with DEX/CRH-test response. J Psychiatr Res. 2004;38(5):453–65.

30. Ciftci TU, Kokturk O, Bukan N, Bilgihan A. The relationship between serum cytokine levels with obesity and obstructive sleep apnea syndrome. Cytokine. 2004;28(2):87–91.

31. Kim Y-K, Na K-S, Myint A-M, Leonard BE. The role of pro-inflammatory cytokines in neuroinflammation, neurogenesis and the neuroendocrine system in major depression. Prog Neuro-Psychopharmacol Biol Psychiatry. 2016;4(64):277–84.

32. Vgontzas AN, Tan TL, Bixler EO, Martin LF, Shubert D, Kales A. Sleep apnea and sleep disruption in obese patients. Arch Intern Med. 1994;154(15):1705–11.

33. Schwartz AR, Patil SP, Laffan AM, Polotsky V, Schneider H, Smith PL. Obesity and obstructive sleep apnea. Proc Am Thorac Soc. 2008;5(2):185–92.

34. Faith MS, Matz PE, Jorge MA. Obesity–depression associations in the population. J Psychosom Res. 2002;53(4):935–42.

35. Luppino FS, de Wit LM, Bouvy PF, Stijnen T, Cuijpers P, Penninx BWJH, et al. Overweight, obesity, and depression: a systematic review and meta-analysis of longitudinal studies. Arch Gen Psychiatry. 2010;67(3):220–9.

36. Stunkard AJ, Faith MS, Allison KC. Depression and obesity. Biol Psychiatry. 2003;54(3):330–7.

37. A prospective study of the role of depression in the development and persistence of adolescent obesity | American Academy of Pediatrics [Internet]. [cited 2020 Sep 5]. Available from: https://pediatrics.aappublications.org/content/110/3/497.short.

38. Dixon JB, Dixon ME, O'Brien PE. Depression in association with severe obesity: changes with weight loss. Arch Intern Med. 2003;163(17):2058–65.

39. Akashiba T, Kawahara S, Akahoshi T, Omori C, Saito O, Majima T, et al. Relationship between quality of life and mood or depression in patients with severe obstructive sleep apnea syndrome. Chest. 2002;122(3):861–5.

40. Shapiro GK, Shapiro CM. Factors that influence CPAP adherence: an overview. Sleep Breath. 2010;14(4):323–35.

41. Marti S, Sampol G, Muñoz X, Torres F, Roca A, Lloberes P, et al. Mortality in severe sleep apnoea/hypopnoea syndrome patients: impact of treatment. Eur Respir J. 2002;20(6):1511–8.

42. Ip MSM, Tse H-F, Lam B, Tsang KWT, Lam W-K. Endothelial function in obstructive sleep apnea and response to treatment. Am J Respir Crit Care Med. 2004;169(3):348–53.

43. Parish JM, Lyng PJ. Quality of life in bed partners of patients with obstructive sleep apnea or hypopnea after treatment with continuous positive airway pressure. Chest. 2003;124(3):942–7.

44. Baron KG, Smith TW, Czajkowski LA, Gunn HE, Jones CR. Relationship quality and CPAP adherence in patients with obstructive sleep apnea. Behav Sleep Med. 2009;7(1):22–36.

45. Leger D, Bayon V, Laaban JP, Philip P. Impact of sleep apnea on economics. Sleep Med Rev. 2012;16(5):455–62.

46. Habukawa M, Uchimura N, Kakuma T, Yamamoto K, Ogi K, Hiejima H, et al. Effect of CPAP treatment on residual depressive symptoms in patients with major depression and coexisting sleep apnea: contribution of daytime sleepiness to residual depressive symptoms. Sleep Med. 2010;11(6):552–7.

47. Weaver TE, Kribbs NB, Pack AI, Kline LR, Chugh DK, Maislin G, et al. Night-to-night variability in CPAP use over the first three months of treatment. Sleep. 1997;20(4):278–83.

48. El-Sherbini AM, Bediwy AS, El-Mitwalli A. Association between obstructive sleep apnea (OSA) and depression and the effect of continuous positive airway pressure (CPAP) treatment. Neuropsychiatr Dis Treat. 2011;7:715–21.

49. Sin DD, Mayers I, Man GCW, Pawluk L. Long-term compliance rates to continuous positive airway pressure in obstructive sleep apnea: a population-based study. Chest. 2002;121(2):430–5.

50. Reeves-Hoche MK, Meck R, Zwillich CW. Nasal CPAP: an objective evaluation of patient compliance. Am J Respir Crit Care Med. 1994;149(1):149–54.

51. Rotenberg BW, Murariu D, Pang KP. Trends in CPAP adherence over twenty years of data collection: a flattened curve. J Otolaryngol Head Neck Surg [Internet]. 2016 [cited 2020 Sep 5];45. Available from: https://www.ncbi.nlm.nih.gov/pmc/articles/PMC4992257/.

52. Kendler KS, Karkowski LM, Prescott CA. Causal relationship between stressful life events and the onset of major depression. AJP. 1999;156(6):837–41.

53. DiMatteo MR, Lepper HS, Croghan TW. Depression is a risk factor for noncompliance with medical treatment: meta-analysis of the effects of anxiety and depression on patient adherence. Arch Intern Med. 2000;160(14):2101–7.

54. Law M, Naughton M, Ho S, Roebuck T, Dabscheck E. Depression may reduce adherence during CPAP titration trial. J Clin Sleep Med. 2014;10(02):163–9.

55. Edinger JD, Carwile S, Miller P, Hope V, Mayti C. Psychological status, syndromatic measures, and compliance with nasal CPAP therapy for sleep apnea. Percept Mot Skills. 1994;78(3_suppl):1116–8.

56. Katon WJ. Clinical and health services relationships between major depression, depressive symptoms, and general medical illness. Biol Psychiatry. 2003;54(3):216–26.

57. Stepnowsky CJ, Bardwell WA, Moore PJ, Ancoli-Israel S, Dimsdale JE. Psychologic correlates of compliance with continuous positive airway pressure. Sleep. 2002;25(7):758–62.

58. Benassi VA, Sweeney PD, Dufour CL. Is there a relation between locus of control orientation and depression? J Abnorm Psychol. 1988;97(3):357–67.

59. O'Connor Christian SL, Aloia MS. Chapter 18 - Motivational enhancement therapy: motivating adherence to positive airway pressure. In: Perlis M, Aloia M, Kuhn B, editors. Behavioral treatments for sleep disorders [Internet]. San Diego: Academic Press; 2011 [cited 2020 Sep 1]. p. 169–81. (Practical Resources for the Mental Health Professional). Available from: http://www.sciencedirect.com/science/article/pii/B9780123815224000183.

60. Bartlett D. Chapter 21 - Cognitive behavioral therapy to increase adherence to continuous positive airway: model I: psycho-education. In: Perlis M, Aloia M, Kuhn B, editors. Behavioral treatments for sleep disorders [Internet]. San Diego: Academic Press; 2011 [cited 2020 Sep 1]. p. 211–4. (Practical Resources for the Mental Health Professional). Available from: http://www.sciencedirect.com/science/article/pii/B9780123815224000213.

61. Bartlett D. Chapter 22 - Cognitive behavioral therapy to increase adherence to continuous positive airway: model II: modeling. In: Perlis M, Aloia M, Kuhn B, editors. Behavioral treatments for sleep disorders [Internet]. San Diego: Academic Press; 2011 [cited 2020 Sep 1]. p. 215–21. (Practical Resources for the Mental Health Professional). Available from: http://www.sciencedirect.com/science/article/pii/B9780123815224000225.

Adherence with Treatment for Sleep Apnea in Patients with Comorbid Post-traumatic Stress Disorder

Ripu D. Jindal and Kawish Garg

Exposure to trauma can sometimes lead to the development of post-traumatic stress disorder (PTSD) for which the presenting symptoms include re-experiencing the trauma, distressing dreams, flashbacks, hypervigilance, and difficulty falling and staying asleep [1]. In the National Comorbidity Survey, lifetime prevalence of PTSD was estimated to be 7.8% [2]. Greater prevalence was noted in sub-populations such as men who saw combat and women who experienced sexual trauma. In the national Vietnam Readjustment study, 15.2 of men and 8.5% of women who served in Vietnam were found to suffer from PTSD 15 or more years after their military service [3]. Among US servicemen and servicewomen returning from more recent deployments, prevalence rates were estimated to be 31% for men and 27% for women [4]. PTSD has been shown to be highly consequential with increased risk of developing physical and other mental health problems [5] and increased healthcare utilization [6].

Sleep disturbances are considered as hallmark symptom of PTSD [7, 8]. Common sleep disturbances in PTSD include insomnia and nightmares. There is also evidence that sleep-related breathing disorder, parasomnia behaviors, and sleep-related movement disorders are more common in patients with PTSD [9]. When left untreated, sleep disturbances in PTSD can be persistent. In one study, those who experienced an avalanche continued to report sleep disturbances at 16-year follow-up [10]. Moreover, unless the sleep disturbances in PTSD are specifically targeted for treatment, those can be persistent despite treatment. In a study of 108 active-duty US Army soldiers who met criteria for PTSD after at least one deployment in support of wars in Iraq and Afghanistan, insomnia was the most frequently reported symptom before and after treatment for PTSD [[11]]. Among participants who did not meet criteria for PTSD, 57% continued to report insomnia. Similarly, in a Canadian study, cognitive behavioral therapy (CBT) had a favorable impact on sleep in patients with PTSD, but a majority of participants continued to suffer from residual sleep difficulties after treatment [12]. Furthermore, persistent sleep difficulties were associated with more severe symptoms of PTSD, depression, and anxiety after treatment. Notably, CBT used in the study was not designed specifically to target insomnia symptoms but included psychoeducation about PTSD, anxiety management techniques, cognitive restructuring, prolonged exposure, and relapse prevention. In contrast, multicomponent CBT tailored to treat insomnia, i.e., cognitive behavioral therapy for insomnia (CBTi), fares much better in addressing sleep disturbances in PTSD [13].

20.1 Treatment Choices in PTSD

Available treatments for PTSD leave much to be desired [14]. Only two medications are approved by the Food and Drug Administration to treat PTSD, and both of those, sertraline and paroxetine, are not known to address the sleep difficulties in PTSD. Prazosin, which showed promise in early studies, failed to outperform placebo in a larger phase 3 trial [15]. And antipsychotic agents offer only a modest benefit in addressing the sleep difficulties of PTSD [16]. Because of the many unappealing side effects associated with the use of antipsychotic agents [17], risk-benefit calculus does not seem to favor the use of these agents to address sleep difficulties in PTSD in patients who have not developed psychosis.

20.2 Sleep Apnea in Patients with PTSD

In a study of 159 veterans of recent conflicts in Iraq and Afghanistan, 69.2% screened to be at high risk for obstructive sleep apnea (OSA) on the Berlin Questionnaire. Furthermore, the severity of PTSD symptoms was associated

R. D. Jindal (✉)
Birmingham VA Medical Center, University of Alabama at Birmingham, Birmingham, AL, USA
e-mail: ripu.jindal@va.gov

K. Garg
Geisinger Holy Spirit Hospital, Camp Hill, PA, USA

with greater risk for the screening positive for OSA on the questionnaire [18]. Notably, even younger and leaner participants seemed to screen positive on the questionnaire.

Obstructive sleep apnea is consistently more prevalent in patients with PTSD across different studies, even though prevalence rates vary considerably from one study to another. A recent meta-analysis yielded a pooled prevalence rate of 75.7% in patients with PTSD when using an apnea hypopnea index (AHI) cut-off of 5 or more and 43.6% for the AHI cut-off of 10 or more. Furthermore, the subgroup analysis indicated that there was a difference in the prevalence of OSA in veterans with PTSD compared to non-veterans and mixed samples [19]. The meta-analysis also suggested that patients with PTSD had lower rates of adherence to CPAP therapy.

20.3 Impact of Positive Pressure Therapy on PTSD

The benefits of treating sleep apnea are so well-established that ethical concerns prevent withholding treatment for the sake of truly randomized trials that would allow definitive causal inferences. That said, data at hand suggest that compliance with positive pressure therapy (PAP) for OSA is associated with improvement in the severity of PTSD symptoms.

20.3.1 Evidence from Retrospective Chart Reviews

A retrospective study of 148 veterans with PTSD and newly diagnosed OSA, and a control group of those without PTSD, suggested that those with PTSD had lesser compliance [20]. Both the groups were comparable in their demographic profiles, though the rates of depression, nightmares, alcohol, and substance abuse issues were predictably greater in the PTSD group. Consistent with results from prior studies, there was lesser sleep efficiency and greater frequency of arousals in the PTSD group. PTSD predicted poorer CPAP adherence at 1-month follow-up. The decrease was detected in terms of proportion of participants who used CPAP for more than 4 hours on at least 70% of the nights, the average use per night, and percentage of nights with more than 4 hours of use. Additionally, nightmares predicted lesser treatment adherence at 30-day follow-up, whereas subjective sleepiness predicted greater compliance. Though the study design does not allow causal inferences, the results do raise the possibility that addressing daytime sleepiness with a stimulant medication may take away some of the motivation for complying with PAP therapy. Reducing the frequency and severity of nightmares remains a challenge [21]. As we plot our way forward, there may be merit in more focused approaches that aim to contain the impact of nightmares on PAP adherence.

A second retrospective study examined compliance with PAP therapy in active-duty soldiers and, consistent with the results from the earlier retrospective chart review, suggested that those with PTSD had lesser compliance with PAP therapy [22]. The authors also reported greater use of PAP in those taking "sedative" medications, i.e., benzodiazepines, non-benzodiazepines, or "atypical" antipsychotic agents, and a trend toward higher rate of insomnia among those with PTSD. The findings were not surprising in light of a previous report that sleep maintenance insomnia predicted poor PAP compliance [23]. The retrospective nature of the study was an important limitation of the study, but the data suggested the possibility that use of sedating medications may help improve some of the poor adherence to CPAP therapy in those with PTSD.

A third retrospective chart review compared frequency of nightmares before and after PAP treatment in 69 veterans with PTSD and sleep apnea [24]. The average numbers of nightmares per week at the two time-points were 10.32 and 5.26, respectively. Furthermore, compliance with PAP seemed to predict the apparent reduction in the frequency of nightmares. Although, in the absence of a control group, regression to the mean cannot be ruled out, the magnitude of the observed reduction suggests that some of it indeed reflects benefit stemming from treatment.

A fourth retrospective chart review examined data from 96 patients with comorbid sleep apnea and PTSD who failed continuous PAP therapy (CPAP) due to expiratory pressure intolerance or complex sleep apnea or both and underwent manual titration with bilevel-auto or adaptive servo-ventilation (ASV) [25] . The two advanced PAP therapies were associated with improvement in insomnia severity for both compliant and partial users. The investigators called for controlled trials to assess the impact of advanced PAP therapies on adherence and sleep and alertness outcomes.

20.3.2 Evidence from Prospective Studies

In a prospective study of combat veterans with PTSD and sleep apnea, average duration of PAP usage per night predicted decrease in the severity of PTSD symptoms after 3 months of PAP therapy [26]. The results were also notable because the two predominant reasons reported for PAP non-adherence were mask discomfort (33%) and claustrophobia (28%). The prospective nature of the study design was an important strength, but it was still limited by the lack of a control group.

A case-controlled observational cohort study at an academic military medical center examined 200 consecutive patients with PTSD, 50 patients with OSA but without

PTSD, and healthy controls without either PTSD or OSA [27]. In consistency with the results from retrospective studies, patients with PTSD were found to be less adherent after 4 weeks after initiation of PAP therapy. Group differences were detected in terms of percentage of nightly use, as well as the minutes per night usage. Furthermore, resolution of sleepiness and improvements in functional outcomes were poorer in the PTSD group even in the subgroup that showed comparable adherence. The results need to be interpreted in light of the inherent limitation of an observational cohort study design, but the study findings call for randomized clinical trials that compare PAP therapy with "enriched" interventions that combine PAP with pharmacological and non-pharmacological interventions.

A second prospective study detected reduction in the severity of PTSD symptoms during first 6 months of use of PAP therapy [28]. Although severity of PTSD symptoms was the primary outcome variable, the study also documented low compliance with PAP therapy in the participants. The lack of a control group was a notable limitation of the study; however, inclusion of newly diagnosed "PAP-naïve" patients with sleep apnea was an important innovation. Controlling for the "noise" of disease chronicity made the results more definitive, yet less generalizable.

In a third prospective study, compliance with PAP over 6 months predicted decrease in the severity of PTSD [29]. The diagnosis of PTSD was made via chart review on basis of scores on the PTSD checklist scale [30]. Interestingly, in those who scored lower on the PTSD checklist scale, and did not meet the cut-off score for the diagnosis of PTSD, poor compliance with PAP predicted increase in the severity of PTSD symptoms, which possibly reflected disease progression to overt PTSD. The limitations of the study design precluded causal inference, but the results provided a strong reason for follow-up investigations.

A crossover trial evaluating PAP versus mandibular advancement (MAD) demonstrated with PAP was more efficacious than MAD at improving sleep apnea; severity of PTSD symptoms improved during both treatment modalities; and the reported adherence to MAD was greater than to PAP [31]. The results suggested that MAD offers a viable alternative for veterans with sleep apnea and PTSD who are nonadherent to PAP.

A recent randomized crossover trial compared auto-titrating-PAP to SensAwake™, which was described as a wake-sensing PAP algorithm that lowers pressure in response to wakefulness, in treating comorbid sleep apnea and PTSD [32]. The assigned treatment was crossed over after 4 weeks. After adjustment for the differences in Epworth Sleepiness scores at baseline, PAP adherence was greater in SensAwake group after 4 weeks, however, SenseAwake by actual assignment did not show any effect on the outcome variables. The results seem to reflect a common drawback of the crossover trials: i.e. effects of initially assigned treatment can "carryover" and alter the response to subsequent treatment/s. Since a "washout" was not option, restricting outcome measurements to the latter part of each treatment period may have enabled the investigators detect a difference between the treatments. The results provide a strong reason to investigate SensAwake™ as a way to address pressure intolerance in patients with PTSD.

20.3.3 The National Adaptive Trial for PTSD-Related Insomnia (NAP)

NAP is a phase 3 clinical trial in PTSD and is sponsored by the VA Office of Research and Development (ClinicalTrials.gov Identifier: NCT03668041). It aims to test three sedating medications, i.e., trazodone, eszopiclone, and gabapentin, against placebo in addressing the sleep disturbances in veterans with PTSD. NAP offers important advancements over previous phase 3 clinical trials of PTSD, including two that are pertinent to this discussion. One, severity of insomnia has been chosen as the only primary outcome variable. The usually chosen outcome variable, the Clinician-Administered PTSD Scale (CAPS) score, has been relegated to being one of the eight secondary outcome variables. To our knowledge, this is the first phase 3 trial that aims to specifically target sleep disturbances in PTSD.

Two, uncontrolled sleep-disordered breathing, which the investigators are defining as an apnea-hypopnea index of 10 or more, is part of the exclusion criteria for the NAP trial. Given the high prevalence of sleep apnea among patients with PTSD, those with sleep apnea will be clinically treated to an AHI of less than 10 before they can be randomized to one of the study arms. The investigators will continue to monitor adherence and response to PAP therapy during the randomized phase. This is important since all the three drugs under investigation in the NAP trial have been previously shown to positively or negatively influence sleep-disordered breathing in small clinical trials. It remains to be seen whether these advancements become the "industry standard" for clinical trials of PTSD.

20.4 Conclusions

PTSD is a common condition with high morbidity and mortality. Sleep disturbances have been called the hallmark symptoms in PTSD, but are usually difficult to treat. Insomnia, sleep-disordered breathing, and sleep-related movement disorders are all more common in patients with PTSD than the general population. Furthermore, there are data to suggest that PTSD impairs treatment adherence to PAP therapy; and successful treatment of sleep apnea contributes to overall improvement in PTSD symptoms. However, ethical concerns preclude withholding treatment for sleep apnea for research purposes, which makes it difficult to ascertain whether treatment of sleep apnea improves PTSD symptoms. That said, we still have the option of comparing "enriched PAP plus" treatments against PAP therapy alone. Such enrichment can take the form of pharmacological and non-pharmacological interventions. Given the concerns about the safety of long-term use of benzodiazepines and the so-called "z" drugs, there is merit in investigating whether short-term use of one of these medications can be useful in kick-starting better adherence to PAP. Similarly, non-pharmacological interventions such as CBTi need to be investigated in combination with PAP therapy. There is also a need to systematically investigate whether more advanced PAP modes such as the bilevel-PAP are superior to CPAP in patients with PTSD and whether this possible superiority would justify the additional costs associated with the use of advanced PAP modes.

Given the paucity of good treatment options in the treatment of PTSD, it is still reasonable to randomize patients with PTSD to placebo or other sham "control" arms. The challenges are plenty, but we are encouraged to see insomnia severity index as the only primary outcome variable in an upcoming phase 3 clinical trial in PTSD.

As the research findings catch up with the clinical need to have answers, the clinicians will do well to pay extra attention to adherence to treatment for OSA in patients with comorbid PTSD. For non-psychiatrist sleep medicine practitioners, we recommend working closely with their psychiatrist colleagues to optimize treatments for patients with comorbid OSA and PTSD. For sleep medicine practitioners with training in psychiatry, the way forward could be to try to treat both the conditions simultaneously with the hope that breakthrough in treating one condition will trigger a positive spiral.

References

1. American Psychiatric Association. Diagnostic and statistical manual of mental disorders. 5th ed. Arlington: American Psychiatric Association; 2013.
2. Kessler RC, Sonnega A, Bromet E, Hughes M, Nelson CB. Posttraumatic stress disorder in the National Comorbidity Survey. Arch Gen Psychiatry. 1995;52(12):1048–60.
3. Schlenger WE, Kulka RA, Fairbank JA, Hough RL, Jordan BK, Marmar CR, Weiss DS. The prevalence of post-traumatic stress disorder in the Vietnam generation: a multimethod, multisource assessment of psychiatric disorder. J Trauma Stress. 1992;5(3):333–63.
4. Thomas JL, Wilk JE, Riviere LA, McGurk D, Castro CA, Hoge CW. Prevalence of mental health problems and functional impairment among active component and National Guard soldiers 3 and 12 months following combat in Iraq. Arch Gen Psychiatry. 2010;67(6):614–23.
5. Asnaani A, Reddy MK, Shea MT. The impact of PTSD symptoms on physical and mental health functioning in returning veterans. J Anxiety Disord. 2014;28(3):310–7.
6. Tuerk PW, Wangelin B, Rauch SA, Dismuke CE, Yoder M, Myrick H, Eftekhari A, Acierno R. Health service utilization before and after evidence-based treatment for PTSD. Psychol Serv. 2013;10(4):401–9.
7. Ross RJ, Ball WA, Sullivan KA, Caroff SN. Sleep disturbance as the hallmark of posttraumatic stress disorder. Am J Psychiatry. 1989;146(6):697–707.
8. Germain A. Sleep disturbances as the hallmark of PTSD: where are we now? Am J Psychiatry. 2013;170(4):372–82.
9. Baird T, McLeay S, Harvey W, Theal R, Law D, O'Sullivan R, Initiative P. Sleep disturbances in Australian Vietnam veterans with and without posttraumatic stress disorder. J Clin Sleep Med. 2018;14(5):745–52.
10. Thordardottir EB, Valdimarsdottir UA, Hansdottir I, Hauksdottir A, Dyregrov A, Shipherd JC, Elklit A, Resnick H, Gudmundsdottir B. Sixteen-year follow-up of childhood avalanche survivors. Eur J Psychotraumatol. 2016;7:30995.
11. Pruiksma KE, Taylor DJ, Wachen JS, Mintz J, Young-McCaughan S, Peterson AL, Yarvis JS, Borah EV, Dondanville KA, Litz BT, Hembree EA, Resick PA. Residual sleep disturbances following PTSD treatment in active duty military personnel. Psychol Trauma. 2016;8(6):697–701.
12. Belleville G, Guay S, Marchand A. Persistence of sleep disturbances following cognitive-behavior therapy for posttraumatic stress disorder. J Psychosom Res. 2011;70(4):318–27.
13. Talbot LS, Maguen S, Metzler TJ, Schmitz M, McCaslin SE, Richards A, Perlis ML, Posner DA, Weiss B, Ruoff L, Varbel J, Neylan TC. Cognitive behavioral therapy for insomnia in posttraumatic stress disorder: a randomized controlled trial. Sleep. 2014;37(2):327–41.
14. Krystal JH, Davis LL, Neylan TC, A. R. M, Schnurr PP, Stein MB, Vessicchio J, Shiner B, Gleason TD, Huang GD. It is time to address the crisis in the pharmacotherapy of posttraumatic stress disorder: a consensus statement of the PTSD Psychopharmacology Working Group. Biol Psychiatry. 2017;82(7):e51–9.
15. Raskind MA, Peskind ER, Chow B, Harris C, Davis-Karim A, Holmes HA, Hart KL, McFall M, Mellman TA, Reist C, Romesser J, Rosenheck R, Shih MC, Stein MB, Swift R, Gleason T, Lu Y, Huang GD. Trial of Prazosin for post-traumatic stress disorder in military veterans. N Engl J Med. 2018;378(6):507–17.
16. Krystal JH, Pietrzak RH, Rosenheck RA, Cramer JA, Vessicchio J, Jones KM, Huang GD, Vertrees JE, Collins J, Krystal AD, G. Veterans Affairs Cooperative Study. Sleep disturbance in chronic military-related PTSD: clinical impact and response to adjunctive risperidone in the Veterans Affairs cooperative study #504. J Clin Psychiatry. 2016;77(4):483–91.
17. Jindal RD, Keshavan MS. Classifying antipsychotic agents : need for new terminology. CNS Drugs. 2008;22(12):1047–59.
18. Colvonen PJ, Masino T, Drummond SP, Myers US, Angkaw AC, Norman SB. Obstructive sleep apnea and posttraumatic stress disorder among OEF/OIF/OND veterans. J Clin Sleep Med. 2015;11(5):513–8.
19. Zhang Y, Weed JG, Ren R, Tang X, Zhang W. Prevalence of obstructive sleep apnea in patients with posttraumatic stress disorder and its impact on adherence to continuous positive airway pressure therapy: a meta-analysis. Sleep Med. 2017;36:125–32.
20. El-Solh AA, Ayyar L, Akinnusi M, Relia S, Akinnusi O. Positive airway pressure adherence in veterans with posttraumatic stress disorder. Sleep. 2010;33(11):1495–500.
21. Waltman SH, Shearer D, Moore BA. Management of post-traumatic nightmares: a review of pharmacologic and nonpharmacologic treatments since 2013. Curr Psychiatry Rep. 2018;20(12):108.

22. Collen JF, Lettieri CJ, Hoffman M. The impact of posttraumatic stress disorder on CPAP adherence in patients with obstructive sleep apnea. J Clin Sleep Med. 2012;8(6):667–72.

23. Wickwire EM, Smith MT, Birnbaum S, Collop NA. Sleep maintenance insomnia complaints predict poor CPAP adherence: a clinical case series. Sleep Med. 2010;11(8):772–6.

24. Tamanna S, Parker JD, Lyons J, Ullah MI. The effect of continuous positive air pressure (CPAP) on nightmares in patients with posttraumatic stress disorder (PTSD) and obstructive sleep apnea (OSA). J Clin Sleep Med. 2014;10(6):631–6.

25. Krakow BJ, McIver ND, Obando JJ, Ulibarri VA. Changes in insomnia severity with advanced PAP therapy in patients with posttraumatic stress symptoms and comorbid sleep apnea: a retrospective, nonrandomized controlled study. Mil Med Res. 2019;6(1):15.

26. El-Solh AA, Vermont L, Homish GG, Kufel T. The effect of continuous positive airway pressure on post-traumatic stress disorder symptoms in veterans with post-traumatic stress disorder and obstructive sleep apnea: a prospective study. Sleep Med. 2017;33:145–50.

27. Lettieri CJ, Williams SG, Collen JF. OSA syndrome and posttraumatic stress disorder: clinical outcomes and impact of positive airway pressure therapy. Chest. 2016;149(2):483–90.

28. Orr JE, Smales C, Alexander TH, Stepnowsky C, Pillar G, Malhotra A, Sarmiento KF. Treatment of OSA with CPAP is associated with improvement in PTSD symptoms among veterans. J Clin Sleep Med. 2017;13(1):57–63.

29. Ullah MI, Campbell DG, Bhagat R, Lyons JA, Tamanna S. Improving PTSD symptoms and preventing progression of subclinical PTSD to an overt disorder by treating comorbid OSA with CPAP. J Clin Sleep Med. 2017;13(10):1191–8.

30. Wortmann JH, Jordan AH, Weathers FW, Resick PA, Dondanville KA, Hall-Clark B, Foa EB, Young-McCaughan S, Yarvis JS, Hembree EA, Mintz J, Peterson AL, Litz BT. Psychometric analysis of the PTSD Checklist-5 (PCL-5) among treatment-seeking military service members. Psychol Assess. 2016;28(11):1392–403.

31. El-Solh AA, Homish GG, Ditursi G, Lazarus J, Rao N, Adamo D, Kufel T. A randomized crossover trial evaluating continuous positive airway pressure versus mandibular advancement device on health outcomes in veterans with posttraumatic stress disorder. J Clin Sleep Med. 2017;13(11):1327–35.

32. Holley A, Shaha D, Costan-Toth C, Slowik J, Robertson BD, Williams SG, Terry S, Golden D, Andrada T, Skeete S, Sheikh K, Butler G, Collen JF. A randomized, placebo-controlled trial using a novel PAP delivery platform to treat patients with .OSA and comorbid PTSD. Sleep Breath. 2020;24(3):1001–9.

Relevance of CPAP in Ophthalmic Disease

21

Tavé A. van Zyl, Bobeck S. Modjtahedi, and Louis T. van Zyl

21.1 Introduction

Obstructive sleep apnea (OSA) is a common condition characterized by repetitive episodes of partial or complete collapse of the upper airway during sleep, leading to hypoxemia and recurrent arousal accompanied by sympathoactivation [1]. OSA carries many systemic sequelae and has been shown to be an independent risk factor for conditions such as hypertension and type 2 diabetes mellitus [2, 3]. The gold standard for diagnosis and classification of OSA is in-lab polysomnography (PSG), which enables quantification of obstructive respiratory events during sleep [4]. The apneic-hypopneic index (AHI) represents the number of these events occurring per hour, where an AHI of 5–15 is considered mild OSA, 15–30 moderate OSA, and >30 severe OSA. The first-line therapy for OSA is continuous positive airway pressure (CPAP).

Given its wide-ranging implications on vascular health and tissue oxygenation, OSA's potential impact on the eye – a highly metabolic, vascularized extension of the central nervous system – seems intuitive and has been the focus of extensive investigation [5–7]. In this chapter, we will briefly review the most commonly described associations between OSA and ophthalmic disease, with a particular emphasis on the potential for CPAP to mitigate the incidence and morbidity of these ophthalmic conditions. We will also discuss potential ocular adverse effects associated with CPAP use and considerations on how to approach these in patients in whom CPAP is indicated.

21.2 Ophthalmic Disease Associations with Obstructive Sleep Apnea and the Role of CPAP

21.2.1 Non-arteritic Anterior Ischemic Optic Neuropathy (NAION)

NAION is a non-inflammatory, non-vasculitic microvascular infarction of the anterior portion of the optic nerve [8]. Endothelial dysfunction and impaired autoregulation of the posterior ciliary arteries supplying this tissue have been implicated in its pathogenesis, which remains incompletely understood [9]. Major risk factors include increased age, male sex, white race, hypertension, diabetes (with evidence of end organ damage), and hypercoagulable states [10]. A structurally crowded optic disc, characterized by a small cup-to-disc ratio, has also been recognized as a key predisposing factor [11].

Evidence supporting a significant association between NAION and OSA consists of several case-control studies, as well as both prospective and retrospective cohort studies, reporting either an increased prevalence of OSA among NAION patients or increased incidence rates of NAION within OSA cohorts [12–19]. These studies are systematically reviewed elsewhere [5, 7].

The role of CPAP therapy in reducing the risk of NAION was explored in a large, retrospective cohort study utilizing billing records of 2,259,061 individuals within a managed care network in the United States [20]. After adjusting for confounding influences, the authors found that patients with OSA receiving CPAP therapy did not have an increased hazard for NAION compared to patients without OSA, while those with untreated OSA had a 16% increased hazard of NAION (HR 1.16; 95% CI, 1.1 to 1.33). While neither OSA severity nor CPAP adherence was addressed in this study, the documentation of CPAP therapy in the medical record appeared to demonstrate a protective effect.

CPAP non-adherence, defined as CPAP use for ≤3 hours per night, has been identified as a strong risk factor for

T. A. van Zyl (✉)
Department of Ophthalmology and Visual Science, Yale School of Medicine, New Haven, CT, USA
e-mail: tave.vanzyl@yale.edu

B. S. Modjtahedi
Department of Ophthalmology, Southern California Permanente Medical Group, Baldwin Park, CA, USA

L. T. van Zyl
Queen's University, Kingston, ON, Canada

© The Author(s), under exclusive license to Springer Nature Switzerland AG 2022
C. M. Shapiro et al. (eds.), *CPAP Adherence*, https://doi.org/10.1007/978-3-030-93146-9_21

second eye involvement in NAION. In a prospective cohort study of 89 patients with a history of NAION in one eye and PSG-confirmed OSA, Aptel and colleagues found an increased risk of bilateral sequential NAION among patients with severe OSA (AHI >30) who were noncompliant with CPAP treatment (HR 5.54, P = 0.04) [17]. Similarly, Chang and colleagues' retrospective chart review (n = 119) of patients with unilateral NAION reported significantly elevated risk of second eye involvement among CPAP nonadherent patients with either moderate (AHI ≥15) or severe (AHI >30) OSA (HR 4.50, P = 0.0015) [21].

21.3 Papilledema and Idiopathic Intracranial Hypertension (IIH)

Papilledema refers to optic disc edema resulting from elevated intracranial pressure of any etiology. IIH, the idiopathic form of pseudotumor cerebri, is a vision-threatening condition characterized by increased intracranial pressure in the absence of identifiable cause (such as tumor, dural venous thrombosis, medication, etc.), leading to compression of the optic nerves by cerebrospinal fluid (CSF) within their optic sheaths [22]. Untreated IIH can result in optic nerve atrophy and irreversible vision loss. Typical symptoms include headache (often worse in the morning), pulsatile tinnitus, and transient visual obscurations. The majority of adult IIH patients are overweight females of childbearing age; in pediatric populations, the association with gender and obesity remains significant only in pubertal patients [23].

Evidence linking OSA with papilledema and IIH is derived from small case series, retrospective cohorts, and observational studies [20, 24–28], which have been reviewed elsewhere [7]. The hypothesized mechanism by which OSA promotes papilledema, supported by evidence from studies utilizing invasive nocturnal CSF monitoring, is that hypercapneic cerebral vasodilation leads to decreased vascular resistance and secondarily increased intracranial blood volume which raises intracranial pressure (ICP) [29, 30]. Additionally, the increased systemic blood pressure, heart rate, and sympathetic tone associated with termination of an obstructive respiratory event has also been associated with a spike in ICP [31]. Even intermittently elevated nocturnal ICP can lead to papilledema [28].

Stein et al.'s previously mentioned retrospective cohort study of 2.2 million individuals within a managed care network in the United States found increased hazard of both papilledema and IIH among patients with OSA [20]. When patients with OSA were separately compared to non-OSA patients based on CPAP treatment status, the authors found that those with treated OSA had a lower hazard of developing IIH (adjusted HR 1.50 [95% CI 0.56 to 4.03]) than those with untreated OSA (2.03 [95% CI 1.65 to 2.49). In contrast to the protective effect of CPAP seen in IIH, and also in contrast to a smaller case series reporting resolution of papilledema with CPAP therapy [24], CPAP did not appear protective for papilledema in this cohort: when compared to patients without OSA, the hazard for developing papilledema was higher in patients with treated OSA than in patients with untreated OSA (adjusted HR 2.05 [95% CI 1.19 to 3.56] for treated versus 1.29 [95% CI 1.10 to 1.50] untreated). These observations must be interpreted with caution, as the treated and untreated OSA cohorts were not compared to each other, but rather to the control cohort without OSA. The lack of CPAP adherence data or OSA severity classification renders these results even more difficult to interpret; for example, it is possible that if OSA patients had higher baseline AHI values than untreated OSA patients, then poor CPAP adherence within this group may have resulted in more papilledema, thereby skewing the results. Despite these gaps, the observations support the primary observation of increased risk of IIH and papilledema among all OSA patients, regardless of treatment status.

21.3.1 Diabetic Retinopathy (DR)

Diabetic retinopathy and diabetic macular edema are leading causes of visual impairment and blindness in working-age adults and represent common microvascular complications of diabetes mellitus (DM) [32]; one in three patients with DM has a form of DR [33]. OSA and DM share many overlapping risk factors, the most prominent one being obesity. Patients with DR have been found to have higher rates of OSA than those without DR, and patients with OSA and DM are more likely to develop DR or experience more rapid progression [6, 34].

Over the past decade, a few clinical studies have addressed the role of CPAP therapy in mitigating DR risk or DR severity. In an observational, prospective longitudinal study of 230 patients with DR (as graded by retinal photographs) and OSA (diagnosed by home PSG), Altaf and colleagues identified OSA as an independent risk factor for DR progression (odds ratio, 5.2; 95% CI confidence interval, 1.2–23.0; P = 0.03) [35]. While not a focus of the study, the authors report that patients with high CPAP compliance, defined as ≥4 hours per night on >70% of nights, had lower rates of progression to advanced DR than untreated or noncompliant groups. Notably, the sample size available for this subanalysis was very limited: among 164 patients in the analysis, 38 patients had moderate to severe OSA, and only 15 were CPAP-compliant.

A small, prospective, uncontrolled study of 54 eyes of 28 patients examined whether CPAP compliance was associated with visual acuity outcomes in OSA patients with

DR and clinically significant macular edema [36]. High CPAP compliance was defined as continuous use of ≥ 2.5 hrs./night as determined via the CPAP machine's internal recording device. Clinically significant macular edema was defined as macular edema involving the fovea as documented on optical coherence tomography (OCT) and OSA by an oxygen desaturation index (ODI) ≥ 10 or AHI ≥ 15. A multivariate analysis controlling for duration of diabetes and systolic blood pressure showed that after 6 months of therapy, high CPAP compliance was associated with improvement in visual acuity versus low compliance (mean change in logMAR -0.11, 95% CI -0.21 to -0.002; $p = 0.047$). No statistical differences were noted between the groups in terms of anatomical improvement (measured by central subfield thickness on OCT) or DR severity score.

The positive results reported by Mason et al. were not replicated in a larger, multicenter, randomized control trial, the Retinopathy and concurrent Obstructive Sleep Apnoea (ROSA) trial (ISRCTN number 95411896) [37]. In this study, 131 patients with severe OSA (ODI ≥ 20 or AHI ≥ 30) and central macular edema were randomized to either standard ophthalmic care with nasal CPAP or standard ophthalmic care without CPAP, over a 12-month period. In multivariate analysis, there was no statistically significant improvement in visual acuity or change in macular thickness or DR severity among patients in the CPAP group versus control. During the study period, CPAP download data revealed overall poor compliance rates at each of the time points (3, 6, 12 months), where less than 30% of patients demonstrated ≥ 4 hours of continuous on $\geq 60\%$ of the nights.

21.3.2 Retinal Vein Occlusion (RVO)

Venous occlusive disorders of the retina, characterized by impaired venous return from the retinal circulation, represent the second leading cause of retinal vascular blindness after diabetic retinopathy [38]. RVOs are classified based on location of the obstruction, i.e., branch retinal vein occlusion (BRVO), hemiretinal vein occlusion (HRVO), or central retinal artery occlusion (CRVO). While age and typical atherosclerotic risk factors have been associated with all types of RVOs, compression of a retinal venule by a thickened and sclerotic arteriole at a crossing point within the retina is most often implicated in cases of BRVO, whereas additional risk factors such as hypercoagulable states or glaucoma may play a more prominent role in HRVO and CRVO.

Given the relationship between systemic vascular risk factors and RVO, OSA's proposed contributions to endothelial dysfunction, hemodynamic changes, and a proinflammatory milieu are likely to extend to the retinal vasculature. Indeed, significantly increased prevalence (up to 96%) of OSA has been reported among patients with RVO to the point that it has been suggested that all patients with RVO should be screened for OSA [39–42]. In a retrospective matched cohort study of 5965 patients with OSA and 29,669 controls, Chou and colleagues reported an adjusted hazard ratio of 1.94 (95% CI 1.03 to 3.65) of incident RVO [43]. The role of CPAP therapy and its influence on incidence rates or severity of RVO has not been reported.

21.3.3 Central Serous Chorioretinopathy (CSC)

CSC is an incompletely understood retinal condition characterized by focal, serous detachment of the retina associated with dysfunction of the underlying retinal pigment epithelium and thickened choroid [44]. Patients with CSC are typically working-aged males with type A personalities in high stress occupations, who present to clinic with new onset blurry and/or distorted central vision in one or both eyes. While acute episodes of CSC typically resolve without treatment within 4 months, chronic CSC is not rare and may lead to permanent scarring in the retina. Although the precise pathophysiology remains unknown, a prominent role for glucocorticoids and mineralocorticoids has emerged. Additional risk factors include smoking, emotional stress, systemic or topical steroid use, diseases with increased endogenous steroids, alcohol use, pregnancy, and untreated hypertension.

Numerous case-control studies and case series have explored the link between OSA and CSC, with conflicting results. In a systematic review and meta-analysis including 7238 patients (1479 with CSC and 5759 controls) from 6 studies, Wu and colleagues found that patients with CSC were more likely to have OSA (odds ratio, 1.56; 95% CI, 1.16–2.10) [45]. In a subsequent, population-based cohort study, Pei-Kang and colleagues analyzed records from 10,753 OSA patients (confirmed with PSG) and 322,590 control subjects in the Taiwan National Health Insurance Database [46]. After adjusting for age, gender, residency, income level, and comorbidities, the investigators found a significantly higher incidence rate of CSC in OSA patients compared with control participants (adjusted incident rate ratio for probable SA: 1.2 [95% CI: 1.1–1.4], $P < 0.0001$). The investigators further examined the role of CPAP therapy by dividing the OSA cohort into those with documentation of CPAP titration versus those without. They found that those in the CPAP group had a significantly decreased CSC incidence rate compared to those in the non-CPAP group (adjusted IRR [95% CI]: 0.5 [0.4–0.6], $P < 0.0001$). Due to the nature of the study, the investigators did not control for CPAP compliance or OSA severity.

21.3.4 Glaucoma and Intraocular Pressure (IOP)

Glaucoma represents a heterogeneous group of ophthalmic diseases characterized by a final common pathway of progressive excavation and degeneration of the optic nerve and characteristic visual field defects, which can lead to blindness [47]. Raised intraocular pressure (IOP), while not a diagnostic criterion, is associated with disease progression and remains the only modifiable risk factor.

Considerable controversy exists in the literature regarding the association between glaucoma (both normal-tension and high-tension types) and OSA. The largest studies to date examining this association have reported negative results [20, 48]; a recent systematic review determined that there was insufficient evidence to support a causative association [7]. Conflicting findings among other studies can be attributable to their small sample size, lack of PSG-based diagnosis, and failure to control for confounding variables. Identifying the relationship between OSA and glaucoma is made challenging by glaucoma's incompletely understood mechanisms and difficulty adjusting for confounders. Although Stein and colleagues found a relationship between OSA (regardless of treatment status) and glaucoma on univariate analysis, this relationship was not statistically significant after adjusting for confounding variables. The authors also specifically explored an association between normal-tension glaucoma and OSA but did not find one in either their adjusted or unadjusted models.

There is less work published regarding the role of CPAP therapy on glaucoma and IOP. In a unique interventional case series, Kiekens and colleagues measured diurnal IOP (i.e., every 2 hours throughout a 24-hour period, with patients always in a supine position) in 21 patients with newly diagnosed sleep apnea who had an AHI >20 and microarousal index ≥30 [49]. One of these patients carried a pre-existing diagnosis of glaucoma (normal tension type) with advanced visual field loss, and four additional patients were found on screening ophthalmic exam to have baseline IOP above statistically normal levels (i.e., ocular hypertension). One month after CPAP initiation, mean IOPs were significantly higher than at baseline. The authors also found significant nocturnal IOP elevation among all patients during CPAP application, which resolved 30 minutes following removal of the CPAP device. Shortcomings of this study included its small sample size and lack of control group. It is also unclear how much the CPAP mask itself contributed to IOP elevation versus the positive airway pressure and whether different masks may have different effects on IOP. Finally, IOP homeostasis is known to be impaired in patients with ocular hypertension and/or glaucoma; therefore, observations in normal subjects cannot be applied to or mixed with those in patients with the disease.

To further address the purported effect of CPAP on IOP, Cohen and colleagues performed a prospective study in 51 newly diagnosed OSA patients without glaucoma [50]. While the investigators observed nocturnal elevation of IOP in both CPAP and non-CPAP groups, there was no statistically significant difference between groups. The suggestion that OSA itself (independent of CPAP use) raises nocturnal IOP beyond expected levels is consistent with findings from Carnero, who found nocturnal IOP elevation in 20 non-glaucomatous patients with OSA who were not receiving CPAP in a prospective study using continuous IOP monitoring using a contact lens sensor [51]. Further studies are needed to clarify the association between OSA, IOP, and CPAP.

21.4 Ophthalmic Adverse Events and Considerations in Patients on CPAP Therapy

21.4.1 Dry Eye and Floppy Eyelid Syndrome

Dry eye syndrome is a very common ophthalmic condition with that increases in prevalence with age [52]. Symptoms include burning sensation, tearing, grittiness, foreign body sensation, and blurred vision that improves with blinking. The pathophysiology is multifactorial, and both systemic and environmental factors play a role. While there is very little published evidence that appropriate CPAP use directly worsens dry eye symptoms, there are a few relevant aspects to consider in patients with OSA on CPAP.

First, an ill-fitting CPAP mask may leak air and direct it toward the eyes, leading to evaporative desiccation of the ocular surface, especially in patients with nocturnal lagophthalmos. In extreme cases, this may lead to severe corneal and conjunctival infections [53].

Second, normal anatomy is such that a patent nasolacrimal system connects the nasal passages to the tear ducts, which are situated in the medial aspects of the eyelid margin; retrograde pressurized air flow may in this situation be directed toward the ocular surface even in the absence of mask leaks. This has been described in a case series and termed CPAP-associated retrograde air escape via the nasolacrimal system (CRANS) [54]. While CRANS is rare in patients with normal anatomy, up to 70% of patients who have had surgery to address epiphora (i.e., dacryocystorhinostomy, DCR) commonly experience nasolacrimal air regurgitation, and this may significantly impact CPAP compliance rates [55]. A cadaveric model study was unable to replicate CRANS in unoperated nasolacrimal systems at pressures as high as 30 cm H_2O; in post-surgical models, the authors found that initial pressures of 16 cm H_2O were required to cause air regurgitation [56]. Once air regurgitation was achieved, the CPAP pressure could be reduced to 6.5–8 cm H_2O to maintain air flow through the system.

Finally, floppy eyelid syndrome (FES) is a condition in which severe lid laxity leads to nocturnal lagophthalmos and ocular surface disease. While FES is not common in patients with OSA, patients with FES have been noted to have an increased incidence of OSA; FES can be diagnosed relatively easily in the office with a simple physical exam and should be considered in OSA patients with dry eye complaints. Evidence for the association between FES and OSA is reviewed elsewhere [37].

21.4.2 Postoperative Considerations After Ophthalmic Surgery

Patients who have undergone intraocular surgery, such as cataract extraction, glaucoma surgery, or vitrectomy, are most likely to present with vision-threatening bacterial intraocular infections (i.e., endophthalmitis) within the first 7 days postoperatively [57]. While rare, endophthalmitis usually leads to devastating loss of vision and, in some cases, loss of the eye. The risk of bacterial seeding is highest prior to epithelialization of the incisions and also if they are compromised mechanically. It is not uncommon for ophthalmic surgeons to recommend a CPAP hiatus immediately postoperatively for up to 7 days; joint management with a sleep specialist is ideal in these situations. While there are no reports in the literature of early postoperative endophthalmitis directly attributable to CPAP use, a case of late-onset endophthalmitis due to *S. mitis* was reported in a patient with a history of glaucoma surgery (trabeculectomy) using CPAP [58]. This case highlights the important point that patients with a history of incisional glaucoma surgery, especially trabeculectomy with adjunctive use of mitomycin C, are at lifelong risk of devastating infection, and any chronic therapy or habits must be carefully considered.

21.5 Conclusion

OSA has been linked to a variety of ophthalmic conditions that affect tissues fundamentally important for vision including the optic nerve and retina. Many of these conditions share common risk factors with OSA or may represent manifestations of similar pathogenic pathways. While evidence supporting the use of CPAP to reduce the risk or severity of these conditions is insufficient for a class 1 recommendation, this does not preclude a general discussion about the potential ocular health benefits of treating OSA and adopting healthy lifestyle habits. As many patients consider blindness to be the worst ailment that could happen to them relative to losing memory, speech, hearing, or a limb [59], educating

them about the potential sight-threatening conditions that are often comorbid with OSA may provide further impetus for adherence with therapy.

References

1. Bisogni V, Pengo MF, Maiolino G, Rossi GP. The sympathetic nervous system and catecholamines metabolism in obstructive sleep apnoea. J Thorac Dis [Internet]. 2016;8(2):243–54. Available from: http://www.ncbi.nlm.nih.gov/pubmed/26904265.
2. Mansukhani MP, Kara T, Caples SM, Somers VK. Chemoreflexes, Sleep Apnea, and Sympathetic Dysregulation. Curr Hypertens Rep [Internet]. 2014;16(9):476. Available from: http://link.springer.com/10.1007/s11906-014-0476-2.
3. Qie R, Zhang D, Liu L, Ren Y, Zhao Y, Liu D, et al. Obstructive sleep apnea and risk of type 2 diabetes mellitus: a systematic review and dose-response meta-analysis of cohort studies. J Diabetes [Internet]. 2020;12(6):455–64. Available from: https://onlinelibrary.wiley.com/doi/abs/10.1111/1753-0407.13017.
4. Qaseem A, Kansagara D, Forciea MA, Cooke M, Denberg TD. Management of chronic insomnia disorder in adults: a clinical practice guideline from the American College of Physicians. Ann Intern Med [Internet]. 2016;165(2):125–33. Available from: http://annals.org/article.aspx?doi=10.7326/M15-2175.
5. Huon L-K, Liu SY-C, Camacho M, Guilleminault C. The association between ophthalmologic diseases and obstructive sleep apnea: a systematic review and meta-analysis. Sleep Breath [Internet]. 2016;20(4):1145–54. Available from: http://link.springer.com/10.1007/s11325-016-1358-4.
6. West SD, Turnbull C. Obstructive sleep apnoea. Eye [Internet]. 2018;32(5):889–903. Available from: http://www.nature.com/articles/s41433-017-0006-y.
7. Wong B, Fraser CL. Obstructive sleep apnea in neuro-ophthalmology. J Neuro Ophthalmol [Internet]. 2019;39(3):370–9. Available from: https://journals.lww.com/10.1097/WNO.0000000000000728.
8. Biousse V, Newman NJ. Ischemic optic neuropathies. Campion EW, editor. N Engl J Med [Internet]. 2015;372(25):2428–36. Available from: http://www.nejm.org/doi/10.1056/NEJMra1413352.
9. Arnold AC. Pathogenesis of nonarteritic anterior ischemic optic neuropathy. J Neuro Ophthalmol [Internet]. 2003;23(2):157–63. Available from: http://journals.lww.com/00041327-200306000-00012.
10. Cestari DM, Gaier ED, Bouzika P, Blachley TS, De Lott LB, Rizzo JF, et al. Demographic, systemic, and ocular factors associated with nonarteritic anterior ischemic optic neuropathy. Ophthalmology [Internet]. 2016;123(12):2446–55. Available from: https://linkinghub.elsevier.com/retrieve/pii/S0161642016309149.
11. Jonas JB, Xu L. Optic disc morphology in eyes after nonarteritic anterior ischemic optic neuropathy. Invest Ophthalmol Vis Sci. 1993;34(7):2260–5.
12. Mojon DS. Association Between Sleep Apnea Syndrome and Nonarteritic Anterior Ischemic Optic Neuropathy. Arch Ophthalmol [Internet]. 2002;120(5):601. Available from: http://archopht.jamanetwork.com/article.aspx?doi=10.1001/archopht.120.5.601.
13. Palombi K, Renard E, Levy P, Chiquet C, Deschaux C, Romanet JP, et al. Non-arteritic anterior ischaemic optic neuropathy is nearly systematically associated with obstructive sleep apnoea. Br J Ophthalmol [Internet]. 2006;90(7):879–82. Available from: https://bjo.bmj.com/lookup/doi/10.1136/bjo.2005.087452.
14. Li J, McGwin G, Vaphiades MS, Owsley C. Non-arteritic anterior ischaemic optic neuropathy and presumed sleep apnoea syndrome screened by the Sleep Apnea scale of the Sleep

Disorders Questionnaire (SA-SDQ). Br J Ophthalmol [Internet]. 2007;91(11):1524–7. Available from: https://bjo.bmj.com/lookup/doi/10.1136/bjo.2006.113803.

15. Bilgin G, Koban Y, Arnold AC. Nonarteritic anterior ischemic optic neuropathy and obstructive sleep apnea. J Neuro Ophthalmol [Internet]. 2013;33(3):232–4. Available from: https://journals.lww.com/00041327-201309000-00005.

16. Arda H, Birer S, Aksu M, Ismailogulları S, Karakucuk S, Mirza E, et al. Obstructive sleep apnoea prevalence in non-arteritic anterior ischaemic optic neuropathy. Br J Ophthalmol [Internet]. 2013;97(2):206–9. Available from: https://bjo.bmj.com/lookup/doi/10.1136/bjophthalmol-2012-302598.

17. Aptel F, Khayi H, Pépin J-L, Tamisier R, Levy P, Romanet J-P, et al. Association of nonarteritic ischemic optic neuropathy with obstructive sleep apnea syndrome. JAMA Ophthalmol [Internet]. 2015;133(7):797. Available from: http://archopht.jamanetwork.com/article.aspx?doi=10.1001/jamaophthalmol.2015.0893.

18. Yang HK, Park SJ, Byun SJ, Park KH, Kim J-W, Hwang J-M. Obstructive sleep apnoea and increased risk of non-arteritic anterior ischaemic optic neuropathy. Br J Ophthalmol [Internet]. 2019;103(8):1123–8. Available from: https://bjo.bmj.com/lookup/doi/10.1136/bjophthalmol-2018-312910.

19. Sun M-H, Lee C-Y, Liao YJ, Sun C-C. Nonarteritic anterior ischaemic optic neuropathy and its association with obstructive sleep apnoea: a health insurance database study. Acta Ophthalmol [Internet]. 2019;97(1):e64–70. Available from: http://doi.wiley.com/10.1111/aos.13832.

20. Stein JD, Kim DS, Mundy KM, Talwar N, Nan B, Chervin RD, et al. The association between glaucomatous and other causes of optic neuropathy and sleep apnea. Am J Ophthalmol [Internet]. 2011;152(6):989–998.e3. Available from: https://linkinghub.elsevier.com/retrieve/pii/S0002939411003709.

21. Chang MY, Keltner JL. Risk factors for fellow eye involvement in nonarteritic anterior ischemic optic neuropathy. J Neuro Ophthalmol [Internet]. 2019;39(2):147–52. Available from: https://journals.lww.com/00041327-201906000-00001.

22. Ahmad SR, Moss HE. Update on the diagnosis and treatment of idiopathic intracranial hypertension. Semin Neurol [Internet]. 2019;39(06):682–91. Available from: http://www.thieme-connect.de/DOI/DOI?10.1055/s-0039-1698744.

23. Gaier ED, Heidary G. Pediatric idiopathic intracranial hypertension. Semin Neurol [Internet]. 2019;39(06):704–10. Available from: http://www.thieme-connect.de/DOI/DOI?10.1055/s-0039-1698743.

24. Lee AG, Golnik K, Kardon R, Wall M, Eggenberger E, Yedavally S. Sleep apnea and intracranial hypertension in men. Ophthalmology [Internet]. 2002;109(3):482–5. Available from: https://linkinghub.elsevier.com/retrieve/pii/S0161642001009873.

25. Bruce BB, Kedar S, Van Stavern GP, Monaghan D, Acierno MD, Braswell RA, et al. Idiopathic intracranial hypertension in men. Neurol Int. 2009;72(4):304–9. Available from: http://www.neurology.org/cgi/doi/10.1212/01.wnl.0000333254.84120.f5.

26. Marcus DM, Lynn J, Miller JJ, Chaudhary O, Thomas D, Chaudhary B. Sleep disorders: a risk factor for Pseudotumor Cerebri? J Neuro Ophthalmol [Internet]. 2001;21(2):121–3. Available from: http://journals.lww.com/00041327-200100020-00014.

27. Peter L, Jacob M, Krolak-Salmon P, Petitjean T, Bastuji H, Grange J-D, et al. Prevalence of papilloedema in patients with sleep apnoea syndrome: a prospective study. J Sleep Res [Internet]. 2007;16(3):313–8. Available from: http://doi.wiley.com/10.1111/j.1365-2869.2007.00598.x.

28. Purvin VA. Papilledema and obstructive sleep apnea syndrome. Arch Ophthalmol [Internet]. 2000;118(12):1626. Available from: http://archopht.jamanetwork.com/article.aspx?doi=10.1001/archopht.118.12.1626m.

29. Sugita Y, Iijima S, Teshima Y, Shimizu T, Nishimura N, Tsutsumi T, et al. Marked episodic elevation of cerebrospinal fluid pressure during nocturnal sleep in patients with sleep apnea hypersomnia syndrome. Electroencephalogr Clin Neurophysiol [Internet]. 1985;60(3):214–9. Available from: https://linkinghub.elsevier.com/retrieve/pii/0013469485900331.

30. Kirkpatrick PJ, Meyer T, Sarkies N, Pickard JD, Whitehouse H, Smielewski P. Papilloedema and visual failure in a patient with nocturnal hypoventilation. J Neurol Neurosurg Psychiatry [Internet]. 1994;57(12):1546–7. Available from: https://jnnp.bmj.com/lookup/doi/10.1136/jnnp.57.12.1546.

31. Wall M, Purvin V. Idiopathic intracranial hypertension in men and the relationship to sleep apnea. Neurol Int. 2009;72(4):300–1. Available from: http://www.neurology.org/cgi/doi/10.1212/01.wnl.0000336338.97703.fb.

32. Lee R, Wong TY, Sabanayagam C. Epidemiology of diabetic retinopathy, diabetic macular edema and related vision loss. Eye Vis [Internet]. 2015;2(1):17. Available from: http://www.eandv.org/content/2/1/17.

33. Yau JWY, Rogers SL, Kawasaki R, Lamoureux EL, Kowalski JW, Bek T, et al. Global prevalence and major risk factors of diabetic retinopathy. Diabetes Care [Internet]. 2012;35(3):556–64. Available from: http://care.diabetesjournals.org/cgi/doi/10.2337/dc11-1909.

34. Zhu Z, Zhang F, Liu Y, Yang S, Li C, Niu Q, et al. Relationship of obstructive sleep apnoea with diabetic retinopathy: a meta-analysis. Biomed Res Int [Internet]. 2017;2017:1–5. Available from: https://www.hindawi.com/journals/bmri/2017/4737064/.

35. Altaf QA, Dodson P, Ali A, Raymond NT, Wharton H, Fellows H, et al. Obstructive sleep apnea and retinopathy in patients with type 2 diabetes. A longitudinal study. Am J Respir Crit Care Med [Internet]. 2017;196(7):892–900. Available from: http://www.atsjournals.org/doi/10.1164/rccm.201701-0175OC.

36. Mason RH, Kiire CA, Groves DC, Lipinski HJ, Jaycock A, Winter BC, et al. Visual improvement following continuous positive airway pressure therapy in diabetic subjects with clinically significant macular oedema and obstructive sleep apnoea: proof of principle study. Theatr Res Int. 2012;84(4):275–82. Available from: https://www.karger.com/Article/FullText/334090.

37. West SD, Prudon B, Hughes J, Gupta R, Mohammed SB, Gerry S, et al. Continuous positive airway pressure effect on visual acuity in patients with type 2 diabetes and obstructive sleep apnoea: a multicentre randomised controlled trial. Eur Respir J [Internet]. 2018;52(4):1801177. Available from: http://erj.ersjournals.com/lookup/doi/10.1183/13993003.01177-2018.

38. Ip M, Hendrick A. Retinal vein occlusion review. Asia Pacif J Ophthalmol (Philadelphia, PA) [Internet]. 2019;7(1):40–5. Available from: https://journals.lww.com/apjoo/Fulltext/2018/01000/Retinal_Vein_Occlusion_Review.7.aspx.

39. Leroux les Jardins G, Glacet-Bernard A, Lasry S, Housset B, Coscas G, Soubrane G. [Retinal vein occlusion and obstructive sleep apnea syndrome] Occlusion veineuse rétinienne et syndrome d'apnée du sommeil. J Fr Ophtalmol [Internet]. 2009;32(6):420–4. Available from: https://linkinghub.elsevier.com/retrieve/pii/S0181551209001867.

40. Glacet-Bernard A. Obstructive sleep apnea among patients with retinal vein occlusion. Arch Ophthalmol [Internet]. 2010;128(12):1533. Available from: http://archopht.jamanetwork.com/article.aspx?doi=10.1001/archophthalmol.2010.272.

41. Kwon HJ, Kang EC, Lee J, Han J, Song WK. Obstructive sleep apnea in patients with branch retinal vein occlusion: a preliminary study. Korean J Ophthalmol [Internet]. 2016;30(2):121. Available from: http://ekjo.org/journal/view.php?doi=10.3341/kjo.2016.30.2.121.

42. Felfeli T, Alon R, Al Adel F, Shapiro CM, Mandelcorn ED, Brent MH. Screening for obstructive sleep apnea amongst patients with retinal vein occlusion. Can J Ophthalmol [Internet]. 2020;55(4):310–6. Available from: https://linkinghub.elsevier.com/retrieve/pii/S0008418219312943.

43. Chou K-T, Huang C-C, Tsai D-C, Chen Y-M, Perng D-W, Shiao G-M, et al. Sleep apnea and risk of retinal vein occlusion: a nationwide population-based study of Taiwanese. Am J Ophthalmol [Internet]. 2012;154(1):200–205.e1. Available from: http://www.ncbi.nlm.nih.gov/pubmed/22464364.

44. Kaye R, Chandra S, Sheth J, Boon CJF, Sivaprasad S, Lotery A. Central serous chorioretinopathy: an update on risk factors, pathophysiology and imaging modalities. Prog Retin Eye Res [Internet]. 2020;79:100865. Available from: https://linkinghub.elsevier.com/retrieve/pii/S1350946220300379

45. Wu CY, Riangwiwat T, Rattanawong P, Nesmith BLW, Deobhakta A. Association of obstructive sleep apnea with central serous chorioretinopathy and choroidal thickness. Retina [Internet]. 2018;38(9):1642–51. Available from: http://www.ncbi.nlm.nih.gov/pubmed/29474303.

46. Liu P-K, Chang Y-C, Tai M-H, Tsai R-K, Chong I-W, Wu K-Y, et al. The association between central serous chorioretinopathy and sleep apnea. Retina [Internet]. 2020;40(10):2034–44. Available from: https://journals.lww.com/10.1097/IAE.0000000000002702.

47. Weinreb RN, Leung CKS, Crowston JG, Medeiros FA, Friedman DS, Wiggs JL, et al. Primary open-angle glaucoma. Nat Rev Dis Prim [Internet]. 2016;2(1):16067. Available from: http://www.nature.com/articles/nrdp201667.

48. Girkin CA. Is there an association between pre-existing sleep apnoea and the development of glaucoma? Br J Ophthalmol [Internet]. 2006;90(6):679–81. Available from: http://www.ncbi.nlm.nih.gov/pubmed/16481379.

49. Kiekens S, Veva De Groot, Coeckelbergh T, Tassignon M-J, van de Heyning P, Wilfried De Backer, et al. Continuous positive airway pressure therapy is associated with an increase in intraocular pressure in obstructive sleep apnea. Investig Opthalmology Vis Sci [Internet]. 2008;49(3):934. Available from: http://iovs.arvojournals.org/article.aspx?doi=10.1167/iovs.06-1418.

50. Cohen Y, Ben-Mair E, Rosenzweig E, Shechter-Amir D, Solomon AS. The effect of nocturnal CPAP therapy on the intraocular pressure of patients with sleep apnea syndrome. Graefe's Arch Clin Exp Ophthalmol [Internet]. 2015;253(12):2263–71. Available from: http://link.springer.com/10.1007/s00417-015-3153-5.

51. Carnero E, Bragard J, Urrestarazu E, Rivas E, Polo V, Larrosa JM, et al. Continuous intraocular pressure monitoring in patients with obstructive sleep apnea syndrome using a contact lens sensor. Rowley JA, editor. PLoS One [Internet]. 2020;15(3):e0229856. Available from: https://dx.plos.org/10.1371/journal.pone.0229856.

52. Farrand KF, Fridman M, Stillman IÖ, Schaumberg DA. Prevalence of diagnosed dry eye disease in the United States among adults aged 18 years and older. Am J Ophthalmol [Internet]. 2017;182:90–8. Available from: http://www.ncbi.nlm.nih.gov/pubmed/28705660.

53. Harrison W, Pence N, Kovacich S. Anterior segment complications secondary to continuous positive airway pressure machine treatment in patients with obstructive sleep apnea. Optom - J Am Optom Assoc [Internet]. 2007;78(7):352–5. Available from: https://linkinghub.elsevier.com/retrieve/pii/S1529183907001169.

54. Singh NP, Walker RJE, Cowan F, Davidson AC, Roberts DN. Retrograde air escape via the nasolacrimal system. Ann Otol Rhinol Laryngol [Internet]. 2014;123(5):321–4. Available from: http://journals.sagepub.com/doi/10.1177/0003489414525924.

55. Vicinanzo MG, Allamneni C, Compton CJ, Long JA, Nabavi CB. The prevalence of air regurgitation and its consequences after conjunctivodacryocystorhinostomy and dacryocystorhinostomy in continuous positive airway pressure patients. Ophthalmic Plast Reconstr Surg [Internet]. 2015;31(4):269–71. Available from: https://journals.lww.com/00002341-201507000-00003.

56. Blandford AD, Cherfan DG, Drake RL, McBride JM, Hwang CJ, Perry JD, Cheng OT. Continuous positive airway pressure thresholds for nasolacrimal air regurgitation in a cadaveric model. Ophthal Plast Reconstr Surg [Internet]. 2018;34(5):440–2. Available from: Journals@Ovid Ovid Full Text.

57. Grzybowski A, Kuklo P, Pieczynski J, Beiko G. A review of preoperative manoeuvres for prophylaxis of endophthalmitis in intraocular surgery. Curr Opin Ophthalmol [Internet]. 2016;27(1):9–23. Available from: http://journals.lww.com/00055735-201601000-00004.

58. Berg EJ, Davies JB, Buboltz MR, Samuelson TW. Late-onset bleb-associated endophthalmitis and continuous positive airway pressure. Am J Ophthalmol Case Reports [Internet]. 2018;10:87–90. Available from: https://linkinghub.elsevier.com/retrieve/pii/S245199361730169X.

59. Scott AW, Bressler NM, Ffolkes S, Wittenborn JS, Jorkasky J. Public attitudes about eye and vision health. JAMA Ophthalmol [Internet]. 2016;134(10):1111. Available from: http://archopht.jamanetwork.com/article.aspx?doi=10.1001/jamaophthalmol.2016.2627.

CPAP Adherence and Bariatric Surgery Patients

22

Raed Hawa

Box 22.1: Clinical Vignette

Rebecca is a 45-year-old married woman who has a long-standing history of obesity. She is 5′3″ and 235 lbs. (BMI = 41.6 kg/m^2). She has hypertension and type II diabetes, as well as recurrent knee problems and a history of a major depressive disorder. She has constantly felt tired and depressed during the day, and her antidepressant medication was of modest help. Because of concerns about her weight contributing to her health problems, including knee difficulties and diabetes, she was referred to a surgeon for possible consideration of bariatric surgery. Before considering surgery, the surgeon wanted her to be screened for obstructive sleep apnea.

On referral, she completed an overnight polysomnogram that showed an apnea-hypopnea index (AHI) of 85 events per hour, with oxygen saturation dropping to a minimum of 81% during a total sleep time of 5 hours and 49 minutes. Events were more severe in REM sleep. After discussing these results with her sleep specialist, she was started on a trial of CPAP that seemed to help subjectively. Rebecca had a CPAP titration study that demonstrated optimal apnea control at a pressure of 12 cmH$_2$O.

After having bariatric surgery and adjusting her diet, Rebecca went on to lose 70 lbs. bringing her weight down to 165 lbs. with a BMI of 29.2 kg/m^2. At times, she felt the CPAP machine was getting cumbersome and was blowing too much air for her, so she stopped using it 5 months postoperatively. At the advice of her family doctor, she visited the sleep specialist to consider her options.

22.1 Apnea and CPAP

Obstructive sleep apnea is a common disorder affecting 3–9% of the general population and is well demonstrated to be a risk factor for resistant hypertension, cardiovascular disease, neurological disease, and all-cause mortality [1]. OSA has known effects on decreasing economic outcomes and worsening quality of life and is also a source of daytime somnolence, fatigue, and motor vehicle accidents [1, 2]. Since the pervasive health effects of untreated OSA are so well described, practice parameters published by the American Academy of Sleep Medicine (AASM) recommend that CPAP should be considered as both a first-line and gold-standard treatment for OSA; many prominent published studies make similar statements [3–5].

Despite numerous advances in CPAP machine dynamics including quieter and lighter pumps, softer masks, and improved portability, use of CPAP continues to be a problem frequently encountered in clinicians' offices and sleep clinics, with adherence rates generally ranging from 30% to 60% [6, 7]. There are many reasons for this problem including feeling uncomfortable using a machine or wearing a mask, lack of convenience dealing with machine and tubings, claustrophobia, and cost [2]. It is also observed that many patients who initially struggle with adherence frequently remain nonadherent and eventually abandon the machine altogether, with consequent return of symptoms and OSA-specific adverse consequences.

22.2 Apnea and Obesity

The prevalence of obstructive sleep apnea (OSA) in obesity ranges from 39% to 98% [8–11]. The highest rates are seen in those with a body mass index (BMI) >40 kg/ m^2 [11]. Prevalence rates and measures of disease severity (apnea-hypopnea index, oxygen desaturations) increase several folds with increasing weight and BMI.

R. Hawa (✉)
Faculty of Medicine, University of Toronto, Toronto, ON, Canada

University Health Network, Toronto, ON, Canada
e-mail: raed.hawa@uhn.ca

Among patients being considered for bariatric surgery, the prevalence of OSA ranges between 64% and 100% [12–18]. Increasing BMI, age, and male gender have been suggested as predictors of likelihood of OSA in bariatric surgery candidates [12]. STOP-Bang is a validated tool that is commonly used for apnea screening in patients with obesity or patients considered for bariatric surgery [19]. Research has found that OSA improved following surgical weight loss but not necessarily resolved OSA [14].

22.3 CPAP and Bariatric Surgery Patients

CPAP adherence is a challenge in the management of apnea in patients undergoing bariatric surgery, similar to CPAP adherence challenges experienced in the general population who have OSA. Unfortunately, literature on CPAP adherence in the bariatric population is sparse. Available literature reports lower rates of CPAP adherence in the bariatric patient cohorts that in the general OSA population [20, 21].

A study demonstrated that in an urban tertiary care academic medical center, a high proportion of presurgical patients that underwent polysomnographic evaluation had severe OSA [20]. Overall CPAP use during the first 30 days of perioperative period was extremely low compared to known CPAP adherence at their institution, as well as compared to the reported national averages of 4.7 hours/night.

Another study evaluated 349 patients referred for polysomnography (PSG) prior to bariatric surgery and found that 33% of the patients had severe apnea, 18% had moderate apnea, 32% had mild apnea, and 17% had no apnea [21]. At a median of 11 months after bariatric surgery, mean body mass index (BMI) was reduced to 38 +/− 1 kg/m^2 ($P < 0.01$ vs 56 +/− 1 kg/m^2 preoperatively), and the mean RDI decreased to 15 +/− 2 ($P < 0.01$ vs 51 +/− 4 preoperatively) in 101 patients who underwent postoperative PSG. However, the use of CPAP machine had declined with the number of patients using CPAP reducing from 83 patients preoperatively to 31 patients approximately 1 year postoperatively.

A prospective study was conducted of 25 severely obese patients (17 men, 8 women with average BMI of 52.7 kg/m^2) with paired diagnostic PSG and questionnaire studies; the first prior to bariatric surgery and the second at least 1 year later [22]. Patients with a moderate sleep apnea and a baseline apnea-hypopnea index (AHI) >25 events per hour were included. The second PSG study was conducted at least 1 year after surgery, and mean percentage of excess weight loss and actual weight loss were 50.1+/−15% (range 24–80%) and 44.9+/−22 kg (range 18–103 kg), respectively. There was a significant fall in AHI from 61.6+/−34 to 13.4+/−13, improved sleep architecture with increased REM and stage III and IV sleep, and decreased daytime sleepiness. CPAP use decreased from 14 patients preoperatively to 4 patients at the final annual follow-up. Overall, CPAP use

appeared to decline dramatically in the months following bariatric surgery as weight loss goals were achieved.

Another study showed that 36% of the patients showed good compliance to CPAP (more than 4 hours for at least 70% of the nights) in the month prior to bariatric surgery [23]. Patients who were older were more compliant. A follow-up study of 121 patients who were diagnosed with OSA and prescribed CPAP prior to bariatric surgery showed that roughly half of the patients were compliant with CPAP prior to surgery and only 15 patients continued to use CPAP with only 2 patients followed up for a repeat sleep study. Possible reasons suggested for nonadherence included nasal discomfort, cost, and lack of knowledge [24].

In one retrospective cross-sectional study of 826 bariatric patients screened for OSA between 2013 and 2015, patients used their CPAP >75% of the nights, and the mean usage was 4 hours +/− 2 hours [25]. Humidification of the CPAP machine (and not CPAP pressure, OSA severity, demographics, or anthropometrics) was the only factor associated with increased CPAP adherence.

22.4 Promoting CPAP Adherence

Factors: Sawyer [26] summarized a number of studies to better understand patients' decisions to adhere to CPAP treatment and was able to identify a number of factors that influence or predict CPAP use. These studies can be categorized as examining the following factors: (1) disease and patient characteristics (disease severity, sleepiness; mood, race); (2) treatment titration procedures (AutoPAP); (3) technological device factors and side effects (heated humidification and claustrophobia); and (4) psychological and social factors (self-efficacy, outcome expectation, risk perception, and presence of partner).

Intervention: Based on the clinical experience of sleep specialists working in the area of sleep medicine and the available literature [6, 27–31], critical components of intervention strategies to promote CPAP adherence in the OSA population include (1) patient education about OSA, including diagnostic information, symptoms, CPAP treatment, and treatment response; (2) guidance for troubleshooting common problems and experiences with CPAP; (3) assisted initial exposure to CPAP; (4) inclusion of support person(s) during early treatment education and exposure (e.g., spouse, bed partner, social support); (5) interface opportunities with other CPAP-treated OSA persons; and (6) follow-up during first weeks of CPAP treatment including medical follow-up and other behavioral interventions (cognitive therapy, motivational therapy). Although these components are based on a relatively small number of intervention studies in adult samples, there is consistency from these studies to support these components.

In addition to the above strategies, and based on the limited literature available [23–25] and cited in this chapter, specific intervention approaches to promote more CPAP adherence in the bariatric patient population include (1) the use of autotitrating PAP units for apnea treatment of bariatric patients; (2) the use of a humidification system for the PAP machine; (3) making sure that the level of apnea is reassessed post surgery to ensure appropriate treatment as needed (decrease pressure requirements post weight loss); (4) education to improve knowledge; and (5) support and follow-up of patients post bariatric surgery.

22.5 Why APAP?

OSA severity has been shown to decrease significantly with surgical weight loss where it is reported that a 10% weight reduction leads to around 26% reduction in the respiratory disturbance index [32]. Also CPAP requirements do decrease as the patients lose weight post surgery – mostly in the first year post bariatric surgery. This is notable, as prior CPAP settings may be higher than required to ablate residual sleep disordered breathing following weight loss. Intolerance to an inappropriately high pressure may promote abandonment of therapy. Ultimately, a multi-pronged approach to optimizing sleep in this population, focusing on sleep quantity, quality, and CPAP adherence, may improve clinical outcomes. Since CPAP pressure requirements change considerably in bariatric surgery patients undergoing rapid weight loss, autotitrating PAP devices have promise for facilitating the management of CPAP therapy during this time. Consideration should be given to the use of autotitrating PAP units as the treatment of choice in these patients [33, 34].

Box 22.2: Case Follow-Up

The sleep physician suggested an autotitrating PAP (APAP). A trial of APAP was initiated at home (minimum EPAP = 6, maximum IPAP = 25 cm of water pressure with a maximum pressure support of 6 cm of water pressure). Rebecca felt her symptoms significantly improved within few days of trying the APAP. She was able to sleep through the night on most nights, and consequently get up earlier, and had more energy during the day. She no longer dozed during the day and even seemed to be in a better mood with people, being more patient and upbeat. Her shortness of breath during the day also improved markedly.

One year post surgery, the patient had concerns that the machine is not working as she has been feeling tired when waking up in the morning. She also reported feeling sleepy during the day. By then Janet's weight has gone down to 145 lbs. with a BMI of 25.7 kg/m^2. A diagnostic polysomnography study was recommended. This time her AHI was 4 events per hour with oxygen saturation dropping to a minimum of 91%, and mean oxygen saturation stayed at 95% during a total sleep time of 6 hours and 53 minutes. She was relieved to hear that her sleep disordered breathing was cured. She stopped using the APAP, and her sleep has improved and her daytime sleepiness was gone.

22.6 Conclusion

CPAP adherence is a challenge in the management of obstructive sleep apnea (OSA), particularly in patients undergoing bariatric surgery. Literature on CPAP adherence in this population is sparse; however it suggests that CPAP use appears to decline dramatically in the months following bariatric surgery. Critical components of intervention strategies have been proposed and are shared in this chapter to promote CPAP adherence in this population.

References

1. Young T, Peppard PE, Gottlieb DJ. Epidemiology of obstructive sleep apnea: a population health perspective. Am J Respir Crit Care Med. 2002;165(9):1217–39.
2. Aurora RN, Casey KR, Kristo D, Auerbach S, Bista SR, Chowdhuri S, Karippot A, Lamm C, Ramar K, Zak R, Morgenthaler TI. Practice parameters for the surgical modifications of the upper airway for obstructive sleep apnea in adults. Sleep. 2010;33(10):1408–13.
3. Gay P, Weaver T, Loube D, Iber C. Evaluation of positive airway pressure treatment for sleep related breathing disorders in adults. Sleep. 2006;29(3):381–401.
4. Morgenthaler TI, Aurora RN, Brown T, Zak R, Alessi C, Boehlecke B, Chesson AL Jr, Friedman L, Kapur V, Maganti R, Owens J. Practice parameters for the use of autotitrating continuous positive airway pressure devices for titrating pressures and treating adult patients with obstructive sleep apnea syndrome: an update for 2007. Sleep. 2008;31(1):141–7.
5. Yaremchuk K, Tacia B, Peterson E, Roth T. Change in Epworth sleepiness scale after surgical treatment of obstructive sleep apnea. Laryngoscope. 2011;121(7):1590–3.
6. Weaver TE, Sawyer AM. Adherence to continuous positive airway pressure treatment for obstructive sleep apnea: implications for future interventions. Indian J Med Res. 2010;131:245.
7. Weaver TE, Grunstein RR. Adherence to continuous positive airway pressure therapy: the challenge to effective treatment. Proc Am Thorac Soc. 2008;5(2):173–8.
8. Cowan DC, Livingston E. Obstructive sleep apnoea syndrome and weight loss. Sleep Disord. 2012;2012:163296.
9. Resta O, Foschino-Barbaro MP, Legari G, Talamo S, Bonfitto P, Palumbo A, Minenna A, Giorgino R, De Pergola G. Sleep-related breathing disorders, loud snoring and excessive daytime sleepiness in obese subjects. Int J Obes. 2001;25(5):669–75.
10. Sergi M, Rizzi M, Comi AL, Resta O, Palma P, De Stefano A, Comi D. Sleep apnea in moderate-severe obese patients. Sleep Breath. 1999;3(2):47–52.

11. Valencia-Flores M, Orea A, Castano VA, Resendiz M, Rosales M, Rebollar V, Santiago V, Gallegos J, Campos RM, González J, Oseguera J. Prevalence of sleep apnea and electrocardiographic disturbances in morbidly obese patients. Obes Res. 2000;8(3):262–9.

12. Carneiro G, Flório RT, Zanella MT, Pradella-Hallinan M, Ribeiro-Filho FF, Tufik S, Togeiro SM. Is mandatory screening for obstructive sleep apnea with polysomnography in all severely obese patients indicated? Sleep Breath. 2012;16(1):163–8.

13. Frey WC, Pilcher J. Obstructive sleep-related breathing disorders in patients evaluated for bariatric surgery. Obes Surg. 2003;13(5):676–83.

14. Lettieri CJ, Eliasson AH, Greenburg DL. Persistence of obstructive sleep apnea after surgical weight loss. J Clin Sleep Med. 2008;4(4):333–8.

15. O'Keeffe T, Patterson EJ. Evidence supporting routine polysomnography before bariatric surgery. Obes Surg. 2004;14(1):23–6.

16. Ravesloot MJ, Hilgevoord AA, Van Wagensveld BA, De Vries N. Assessment of the effect of bariatric surgery on obstructive sleep apnea at two postoperative intervals. Obes Surg. 2014;24(1):22–31.

17. Sareli AE, Cantor CR, Williams NN, Korus G, Raper SE, Pien G, Hurley S, Maislin G, Schwab RJ. Obstructive sleep apnea in patients undergoing bariatric surgery—a tertiary center experience. Obes Surg. 2011;21(3):316–27.

18. Sharkey KM, Orff HJ, Tosi C, Harrington D, Roye GD, Millman RP. Subjective sleepiness and daytime functioning in bariatric patients with obstructive sleep apnea. Sleep Breath. 2013;17(1):267–74.

19. Chung F, Yang Y, Liao P. Predictive performance of the STOP-Bang score for identifying obstructive sleep apnea in obese patients. Obes Surg. 2013;23(12):2050–7.

20. Guralnick AS, Pant M, Minhaj M, Sweitzer BJ, Mokhlesi B. CPAP adherence in patients with newly diagnosed obstructive sleep apnea prior to elective surgery. J Clin Sleep Med. 2012;8(5):501–6.

21. Haines KL, Nelson LG, Gonzalez R, Torrella T, Martin T, Kandil A, Dragotti R, Anderson WM, Gallagher SF, Murr MM. Objective evidence that bariatric surgery improves obesity-related obstructive sleep apnea. Surgery. 2007;141(3):354–8.

22. Dixon JB, Schachter LM, O'Brien PE. Polysomnography before and after weight loss in obese patients with severe sleep apnea. Int J Obes. 2005;29(9):1048–54.

23. Dotan Y, Clarke T, Michael E, Rohit S, Lewis J, Kristen R, Sydney C, Daraz Y, Vega Sanchez ME, Jaffe F, Krachman SL. Compliance of patients with obstructive sleep apnea undergoing bariatric surgery to CPAP and effect on outcome. Am J Respir Crit Care Med. 2018;197:A3978.

24. Nguyen RT, Hassan S, Adrah R, Gu S, Nguyen S, Zaman M. PSG and CPAP use before and after bariatric surgery: a five year cohort study. Sleep. 2017;40:A206.

25. Cho PS, Hetherington JP, Kirby R, Lee KK. Determinants of CPAP compliance in bariatric patients with obstructive sleep apnoea. Eur Respir J. 2017;50(61):PA2284.

26. Sawyer AM, Gooneratne NS, Marcus CL, Ofer D, Richards KC, Weaver TE. A systematic review of CPAP adherence across age groups: clinical and empiric insights for developing CPAP adherence interventions. Sleep Med Rev. 2011;15(6):343–56.

27. Kohler M, Smith D, Tippett V, Stradling JR. Predictors of long-term compliance with continuous positive airway pressure. Thorax. 2010;65(9):829–32.

28. Meslier N, Lebrun T, Grillier-Lanoir V, Rolland N, Henderick C, Sailly JC, Racineux JL. A French survey of 3,225 patients treated with CPAP for obstructive sleep apnoea: benefits, tolerance, compliance and quality of life. Eur Respir J. 1998;12(1):185–92.

29. Wells RD, Freedland KE, Carney RM, Duntley SP, Stepanski EJ. Adherence, reports of benefits, and depression among patients treated with continuous positive airway pressure. Psychosom Med. 2007;69(5):449–54.

30. Hoffstein V, Viner S, Mateika S, Conway J. Treatment of obstructive sleep apnea with nasal continuous positive airway pressure. Am Rev Respir Dis. 1992;145(841):e5.

31. Massie CA, Hart RW, Peralez K, Richards GN. Effects of humidification on nasal symptoms and compliance in sleep apnea patients using continuous positive airway pressure. Chest. 1999;116(2):403–8.

32. Foster GD, Borradaile KE, Sanders MH, Millman R, Zammit G, Newman AB, Wadden TA, Kelley D, Wing RR, Pi-Sunyer FX, Reboussin D. A randomized study on the effect of weight loss on obstructive sleep apnea among obese patients with type 2 diabetes: the sleep AHEAD study. Arch Intern Med. 2009;169(17):1619–26.

33. Lankford DA, Proctor CD, Richard R. Continuous positive airway pressure (CPAP) changes in bariatric surgery patients undergoing rapid weight loss. Obes Surg. 2005;15(3):336–41.

34. Massie CA, Hart RW. Changes in continuous positive airway pressure (CPAP) during the first six months following bariatric surgery. Sleep Diagnosis Therapy. 2007;2(1):27–32.

CPAP Adherence in Pregnancy

23

Ela Kadish and Noah Gilad

23.1 Sleep Disorders in Pregnancy

Alteration in sleep is a common finding among pregnant women, and many women complain about changes in sleep duration and quality which can be a result of changes in sleep patterns and physiological changes associated with pregnancy. The sleep pattern changes are associated with sleep fragmentation and can predispose pregnant women to the development of sleep disordered breathing (SDB) [1, 2]. Non-respiratory physical changes, such as weight gain, can also result in the development of SDB as it increases the prevalence of obesity in pregnant women, which in turn increase the risk of developing OSA.

The exact prevalence of SDB in pregnancy, diagnosed by polysomnography (PSG), is not established. Large prospective studies with precise definitions of SDB and estimated prevalence are lacking. That said, many studies have shown an increase incident of snoring, nocturnal hypoxemia, and obstructive sleep apnea (OSA) among pregnant women [3–9].

The diagnosis of OSA is obtained by the demonstration of at least five obstructive respiratory events (apneas, hypopneas, or respiratory effort-related arousals) per hour of sleep in the presence of sleep-related symptoms or comorbidities or 15 or more obstructive respiratory events per hour of sleep [10]. Clinically, OSA is manifested by the occurrence of daytime sleepiness, loud snoring, witnessed breathing interruptions, or awakening due to gasping or choking.

The prevalence of OSA with apnea-hypopnea index (AHI) greater than 5 has been reported to be 3.6% in early pregnancy and 8.3% in mid-pregnancy [9].

Many studies suggest that snoring occurs in 14% to 45% of pregnant women [3–5] as opposed to 4% of premenopausal, nonpregnant women. A study of 502 pregnant women found that 23% of the study population reported regular snoring [6]. Since it has been shown that women in general tend to under-report snoring on questionnaires [11], these numbers may well be an underestimation of the true incidence of snoring among pregnant women.

Marked nocturnal hypoxemia (SaO2 of less than 95%) was demonstrated in a study involving 28 pregnant normotensive and hypertensive women at more than 35 weeks gestation [8].This result is consistent with previous findings that showed a small but significant reduction in SaO2 during pregnancy at the third trimester, compared with postpartum studied in the same individuals [7].

Symptoms of daytime hypersomnolence increase progressively during pregnancy [12–14] with reported abnormally high Epworth Sleepiness Scale (ESS) scores in close to 25% of pregnant women [14].

23.2 Chemical/Hormonal Changes During Pregnancy

During pregnancy, the respiratory system changes to meet the increased demand. These changes include hormonal, mechanical and volume adaptations, and may be the underlying cause of SDB.

23.2.1 Chest and Volume Changes

The functional residual capacity (FRC) is reduced by approximately 20% due to the rising diaphragm position that is being pushed upward by the enlarged uterus [15–17]. This reduction with the combination of the physiological FRC reduction during sleep can cause decreased oxygenation which worsens the arterial/oxygen gradient [18]. During pregnancy, a compensatory mechanism mediated by progesterone elevation causes a right shift of the oxyhemoglobin desaturation curve, which may improve oxygenation temporarily [19].

E. Kadish (✉)
Hebrew University of Jerusalem, Jerusalem, Israel

N. Gilad
University of Toronto, Toronto, ON, Canada

© The Author(s), under exclusive license to Springer Nature Switzerland AG 2022
C. M. Shapiro et al. (eds.), *CPAP Adherence*, https://doi.org/10.1007/978-3-030-93146-9_23

In keeping with the upregulation of central respiratory drive, there is increased diaphragmatic effort leading to greater negative inspiratory pressures at the level of the upper airway. This may be related to an increased tendency for the upper airway to collapse during sleep [17].

Potential desaturations that can occur in the supine position may be secondary to positionally induced changes in cardiac output and/or early airway closure during tidal breathing secondary to reduced pharyngeal size and increased airway collapsibility [20].

23.2.2 Hormonal Changes

While progesterone improves placental oxygenation, it also markedly upregulates ventilatory drive at the level of the central chemoreceptors that lead to respiratory alkalosis which can cause central apneas during non-rapid eye movement sleep [18]. In addition, prostaglandin F2α increases airway resistance by bronchial smooth muscle and may cause relative bronchoconstriction [20].

23.2.3 Upper Airway Changes

Reduced pharyngeal dimensions during pregnancy has been demonstrated using the Mallampati score [21]. Patency of the upper airway is well-known to be an important predictor of the presence and severity of SDB, with reduced dimensions of the pharynx being strongly associated with obstructive sleep apnea [22]. In addition, there are significant changes to the mucosa of the nasopharynx and oropharynx during pregnancy. The mucosal changes in the upper airway include hyperemia, edema, leakage of plasma into the stroma, glandular hypersecretion, increased phagocytic activity, and increased mucopolysaccharide content. All of these result in nasal congestion, often called rhinitis of pregnancy, that can worsen OSA symptoms [23].

23.3 The Effects of Sleep Disorders on Pregnancy Outcomes

The association between SDB symptoms and adverse gestational outcomes has been consistently demonstrated over multiple studies and is correlated with gestational hypertensive disorders [3–6, 24], preeclampsia [6], and gestational diabetes [25]. In addition, preexisting sleep-related hypoventilation has shown to potentially impose additional stress on pregnant woman and the fetus [26]. Therefore, accurate diagnosis and quick intervention are crucial in order to improve maternal and fetal outcomes.

23.3.1 Endothelium Insult

Pregnancies complicated by OSA are at an increased risk for preeclampsia and hypertensive disorders [4–6, 27, 28]. Periods of hypoxia and hypercapnia in OSA result in sympathetic activation, with elevated catecholamines. Baroreceptor sensitivity may also be altered, resulting in sustained hypertension [29]. OSA directly affects the vascular endothelium by promoting inflammation and oxidative stress while decreasing NO availability and repair capacity [30]. Similar mechanisms are known to occur during trophoblastic implantation insults. Yinon et al. [28] found that pregnant women with preeclamptic toxemia (PET) had a significantly higher respiratory disturbance index (RDI) and lower endothelial function index (EFI) than those without hypertensive pregnancies. Blood pressure was significantly correlated with RDI and with EFI. EFI tended to correlate with RDI. Dysregulation of pro- and antiangiogenic factors is thought to be causally linked to the condition. Before and during PET, maternal serum concentrations of antiangiogenic soluble fms-like tyrosine kinase-1 (sFlt-1) were increased and levels of pro-angiogenic placental growth factor (PlGF) were decreased. In 2002, Levine et al. [31] showed that the sFlt1/PlGF ratio was associated with the clinical diagnosis of preeclampsia. Participants with gestational hypertension had moderately elevated sFlt1/PlGF ratios, whereas participants with preeclampsia had markedly elevated sFlt1/PlGF ratios compared with participants who had no hypertensive disorder. Another study showed that in women with suspected preeclampsia before 34 weeks of gestation, the presence of a higher circulating sFlt1/PlGF ratio predicted adverse outcomes occurring within 2 weeks [32]. The same endothelial dysfunction was found in pregnant women with OSA [33]. Specifically, the ratio of VEGF-R1 and PlGF was significantly higher in pregnant women with OSA compared to controls, even after adjusting for gestational age, BMI, and chronic hypertension when women with preeclampsia were excluded from the analyses. It has also been shown that the use of CPAP can eliminate the nocturnal increments in blood pressure in pregnant women with OSA and PET [34]. Furthermore, in pregnant women with hypertension and chronic snoring, nasal CPAP use during the first 8 weeks of pregnancy combined with standard prenatal care is associated with better blood pressure control and improved pregnancy outcomes [35].

An alternative explanation would be that preeclampsia might lead to the development of OSA; women with preeclampsia have lower oncotic pressures than normal pregnant women, have a larger neck circumference and a smaller upper airway size [36]. Additional studies are needed to evaluate this theory further.

23.3.2 Metabolic/Inflammatory Mechanism

Multiple studies have demonstrated an association between SDB, diabetes mellitus, and abnormal glucose metabolism outside of pregnancy. OSA has been linked to decreased insulin sensitivity [37], with the degree of SDB severity correlated with insulin resistance [38–41]. These findings were independent of age, BMI at delivery, multifetal pregnancy, and smoking (adjusted odds ratio [OR] 2.1, 95% CI 1.3–3.4) [4]. When snoring, gasping, and apnea symptoms were combined, the association was stronger (adjusted OR 4.0, 95% CI 1.4–11.1) suggesting that the association was greater with a higher likelihood of OSA [4].

Hypoxia and sleep fragmentation may increase cortisol secretion with abnormalities in insulin and glucose metabolism. This continued cortisol secretion reduces glucocorticoid receptor sensitivity, resulting in chronic hypothalamic-pituitary-adrenal axis activation [29]. Izic-Balserak and Pien [42] suggest a model in which habitual poor sleep quality or short sleep duration (SSD), specifically insufficient slow wave sleep (SWS), can lead to impaired glucose tolerance. As has been described in sleep deprivation studies, SSD and decreased SWS may augment the inflammatory response by increasing circulating concentrations of interleukin-6 (IL-6), tumor necrosis factor alpha (TNF-alpha), and C-reactive protein (CRP), which are involved in the pathogenesis of insulin resistance and type 2 diabetes. It is possible that the physiological increase in insulin resistance during pregnancy, when compounded by OSA, might lead to less favorable obstetrical outcomes. In a study using rats, gestational intermittent hypoxia altered offspring response to a subsequent postnatal inflammatory challenge, increased their ventilation and lowered their hypoxic ventilatory responses [43].

Studies evaluating the association between SDB symptoms and fetal outcomes are scarce, with inconsistent results. Definitions of outcomes may contribute to the inconsistencies, and further studies to clarify these observations are needed.

23.4 CPAP Intervention

Despite the lack of research on the subject, it remains reasonable to treat pregnant patients with the same indications as nonpregnant patients. All women should consider behavioral modifications prior to other methods of intervention. However, due to the fact that weight loss is the recommended change in the general population and is not as practical in pregnant women, other methods should be considered.

CPAP with good adherence might significantly improve the gestational results of those who develop gestational OSA and is the first-line treatment of OSA. It reduces the frequency of respiratory events during sleep, limits hypoxic episodes, decreases daytime hypersomnolence, and improves quality of life [44, 45]. The diagnosis and severity of the condition should be well established before making decisions regarding management, and be reevaluated as the pregnancy progresses. The predictable weight gain during pregnancy might cause an increase in pressure requirements by 1–2 cm [46]. The general first night effect may mask sleep apnea in pregnancy and may be an argument for doing full polysomnography in a home environment.

Nocturnal CPAP treatment has been shown to improve blood pressure in all sleep stages in a group of women with severe preeclampsia compared with nontreatment in the same patients [34].

Both the acute and chronic effects of CPAP have been studied in subgroups of pregnant patients. Successful treatment of OSA has been shown to lead to many clinical improvements, including better quality of life, decreased daytime sleepiness, lower blood pressure [35, 44, 45, 47–50], decreased vascular morbidity and mortality [34, 51–53], improvement in gestational diabetes [54], and improved fetal outcomes when compared with controls [35]. Treatment of OSA has also been shown to result in a reduction in healthcare utilization [55, 56].

In conclusion, the physiological changes that women encounter during pregnancy place pregnant women at an increased risk for SDB. When a pregnant woman has SDB, she is at a higher risk for adverse obstetrical outcomes. Therefore, SDB assessment, accurate diagnosis, effective treatment, and high adherence to treatment is crucial in this short but important period. The use of CPAP is generally safe and well tolerated during pregnancy. It may be initiated after an in-laboratory titration, or one can prescribe an auto-titrating device. The latter may be better suited to pregnant women, because it allows the clinician to increase the range of therapeutic pressure during the course of pregnancy.

References

1. Bourjeily G, Ankner G, Mohsenin V. Sleep-disordered breathing in pregnancy. Clin Chest Med. 2011;32(1):175–89.
2. Kryger MH, Roth T, Dement WC. (2011). Principles and practice of sleep medicine, Philadelphia, Baskı.
3. Ursavas A, Karadag M, Nalc   N, Ercan I, Gozu RO. Self-reported snoring, maternal obesity and neck circumference as risk factors for pregnancy-induced hypertension and preeclampsia. Respiration. 2008;76(1):33–9.
4. Bourjeily G, Raker CA, Chalhoub M, Miller MA. Pregnancy and fetal outcomes of symptoms of sleep-disordered breathing. Eur Respir J. 2010;36(4):849–55.
5. Calaora-Tournadre D, Ragot S, Meurice JC, Pourrat O, D'Halluin G, Magnin G, Pierre F. Obstructive sleep apnea syndrome during pregnancy: prevalence of main symptoms and relationship with pregnancy induced-hypertension and intra-uterine growth retardation. La Revue de medecine interne. 2006;27(4):291–5.

6. Franklin KA, Holmgren PÅ, Jönsson F, Poromaa N, Stenlund H, Svanborg E. Snoring, pregnancy-induced hypertension, and growth retardation of the fetus. Chest. 2000;117(1):137–41.

7. Hertz G, Fast A, Feinsilver SH, Albertario CL, Schulman H, Fein AM. Sleep in normal late pregnancy. Sleep. 1992;15(3):246–51.

8. Bourne T, Ogilvy AJ, Vickers R, Williamson K. Nocturnal hypoxaemia in late pregnancy. Br J Anaesth. 1995;75(6):678–82.

9. Facco FL, Parker CB, Reddy UM, Silver RM, Koch MA, Louis JM, et al. Association between sleep-disordered breathing and hypertensive disorders of pregnancy and gestational diabetes mellitus. Obstet Gynecol. 2017;129(1):31.

10. Adult Obstructive Sleep Apnea Task Force of the American Academy of Sleep Medicine. Clinical guideline for the evaluation, management and long-term care of obstructive sleep apnea in adults. J Clin Sleep Med. 2009;5(3):263–76.

11. Redline S, Kump K, Tishler PV, Browner ILENE, Ferrette V. Gender differences in sleep disordered breathing in a community-based sample. Am J Respir Crit Care Med. 1994;149(3):722–6.

12. Leung PL, Hui DSC, Leung TN, Yuen PM, Lau TK. Sleep disturbances in Chinese pregnant women. BJOG. 2005;112(11):1568–71.

13. Pien GW, Fife D, Pack AI, Nkwuo JE, Schwab RJ. Changes in symptoms of sleep-disordered breathing during pregnancy. Sleep. 2005;28(10):1299–305.

14. Bourjeily G, Raker C. Epworth sleepiness score in pregnancy. American Thoracic Society in Toronto. 2008.

15. Jordan AS, McSharry DG, Malhotra A. Adult obstructive sleep apnoea. Lancet. 2014;383(9918):736–47.

16. Bixler EO, Vgontzas AN, Lin HM, Ten Have T, Rein J, Vela-Bueno A, Kales A. Prevalence of sleep-disordered breathing in women: effects of gender. Am J Respir Crit Care Med. 2001;163(3):608–13.

17. Louis JM, Mogos MF, Salemi JL, Redline S, Salihu HM. Obstructive sleep apnea and severe maternal-infant morbidity/mortality in the United States, 1998-2009. Sleep. 2014;37(5):843–9.

18. Pien GW, Pack AI, Jackson N, Maislin G, Macones GA, Schwab RJ. Risk factors for sleep-disordered breathing in pregnancy. Thorax. 2014;69(4):371–7.

19. Pamidi S, Marc I, Simoneau G, Lavigne L, Olha A, Benedetti A, et al. Maternal sleep-disordered breathing and the risk of delivering small for gestational age infants: a prospective cohort study. Thorax. 2016;71(8):719–25.

20. O'Brien LM, Bullough AS, Owusu JT, Tremblay KA, Brincat CA, Chames MC, et al. Snoring during pregnancy and delivery outcomes: a cohort study. Sleep. 2013;36(11):1625–32.

21. Fung AM, Wilson DL, Lappas M, Howard M, Barnes M, O'Donoghue F, et al. Effects of maternal obstructive sleep apnoea on fetal growth: a prospective cohort study. PLoS One. 2013;8(7):e68057.

22. Brown NT, Turner JM, Kumar S. The intrapartum and perinatal risks of sleep-disordered breathing in pregnancy: a systematic review and metaanalysis. Am J Obstet Gynecol. 2018;219(2):147–61.

23. Sharma SK, Nehra A, Sinha S, Soneja M, Sunesh K, Sreenivas V, Vedita D. Sleep disorders in pregnancy and their association with pregnancy outcomes: a prospective observational study. Sleep Breath. 2016;20(1):87–93.

24. Pérez-Chada DANIEL, Videla AJ, O'Flaherty ME, Majul C, Catalini AM, Caballer CA, Franklin KA. Snoring, witnessed sleep apnoeas and pregnancy-induced hypertension. Acta Obstet Gynecol Scand. 2007;86(7):788–92.

25. Pamidi S, Pinto LM, Marc I, Benedetti A, Schwartzman K, Kimoff RJ. Maternal sleep-disordered breathing and adverse pregnancy outcomes: a systematic review and metaanalysis. Am J Obstet Gynecol. 2014;210(1):52–e1.

26. Ayyar L, Shaib F, Guntupalli K. Sleep-disordered breathing in pregnancy. Sleep Med Clin. 2018;13(3):349–57.

27. Louis JM, Auckley D, Sokol RJ, Mercer BM. Maternal and neonatal morbidities associated with obstructive sleep apnea complicating pregnancy. Am J Obstet Gynecol. 2010;202(3):261–e1.

28. Yinon D, Lowenstein L, Suraya S, Beloosesky R, Zmora O, Malhotra A, Pillar G. Pre-eclampsia is associated with sleep-disordered breathing and endothelial dysfunction. Eur Respir J. 2006;27(2):328–33.

29. Fung AM, Wilson DL, Barnes M, Walker SP. Obstructive sleep apnea and pregnancy: the effect on perinatal outcomes. J Perinatol. 2012;32(6):399–406.

30. Jelic S, Padeletti M, Kawut SM, Higgins C, Canfield SM, Onat D, et al. Clinical perspective. Circulation. 2008;117(17):2270–8.

31. Levine RJ, Maynard SE, Qian C, Lim KH, England LJ, Yu KF, et al. Circulating angiogenic factors and the risk of preeclampsia. N Engl J Med. 2004;350(7):672–83.

32. Rana S, Powe CE, Salahuddin S, Verlohren S, Perschel FH, Levine RJ, et al. Angiogenic factors and the risk of adverse outcomes in women with suspected preeclampsia. Circulation. 2012;125(7):911–9.

33. Bourjeily G, Curran P, Butterfield K, Maredia H, Carpenter M, Lambert-Messerlian G. Placenta-secreted circulating markers in pregnant women with obstructive sleep apnea. J Perinat Med. 2015;43(1):81–7.

34. Edwards N, Blyton DM, Kirjavainen T, Kesby GJ, Sullivan CE. Nasal continuous positive airway pressure reduces sleep-induced blood pressure increments in preeclampsia. Am J Respir Crit Care Med. 2000;162(1):252–7.

35. Poyares D, Guilleminault C, Hachul H, Fujita L, Takaoka S, Tufik S, Sass N. Pre-eclampsia and nasal CPAP: part 2. Hypertension during pregnancy, chronic snoring, and early nasal CPAP intervention. Sleep Med. 2007;9(1):15–21.

36. Izci B, Vennelle M, Liston WA, Dundas KC, Calder AA, Douglas NJ. Sleep-disordered breathing and upper airway size in pregnancy and post-partum. Eur Respir J. 2006;27(2):321–7.

37. Theorell-Haglöw J, Berne C, Janson C, Lindberg E. Obstructive sleep apnoea is associated with decreased insulin sensitivity in females. Eur Respir J. 2008;31(5):1054–60.

38. Matthews DR, Hosker JP, Rudenski AS, Naylor BA, Treacher DF, Turner RC. Homeostasis model assessment: insulin resistance and β-cell function from fasting plasma glucose and insulin concentrations in man. Diabetologia. 1985;28(7):412–9.

39. Otake K, Sasanabe R, Hasegawa R, Banno K, Hori R, Okura Y, et al. Glucose intolerance in Japanese patients with obstructive sleep apnea. Intern Med. 2009;48(21):1863–8.

40. Peled N, Kassirer M, Shitrit D, Kogan Y, Shlomi D, Berliner AS, Kramer MR. The association of OSA with insulin resistance, inflammation and metabolic syndrome. Respir Med. 2007;101(8):1696–701.

41. Punjabi NM, Beamer BA. Alterations in glucose disposal in sleep-disordered breathing. Am J Respir Crit Care Med. 2009;179(3):235–40.

42. Izci-Balserak B, Pien GW. The relationship and potential mechanistic pathways between sleep disturbances and maternal hyperglycemia. Curr Diab Rep. 2014;14(2):459.

43. Johnson SM, Randhawa KS, Epstein JJ, Gustafson E, Hocker AD, Huxtable AG, et al. Gestational intermittent hypoxia increases susceptibility to neuroinflammation and alters respiratory motor control in neonatal rats. Respir Physiol Neurobiol. 2018;256:128–42.

44. Giles TL, Lasserson TJ, Smith B, White J, Wright JJ, Cates CJ. Continuous positive airways pressure for obstructive sleep apnoea in adults. Cochrane Database Syst Rev. 2006;1:CD001106.

45. Patel SR, White DP, Malhotra A, Stanchina ML, Ayas NT. Continuous positive airway pressure therapy for treating gess in a diverse population with obstructive sleep apnea: results of a meta-analysis. Arch Intern Med. 2003;163(5):565–71.

46. Bourjeily G. Sleep disorders in pregnancy. Obstetr Med. 2009;2(3):100–6.

47. D'Ambrosio C, Bowman T, Mohsenin V. Quality of life in patients with obstructive sleep apnea: effect of nasal continuous positive airway pressure—a prospective study. Chest. 1999;115(1):123–9.

48. Gay P, Weaver T, Loube D, Iber C. Evaluation of positive airway pressure treatment for sleep related breathing disorders in adults. Sleep. 2006;29(3):381–401.

49. Sullivan C, Berthon-Jones M, Issa F, Eves L. Reversal of obstructive sleep apnoea by continuous positive airway pressure applied through the nares. Lancet. 1981;317(8225):862–5.

50. Guilleminault C, Palombini L, Poyares D, Takaoka S, Huynh NTL, El-Sayed Y. Pre-eclampsia and nasal CPAP: part 1. Early intervention with nasal CPAP in pregnant women with risk-factors for pre-eclampsia: preliminary findings. Sleep Med. 2007;9(1):9–14.

51. Marin JM, Carrizo SJ, Vicente E, Agusti AG. Long-term cardiovascular outcomes in men with obstructive sleep apnoea-hypopnoea with or without treatment with continuous positive airway pressure: an observational study. Lancet. 2005;365(9464):1046–53.

52. Shah NA, Yaggi HK, Concato J, Mohsenin V. Obstructive sleep apnea as a risk factor for coronary events or cardiovascular death. Sleep Breath. 2010;14(2):131–6.

53. Yaggi HK, Concato J, Kernan WN, Lichtman JH, Brass LM, Mohsenin V. Obstructive sleep apnea as a risk factor for stroke and death. N Engl J Med. 2005;353(19):2034–41.

54. Pamidi S, Kimoff RJ. Maternal sleep-disordered breathing. Chest. 2018;153(4):1052–66.

55. Bahammam A, Delaive K, Ronald J, Manfreda J, Roos L, Kryger MH. Health care utilization in males with obstructive sleep apnea syndrome two years after diagnosis and treatment. Sleep. 1999;22(6):740–7.

56. Kapur VK, Alfonso-Cristancho R. Just a good deal or truly a steal? Medical cost savings and the impact on the cost-effectiveness of treating sleep apnea. Sleep. 2009;32(2):135.

Pathophysiology of Obstructive Sleep Apnea in Children

Relevance to Treatment Approaches

Ian MacLusky

Historically, for the majority of children with obstructive sleep apnea syndrome (OSAS), the etiology (and hence treatment) was nasal obstruction due to adenoid hypertrophy. Adenoidectomy (usually with tonsillectomy) has been the primary treatment modality, usually with a high degree of therapeutic success [1]. Obstructive sleep apnea syndrome is, however, a heterogeneous condition, especially in children, with a marked variability in both presentation and clinical severity [2]. Even with similar degrees of adenoid hypertrophy, the presence and severity of obstructive sleep apnea is highly variable, arising as a consequence of a combination of multiple factors (below), with only a loose correlation between adenotonsillar size [3] and severity of OSAS. Consequently, though adenoidectomy is an effective treatment for the majority of children with obstructive sleep apnea, approximately 20% of children will have persisting OSAS post adenotonsillectomy [4–6], the precise number depending upon the exact definition of "success" [1, 4, 6], age and severity of OSAS at time of surgery [7], duration of follow-up [8], as well as presence of other associated conditions, such as obesity [7, 9] or craniofacial anatomy [4], with ongoing debate regarding the long-term success rate [8, 10]. Consequently, the increasing numbers of children with obesity, as well as increased recognition in other, high-risk groups, such as Down's syndrome, has resulted in increasing numbers of children with OSAS for whom adenoidectomy is either ineffective [7] or not a therapeutic option [9]. For these children continuous positive airway pressure (CPAP), by using positive pressure to "stent" open the airway during inspiration (using either nasal or full-face mask), remains the primary treatment alternative [2, 4, 9]. However, although nasal CPAP has a proven effectiveness [11], as discussed in the other chapters of this book, there are, however, significant technical issues, as well as problems with both short-

and long-term compliance, that limit its use in children. It should be noted that, despite this, one of the advantages of CPAP is that it is an undoable therapy (compared to surgical intervention) and hence is amenable to a therapeutic trial. If well tolerated, and effective, they can persevere, but if ineffective, or poorly tolerated, can simply be discontinued, and alternative treatment options considered.

1. Compliance. Compliance with CPAP therapy remains an ongoing issue, even in adults. Compounding this is a child's ability to understand the necessity for CPAP (though compliance is actually better in children with developmental delay [12]), as well as the fact that children normally wake up and move several times during the night, resulting in repeated episodes of dislodgment, leading to sleep fragmentation not only of the child, but the whole family [13]. Consequently, long-term compliance is generally only around 50% of those in whom CPAP is prescribed [9, 12], the precise rate again being somewhat dependent upon definition of treatment success [14].
2. "Side effects"
   (a) Skin breakdown. There is very little soft tissue over the nasion and forehead, persistent pressure from nasal CPAP frequently been associated skin breakdown at these sites [15]. Improved mask design, as well as judicious skincare, can minimize this risk, but not completely abolish this risk.
   (b) Long-term nasal CPAP has been associated with significant craniofacial remodeling [16] (primarily in younger children), resulting in maxillary retrusion, with not only adverse impact on dentition but also narrowing of nasopharynx, potentially perpetuating OSAS.
3. Duration of therapy.

Although nasal CPAP is usually an effective treatment, it is not "curative" – it is only effective if worn. The question is therefore how long is treatment going to be required,

I. MacLusky (✉)
Department of Pediatrics, Children's Hospital of Eastern Ontario, University of Ottawa, Ottawa, ON, Canada
e-mail: imaclusky@cheo.on.ca

© The Author(s), under exclusive license to Springer Nature Switzerland AG 2022
C. M. Shapiro et al. (eds.), *CPAP Adherence*, https://doi.org/10.1007/978-3-030-93146-9_24

with neither parents nor child looking forward to lifelong CPAP therapy. It is therefore important in children, if at all possible, to treat the underlying etiology, with CPAP, if required, used as a temporizing device until the child has outgrown their OSAS or a definitive treatment becomes available.

Consequently, CPAP, particularly for long-term use, is a less than ideal treatment for children with OSAS, and alternative therapies should be considered. Given the marked heterogeneity of the patient population, an understanding of the pathophysiology of OSAS in children is useful to be able to identify the specific cause(s) in individual children [17] and hence hopefully allow for a tailored treatment approach. Complicating this, however, is the fact that the alternative therapies have their own problems, both in terms of effectiveness and potential side effects. Treatment decisions therefore need to be based on a balance between both short- and long-term morbidity associated with untreated OSAS [2] versus the risks associated with treatment [4, 9], though admittedly these issues are frequently hard to quantify any one child. This chapter will briefly review the pathophysiology of OSAS in children, with reference to alternative treatment options, with more detailed reviews available [4, 6, 18].

24.1 Pathophysiology of OSAS in Children

The presence and severity of OSAS in children arises as a complex interplay of processes both causing increased upper airway resistance, reduction in oropharyngeal diameter, increased collapsibility of oropharynx, and blunted arousal response to upper obstruction [17].

1. Nasal obstruction.
   (a) Adenoid hypertrophy. As noted, although adenoid hypertrophy is historically the primary cause of OSAS in children, there is limited correlation between adenoid size and presence and severity of OSAS. Part of the explanation is due to variability in cross-sectional diameter of the nasopharynx, with children with reduced nasopharyngeal diameter obviously, being at increased risk [17, 19].
   (b) Other causes of nasal obstruction (nasal septal deviation, allergic rhinitis). Airway resistance is proportional to the fourth power of the radius – halving the diameter causing a 16-fold increase in airway resistance [20]. As a consequence, in children (with small nasal diameter) even a small additional reduction (such as due to mucosal edema due to parental smoking/allergic rhinitis) can cause a significant increase in the upper airway resistance.
   (c) Hard palate. Patients with high arched or narrow hard palates, by causing narrowing in his loss of volume

of the nasopharynx, are at increased risk of obstructive sleep apnea.
   (d) Maxillary hypoplasia – there are a number of syndromes in which maxillary hypoplasia is a frequent component (Crouzon's/Apert's). Inevitably a change in maxillary structure that leads to loss of cross-sectional diameter of the nasopharynx (above) will be associated with an increased risk of OSAS.
   (e) "Adenoid facies." Chronic nasal obstruction is associated with chronic, mouth breathing, and a classic facial pattern, with high arched palate, narrow maxillary arch, and class II malocclusion [21]. Although it is unclear whether the "adenoid facies" is a cause, or a consequence of the chronic nasal obstruction [21], mouth breathing, due to associated changes in airway anatomy, might potentially propagate the OSAS [22]. Moreover, by bypassing the nasal obstruction, mouth breathing might potentially lead to a "false-negative" polysomnography – absence of significant obstructive sleep apnea inferring the absence of any significant airway occlusion.
2. Loss of volume of oropharynx. As noted, OSAS is typically multifactorial, arising as not simply as a result of upper airway (nasal) obstruction but also dependent upon a combination of retropositioning of the tongue base (retrognathia, inferior positioning of the hyoid bone), crowding of the oropharynx (obesity), loss of oromotor tone, and decreased sensory response [10] and blunted arousal response (below) all contributing to the risk of developing OSAS in any one child [19]. Increased collapsibility appears to arise as a result of both reduction in tissue tone [2] and reduction in laryngeal dilator muscle tone [23]. Consequently, in patients with lower oropharyngeal volume, and lower tissue tone, reduced negative pressures are required to cause collapse of oropharynx (pCrit), with correlation both with severity of OSAS and CPAP pressures necessary for correction [24].
   (a) Obesity. As with adults, the increasing incidence of obesity in children is an increasing cause of OSAS in children, resulting in a changing pattern of disease [10, 25]. Obesity is believed to increase the risk of OSAS not simply by change in upper airway anatomy (with correlation of neck size and OSAS risk [26]) but also adversely affect respiratory mechanics and (at least in adults) respiratory drive [25].
   (b) Posterior positioning of tongue base. Either enlargement or posterior displacement of the tongue will cause narrowing of the hypopharynx and hence increased risk of OSAS [19].
      (i) Mandibular size. Multiple studies have shown an association between both mandibular size, relative position of mandible in relation to maxilla and cranial base, and increasing risk of

OSAS [19]. Loss of volume or oropharynx, with retropositioning of tongue base, causes crowding of posterior oropharynx and hence potentiating risk of OSAS (above). Micrognathia is associated with multiple genetic syndromes.

(ii) Macroglossia. In any condition in which there is "overgrowth" of the tongue relative to the oropharynx (Down's syndrome, Beckwith-Wiedemann syndrome), causing crowding of the posterior oropharynx is inevitably associated with increasing risk of OSAS.

Consequently, there is a correlation between both mandibular size, relative tongue size, and risk of OSAS [27]. Three-dimensional MRI has been used to objectively assess airway anatomy (awake and asleep) [28], but is obviously difficult to use in routine clinical practice. Clinical assessment supported by lateral face Xray can, however, provide significant clinical information on facial anatomy, and ororopharyngeal and nasopharyngeal airway patency [19, 29], and is more readily available.

3. Reduced tone of oropharynx. OSAS arises as a consequence of a combination of upper airway obstruction, blunted arousal response (below), loss of volume of oropharynx, and increased oropharyngeal collapsibility. Increased collapsibility appears to arise as a result of both reduction in tissue tone [2] and reduction in laryngeal dilator muscle activity [23, 30]. Consequently, in patients with lower oropharyngeal volume, and lower tissue tone, reduced negative pressures are required to cause collapse of oropharynx (pCrit), with correlation both with severity of OSAS and CPAP pressures necessary for correction [24].

(a) Reduced tissue tone. As noted, obesity is increasingly a factor in the development of OSAS in children.

(b) Reduced sensory appreciation. At least in adults, there is evidence of not only chronic inflammation but also sensory denervation of upper airway receptors [31], potentially contributing to the blunted arousal response seen in patients with chronic OSAS [32].

(c) Reduction in motor tone. Maintenance of airway patency (and reopening of upper airway post closure) requires a coordinated activation of laryngeal dilators. As noted, the pressure required to cause airway collapse (pCrit) is reduced in individuals with OSAS, suggestive of reduced oromotor tone (also explaining the predilection for OSAS in REM sleep, which is associated with reduced laryngeal muscle tone [33]). Patients with diffuse reduction in skeletal muscle tone (spinal muscle atrophy, muscular dystrophies) are obviously at increased risk of OSAS, though typi-

cally present more with obstructive hypoventilation, rather than overt apneas [34]. Of note, disorders involving brainstem respiratory nuclei (such as Arnold-Chiari malformation [35]) may not only produce central sleep apnea but also obstructive sleep apnea, presumably due to dysfunction in 9th, 10th, and 11th cranial nerve nuclei, resulting in decreased sensory/oromotor control of pharyngeal dilators [36].

4. Arousal response. The role of cortical arousal, and hence sleep fragmentation, in the spectrum of OSAS is complex [32]. Classically, with collapse of the upper airway causing obstruction, resolution is dependent upon return of normal upper airway motor tone, but with resulting sleep fragmentation [37]. In patients with OSAS, there is evidence of adaptation of the upper airway dilator muscles, with hypo responsiveness of upper airway sensory fibers [31], and hence blunting of arousal threshold. There is, however, significant variability in the arousal threshold between different individuals – the degree (and duration) of obstruction that is required to trigger an arousal [38], particularly in children in whom partial obstruction tending to result in hypopneas rather than overt apneas [17]. As well, in some children partial obstruction may trigger an arousal before development of either hypopnea or apnea. This will result in significant sleep fragmentation, in the absence of overt obstructive sleep apnea – termed by Guilleminault et al. "upper airway resistance syndrome" (UARS) [2, 39]. This might explain the divergence between clinical severity as assessed by parents, compared to the OAHI score on polysomnography [2]. Consequently the "gold standard" evaluation of sleep-disordered breathing by polysomnography should therefore be taken as one (though significant) component in the overall assessment of OSAS severity.

24.2 Treatment Options

1. Adenotonsillectomy.
2. Nasal CPAP.
3. Elimination of environmental factors, such as irritants/allergens (parental smoking, cat dander, house dust mite allergen) that might be contributing to nasal obstruction [40].
4. Topical nasal steroids are frequently prescribed, even in children with obvious adenoid hypertrophy, as "a therapeutic trial." The precise effectiveness of this therapy (especially long-term) remains a matter of debate [4] and is probably dependent upon issues in addition to adenoid hypertrophy (allergic rhinitis). Topical nasal steroids are safe and can certainly be used as a temporizing treatment,

until more definitive treatment (adenoidectomy), or in children with milder degrees of or seasonal OSAS.

5. Leukotriene antagonists. Leukotrienes are key inflammatory mediators in the respiratory system. Cysteinyl leukotriene receptor-1 expression is elevated in the tonsillar tissues of children with OSAS [41] and has been implicated in adenotonsillar hypertrophy. Use of the leukotriene receptor antagonist montelukast appears to have an at least short-term, therapeutic effect in children with mild OSAS [42].

6. Orthodontic treatment. Narrowing of the hard palate, by reducing nasopharyngeal volume, and mandibular hypoplasia, by causing posterior placement of tongue, and loss of oropharyngeal volume are both associated with increased risk for OSAS. A variety of orthodontic approaches have been suggested as a means for correcting these anatomical issues [43], used alone or in combination with adenotonsillectomy [44].

   (a) Rapid maxillary expansion (RME), using an orthodontic device to cause political widening, with flattening of the palatal arch, and inferior displacement of the maxilla, by increasing cross-sectional diameter of the nares appears to be an effective therapy in selected patients [45], with potential long-term benefit.

   (b) Orthopedic mandibular advancement (OMA). For the majority of children with small or reclusive mandibles, particularly when associated with specific syndromes, mandibular advancement surgery remains the primary treatment modality [46]. Nonsurgical devices have been suggested, but there is limited evidence to support the effectiveness of this approach [19].

In summary, although there is evidence of benefit, the studies available to date have been heterogeneous in both design and patient population, and it is therefore difficult to derive any generalized conclusions [43].

5. Weight loss. Childhood obesity is an ever-increasing problem worldwide, leading to a shift in both etiology and clinical spectrum for pediatric OSAS [2, 25]. Moreover, not only does obesity increase risk of OSAS in children; it also (if present) reduces success rate for adenotonsillectomy, even in patients with significant adenotonsillar hypertrophy [25]. Although weight loss in these children will lead to improvement in their sleep-disordered breathing [47], weight loss programs require intensive and ongoing intervention, though, even then, with limited long-term success [48, 49]. Thus, many children with morbid obesity as the primary etiology are faced with the prospect of requiring lifelong nasal CPAP for management of their obstructive sleep apnea, which is obviously a far from satisfactory outcome.

6. Supplemental oxygen. Supplemental oxygen, by increasing intrapulmonary oxygen, will reduce severity of desaturations [50], but may result in more prolonged apneas [51], and potential hypercapnia, and is therefore not recommended as a routine treatment [4, 50].

7. Myofunctional therapy. As noted, reduction in oromotor muscle tone appears to be a significant contributor to risk of OSAS. A series of oropharyngeal exercises have been developed to improve upper airway muscle tone [52], which do appear to have a significant (though variable) therapeutic benefit [53]. The long-term effectiveness, as well as patient selection, for this therapy, however, remains to be clarified.

8. Other surgical options. A variety of alternative surgical approaches have been suggested, such as tongue reduction surgery and maxilla and mandibular advancement/reconstruction [18]. Evidence for their success is somewhat anecdotal, being used in very specific clinical situations (most commonly children with craniofacial syndromes), usually within tertiary care centers, where other, more "conventional" treatment options have been exhausted [54].

9. Tracheostomy. If none of the above is effective, or an option, in patients with severe OSAS, tracheostomy (by bypassing the site of the obstruction) may be the only remaining treatment option. Given the known risks (both short and long term) associated with tracheostomy, as well as the resulting marked increase in caregiver workload and training required, it is usually considered only in the more severe cases, where other treatment options have been excluded [24].

10. Do nothing. Given the issues with long-term CPAP therapy, sometimes, particularly in children with mild OSAS, the question then is whether treatment (such as CPAP) is actually causing more harm than the disease (OSAS), especially since, in a significant number of children, the OSAS will resolve with age and time [1, 55]. This has to be balanced against the concerns that there does appear to be a critical age (early childhood) when sleep fragmentation may have a long-term impact on neurocognitive development and learning [56], even once the OSAS has resolved [9, 57]. Consequently, if therapy is indeed to be instituted, it should probably be started in early childhood, rather deferring until it is obvious that spontaneous resolution is not going to occur.

In summary, the large number of available treatments for pediatric OSAS testifies to both the heterogeneity of the syndrome and that no single treatment is universally effective. Although nasal CPAP has a high degree of success (if worn), given both short- and long-term issues associated with CPAP therapy, consideration should be made for treatment options other than nasal CPAP. This requires an appreciation of the precise pathophysiology behind the development of OSAS in any specific child, with a tailored approach to therapy depending upon the child's individual circumstances.

References

1. Marcus CL, Moore RH, Rosen CL, Giordani B, Garetz SL, Taylor HG, et al. A randomized trial of adenotonsillectomy for childhood sleep apnea. N Engl J Med. 2013;368(25):2366–76.
2. Dehlink E, Tan HL. Update on paediatric obstructive sleep apnoea. J Thorac Dis. 2016;8(2):224–35.
3. Wang J, Zhao Y, Yang W, Shen T, Xue P, Yan X, et al. Correlations between obstructive sleep apnea and adenotonsillar hypertrophy in children of different weight status. Sci Rep. 2019;9(1):11455.
4. Lipton AJ, Gozal D. Treatment of obstructive sleep apnea in children: do we really know how? Sleep Med Rev. 2003;7(1):61–80.
5. Tauman R, Gulliver TE, Krishna J, Montgomery-Downs HE, O'Brien LM, Ivanenko A, et al. Persistence of obstructive sleep apnea syndrome in children after adenotonsillectomy. J Pediatr. 2006;149(6):803–8.
6. Kaditis AG, Alonso Alvarez ML, Boudewyns A, Alexopoulos EI, Ersu R, Joosten K, et al. Obstructive sleep disordered breathing in 2- to 18-year-old children: diagnosis and management. Eur Respir J. 2016;47(1):69–94.
7. Bhattacharjee R, Kheirandish-Gozal L, Spruyt K, Mitchell RB, Promchiarak J, Simakajornboon N, et al. Adenotonsillectomy outcomes in treatment of obstructive sleep apnea in children: a multicenter retrospective study. Am J Respir Crit Care Med. 2010;182(5):676–83.
8. Huang YS, Guilleminault C, Lee LA, Lin CH, Hwang FM. Treatment outcomes of adenotonsillectomy for children with obstructive sleep apnea: a prospective longitudinal study. Sleep. 2014;37(1):71–6.
9. Marcus CL, Brooks LJ, Draper KA, Gozal D, Halbower AC, Jones J, et al. Diagnosis and management of childhood obstructive sleep apnea syndrome. Pediatrics. 2012;130(3):e714–55.
10. Huang YS, Guilleminault C. Pediatric obstructive sleep Apnea: where do we stand? Adv Otorhinolaryngol. 2017;80:136–44.
11. Waters KA, Everett FM, Bruderer JW, Sullivan CE. Obstructive sleep apnea: the use of nasal CPAP in 80 children. Am J Respir Crit Care Med. 1995;152(2):780–5.
12. Hawkins SM, Jensen EL, Simon SL, Friedman NR. Correlates of Pediatric CPAP adherence. J Clin Sleep Med. 2016;12(6):879–84.
13. Marcus CL, Ward SL, Mallory GB, Rosen CL, Beckerman RC, Weese-Mayer DE, et al. Use of nasal continuous positive airway pressure as treatment of childhood obstructive sleep apnea. J Pediatr. 1995;127(1):88–94.
14. Sawyer AM, Gooneratne NS, Marcus CL, Ofer D, Richards KC, Weaver TE. A systematic review of CPAP adherence across age groups: clinical and empiric insights for developing CPAP adherence interventions. Sleep Med Rev. 2011;15(6):343–56.
15. Alqahtani JS, Worsley P, Voegeli D. Effect of humidified noninvasive ventilation on the development of facial skin breakdown. Respir Care. 2018;63(9):1102–10.
16. Li KK, Riley RW, Guilleminault C. An unreported risk in the use of home nasal continuous positive airway pressure and home nasal ventilation in children: mid-face hypoplasia. Chest. 2000;117(3):916–8.
17. Katz ES, D'Ambrosio CM. Pathophysiology of pediatric obstructive sleep apnea. Proc Am Thorac Soc. 2008;5(2):253–62.
18. Randerath WJ, Verbraecken J, Andreas S, Bettega G, Boudewyns A, Hamans E, et al. Non-CPAP therapies in obstructive sleep apnoea. Eur Respir J. 2011;37(5):1000–28.
19. Sutherland K, Lee RW, Cistulli PA. Obesity and craniofacial structure as risk factors for obstructive sleep apnoea: impact of ethnicity. Respirology. 2012;17(2):213–22.
20. Hurley JJ, Hensley JL. Physiology, airway resistance. Treasure Island: StatPearls; 2021.
21. Elluru RG. Adenoid facies and nasal airway obstruction: cause and effect? Arch Otolaryngol Head Neck Surg. 2005;131(10):919–20.
22. Kim EJ, Choi JH, Kim KW, Kim TH, Lee SH, Lee HM, et al. The impacts of open-mouth breathing on upper airway space in obstructive sleep apnea: 3-D MDCT analysis. Eur Arch Otorhinolaryngol. 2011;268(4):533–9.
23. Marcus CL, Keenan BT, Huang J, Yuan H, Pinto S, Bradford RM, et al. The obstructive sleep apnoea syndrome in adolescents. Thorax. 2017;72(8):720–8.
24. Landry SA, Joosten SA, Eckert DJ, Jordan AS, Sands SA, White DP, et al. Therapeutic CPAP level predicts upper airway collapsibility in patients with obstructive sleep Apnea. Sleep. 2017;40(6):zsx056.
25. Arens R, Muzumdar H. Childhood obesity and obstructive sleep apnea syndrome. J Appl Physiol (1985). 2010;108(2):436–44.
26. Kawaguchi Y, Fukumoto S, Inaba M, Koyama H, Shoji T, Shoji S, et al. Different impacts of neck circumference and visceral obesity on the severity of obstructive sleep apnea syndrome. Obesity (Silver Spring). 2011;19(2):276–82.
27. Chi L, Comyn FL, Mitra N, Reilly MP, Wan F, Maislin G, et al. Identification of craniofacial risk factors for obstructive sleep apnoea using three-dimensional MRI. Eur Respir J. 2011;38(2):348–58.
28. Fleck RJ, Shott SR, Mahmoud M, Ishman SL, Amin RS, Donnelly LF. Magnetic resonance imaging of obstructive sleep apnea in children. Pediatr Radiol. 2018;48(9):1223–33.
29. Shintani T, Asakura K, Kataura A. Evaluation of the role of adenotonsillar hypertrophy and facial morphology in children with obstructive sleep apnea. ORL J Otorhinolaryngol Relat Spec. 1997;59(5):286–91.
30. Ayuse TKJ, Sanuki T, Kurata S, Okayasu I. Pathogenesis of upper airway obstruction and mechanical intervention during sedation and sleep. J Dental Sleep Med. 2016;3(1):11–9.
31. Boyd JH, Petrof BJ, Hamid Q, Fraser R, Kimoff RJ. Upper airway muscle inflammation and denervation changes in obstructive sleep apnea. Am J Respir Crit Care Med. 2004;170(5):541–6.
32. Eckert DJ, Younes MK. Arousal from sleep: implications for obstructive sleep apnea pathogenesis and treatment. J Appl Physiol (1985). 2014;116(3):302–13.
33. Huang J, Karamessinis LR, Pepe ME, Glinka SM, Samuel JM, Gallagher PR, et al. Upper airway collapsibility during REM sleep in children with the obstructive sleep apnea syndrome. Sleep. 2009;32(9):1173–81.
34. Suresh S, Wales P, Dakin C, Harris MA, Cooper DG. Sleep-related breathing disorder in Duchenne muscular dystrophy: disease spectrum in the paediatric population. J Paediatr Child Health. 2005;41(9–10):500–3.
35. Selvadurai S, Al-Saleh S, Amin R, Zweerink A, Drake J, Propst EJ, et al. Utility of brain MRI in children with sleep-disordered breathing. Laryngoscope. 2017;127(2):513–9.
36. Leu RM. Sleep-related breathing disorders and the Chiari 1 malformation. Chest. 2015;148(5):1346–52.
37. Remmers JE, deGroot WJ, Sauerland EK, Anch AM. Pathogenesis of upper airway occlusion during sleep. J Appl Physiol Respir Environ Exerc Physiol. 1978;44(6):931–8.
38. Marcus CL, Moreira GA, Bamford O, Lutz J. Response to inspiratory resistive loading during sleep in normal children and children with obstructive apnea. J Appl Physiol (1985). 1999;87(4):1448–54.
39. Bao G, Guilleminault C. Upper airway resistance syndrome--one decade later. Curr Opin Pulm Med. 2004;10(6):461–7.
40. Kohler M, Bloch KE, Stradling JR. The role of the nose in the pathogenesis of obstructive sleep apnoea and snoring. Eur Respir J. 2007;30(6):1208–15.

41. Kaditis AG, Ioannou MG, Chaidas K, Alexopoulos EI, Apostolidou M, Apostolidis T, et al. Cysteinyl leukotriene receptors are expressed by tonsillar T cells of children with obstructive sleep apnea. Chest. 2008;134(2):324–31.

42. Goldbart AD, Greenberg-Dotan S, Tal A. Montelukast for children with obstructive sleep apnea: a double-blind, placebo-controlled study. Pediatrics. 2012;130(3):e575–80.

43. Huynh NT, Desplats E, Almeida FR. Orthodontics treatments for managing obstructive sleep apnea syndrome in children: a systematic review and meta-analysis. Sleep Med Rev. 2016;25:84–94.

44. Templier L, Rossi C, Miguez M, Perez JC, Curto A, Albaladejo A, et al. Combined surgical and orthodontic treatments in children with OSA: a systematic review. J Clin Med. 2020;9(8):2387.

45. Camacho M, Chang ET, Song SA, Abdullatif J, Zaghi S, Pirelli P, et al. Rapid maxillary expansion for pediatric obstructive sleep apnea: a systematic review and meta-analysis. Laryngoscope. 2017;127(7):1712–9.

46. Noller MW, Guilleminault C, Gouveia CJ, Mack D, Neighbors CL, Zaghi S, et al. Mandibular advancement for pediatric obstructive sleep apnea: a systematic review and meta-analysis. J Craniomaxillofac Surg. 2018;46(8):1296–302.

47. Verhulst SL, Franckx H, Van Gaal L, De Backer W, Desager K. The effect of weight loss on sleep-disordered breathing in obese teenagers. Obesity (Silver Spring). 2009;17(6):1178–83.

48. Zolotarjova J, Ten Velde G, Vreugdenhil ACE. Effects of multidisciplinary interventions on weight loss and health outcomes in children and adolescents with morbid obesity. Obes Rev. 2018;19(7):931–46.

49. Styne DM, Arslanian SA, Connor EL, Farooqi IS, Murad MH, Silverstein JH, et al. Pediatric obesity-assessment, treatment, and prevention: an Endocrine Society clinical practice guideline. J Clin Endocrinol Metab. 2017;102(3):709–57.

50. Brouillette RT, Waters K. Oxygen therapy for pediatric obstructive sleep apnea syndrome: how safe? How effective? Am J Respir Crit Care Med. 1996;153(1):1–2.

51. Mehta V, Vasu TS, Phillips B, Chung F. Obstructive sleep apnea and oxygen therapy: a systematic review of the literature and meta-analysis. J Clin Sleep Med. 2013;9(3):271–9.

52. Guimaraes KC, Drager LF, Genta PR, Marcondes BF, Lorenzi-Filho G. Effects of oropharyngeal exercises on patients with moderate obstructive sleep apnea syndrome. Am J Respir Crit Care Med. 2009;179(10):962–6.

53. Bandyopadhyay A, Kaneshiro K, Camacho M. Effect of myofunctional therapy on children with obstructive sleep apnea: a meta-analysis. Sleep Med. 2020;75:210–7.

54. Cohen SR, Simms C, Burstein FD, Thomsen J. Alternatives to tracheostomy in infants and children with obstructive sleep apnea. J Pediatr Surg. 1999;34(1):182–6. discussion 7.

55. Venekamp RP, Hearne BJ, Chandrasekharan D, Blackshaw H, Lim J, Schilder AG. Tonsillectomy or adenotonsillectomy versus non-surgical management for obstructive sleep-disordered breathing in children. Cochrane Database Syst Rev. 2015;10:CD011165.

56. Galland B, Spruyt K, Dawes P, McDowall PS, Elder D, Schaughency E. Sleep disordered breathing and academic performance: a meta-analysis. Pediatrics. 2015;136(4):e934–46.

57. Gozal D. Obstructive sleep apnea in children: implications for the developing central nervous system. Semin Pediatr Neurol. 2008;15(2):100–6.

PAP Management and Adherence for Children and Adolescents with OSAS

Anna C. Bitners and Raanan Arens

25.1 Introduction

Obstructive sleep apnea syndrome (OSAS) is a respiratory disorder characterized by recurrent partial or complete airway obstruction during sleep leading to sleep fragmentation and ventilation abnormalities. The estimated prevalence rate of OSAS in childhood ranges from 1.2% to 5.7%, peaks between 2 and 8 years of age, and is usually associated with adenotonsillar hypertrophy [1]; however, OSAS can occur in children of all ages, even children with normal size tonsils and adenoids, including those who have undergone adenotonsillectomy (AT). As early as the neonatal period, underlying conditions such as craniofacial anomalies affecting upper airway structure and neurological disorders affecting upper airway neuromotor tone may lead to airway obstruction during sleep. Later onset of symptoms, particularly when associated with obesity, may be seen during school-age and adolescent years, and in some populations the incidence may exceed 50% [2]. The process of diagnosing childhood OSAS continues to progress as more morbidities are recognized and more evolved diagnostic methodologies become available [3].

The American Academy of Pediatrics (AAP) recommends routine screening for OSAS at each health maintenance visit [1]. Nocturnal symptoms include snoring, gasping, respiratory pauses, and restless sleep. Daytime sleepiness is less common in children; however, chronic sleep deprivation and intermittent hypoxia associated with OSAS may lead to behavioral problems and neurocognitive impairments. Polysomnography is the gold standard for the diagnosis of OSAS and establishes both the presence and severity of the disorder.

The AAP recommends AT as the first-line treatment for OSAS [1]. This recommendation is supported by the results of a large randomized clinical trial which found that surgical intervention with AT was associated with significant improvements in behavior, quality of life, and polysomnographic findings as compared to watchful waiting [4]. While AT improves respiratory parameters, it is not universally curative, and as many as 70% of children still exhibit residual disease following surgery [5]. This statistic is predicted on the population being served and will differ depending on the referral base and if the facility is a tertiary care center.

For persistent OSAS following surgery, positive airway pressure (PAP) therapy is recommended [1]. PAP therapy may also be used in cases where AT is not indicated, such as in children with non-obstructive tonsils and/or adenoid and those with OSAS due to comorbid conditions such as craniofacial abnormalities restricting upper airway size or neurologic disorders increasing upper airway collapsibility [6]. In addition to AT and PAP, adjunctive therapies such as intranasal corticosteroids and weight loss (for overweight or obese children) may also be indicated. A summary of management strategies for children with OSAS is presented in Table 25.1.

25.2 Indications for PAP

PAP may be indicated for OSAS—and other forms of sleep disordered breathing—in a variety of clinical scenarios including management of residual OSAS following AT, OSAS associated with obesity, craniofacial anomalies, genetic disorders affecting upper airway structure and function during sleep, and OSAS in infancy. Each of these will be discussed in further detail.

25.2.1 Residual OSAS Following AT

A common indication for PAP in otherwise healthy children with OSAS is for the management of residual OSAS following AT. Only 27.2% of children experience complete resolution of OSAS following surgery [5]. When persistent OSAS

A. C. Bitners · R. Arens (✉)
Division of Respiratory and Sleep Medicine, Department of Pediatrics, Children's Hospital at Montefiore, Albert Einstein College of Medicine, Bronx, NY, USA
e-mail: abitner2@jhmi.edu; raanan.arens@einsteinmed.edu

C. M. Shapiro et al. (eds.), *CPAP Adherence*, https://doi.org/10.1007/978-3-030-93146-9_25

Table 25.1 Management of the child with OSAS

Otherwise healthy children

Mild OSAS	Moderate OSAS	Severe OSAS
AT vs watchful waiting for 6 months Intranasal corticosteroid Weight management, if overweight/obese	Specialist referral (e.g., sleep medicine, otolaryngology) AT PAP therapy Weight management, if overweight/obese	Specialist referral (e.g., sleep medicine, otolaryngology) Cardiology evaluation AT with overnight observation PAP therapy Weight management, if overweight/obese

Children with complex comorbidities

Mild OSAS	Moderate OSAS	Severe OSAS
Specialist referral (e.g., sleep medicine, otolaryngology) AT Intranasal corticosteroid Weight management, if overweight/obese	Specialist referral (e.g., sleep medicine, otolaryngology) AT with overnight observation Other airway and/or craniofacial surgery PAP therapy Weight management, if overweight/obese	Specialist referral (e.g., sleep medicine, otolaryngology, craniofacial team) Cardiology evaluation AT with overnight observation Other airway and/or craniofacial surgery PAP therapy Weight management, if overweight/obese

Children with residual OSAS following AT

Mild OSAS	Moderate OSAS	Severe OSAS
Intranasal corticosteroid Weight management, if overweight/obese	PAP therapy Weight management, if overweight/obese	PAP therapy Weight management, if overweight/obese Secondary surgical intervention Tracheostomy

Modified from Bitners and Arens [79]

AT adenotonsillectomy, *OSAS* obstructive sleep apnea syndrome, *PAP* positive airway pressure

is suspected, a repeat polysomnogram should be performed to confirm the diagnosis. While there is no absolute apnea-hypopnea index (AHI) cutoff, treatment of residual OSAS may be indicated if the postoperative AHI is above 5 events/hour. Risk factors associated with persistent OSAS following surgery include age >7 years, severe disease, asthma, and obesity [5, 7]. In the immediate postoperative period, children are at risk for respiratory complications and oxygen desaturations—particularly those with age <2 years, craniofacial anomalies, hypotonia, obesity, and high-risk PSG findings [8, 9]. These patients may require overnight observation following surgery for monitoring and can be treated effectively with PAP if oxygen desaturation occurs [8].

25.2.2 OSAS Associated with Obesity

Obesity itself increases the risk of OSAS more than fourfold [10]. With the current epidemic of childhood obesity, the number of children affected by residual OSAS following surgery is significant and likely to rise. The exact reason for

persistent OSAS in that population is multifactorial and includes anatomical risk factors such as increased size of the parapharyngeal fat pads and increased visceral adiposity which reduce upper airway size and stability during sleep [2]. As with non-obese children, AT is considered first-line therapy; however, OSAS may persist in up to 76% of children following surgery [11]. This may be due in part to residual adenotonsillar tissue and/or increased volume of the soft palate which have been observed following AT in children with obesity [12].

25.2.3 OSAS Associated with Craniofacial Anomalies

Children with conditions which affect development of the facial skeleton are at increased risk of developing OSAS. While AT may be useful in widening the upper airway, it is not always considered first-line therapy and is rarely sufficient to treat OSAS in these children.

Craniosynostosis is caused by premature closure of one or more cranial sutures. It may be an isolated finding or occur in the context of genetic syndromes such as Apert, Crouzon, or Pfeiffer syndrome. OSAS is present in 40–84% of these children [13–15] and is predominantly due to midface hypoplasia, although choanal atresia and adenotonsillar hypertrophy can also contribute [16]. Surgical management of OSAS—including AT and midface advancement—are not always successful and can be associated with high complication rates [14, 17]. Furthermore, many children remain dependent on PAP or require tracheotomy following surgery [14]. PAP therapy can be used for children awaiting surgery or those who responded only partially to surgical management. Because there is some evidence that OSAS resolves over time [18], PAP therapy should be considered as an alternative to invasive surgical procedures. While PAP is effective in reducing the severity of OSAS [19, 20], its use presents certain challenges. Achieving an appropriate mask fit can be difficult in children. This problem may be exacerbated in children with craniofacial anomalies. PAP adherence in children with craniosynostosis is not well-studied but appears to be high with reported rates of 4/5 (80%) [19] and 10/12 (83%) [20].

Pierre-Robin sequence is characterized by a triad of micrognathia, glossoptosis, and upper airway obstruction which may be accompanied by cleft palate. There is a high prevalence of OSAS at 46–83% [21]. Children with mild upper airway obstruction may be adequately managed with lateral or prone position and nasopharyngeal stenting [22]. If further respiratory support is required, a trial of PAP therapy is warranted. PAP is shown to be effective in children with Pierre-Robin sequence [23, 24] and is a good alternative to invasive surgical treatment, particularly because many children do not require prolonged PAP use [24] and some children experience relief of upper airway obstruction with time [25, 26].

25.2.4 OSAS Associated with Down Syndrome

Up to 70% of children with Down syndrome have OSAS, and about half exhibit severe disease [27]. Risk factors leading to OSAS in children with Down syndrome include midface or mandibular hypoplasia, macroglossia, lingual tonsil hypertrophy, decreased airway neuromotor tone, and hypopharyngeal collapse. AT is considered first-line treatment, but success rates can be as low as 20% [28]. Persistent OSAS may be treated with PAP therapy.

25.2.5 OSAS in Infancy

OSAS can occur in very young children, including in the first year of life. Due to their unique anatomy and physiology, infants are predisposed to obstructive events and desaturations during sleep. This includes high nasal resistance, reduced airway stiffness, increased chest wall compliance, and ventilatory control instability [6, 29]. A propensity for upper airway obstruction can be exacerbated by gastroesophageal reflux, which can lead to upper airway edema and laryngospasm. OSAS in infancy may also develop in the context of craniofacial abnormalities and genetic syndromes, as discussed above. Neuromuscular disorders which affect upper airway tone may also contribute to OSAS. PAP has shown to be effective in improving respiratory parameters for infants with OSAS [30, 31]. Although initiation of PAP therapy may be challenging in this age group, many infants can acclimatize and tolerate PAP therapy well.

25.3 Mechanisms of PAP Ventilation

Simplistically, the upper airway can be modeled as a collapsible tube, whereby obstruction occurs when the pressure surrounding the airway exceeds the pressure within the airway. PAP therapy serves as a pneumatic splint for the soft tissues of the upper airway by maintaining the intraluminal pressure above the airway critical closing pressure (Pcrit), which is the intraluminal pressure required to maintain patency. Children with OSAS have a high Pcrit compared to controls, which explains their propensity for airway collapse during sleep [32, 33]. Studies using magnetic resonance imaging (MRI) in adults demonstrate that effective PAP therapy increases the mean airway cross-sectional area (CSA), minimum airway CSA, and upper airway volume [34, 35] thereby protecting the airway from collapse and obstruction. In addi-

tion to the pneumatic splinting effect, PAP therapy exerts a variety of other effects on the upper airway. For example, effective PAP increases end expiratory lung volume, and the resultant thoracic inflation exerts a tracheal "tug" effect which stiffens the upper airway and reduces its propensity for collapse [36]. Addition benefit with PAP may be derived from anatomic changes to the upper airway soft tissues, including reduced airway edema and decreased thickness of the lateral pharyngeal walls [35].

PAP also has measurable effects on cardiopulmonary physiology. In patients with OSAS, the negative intrathoracic pressure generated during apneas leads to decreased left ventricular filling and stroke volume [37]. CPAP increases intrathoracic pressure with a consequent reduction in ventricular preload and afterload [38]. With time, nocturnal CPAP therapy may confer a cardioprotective effect and has been associated with improved exercise tolerance in adults with heart failure [38] which may be attributable to decreased left ventricular stroke work and myocardial oxygen consumption in PAP users [39].

25.4 Forms of PAP Ventilation

For treatment of OSAS, PAP therapy can be utilized in a variety of modes. Continuous PAP (CPAP) and bilevel PAP (BPAP) are most common, but automatic PAP (APAP) and adaptive servo ventilation (ASV) may also be employed. The various forms of PAP ventilation and their indications are displayed in Table 25.2.

CPAP delivers constant pressure throughout the respiratory cycle. In BPAP, the inspiratory pressure and expiratory pressures are adjusted separately to allow for increased pressure during the inspiratory phase. There is no significant difference in adherence rates between CPAP and BPAP in adults [40] or children [41, 42]. While there are no specific

Table 25.2 Forms of PAP ventilation

Form	Method	Indications
CPAP	Applies continuous pressure during both inspiration and expiration	OSAS due to upper airway obstruction
BPAP	Applies two pressure levels: Inspiratory and expiratory	OSAS with obstructive hypoventilation, non-obstructive hypoventilation
APAP (auto PAP)	Applied pressure is adjusted to the patient's respiration	Positional OSAS, sleep stage-dependent OSAS
ASV	Pressure is adjusted to the patient's respiration to deliver a set ventilation	Complex sleep apnea, central sleep apnea

Modified from Nandalike and Arens [80]
CPAP continuous positive airway pressure, *BPAP* bilevel positive airway pressure, *APAP (Auto PAP)* automatic positive airway pressure, *ASV* adaptive servo ventilation

criteria for use of BPAP in pediatric OSAS, a trial of BPAP may be warranted for children with poor CPAP adherence secondary to pressure intolerance as BPAP provides pressure relief during expiration and may reduce the mean airway pressure during the respiratory cycle. Some children with pressure intolerance may also benefit from using a PAP device with a "ramp" function which slowly increases the pressure and allows children to fall asleep without the full force of therapeutic PAP.

Whether CPAP or BPAP is used, the pressure settings are initially determined during an overnight attended sleep study with PAP titration [43]. Respiratory and sleep parameters are monitored as pressure is increased with the goal of eliminating respiratory events and gas exchange abnormalities while maintaining patient comfort. Titration may be performed on the same night as the initial polysomnogram to diagnose OSAS (split-night study) or during a second full-night study. In children, split night studies are not recommended because it does not allow the child to become acclimatized to the mask prior to usage. Unfamiliarity and discomfort with the mask in this setting may lead to decreased PAP adherence in the future.

Auto-titrating PAP (APAP), also known as auto-adjusting PAP, is an alternative to CPAP or BPAP. Based on the patient's airflow, APAP delivers a variable pressure between two pre-determined set points at the level required to prevent apneas and hypopneas. Pressure is decreased in the absence of obstructive events and increased when obstructions occur, as in REM sleep or with positional changes. APAP is less commonly used, but has been shown to be safe and effective in children [44–46].

25.5 Adherence to PAP Therapy

25.5.1 Defining Adherence

PAP therapy is a highly effective for treatment of OSAS in children across age groups and with a range of underlying pathophysiological mechanisms; however, effectiveness is limited by poor adherence. When PAP is prescribed, it is typically intended to be used every night for the duration of sleep. For a variety of reasons, PAP is often not used for all hours of sleep, but at present there is no standardized definition of adherence to PAP therapy. In the adult literature, studies of CPAP often define adherence as 4 hours per night on at least 70% of nights [47, 48]. This definition emerged after several early studies reported that average nightly CPAP use was approximately 4.7 hours/night [49]. Similarly, studies analyzing adherence rates in children typically define adherence as >4 hours/night for at least 50–70% of nights [50, 51]. This definition has been operationalized in studies investigating the factors associated with adherence to therapy.

Because insurance companies often require adequate adherence as a prerequisite to coverage, adherence surveillance has become standard of care for adults using PAP [40, 52]. While this benchmark is a useful metric for comparing adherence between study groups or across clinical trials, it is important to acknowledge that its clinical significance is not clear. Studies in adults have shown that some benefits of PAP require nightly use of six or more hours/night, which is significantly longer than the 4-hour benchmark used to report adherence. For example, improvement in blood pressure and quality of life require greater than 5.6 and 7.5 hours per night, respectively [53, 54]. Furthermore, improvement in Epworth Sleepiness Scale exhibits a dose-response relationship with CPAP therapy, such that increasing benefit is garnered from additional use [54, 55]. As a further example, in a historical cohort of 871 patients with OSAS, the 5-year survival rate of PAP users with high adherence (>6 hours) was 96.4% as compared to 85.5% in users with low adherence (<1 hour) [56]. A meta-analysis of RCTs later found no relationship between CPAP use and cardiovascular mortality, but some included studies had low CPAP use (<3.5 hours/night) which raises the possibility that poor adherence influenced the findings [57]. There is also growing recognition that OSAS is a heterogenous disorder with a multifaceted pathophysiology and that individual phenotypes may respond differently to treatment [58, 59].

When CPAP was first used in the treatment of OSAS in children, measurement of adherence was limited to patient self-report or parental recall, which may overestimate usage as compared to objective data [60]. Technological advancements have since enabled objective measurement of adherence. PAP machines are now equipped with software which tracks nightly usage as the number of hours that the mask is on and therapeutic pressure is provided. This was developed both to track adherence with PAP and to assess outcomes of treatment on end-organ disease.

25.5.2 Quantifying Adherence

In studies of adults using PAP, reported adherence to PAP therapy ranges from 2.9 to 6.5 hours/night, with many studies reporting 4.4–5.4 hours/night [40]. Reports of % nights used range from 78 to 98%, with many studies reporting use on 81–94% of nights [40]. The percentage of adult patients using CPAP >4 hours per night is 66–73% [61, 62].

In the extant literature, adherence rates for children vary widely depending on the study population and definition of adherence. In a report of 50 children (aged 6 months–18 years), mean daily use of CPAP was 4.7 hours (IQR 1.4–7.0), and mean daily use on days used was 6.4 hours (IQR 3.3–8.3). While sleep requirements vary with age, 4.7 hours is significantly less than optimal sleep duration, suggesting that many children used CPAP for only a portion of the night. There was also high variability between days: 24% of children used CPAP (defined as at least 1 hour/night) on less than half the nights. In a randomized, controlled trial of pressure release (Bi-Flex) compared to CPAP, Marcus et al. noted suboptimal adherence in both groups, with no difference in effectiveness or adherence [60]. In the first month of use, mean daily use of CPAP and Bi-Flex were 3.4 and 3.1 hours, respectively, and declined to 2.1 hours for CPAP and remained 3.1 hours for Bi-Flex in the third month of use. There was also marked variability between patients, with average nightly use during the first month ranging from 1 to 536 minutes/night. Simon et al. reported average daily use of 3.35 hours/night, with participants using CPAP for at least 4 hours/night on only 41% of days [63]. They developed a CPAP-specific questionnaire to identify barriers to adherence and found that not using the machine when away from home and the child not feeling well were the most frequently reported barriers to use.

When interpreting adherence data, it is important to distinguish between "time on" and "time at pressure," the latter being indicative of therapeutic use. In their cohort, DiFeo et al. found that average time with the device on was 4.9 ± 2.7 hours/night, whereas the average time that the device was on and delivering full pressure was 3 ± 3 hours [64]. In a cohort of 141 children, Xanthopoulos et al. measured adherence using three metrics: average use per night (2.94 hours), percentage of days used (74.2%), and duration of use on days used (4.5 hours) [65]. They found that adherence variables were highly correlated with each other, suggesting that children with high adherence tend to use PAP routinely and consistently throughout the night. This observation is supported by the findings of Hawkins et al., who compared average daily use in adherent vs non-adherent children [66]. They defined adherence as >70% nightly use and average usage ≥4 hours/night. Of 140 participants, 69 (49%) were adherent to therapy. The mean daily use was 7.4 hours/night in the adherent group and 1.7 hours/night in the non-adherent group. PAP was used on 94% of nights in the adherent group compared to 52% of nights in the non-adherent group. Overall, studies show that while some children are highly adherent to PAP therapy, there is an overall trend of suboptimal adherence to PAP.

25.6 Factors Predicting and Associated with PAP Adherence

In a review of PAP adherence in children which examined factors influencing PAP use from 16 studies, only three factors were associated with increased PAP usage in more than one study: younger age (5/13 studies, 38%), female sex (2/11 studies, 18.2%), and presence of developmental delay (2/5 studies, 40%) [50]. Another recent systematic review and meta-analysis which evaluated factors associated with adherence similarly identified younger age, female sex, and presence of developmental delay but also found Caucasian race, increased level of maternal education, and higher AHI to be predictive [51]. A meta-analysis was performed for several characteristics revealing on odds ratio (OR) of 1.48 and 1.26 for female sex and Caucasian race, respectively. The mean difference in AHI between adherent and non-adherent groups was 4.32 events/hour.

While individual studies have reported associations with race [64], BMI [67], medical comorbidities [68], mask type [69], device type [68], disease severity [41], duration of PAP use [63], household income [70], and maternal education [64], none of these factors was found to be significant in more than one study [50]. Individual studies have reported increased adherence in children who underwent titration at age < 6 months [70], had caregivers with increased self-efficacy [65] or concern [67], experienced fewer treatment barriers [63], and received monetary assistance in purchasing the machine [68]; however, these factors have only been evaluated by a single study. Further studies exploring these associations are needed to corroborate the findings and assess their generalizability in larger samples. Of note, the factors found to be associated with PAP adherence in children vary considerably from those in adults (Table 25.3). A summary of studies assessing PAP adherence in children and adolescents is presented in Table 25.4.

Because increasing age is routinely associated with decreased PAP use, adolescents are at high risk for PAP non-adherence. O'Donnell et al. found that adolescents age 13–18 years had a mean daily use of just 3.6 hours and used PAP on only 57.9% of nights compared to 74.2% (age 6–12) and 94.6% (age ≤ 5) in younger children [69]. Similarly, DiFeo et al. found that older children and adolescents were less likely to be adherent to therapy after excluding children with developmental delay from the analysis [64]. Poor adherence in this age group may be related to their unique stage of

Table 25.3 Factors which may be associated with PAP adherence in adults and children

Children	Adults
Baseline characteristics	
Younger age [64, 69]	High AHI, ODI [81–83]
Female sex [66, 68]	High Epworth Sleepiness Scale [84]
Developmental delay [66, 70]	
Financial support/resources [68, 70]	Low nasal resistance [85]
	Early PAP adherence [74]
Interventions	
Interdisciplinary intervention programs [75, 76, 78]	Telemonitoring [40]
Behavioral therapy [75, 76, 78]	Device troubleshooting [40]
Token economy [77]	Educational or behavioral interventions [40]

AHI apnea-hypopnea index, ODI oxygen desaturation index

Table 25.4 Factors associated with PAP adherence in children and adolescents

Author/year	N	Study type	Factors associated with adherence	Factors not associated with adherence
DiFeo 2012 [64]	56	Prospective observational	Younger age, maternal education, race, family social support	Sex, obesity status, developmental delay, disease severity, nasal symptoms, sleepiness, child behavior, parental stress, pressure setting
Hawkins 2016 [66]	52	Retrospective review	Female sex, developmental delay	Age, ethnicity, obesity status, disease severity, pressure setting, device mode, insurance status, presence of residual OSAS
Kang 2019 [70]	177	Retrospective review	Developmental delay, higher median neighborhood income, higher PAP pressure, titration at <6 months of age	Not reported
Lynch 2019 [67]	25	Prospective observational	Younger age, lower BMI, higher baseline OSA-18 score, decreased sleep disturbance and decreased caregiver concern after initiation of PAP	Sex, race, household income, maternal education, disease severity, physical symptoms, emotional disturbance, daytime function
Marcus 2006 [60]	21	Randomized double-blind clinical trial	Not reported	Age, sex, race, disease severity, device mode, OSAS symptoms, pressure setting, indication for PAP
Marcus 2012 [42]	56	Randomized double-blind clinical trial	Not reported	Age, obesity status, device mode
Nathan 2013 [68]	51	Retrospective review	Female sex, asthma, genetic syndrome, BPAP (compared to CPAP), funding from social work	Obesity status, disease severity, polysomnogram indices, counseling prior to treatment initiation, air humidification
Nixon 2011 [86]	30	Prospective observational	Smaller difference between initial prescribed pressure and final treatment pressure	Age, sex, disease severity, comorbidities, intellectual disability, socioeconomic status, location of CPAP initiation (home vs hospital)
O'Donnell 2006 [69]	50	Retrospective review	Younger age, nasal mask	Sex, disease severity, prior surgical treatment, typical cognitive ability, psychology referral and support
Simon 2012 [63]	48	Prospective observational, development of screening tool (ABCQ)	Greater length of time prescribed PAP, fewer greater to adherence (as measured by ABCQ score)	Device mode, device brand, mask type, home health-care provider
Uong 2007 [41]	27	Retrospective review	Higher baseline AHI, greater improvement in AHI on PAP	Age, sex, race, BMI, device mode, OSAS symptoms
Xanthopoulos 2017 [65]	141	Retrospective review	Greater caregiver-reported self-efficacy	Caregiver-reported risk perception and outcome expectations. Patient-reported risk perception, outcome expectation, or self-efficacy

development marked by increased autonomy, shifting social pressures, feelings of invincibility, desire to conform to peer group norms, and challenge of authority figures [64]. Accordingly, reasons for PAP non-adherence in adolescents may differ from those for younger children.

Qualitative studies exploring perceptions of PAP use and challenges to adherence in adolescents specifically provide insight into the adherence patterns in this age group. Prashad et al. analyzed semi-structured interviews with adolescent PAP users (age 12–18) and their caregivers [71]. They identified four key issues that played a role in adherence: degree of structure in the home, social reactions, mode of communication among family members, and perception of benefits. Adolescents with high PAP adherence had a stable family structure which incorporated PAP into the family's daily routine and allowed for parental assistance with troubleshooting PAP problems. They described being motivated to use PAP out of personal fear of the consequences of

untreated OSAS and to alleviate caregiver concern. Parents of adolescents with high adherence described using an authoritative—as opposed to authoritarian—parenting style. Based on their findings, the authors suggested that interventional strategies which address health education, offer peer support groups, and provide developmentally appropriate individualized support may be successful in improving adherence in this population. Another qualitative analysis of adolescent PAP users performed by Alebraheem et al. also highlighted the importance of identifying the patient's desired level of family involvement and providing developmentally appropriate support [72]. In their study, participants noted that an adjustment and acclimatization period was important to address issues with PAP and that the perception of challenges to PAP use were emphasized over symptom relief. Based on their findings, the authors suggest that interventions to improve adherence in adolescent PAP users could include anticipatory guidance regarding potential barriers, encouragement of patient-caregiver dialogue regarding challenges, and hospital-moderated peer support forums.

In adults, there is no difference in adherence rates between CPAP and BPAP or CPAP and APAP; however certain patients may prefer BPAP or APAP and tolerate it better [73]. In children, two studies have shown that adherence is greater in CPAP users compared to BPAP users, but the difference was not significant [41, 42]. Similarly, preliminary adherence data in children showed no difference between APAP and CPAP [44].

25.7 Interventions to Improve Adherence

The American Academy of Sleep Medicine recently commissioned an expert task force to conduct a systematic review and meta-analysis of PAP therapy in adults which found that telemonitoring, device troubleshooting, and educational or behavioral interventions were associated with a clinically significant improvement in adherence [73]. Although some of these interventions may also be useful in the pediatric population, the myriad of differences between the pediatric and adult populations imply that findings may not be correlated across age groups. While specific strategies and interventions may vary, there is a general trend—in both adults and children—of improved adherence following behavioral interventions. Particularly because adherence rates in the first days-weeks of therapy predict long-term adherence [74], many interventions target initiation and early utilization of PAP. Although side effects do not predict non-adherence [49], providers should troubleshoot adverse effects with individual patients in order to improve comfort, and this may increase usage for some individuals. Screening for mask discomfort, mask leak, nasal congestion, and eye dryness at clinic visits can identify potential problems which may be impacting adherence. Providing children and their families with psychosocial support (through PAP education and close clinical follow-up) and assistance with troubleshooting (through device adjustments) is key. In pediatrics, a desensitization process can help children accommodate to the mask. Prior to the PAP titration study, parents can introduce their child to the mask at home, while they are participating in an enjoyable activity to allow the child to acclimatize to the mask before the introduction of pressure delivery. If the child experiences discomfort from the mask, a different interface or mask type can be trialed. While the number of studies specifically addressing interventions to improve PAP adherence in children is modest, behavioral interventions, reward tables, and financial support have shown promise.

Several studies have described behavioral interventions and reported on their success in promoting adherence to PAP in children. For example, Harford and colleagues described an interdisciplinary adherence clinical program which used individualized assessment and behavioral intervention to improve adherence [75]. The program was staffed by an interdisciplinary team including a clinical psychologist and respiratory therapist, with supervision from a physician. The initial visit included PAP education, familiarization with the PAP machine, mask selection with desensitization, and assessment of patient/family strengths and barriers to adherence. Initially, patients returned every 2 weeks. Of seven patients who were referred to the program for non-adherence, three (43%) saw improvement in adherence with average use improving from 20.8% to 92.3%. In another behaviorally oriented intervention of children with poor adherence, individualized counseling, recommendations, and behavioral therapy led to improved PAP usage in 75% of participants [76]. Average nightly use in patients whose families participated in a 1.5-hour behavior consultation session increased from 1.7 to 8.6 hours per night. While these studies are modest in size—with 19 and 20 patients, respectively—they demonstrate that relatively brief periods of intensive, individualized behavioral interventions can have a dramatic impact on adherence for some children and their families.

To evaluate the efficacy of utilizing a "token economy" reward system to improve adherence, Mendoza-Ruiz et al. compared usage data from before and after the introduction of a weekly chart that children used to indicate the days they had (green token) or had not (red token) used PAP [77]. The study included six children with poor baseline adherence and a control group for comparison. After 3 weeks using the reward system, average PAP use in the poorly adherence children increased from 4.7 to 6.4 nights/week and from 1.0 to 5.5 hours/night. Although the sample size was small, the increase in hours used per night reached statistical significance. These results suggest that reward systems and token economy can motivate children to accept PAP treatment, although this effect may diminish with increasing age.

Large-scale intervention programs have also been successful in increasing attendance at PAP-related clinical visits. For example, an interdisciplinary intensive PAP program which included 274 patients over 4 years demonstrated success in improving attendance at follow-up visits and titration polysomnograms [78]. This comprehensive PAP program included pre-visit preparation to secure the PAP machine, addition of a psychologist and respiratory therapist into the care team at clinic visits, and follow-up phone calls. After implementation of the enhanced services, the percentage of patients who appeared for a follow-up visit increased from 68% to 81%, and the percentage of children who received a titration polysomnogram rose from 38% to 84%. Although adherence data was not recorded prior to the initiation of the program, children who participated and attended a follow-up visit wore PAP an average of 63.6% nights for an average of 4.3 hours on nights used in the first month. The cost associated with expanded services is an important barrier to widespread implementation of comprehensive intervention programs. A cost analysis using national salary estimates and Medicare reimbursement levels indicated that the program cost was greater than projected reimbursement. To fully cover program costs, the required reimbursement would be 1.92 times the Medicare rate, making it economically unfeasible for some centers. Additionally, the effect of such programs on adherence to PAP use at home is still unknown.

25.8 Summary

PAP therapy is a safe and effective treatment for OSAS in children, particularly those with persistent disease following surgery or OSAS associated with obesity, craniofacial abnormalities, or genetic syndromes. Adherence to therapy remains a significant barrier to adequate treatment. Factors associated with improved adherence in children include younger age, female sex, presence of developmental delay, Caucasian race, increased level of maternal education, and higher AHI. Behavioral interventions are successful in improving adherence, particularly when implemented at initiation and during early utilization of PAP, as early adherence predicts future utilization of therapy.

Funding Dr. Arens is supported by grant number NIH-1R01HL130468-A1 from The National Institutes of Health.

References

1. Marcus CL, Brooks LJ, Draper KA, Gozal D, Halbower AC, Jones J, Schechter MS, Sheldon SH, Spruyt K, Ward SD, Lehmann C, Shiffman RN, American Academy of P. Diagnosis and management of childhood obstructive sleep apnea syndrome. Pediatrics. 2012;130:576–84.
2. Arens R, Muzumdar H. Childhood obesity and obstructive sleep apnea syndrome. J Appl Physiol. 2010;108:436–44.
3. Muzumdar H, Arens R. Diagnostic issues in pediatric obstructive sleep apnea. Proc Am Thorac Soc. 2008;5:263–73.
4. Marcus CL, Moore RH, Rosen CL, Giordani B, Garetz SL, Taylor HG, Mitchell RB, Amin R, Katz ES, Arens R, Paruthi S, Muzumdar H, Gozal D, Thomas NH, Ware J, Beebe D, Snyder K, Elden L, Sprecher RC, Willging P, Jones D, Bent JP, Hoban T, Chervin RD, Ellenberg SS, Redline S, Childhood Adenotonsillectomy T. A randomized trial of adenotonsillectomy for childhood sleep apnea. N Engl J Med. 2013;368:2366–76.
5. Bhattacharjee R, Kheirandish-Gozal L, Spruyt K, Mitchell RB, Promchiarak J, Simakajornboon N, Kaditis AG, Splaingard D, Splaingard M, Brooks LJ, Marcus CL, Sin S, Arens R, Verhulst SL, Gozal D. Adenotonsillectomy outcomes in treatment of obstructive sleep apnea in children: a multicenter retrospective study. Am J Respir Crit Care Med. 2010;182:676–83.
6. Arens R, Marcus CL. Pathophysiology of upper airway obstruction: a developmental perspective. Sleep. 2004;27:997–1019.
7. Imanguli M, Ulualp SO. Risk factors for residual obstructive sleep apnea after adenotonsillectomy in children. Laryngoscope. 2016;126:2624–9.
8. Rosen GM, Muckle RP, Mahowald MW, Goding GS, Ullevig C. Postoperative respiratory compromise in children with obstructive sleep apnea syndrome: can it be anticipated? Pediatrics. 1994;93:784–8.
9. De A, Waltuch T, Gonik NJ, Nguyen-Famulare N, Muzumdar H, Bent JP, Isasi CR, Sin S, Arens R. Sleep and Breathing the first night after Adenotonsillectomy in obese children with obstructive sleep Apnea. J Clin Sleep Med. 2017;13:805–11.
10. Redline S, Tishler PV, Schluchter M, Aylor J, Clark K, Graham G. Risk factors for sleep-disordered breathing in children. Associations with obesity, race, and respiratory problems. Am J Respir Crit Care Med. 1999;159:1527–32.
11. Andersen IG, Holm JC, Homoe P. Obstructive sleep apnea in obese children and adolescents, treatment methods and outcome of treatment – a systematic review. Int J Pediatr Otorhinolaryngol. 2016;87:190–7.
12. Nandalike K, Shifteh K, Sin S, Strauss T, Stakofsky A, Gonik N, Bent J, Parikh SR, Bassila M, Nikova M, Muzumdar H, Arens R. Adenotonsillectomy in obese children with obstructive sleep apnea syndrome: magnetic resonance imaging findings and considerations. Sleep. 2013;36:841–7.
13. Al-Saleh S, Riekstins A, Forrest CR, Philips JH, Gibbons J, Narang I. Sleep-related disordered breathing in children with syndromic craniosynostosis. J Craniomaxillofac Surg. 2011;39:153–7.
14. Bannink N, Nout E, Wolvius EB, Hoeve HL, Joosten KF, Mathijssen IM. Obstructive sleep apnea in children with syndromic craniosynostosis: long-term respiratory outcome of midface advancement. Int J Oral Maxillofac Surg. 2010;39:115–21.
15. Alsaadi MM, Iqbal SM, Elgamal EA, Salih MA, Gozal D. Sleep-disordered breathing in children with craniosynostosis. Sleep Breat = Schlaf & Atmung. 2013;17:389–93.
16. Cielo CM, Marcus CL. Obstructive sleep apnoea in children with craniofacial syndromes. Paediatr Respir Rev. 2015;16:189–96.
17. Saengthong P, Chaitusaney B, Hirunwiwatkul P, Charakorn N. Adenotonsillectomy in children with syndromic craniosynostosis: a systematic review and meta-analysis. Eur Arch Otorhinolaryngol. 2019;276:1555–60.
18. Driessen C, Mathijssen IM, De Groot MR, Joosten KF. Does central sleep apnea occur in children with syndromic craniosynostosis? Respir Physiol Neurobiol. 2012;181:321–5.
19. Gonsalez S, Thompson D, Hayward R, Lane R. Treatment of obstructive sleep apnoea using nasal CPAP in children with craniofacial dysostoses. Childs Nerv Syst. 1996;12:713–9.
20. Jarund M, Dellborg C, Carlson J, Lauritzen C, Ejnell H. Treatment of sleep apnoea with continuous positive airway pressure in children with craniofacial malformations. Scand J Plast Reconstr Surg Hand Surg. 1999;33:67–71.
21. Anderson IC, Sedaghat AR, McGinley BM, Redett RJ, Boss EF, Ishman SL. Prevalence and severity of obstructive sleep apnea and snoring in infants with Pierre Robin sequence. Cleft Palate Craniofac J. 2011;48:614–8.
22. Hsieh ST, Woo AS. Pierre Robin Sequence. Clin Plast Surg. 2019;46:249–59.
23. Leboulanger N, Picard A, Soupre V, Aubertin G, Denoyelle F, Galliani E, Roger G, Garabedian EN, Fauroux B. Physiologic and clinical benefits of noninvasive ventilation in infants with Pierre Robin sequence. Pediatrics. 2010;126:e1056–63.
24. Amaddeo A, Abadie V, Chalouhi C, Kadlub N, Frapin A, Lapillonne A, Leboulanger N, Garabedian EN, Picard A, Fauroux B. Continuous positive airway pressure for upper airway obstruction in infants with Pierre Robin sequence. Plast Reconstr Surg. 2016;137:609–12.
25. Staudt CB, Gnoinski WM, Peltomaki T. Upper airway changes in Pierre Robin sequence from childhood to adulthood. Orthod Craniofac Res. 2013;16:202–13.

26. Ehsan Z, Kurian C, Weaver KN, Pan BS, Huang G, Hossain MM, Simakajornboon N. Longitudinal sleep outcomes in neonates with Pierre Robin sequence treated conservatively. J Clin Sleep Med. 2019;15:477–82.

27. Lee C-F, Lee C-H, Hsueh W-Y, Lin M-T, Kang K-T. Prevalence of obstructive sleep Apnea in children with down syndrome: a meta-analysis. J Clin Sleep Med. 2018;14:867–75.

28. Farhood Z, Isley JW, Ong AA, Nguyen SA, Camilon TJ, LaRosa AC, White DR. Adenotonsillectomy outcomes in patients with Down syndrome and obstructive sleep apnea. Laryngoscope. 2017;127:1465–70.

29. Katz ES, Mitchell RB, D'Ambrosio CM. Obstructive sleep apnea in infants. Am J Respir Crit Care Med. 2012;185:805–16.

30. Guilleminault C, Pelayo R, Clerk A, Leger D, Bocian RC. Home nasal continuous positive airway pressure in infants with sleep- disordered breathing. J Pediatr. 1995;127:905–12.

31. Downey R 3rd, Perkin RM, MacQuarrie J. Nasal continuous positive airway pressure use in children with obstructive sleep apnea younger than 2 years of age. Chest. 2000;117:1608–12.

32. Isono S, Shimada A, Utsugi M, Konno A, Nishino T. Comparison of static mechanical properties of the passive pharynx between normal children and children with sleep-disordered breathing. Am J Respir Crit Care Med. 1998;157:1204–12.

33. Marcus CL, McColley SA, Carroll JL, Loughlin GM, Smith PL, Schwartz AR. Upper airway collapsibility in children with obstructive sleep apnea syndrome. J Appl Physiol. 1994;77:918–24.

34. Schwab RJ, Gupta KB, Gefter WB, Metzger LJ, Hoffman EA, Pack AI. Upper airway and soft tissue anatomy in normal subjects and patients with sleep-disordered breathing. Significance of the lateral pharyngeal walls. Am J Respir Crit Care Med. 1995;152:1673–89.

35. Schwab RJ, Pack AI, Gupta KB, Metzger LJ, Oh E, Getsy JE, Hoffman EA, Gefter WB. Upper airway and soft tissue structural changes induced by CPAP in normal subjects. Am J Respir Crit Care Med. 1996;154:1106–16.

36. Heinzer RC, Stanchina ML, Malhotra A, Fogel RB, Patel SR, Jordan AS, Schory K, White DP. Lung volume and continuous positive airway pressure requirements in obstructive sleep apnea. Am J Respir Crit Care Med. 2005;172:114–7.

37. Arzt M, Bradley TD. Treatment of sleep apnea in heart failure. Am J Respir Crit Care Med. 2006;173:1300–8.

38. Steiner S, Schueller PO, Schannwell CM, Hennersdorf M, Strauer BE. Effects of continuous positive airway pressure on exercise capacity in chronic heart failure patients without sleep apnea. J Physiol Pharmacol. 2007;58(Suppl 5):665–72.

39. Kaye DM, Mansfield D, Naughton MT. Continuous positive airway pressure decreases myocardial oxygen consumption in heart failure. Clin Sci (Lond). 2004;106:599–603.

40. Patil SP, Ayappa IA, Caples SM, Kimoff RJ, Patel SR, Harrod CG. Treatment of adult obstructive sleep Apnea with positive airway pressure: an American Academy of sleep medicine systematic review, meta-analysis, and GRADE assessment. J Clin Sleep Med. 2019;15:301–34.

41. Uong EC, Epperson M, Bathon SA, Jeffe DB. Adherence to nasal positive airway pressure therapy among school-aged children and adolescents with obstructive sleep apnea syndrome. Pediatrics. 2007;120:e1203–11.

42. Marcus CL, Beck SE, Traylor J, Cornaglia MA, Meltzer LJ, DiFeo N, Karamessinis LR, Samuel J, Falvo J, DiMaria M, Gallagher PR, Beris H, Menello MK. Randomized, double-blind clinical trial of two different modes of positive airway pressure therapy on adherence and efficacy in children. J Clin Sleep Med. 2012;8:37–42.

43. Berry RB, Albertario CL, Harding SM, Al E. The AASM manual for the scoring of sleep and associated events: rules, terminology and technical specifications, Version 2.5. 2018.

44. Mihai R, Vandeleur M, Pecoraro S, Davey MJ, Nixon GM. Autotitrating CPAP as a tool for CPAP initiation for children. J Clin Sleep Med. 2017;13:713–9.

45. Khaytin I, Tapia IE, Xanthopoulos MS, Cielo C, Kim JY, Smith J, Matthews EC, Beck SE. Auto-titrating CPAP for the treatment of obstructive sleep apnea in children. J Clin Sleep Med. 2020;16:871–8.

46. Palombini L, Pelayo R, Guilleminault C. Efficacy of automated continuous positive airway pressure in children with sleep-related breathing disorders in an attended setting. Pediatrics. 2004;113:e412–7.

47. Kribbs NB, Pack AI, Kline LR, Smith PL, Schwartz AR, Schubert NM, Redline S, Henry JN, Getsy JE, Dinges DF. Objective measurement of patterns of nasal CPAP use by patients with obstructive sleep apnea. Am Rev Respir Dis. 1993;147:887–95.

48. Pepin JL, Krieger J, Rodenstein D, Cornette A, Sforza E, Delguste P, Deschaux C, Grillier V, Levy P. Effective compliance during the first 3 months of continuous positive airway pressure. A European prospective study of 121 patients. Am J Respir Crit Care Med. 1999;160:1124–9.

49. Sawyer AM, Gooneratne NS, Marcus CL, Ofer D, Richards KC, Weaver TE. A systematic review of CPAP adherence across age groups: clinical and empiric insights for developing CPAP adherence interventions. Sleep Med Rev. 2011;15:343–56.

50. Watach AJ, Xanthopoulos MS, Afolabi-Brown O, Saconi B, Fox KA, Qiu M, Sawyer AM. Positive airway pressure adherence in pediatric obstructive sleep apnea: a systematic scoping review. Sleep Med Rev. 2020;51:101273.

51. Blinder H, Momoli F, Bokhaut J, Bacal V, Goldberg R, Radhakrishnan D, Katz SL. Predictors of adherence to positive airway pressure therapy in children: a systematic review and meta-analysis. Sleep Med. 2020;69:19–33.

52. Berry RB, Wagner MH. Sleep medicine pearls. 3rd ed. Philadelphia: Saunders; 2015. p. 323.

53. Barbe F, Duran-Cantolla J, Capote F, de la Pena M, Chiner E, Masa JF, Gonzalez M, Marin JM, Garcia-Rio F, de Atauri JD, Teran J, Mayos M, Monasterio C, del Campo F, Gomez S, de la Torre MS, Martinez M, Montserrat JM, Spanish S, Breathing G. Long-term effect of continuous positive airway pressure in hypertensive patients with sleep apnea. Am J Respir Crit Care Med. 2010;181:718–26.

54. Weaver TE, Maislin G, Dinges DF, Bloxham T, George CF, Greenberg H, Kader G, Mahowald M, Younger J, Pack AI. Relationship between hours of CPAP use and achieving normal levels of sleepiness and daily functioning. Sleep. 2007;30:711–9.

55. Antic NA, Catcheside P, Buchan C, Hensley M, Naughton MT, Rowland S, Williamson B, Windler S, McEvoy RD. The effect of CPAP in normalizing daytime sleepiness, quality of life, and neuro-cognitive function in patients with moderate to severe OSA. Sleep. 2011;34:111–9.

56. Campos-Rodriguez F, Pena-Grinan N, Reyes-Nunez N, De la Cruz-Moron I, Perez-Ronchel J, De la Vega-Gallardo F, Fernandez-Palacin A. Mortality in obstructive sleep apnea-hypopnea patients treated with positive airway pressure. Chest. 2005;128:624–33.

57. Labarca G, Dreyse J, Drake L, Jorquera J, Barbe F. Efficacy of continuous positive airway pressure (CPAP) in the prevention of cardiovascular events in patients with obstructive sleep apnea: systematic review and meta-analysis. Sleep Med Rev. 2020;52:101312.

58. Eckert DJ, White DP, Jordan AS, Malhotra A, Wellman A. Defining phenotypic causes of obstructive sleep apnea. Identification of novel therapeutic targets. Am J Respir Crit Care Med. 2013;188:996–1004.

59. Carberry JC, Amatoury J, Eckert DJ. Personalized management approach for OSA. Chest. 2018;153:744–55.

60. Marcus CL, Rosen G, Ward SL, Halbower AC, Sterni L, Lutz J, Stading PJ, Bolduc D, Gordon N. Adherence to and effectiveness of

positive airway pressure therapy in children with obstructive sleep apnea. Pediatrics. 2006;117:e442–51.

61. Hudgel DW, Fung C. A long-term randomized, cross-over comparison of auto-titrating and standard nasal continuous airway pressure. Sleep. 2000;23:645–8.

62. Nussbaumer Y, Bloch KE, Genser T, Thurnheer R. Equivalence of autoadjusted and constant continuous positive airway pressure in home treatment of sleep apnea. Chest. 2006;129:638–43.

63. Simon SL, Duncan CL, Janicke DM, Wagner MH. Barriers to treatment of paediatric obstructive sleep apnoea: development of the adherence barriers to continuous positive airway pressure (CPAP) questionnaire. Sleep Med. 2012;13:172–7.

64. DiFeo N, Meltzer LJ, Beck SE, Karamessinis LR, Cornaglia MA, Traylor J, Samuel J, Gallagher PR, Radcliffe J, Beris H, Menello MK, Marcus CL. Predictors of positive airway pressure therapy adherence in children: a prospective study. J Clin Sleep Med. 2012;8:279–86.

65. Xanthopoulos MS, Kim JY, Blechner M, Chang MY, Menello MK, Brown C, Matthews E, Weaver TE, Shults J, Marcus CL. Self-efficacy and short-term adherence to continuous positive airway pressure treatment in children. Sleep. 2017;40:1–7.

66. Hawkins SM, Jensen EL, Simon SL, Friedman NR. Correlates of Pediatric CPAP adherence. J Clin Sleep Med. 2016;12:879–84.

67. Lynch MK, Elliott LC, Avis KT, Schwebel DC, Goodin BR. Quality of life in youth with Obstructive Sleep Apnea Syndrome (OSAS) treated with Continuous Positive Airway Pressure (CPAP) therapy. Behav Sleep Med. 2019;17:238–45.

68. Nathan AM, Tang JP, Goh A, Teoh OH, Chay OM. Compliance with noninvasive home ventilation in children with obstructive sleep apnoea. Singap Med J. 2013;54:678–82.

69. O'Donnell AR, Bjornson CL, Bohn SG, Kirk VG. Compliance rates in children using noninvasive continuous positive airway pressure. Sleep. 2006;29:651–8.

70. Kang EK, Xanthopoulos MS, Kim JY, Arevalo C, Shults J, Beck SE, Marcus CL, Tapia IE. Adherence to positive airway pressure for the treatment of obstructive sleep Apnea in children with developmental disabilities. J Clin Sleep Med. 2019;15:915–21.

71. Prashad PS, Marcus CL, Maggs J, Stettler N, Cornaglia MA, Costa P, Puzino K, Xanthopoulos M, Bradford R, Barg FK. Investigating reasons for CPAP adherence in adolescents: a qualitative approach. J Clin Sleep Med. 2013;9:1303–13.

72. Alebraheem Z, Toulany A, Baker A, Christian J, Narang I. Facilitators and barriers to positive airway pressure adherence for adolescents. A qualitative study. Ann Am Thorac Soc. 2018;15:83–8.

73. Patil SP, Ayappa IA, Caples SM, Kimoff RJ, Patel SR, Harrod CG. Treatment of adult obstructive sleep Apnea with positive airway pressure: an American Academy of sleep medicine clinical practice guideline. J Clin Sleep Med. 2019;15:335–43.

74. Budhiraja R, Parthasarathy S, Drake CL, Roth T, Sharief I, Budhiraja P, Saunders V, Hudgel DW. Early CPAP use identifies subsequent adherence to CPAP therapy. Sleep. 2007;30:320–4.

75. Harford KL, Jambhekar S, Com G, Pruss K, Kabour M, Jones K, Ward WL. Behaviorally based adherence program for pediatric patients treated with positive airway pressure. Clin Child Psychol Psychiatry. 2013;18:151–63.

76. Koontz KL, Slifer KJ, Cataldo MD, Marcus CL. Improving pediatric compliance with positive airway pressure therapy: the impact of behavioral intervention. Sleep. 2003;26:1010–5.

77. Mendoza-Ruiz A, Dylgjeri S, Bour F, Damagnez F, Leroux K, Khirani S. Evaluation of the efficacy of a dedicated table to improve CPAP adherence in children: a pilot study. Sleep Med. 2019;53:60–4.

78. Riley EB, Fieldston ES, Xanthopoulos MS, Beck SE, Menello MK, Matthews E, Marcus CL. Financial analysis of an intensive Pediatric continuous positive airway pressure program. Sleep. 2017;40:1–8.

79. Bitners AC, Arens R. Evaluation and Management of Children with obstructive sleep Apnea syndrome. Lung. 2020;198:257–70.

80. Nandalike K, Arens R. Ventilator support in children with obstructive sleep Apnea syndrome. In: Sterni LM, Carroll JL, editors. Caring for the ventilator dependent child: a clinical guide. New York: Humana Press; 2016.

81. Gay P, Weaver T, Loube D, Iber C, Positive Airway Pressure Task F, Standards of Practice C, American Academy of Sleep M. Evaluation of positive airway pressure treatment for sleep related breathing disorders in adults. Sleep. 2006;29:381–401.

82. Kohler M, Smith D, Tippett V, Stradling JR. Predictors of long-term compliance with continuous positive airway pressure. Thorax. 2010;65:829–32.

83. Riachy M, Najem S, Iskandar M, Choucair J, Ibrahim I, Juvelikian G. Factors predicting CPAP adherence in obstructive sleep apnea syndrome. Sleep Breath = Schlaf & Atmung. 2017;21:295–302.

84. McArdle N, Devereux G, Heidarnejad H, Engleman HM, Mackay TW, Douglas NJ. Long-term use of CPAP therapy for sleep apnea/hypopnea syndrome. Am J Respir Crit Care Med. 1999;159:1108–14.

85. Li HY, Engleman H, Hsu CY, Izci B, Vennelle M, Cross M, Douglas NJ. Acoustic reflection for nasal airway measurement in patients with obstructive sleep apnea-hypopnea syndrome. Sleep. 2005;28:1554–9.

86. Nixon GM, Mihai R, Verginis N, Davey MJ. Patterns of continuous positive airway pressure adherence during the first 3 months of treatment in children. J Pediatr. 2011;159:802–7.

CPAP Adherence in Children with Special Health-Care Needs

26

Anya McLaren-Barnett and Indra Narang

26.1 Sleep Disordered Breathing in Children with Special Health-Care Needs

Children with special health-care needs (CSHCN) is defined as "those who have or at risk for chronic physical, developmental, behavioural, or emotional conditions requiring health and related services of a type or amount beyond that required by children generally" [1]. CSHCN are a particularly vulnerable population that rely on multiple health-care providers and health-care services to enhance their health [2]. The estimated prevalence of this population in the United States is between 12 and 18% [3]. Worldwide, there are an estimated 93 million or 4% of children living with disabilities [4]. Though the population is diverse in terms of the range of levels of functional abilities, they all share the consequences of their conditions, namely, their reliance on medications or therapies, special educational services, or assistive devices or equipment [5].

The most complex CSHCN are described as children with medical complexity (CMC) [6]. CMC children share four characteristics: the presence of one or more complex chronic conditions that are often multisystem and severe; functional limitation that is significant and often reliant on technology such as feeding tubes, NPPV, and/or tracheostomies; high health-care utilization; and significant familial social and financial impact. Important determinants of health outcomes in the CSHCN population include social health determinants such as socioeconomic status [7], accessibility to family-centered care, the availability and adequacy of health insurance coverage, and the presence of a usual source of care available to families when the child is sick [5]. In addition, families of the CSHCN population often require support in coping with the consequences of their children's health conditions. The term children with "typical development" (TD) is used to describe children who do not have special health-care needs.

26.1.1 Prevalence

Within the group of CHSCN particularly within CMC, there are specific populations that are particularly prone to disturbances of sleep, specifically SDB. These include children with neurodevelopmental disorders, genetic conditions, craniofacial anomalies, and neuromuscular disorders. The prevalence of sleep disordered breathing that has been reported in these conditions is outlined in Table 26.1.

26.1.2 Mechanism of SDB

In general, SDB, in particular OSA, results from structural factors that reduce the size of the airway as well as deficits that impair the ability to maintain a patent airway during sleep [41]. The other factors that contribute to SDB in the CSCHN population include craniofacial features, muscle weakness, and obesity. In neurologically impaired children, additional factors include seizures, esophageal reflux, and excessive oral secretions.

26.1.2.1 Craniofacial Features
Craniofacial conditions are highly variable and can exist in isolation or as part of a syndrome [41]. Craniofacial features that increase the risk of OSA include mandibular retrusion, maxillary deficiency or hypoplasia, inferior displacement of the hyoid bone, and cranial base abnormalities [42–45]. These abnormalities can lead to a compromised airway space and increased risk of upper airway collapsibility thus leading to OSA. This may be further exacerbated by increased collapsibility of the upper airway secondary to

A. McLaren-Barnett (✉)
Division of Pediatric Respirology, Department of Pediatrics, McMaster University, Hamilton, ON, Canada
e-mail: mclara1@mcmaster.ca

I. Narang
Sleep Medicine, Division of Respiratory Medicine, Sick Children's Hospital, Toronto, ON, Canada

Table 26.1 Prevalence of sleep disordered breathing in pediatric patients with special needs

Condition	SRBD condition	Prevalence
Neurodevelopmental		
Autism [8–11]	Obstructive sleep apnea	8–58%
Cerebral palsy (CP) [12]	Obstructive sleep apnea	14–15%
Genetic		
Achondroplasia [13–21]	Obstructive sleep apnea	10–87%
	Central sleep apnea	NR
Angelman syndrome [22]	Obstructive sleep apnea	30%
Down syndrome (DS) [23]	Obstructive sleep apnea	30–79%
	Central sleep apnea	12%
	Nocturnal hypoventilation	NR
Prader-Willi syndrome (PWS) [24–26]	Obstructive sleep apnea	0–100%
	Narcolepsy	35%
	Central sleep apnea	12%
Mucopolysaccharidosis (MPS) [27, 28]	Obstructive sleep apnea	69–95%
Rett syndrome [29, 30]	Obstructive sleep apnea	41–69%
	Central sleep apnea	7–8%
Craniofacial		
Treacher Collins syndrome (TCS) [31, 32]	Obstructive sleep apnea	37.5–54%
Pierre Robin sequence (PRS) [33, 34]	Obstructive sleep apnea	80–85%
Crouzon syndrome [35]	Obstructive sleep apnea	64–65%
Neuromuscular		
Duchenne muscular dystrophy (DMD) [36, 37]	Obstructive sleep apnea	31–64%
	Central sleep apnea	34%
	Nocturnal hypoventilation	16–21%
Myotonic dystrophy type 1 [38]	Obstructive sleep apnea	55%
Congenital muscular dystrophies [39]	Central sleep apnea	40%
	Obstructive sleep apnea	10%
	Obstructive and central sleep apnea	15%
Pompe disease [40]	Nocturnal hypoventilation	75%

NR not reported

muscle fatigue (related to the upper airway muscles working constantly against an increased mechanical load), a factor that is not unique to this population [41, 46, 47]. Co-occurring motor dysfunction has been found in children with cleft palate and micrognathia and can further contribute to OSA [48]. Some conditions in which craniofacial features increase OSA prevalence include PRS, TCS, DS, and achondroplasia [42–45].

26.1.2.2 Muscle Weakness

In conditions associated with neuromuscular weakness, diaphragm weakness and REM-related atonia can lead to "pseudocentral" or "diaphragmatic" sleep disordered breathing in which suppression of the intercostal muscle activity and decreased contribution of the ribcage in tidal volume leads to increased burden of breathing for the diaphragm (which is already weak) [49]. Low lung volumes in the supine position during sleep and decreased ventilatory response to hypercarbia (either from neuromuscular weakness in the presence of an intact central drive or from a decrease in chemosensitivity with chronic hypercapnia) can lead to hypoventilation evidenced by increased carbon dioxide (CO_2) levels [49]. Pharyngeal hypotonia or neuropathy as well as bulbar symptoms and low lung volumes contribute to OSA [19, 28, 50–52], for example, in children with CP. Their presentation includes abnormal muscle tone of the upper airway including laryngeal dystonia, severe laryngomalacia due to reduced tone in the supraglottic structures, and concurrent pseudobulbar palsy [53–55]. Epilepsy may further increase the risk of OSA in cerebral palsy, especially in children with more severe CP [56]. The exact etiology by which this occurs is not clear [56].

26.1.2.3 Obesity

Obesity occurs at a higher incidence in the CSHCN posing an additional risk factor for SDB. Youth with CSHCN have an obesity rate of 22% compared with 16% without CSHCN and is an additional risk factor severity of OSA [52, 57]. For example, obesity prevalence is estimated to be 24.6%, 31.2%, and 18.6% in children with autism, DS, and spina bifida, respectively [58]. This is in comparison to obesity rates between 8 and 18.2% in Canadian youth [59]. In children with autism, weight was identified as the only independent predictor of severe OSA in children when compared to other factors such as age, tonsil size, history of allergies, asthma, seizure disorder, gastroesophageal reflux disease, or ADHD [8].

The mechanistic factors involved in OSA in the obese CSHCN population have not been well studied. However, in children with typical development, several anatomic and functional factors contribute to OSA. These include adenotonsillar hypertrophy which may occur at a higher frequency in obese children [60]. Adipose tissue deposited around the pharynx and neck limit airway patency and increase airway resistance both of which are important contributors to the development of OSA in obese youth [61–64]. In addition, there may be other soft tissues that contribute to obstruction of the upper airway such as the soft palate, lateral pharyngeal walls, tongue, and pharyngeal fat pads which have been found to be larger in obese children [64–67]. Functional factors in obese children include altered neuromuscular tone which leads to greater upper airway collapsibility [68]. Additional mechanistic factors include altered chest wall mechanics (reduced lung compliance) and reduced lung volumes which lead to decreased oxygen reserve and increased likelihood of hypoxemia [69, 70]. An important metabolic factor in obesity-related OSA is increased leptin and leptin resistance. Leptin is a satiety hormone that is produced by adipose tissue and plays multiple roles in metabolism, immunity, and inflammation. In obesity, leptin levels are high, and OSA can induce leptin resistance which is thought to impair the regulation of the upper airway and diaphragmatic control [71].

26.1.3 Impact of Untreated OSA

OSA impacts several outcomes in CSHCN that include cardiovascular, behavioral, and metabolic effects in addition to effects on quality of life (QOL) and sudden death.

In children with PWS, growth hormone (GH) may improve OSA in the short term; however mounting evidence suggests that the GH-mediated growth of lymphoid tissue can increase risk of OSA and sudden death [72–79]. There is also an increased risk of sudden death in infants with achondroplasia particularly between the ages of 1 month and 1 year [80, 81]. From a cardiovascular perspective, there is evidence of a direct relationship between elevated pulmonary pressure and upper airway obstruction in children with DS [82–88]. Co-occurring pulmonary hypertension (PHTN) and OSA have been described in children with other conditions including MPS [79, 89, 90], PWS [91], and achondroplasia [92]. Treatment of residual OSA improves nocturnal gas exchange and resolved pulmonary hypertension in these patients [83, 84, 86, 87, 93].

Language development, executive function, and cognitive outcomes (particularly in verbal intelligence quotient and cognitive flexibility) have been found to be worse in DS children with OSA than those without [93–98]. This may be more significant in children with congenital heart disease but improves with OSA treatment [97, 99]. Treatment of OSA with adenotonsillectomy significantly improves behavioral problems, sleep, social communication, attention, and repetitive behaviors in CSHCN [100–102].

Daily life functions, QOL, and parental quality of life are negatively impacted by OSA in DS children [103–105]. Treatment of OSA in this population improves their sleep, mood, and functioning [106]. Similar QOL improvements have been seen in children with cerebral palsy whose OSA is treated in that they experience an improvement in sleep disturbance, daytime functioning, and caregiver concern. Parental QOL score also improves [107, 108]. The presence of OSA may also lead to comorbidities such as metabolic syndrome and hepatic steatosis [109–112] in children.

26.1.4 Therapeutic Interventions

Adenotonsillectomy is the first-line treatment for OSA in children and is usually successful in close to 80% of otherwise healthy children [113]. However, in the CSHCN population there is persistent OSA despite adenotonsillectomy with a requirement for PAP therapy post surgery [37, 94, 114, 115]. Though PAP is the main therapy, there are adjunctive therapeutic interventions frequently used in this population such as uvulopalatopharyngoplasty (UPPP), aggressive management of seizures, esophageal reflux, and excessive oral secretions as well as the application of mandibular distraction and skeletal expansion whenever feasible [50, 108]. Oral appliances or functional orthopedic devices are potential adjunctive therapies; however, their effectiveness is not well established. There may be specific cases such as children with craniofacial anomalies where these devices may serve as auxiliary in the treatment of OSA [116, 117]. The focus of this chapter will be on the use of NPPV in the CHCSN population.

26.1.4.1 PAP

PAP is a common treatment modality in CSHCN who have SDB especially in children in whom the prevalence of OSA may continue to be high despite repeated upper airway surgery [13, 16, 18, 118–121]. PAP describes the delivery of pressurized air to the lungs via an external interface worn on the face. There are two main modes of PAP therapy: continuous positive airway pressure (CPAP) and bilevel positive airway pressure (BiPAP or BPAP). Both CPAP and BPAP are highly efficacious in the treatment of pediatric sleep disordered breathing. Long-term PAP is indicated in children with sleep and respiratory disorders including upper airway obstruction, musculoskeletal weakness and chest wall restriction, chronic lung diseases, central nervous system disorders, and other systemic disorders with respiratory insufficiency [122]. Some of the relative contraindications include failure to protect the upper airway, uncontrolled bulbar dysfunction, significant GERD and aspiration risk, inability to tolerate PAP therapy, lack of sufficient caregiver support in the home, ventilatory dependency that exceeds 16 h/day, inability to find an interface of adequate fit, and recent upper airway or craniofacial surgery [123].

The effectiveness of PAP therapy is limited by poor adherence in the pediatric population [124]. CPAP is most commonly used; however in some children with OSA as well as other sleep disordered breathing conditions, BPAP is also used [125]. PAP significantly improves obstructive apnea-hypopnea index (OAHI), respiratory disturbance index (RDI), oxygen nadir and arousal index. In addition, BPAP improves in daytime and nocturnal symptoms irrespective of mode of ventilation [126, 127]. The use of PAP therapy to treat pediatric OSA improves neurobehavioral function, decreases nocturnal symptoms of sleep disordered breathing, and improves daytime somnolence and school performance, attention, and academic functioning [127–136]. The factors related to suboptimal PAP adherence in children are multifactorial and are explored further below.

26.2 Positive Airway Pressure in Children

There are different modes of PAP therapy used in pediatrics, and these are summarized below in Table 26.2 [137]. CPAP provides a constant distending pressure at a single prescribed pressure level during both inspiratory and expiratory phases of the respiratory cycle [123]. CPAP works by preventing alveolar collapse which leads to an increase in the functional residual capacity (FRC) while minimizing work of breathing by the muscles of inspiration. The overall effect is an improvement in gas exchange in patients with an adequate respiratory drive [138]. CPAP does not provide tidal breathing support, and patients on this therapy must be able to maintain airway patency and have adequate respiratory muscle strength and neurological drive to breathe [138].

BPAP provides a cycling, pre-set pressure support which is higher during inspiration (inspiratory positive airway pressure [IPAP]) than during expiration (expiratory positive airway pressure [EPAP]). The IPAP augments the patient's inspiratory effort and should be delivered in synchrony with the patient's respiratory efforts [139–141]. Provision of IPAP is intended to minimize work of breathing and decrease the respiratory rate as well as the $paCO_2$. EPAP functions to eliminate upper airway obstruction, reduce intrinsic PEEP, and improve oxygenation [124]. BPAP devices provide up to four different modes of ventilation: spontaneous mode, spontaneous/timed mode, pressure control mode, and timed mode. In addition to IPAP and EPAP, other BPAP settings include rate, inspiratory time, and sensitivity [123]. No significant relationship between a particular mode of noninvasive ventilation and adherence has been found [127, 132, 142, 143].

All devices have a water chamber with temperature control for heated humidity or cool passive humidity. In addition, CPAP devices have an in-line heat and moisture exchanger device [137]. PAP devices have features to facilitate sleep onset and acclimatization such as ramp and pressure reduction during exhalation. The ramp setting allows the therapeutic pressure level to be achieved from a subtherapeutic baseline at the time the machine is turned on. This usually occurs over a period of 15–30 minutes. In cases where there is discomfort related to exhaling against a high pressure, there is the option for pressure reduction during exhalation. This is done through the diversion of airflow from the patient once the beginning of exhalation is detected by the machine. Alternatively, the motor speed is reduced to

Table 26.2 The indication and functionality of PAP in children. Reproduced with permission from Parmar et al. [137]

Mode	Primary indication and clinical utility	Functionality
CPAP: fixed pressure CPAP mode	OSA	Distends upper airway preventing pharyngeal collapse
Auto-CPAP: auto-titrating CPAP mode	1. OSA 2. Positional or REM-related OSA 3. PAP therapy acclimatization prior to PSG 4. CPAP patients with sudden change in OSA severity due to surgery or rapid weight change	Auto-adjusting CPAP pressure within a prescribed range, upon detection of upper airway resistance/airflow limitation. Provide higher pressures only when required during varying sleep stages or positions
BPAP-S: spontaneous BPAP mode	1. Patients with OSA who are intolerant to CPAP at high pressures due to discomfort exhaling, not mitigated by comfort features	Two pressures prescribed: higher inspiratory pressure and lower expiratory pressure to provide cycling levels of pressure which is synchronized with the patient breath
Auto-BPAP: auto-titrating spontaneous BPAP mode	1. Positional or REM-related OSA where patient is intolerant to high auto-PAP pressures 2. BPAP therapy acclimatization prior to PSG	Auto-adjusting EPAP level as in Auto-CPAP with a fixed pressure support level allowing for higher pressures upon inhalation. Cycling pressure is synchronized with patient effort
BPAP-ST: spontaneous-timed BPAP mode	1. Children with OSA who present with mixed apnea 2. CPAP emergent central apneas 3. Persistent hypoventilation following resolution of OSA with CPAP	Similar to BPAP-S with the addition of a back-up respiratory rate setting to ensure a minimum number of breaths per minute are delivered
VAPS: volume assured pressure support BPAP mode	1. Obesity hypoventilation syndrome 2. Congenital central hypoventilation syndrome	Auto-titrating pressure support allows delivery of a constant target volume in the presence of changing lung mechanics and patient effort resulting from changes in sleep position or sleep stage

Data from the PAP device can be wirelessly transferred to a cloud-based software system on a daily basis allowing for the patient to view therapy data online via smartphone applications or on the device itself. The physician can remotely monitor cloud-based data or manually download the data from the device via a data card, USB, or data cable. The PAP data available includes usage and efficacy data. Of note is that the algorithms for apnea-hypopnea index (AHI) on current PAP devices are derived from adult criteria so care should be taken when interpreting.

decrease the treatment pressure based on the reduction level that is selected by the clinician [123, 137].

26.2.1 Definition of PAP Adherence

There is variability and inconsistency in the definition of PAP adherence. Data from several seminal papers on PAP adherence in adults in the mid-1990s led to a common assumption that CPAP use of 4 hrs/night on 70% of nights was the clinical and empiric benchmark of PAP adherence [144–147]. However, a threshold of CPAP usage 4 hrs/night may have limited applicability in evaluating health and functional outcomes in this population [144]. In general, it has been observed that increased CPAP usage improves outcomes (e.g., subjective sleepiness, verbal, and executive function) for adults with OSA [144], and similar findings have been reported in children [144].

In children, the optimal definition of PAP adherence is not clear. Parents tend to overestimate their child's PAP usage, and so it is important to obtain objective adherence data when assessing usage [131, 132]. In a systematic review of PAP adherence in pediatric OSA, of 1079 participants from 20 studies, the average adherence that was reported in the studies was less than 60% although adherence was not defined in a homogenous way across the studies [148]. On average, PAP was used 4 hours per night to 5.2 hours per night (non-naïve/existing PAP users). A recent cross-sectional big-data analysis in over 20, 000 children (mean age 13 years +/−3.7 years) showed that only 46.3% were adherent [148]. The criteria for adherence in this study were PAP use for 4 h or more per night on at least 70% of the nights since therapy onset during a consecutive 30-day period during the initial 90 days of use [149]. Further research is needed to define the target CPAP usage in children that optimizes important health outcomes especially as children sleep longer than adults, with variation depending on developmental stage. Thus, average PAP use of 4 hours/night across all age groups is likely significantly below the ideal time needed to optimize the clinical benefit of PAP [124, 144, 150–152].

26.2.2 Interfaces and Devices

The PAP device consists of a machine which provides the airflow and the hose which connects the flow generator (sometimes via an in-line humidifier) to the interface. The routine use of pressure ramping and humification may be an important factor in adherence [153].

Recently, there has been an expansion of available pediatric interfaces, and there continue to be efforts to create new options [154]. However, there are still limitations as it per-

tains to the options for facial masks and headgear [155]. There are four types of PAP interfaces as illustrated in Fig. 26.1: nasal, nasal pillow, oronasal, and total face. More recently, personalized 3D-printed CPAP mask designs have become an option for children with craniofacial anomalies [156]. The choice of interface depends on the characteristics of the patient and include but are not limited to underlying disease age, ventilatory mode, facial characteristics, safety risks (related to the potential development of skin ulcerations, claustrophobia, gastric insufflation, and aspiration), degree of cooperation, and severity of respiratory impairment [138, 141, 157]. Features of an acceptable interface include good adhesion, a low resistance to airflow and lightweight, minimal dead space volume, and minimal pressure on the skin [158]. Accessories to the interface include headgear and chin straps.

An unpleasant initial exposure to PAP can affect early attempts to use therapy and can cause a prolonged period of treatment rejection from both child and caregiver [159]. The main reason for a change in the interface is facial discomfort [155]. In patients with tactile aversions such as children with developmental delay (DD), initial acceptance of the interface is often challenging. Parents should be educated about the significant time investment and patience involved in the successful initiation and maintenance of PAP [160]. Mask fit has been found to be highly predictive of PAP use [149]. PAP use was found to be the lowest in 20, 553 children when the median mask leak (averaged over 90 days) exceeded 24 L/min (282 [43·7%], $p < 0·0001$) [149]. Children that use a face mask as opposed to a nasal mask may take a longer time to be established on PAP [153].

Nasal masks (Fig. 26.1a) are the most commonly used interface in children [122]. This interface rests on the nasal bridge and both sides of the nose. When worn, it allows communication and use of a pacifier and reduces risk of aspiration. In children with high nasal resistance, there is a risk for mouth leak, nasal dryness, bleeding, and skin injury. Nasal pillows (Fig. 26.1b) rest on the inner rim of the nostrils and carries less risk for skin injury because of lack of contact with the nasal bridge as well as less overall contact surface area. The limitations with use are similar as that for the nasal mask. The oronasal mask (Fig. 26.1c) covers the mouth, nose, and part of the chin. It has the advantage of reduced mouth leak but increases aspiration risk and subsequent airway obstruction as well as skin injury. The total face mask (Fig. 26.1d) covers the entire face and has similar limitations as the oronasal mask. However, this interface carries less risk for skin injuries [155].

All noninvasive devices have a built-in or intentional leak to prevent re-breathing of carbon dioxide [123]. The issue of unintentional leak can be addressed with the use of pacifiers in infants and chin straps in older children as well as ensuring adequate interface fit. Ensuring continued proper inter-

Fig. 26.1 Types of PAP interface.
(**a**) Nasal mask. (**b**) Nasal Pillows.
(**c**) Oro-nasal mask (**d**) Full Face Mask

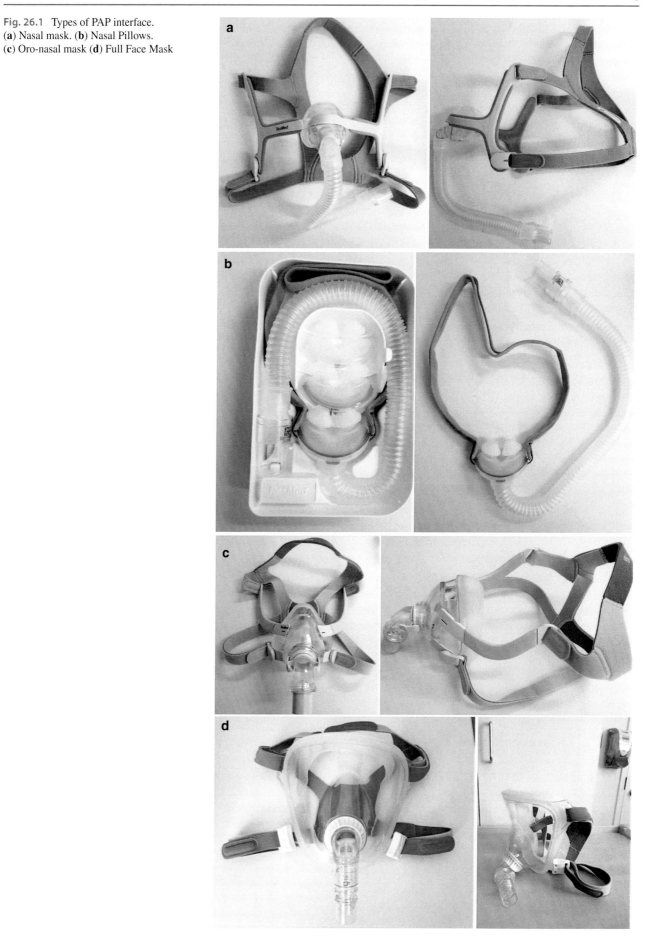

face fit can be achieved through thorough assessment for signs of mask replacement (spotted surfaces, weakened mask structures, loose materials, or poor cushion seal). In some cases, a custom-made interface may be necessary to achieve adequate fit [161]. In children ($n = 62$) treated with NIV at home for at least a month, the level of unintentional leak was not different between patients using a nasal mask or a facial mask. There was no correlation between level of unintentional leak, nocturnal gas exchange, and treatment adherence [142].

Reported complications of PAP use include short-term issues related to the interface such as skin breakdown, skin erythema, nasal congestion, rhinorrhea, epistaxis, feeling of suffocation, conjunctivitis, and rhinitis [123, 124, 126, 131, 132]. In children with single ventricle physiology and/or hypovolemic states, special care must be taken to avoid cardiorespiratory compromise [123]. However, serious complications from PAP use are not frequently reported and do not seem to play a role in PAP adherence [124, 162]. It is important to note that minor side effects may impact adherence [126, 145]. Nasal symptoms tend to be the most frequently reported side effects and interestingly tend to occur more commonly in patients using CPAP than in those using BPAP [124, 126, 127]. A significant long-term complication is that of midfacial bony deformation or hypoplasia thought to be related to long-term mask pressure [163, 164]. This complication is not frequently reported in the literature; however children with underlying craniofacial conditions that are compliant with nasal PAP may be at increased risk of this issue [163]. The apparent rare occurrence of this complication may be related to the relative short duration of assessment in most adherence [132].

In up to 20% of children initiated on PAP, the initial interface is changed because of facial discomfort. Children with underlying maxillofacial deformity issues may require more frequent mask changes [157]. In some cases, custom-made masks are necessary for adequate fit and comfort in children with craniofacial abnormalities [132]. The interface should be changed or modified at the first sign of intolerance, discomfort, and inefficacy of PAP because of leaks or facial deformity [155]. There is limited data on the effect of mask interface on adherence [148]. In one study, better PAP adherence was achieved in children with DS who were changed from nasal to full face mask [153]. In another cohort of CSHCN with OSA ($n = 62$), no significant differences in adherence to PAP was found between nasal cannula, face mask, and nasal mask [142]. Similarly, in a study by Simon and colleagues i($n = 51$) 68% who were labeled as CSHCN, there was no significant difference in adherence between the use of a full face mask versus nasal mask [143].

26.2.3 Current Data and Challenges to Positive Airway Pressure Adherence in Children

Adherence to PAP in children seems to be multifactorial with inconsistency in the identification of predictive factors for adherence across studies [144]. This may be related to the retrospective nature of pediatric studies as well as the small sample sizes (ranging from 29 to 140 patients) [148]. In a comprehensive review of PAP adherence in 46 studies with 3000 participants between these studies from across the globe, the following inclusion criteria were used: age 0–21 years; participants with OSA treated with PAP (including CPAP, APAP, BPAP); studies reporting outcome measures of hours of PAP use or frequency of adherence; and studies reported in English [148]. More than two thirds of the participants had complete PAP use/adherence data. The factors associated with adherence include individual factors, family and social factors, disease and mode of therapy, and PAP technology factors. Children with DD are included in many of the studies looking at PAP adherence. These are reviewed in the following section. The largest dataset of pediatric adherence data comes from the United States where a retrospective cross-sectional analysis of the Airview database was carried out in children between the ages of 4 and 18 years old ($n = 12,699$) from 2014 to 2018 [149]. The criteria for adherence in this study was PAP use for 4 h or more per night on at least 70% of the nights since therapy onset during a consecutive 30-day period during the initial 90 days of use. 61.8% of the cohort used PAP over the 90-day monitoring period with only 46.3% being adherent [149]. The factors that were found to be associated with adherence included younger age, residual AHI, use and onset of patient engagement programs, PAP pressure, and nightly median PAP mask leak [149].

In the few randomized control trials that have assessed adherence in the pediatric population, significantly lower usage among youth has been observed. Marcus et al. compared the effectiveness and adherence of CPAP and BPAP in newly diagnosed OSA children ($n = 29$) that had never used PAP before. The authors arbitrarily defined adherence as >3 h/night of PAP use even though 3 hours of use was noted to be suboptimal by the authors [124]. Of the 29 participants, 1 had a craniofacial anomaly, and 12 (2/3 of the patients) were obese. Eight patients dropped out of the study without providing final downloads despite receiving intensive support (use of free equipment and frequent telephone and clinic follow-up). Adherence outcomes were assessed at 6 months, and no difference was found between the two treatment groups (16 in BPAP group and 13 in CPAP group). Adherence was concluded to be suboptimal at 3.83 ± 3.3 hours/night among the 29 participants. There was also no difference in resolution of OSA (as documented by PSG) between the two modes of pressure delivery [124]. Other randomized controlled trials looking at PAP adherence similarly report poor adherence to PAP irrespective of mode of therapy and the use of shared decision-making tools [125, 128, 165].

As stated earlier the factors that influence PAP use have been explored in mostly retrospective studies. These factors can be categorized into facilitators and barriers to PAP use and adherence and can be further classified into four groups: PAP technology, caregiver/family unit, individual, and disease.

26.2.3.1 Individual Factors

Age
Younger children generally tend to be more adherent to PAP compared to older children [136, 149, 162, 166, 167]. Avis and colleagues found that 3-month CPAP adherence was better among younger (mean age ± SD, 10.7 ± 2.2) vs older children with a mean age of 14.7 ± 1.1 ($t = 5.1$, $P = 0.01$) [166]. O'Donnell et al. found that not only were younger children (6–12 years old vs 13–18 years old) more likely to be adherent to therapy, they were also more likely to accept nasal CPAP (nCPAP) [153]. Of the children that accepted PAP, there was a statistically significant decrease in adherence (% of days nCPAP used and mean daily use on days nCPAP was used) [153].

Sex
In two separate retrospective studies, female gender was significantly associated with PAP adherence [126, 168]. In one study, adherence data for 140 patients was examined – 76 male and 64 female. The average age (±SD) in the adherent and nonadherent groups were 12.0 ± 5.7 years and 12.7 ± 4.7 years, respectively. Females were 1.5 times more adherent to CPAP (60.9% vs 39.5% odds ratio = 2.41, 95%CI = 1.20–4.85; $p = 0.01$).

Underlying Medical Conditions
DD may be associated with better adherence in children. Hawkins and colleagues found a diagnosis of DD was associated with CPAP adherence (OR = 2.55, 95%CI = 1.27–5.13; $p = 0.007$). In this study, DD was defined as any form of non-typical development from mild (e.g., speech delay) to severe (e.g., static encephalopathy). Associated comorbidities and sex were not found to be significant factors influencing adherence [168]. Patients with obesity or atopic illness trended toward poor adherence in this study, but these factors did not reach statistical significance [168]. Kang et al. similarly found that PAP adherence in children with developmental disabilities was better than in those without [169]. Children with DD at both 3- and 6-month timepoints had higher percentage adherence usage compared to children with TD [169].

Race
There are limited data in children on the impact of ethnicity on adherence. In large retrospective studies ($n > 20,000$ participants), participant characteristics such as race were not available for analysis [149]. Smaller studies assessing how race affects adherence have not been well powered. Children who were African American (AA) (33 out of a total of 59 children) had PAP usage of (2.5 ± 2.4 vs 4.2 ± 2.8 h in month-1, $p = 0.021$) at the 1-month assessment timepoint when compared to other races [Caucasian ($n = 20$) and children of more than one race ($n = 3$)]. There was no significant difference in the number of nights that PAP was placed on or the number of hours of use at 3 months [162].

26.2.3.2 Family and Social Factors
DiFeo et al. found that higher number of PAP nights used correlated with a higher level of maternal education ($p = 0.002$) [162]. PAP use is higher for children who have a family member that is on PAP therapy, a higher average nightly hour of PAP use for all nights ($p = 0.04$), and nights used at 3 months ($p = 0.04$) after PAP was initiated [167]. Additional important factors that influence PAP adherence include the structure in the home, social reactions, style of communication (e.g., nagging/fighting, trust or respect, desire to please) within family, and perception of benefits of therapy [170].

Factors that have consistently been associated with non-adherence in children and adults include being asymptomatic of daytime symptoms of SDB, nasal obstruction, low self-efficacy, lack of risk perception, and lower socioeconomic status [171]. In adolescents, home and family structure, style of communication, social reactions and attitudes, adolescent perception of PAP benefits, and design of machine were important factors influencing adherence [170, 172]. Additional factors include the importance of an adjustment period to therapy, individual-specific family support based on the unique needs of adolescents, and perceived challenges to therapy outweighing perception of symptom relief [170, 172].

26.2.3.3 Disease and Mode of Therapy
Subtherapeutic CPAP pressures and hence inadequate treatment of OSA may impact early adherence to therapy [150]. Contrary to the previously described randomized trials described above that did not find any difference in mode of PAP therapy [125, 128, 165], a study in an Australian cohort of children found better adherence with BPAP. In this study 136 children (mostly non-obese) were initiated on PAP therapy (46 BPAP and 90 CPAP) with the intention of long-term use [173]. After exclusion of patients in both arms, 19 BPAP patients had downloadable data at 1 year compared to 17 CPAP patients. Patients in the CPAP and BPAP group were lost to follow-up for a variety of reasons including death ($n = 1$; $n = 5$), transition to adult services

($n = 2$; $n = 5$), lost to follow-up ($n = 10$; $n = 2$), non-tolerant ($n = 4$; $n = 4$), symptom resolution, and no longer using ($n = 16$). Ninety-one percent of BPAP users were adherent (defined as using the machine for ≥ 4 hours/night for 70% of the days) compared with 75% of CPAP users. The authors attribute this difference to the diagnostic profile of the patients with most patients in the BPAP group having neuromuscular and/or central nervous system disorders. However, the significance of these findings should be interpreted with caution due to the low numbers studied. The BPAP group were also older ($9.8 \pm 5.9y$) than the CPAP group ($6.9 \pm 5.5y$), and this could have contributed to their tolerance in terms of greater ability to reason with these children as to the importance of their therapy [173]. The CPAP use (70% adherence rate) in this study was similar to the findings by Uong et al. when compared to BPAP in primarily obese children at follow-up [127].

Children with obesity-related SDB with lower nocturnal oxygen saturation nadir were more likely to adhere to PAP therapy [174]. Subtherapeutic PAP pressures which lead to suboptimal therapy seem to decrease individual motivation to use PAP therapy. Bhattacharjee et al. found that higher PAP pressures had better adherence and that an increased residual AHI specifically of at least 5 events/hour had the lowest PAP use (1822 [55·6%], $p < 0·0001$) which concur with data from other studies [150]. In another study, patients with a higher baseline AHI and a greater change in AHI on PAP were more likely to be adherent [127].

26.2.3.4 PAP Technology

Interventions
Predictors of long-term adherence to PAP are the length of time that the child is prescribed PAP, and the consistent early attempts to use it [143, 150] especially with use of parent and patient engagement programs (PEP). These programs provide real-time daily feedback to patients about their PAP use while simultaneously coaching them based on the data collected. Information can be accessed via a proprietary website or mobile app. The use of a PEP at the initiation of PAP therapy has been associated with increased PAP adherence (63.2%) in children that used this technology [175]. Additionally, children in a patient adherence program are less likely (20.9%) to terminate therapy compared to those not enrolled in a patient engagement program [149]. Better PAP usage of 7 hours per night for 73% of the week for a mean of 18.1 months has been reported in school aged children and adolescents between 7 and 19 years, $n = 46$ [127]. In the PEP, patients can access information related to PAP use time and duration, mask leak, respiratory events per hour of use, and the number of times that the mask is placed and removed. Patients receive suggestions and coaching aimed at troubleshooting issues and encourage usage. Messages are designed to enhance self-management, recognize success through award, and permit patients to identify and solve treatment issues on their own [149].

Behavioral interventions may be beneficial in promoting CPAP adherence [106]. In one study, participants between 1 and 15 years ($n = 20$) self-selected to one of three treatment arms: behavior consultation and recommendation session (CR+), behavior consultation and recommendations plus a course of behavioral therapy (BT), and a group for whom behavior therapy was recommended after consultation but the family did not follow-up (CR-). A behavior consultation consisted of trained staff observing CPAP application, a structured interview about preferences and dislikes of the child, and recommendations for a one-week treatment trial were then provided in the CR+ group. Participants in the first two groups showed higher CPAP use than those in the third group [106]. The CR+ group showed significantly longer PAP usage at posttreatment compared to the CR- group (average of 8.58 hrs vs 0.67 hrs, respectively).

In addition to other forms of behavioral intervention [176, 177], other factors have shown to have a positive impact on PAP adherence. Of note is that these factors were explored in pilot studies with very small numbers. Mendoza-Ruiz and colleagues assessed the effect of a table based on token economy [178]. In this study children ($n = 6$) placed a green or red token to indicate whether CPAP was used or not, respectively. An objective number of nights of use were decided between parent and child, and a reward was chosen. The use of this table was found to be effective in improving CPAP adherence at 1 month [178]. In a study assessing the effect of medical hypnosis on PAP adherence, nine children between 2 and 15 years old had sessions of hypnosis techniques performed by a nurse trained in administering these techniques. Hypnosis techniques based on distraction in the youngest to indirect or direct hypnotic suggestions in older children to obtain a progressive psychocorporal relaxation were employed [161]. All patients studied accepted the interface within three sessions and had a median use of 7.5 h per night at a 6-month assessment timepoint. Access to a pediatric PAP team with expertise in therapeutic education and CPAP/PAP may also lead to better adherence [93, 179, 180]. Access to a respiratory therapist (RT) trained in PAP use at clinic visits [181] and PAP desensitization are additional factors found to have a positive effect on PAP use and adherence [182].

In summary, the pediatric studies assessing PAP adherence in children are limited to mostly retrospective studies with small numbers conducted in centers with differing clinical practices as it pertains to multidisciplinary care. However, findings from these studies suggest that the developmental components of childhood, socioenvironmental factors, initial PAP exposure, and degree of SDB are important factors in pediatric PAP adherence.

Table 26.3 Summary of the findings from studies assessing adherence in CSHCN

Authors	N	Age	Study design	% CSHCN	Adherence definition	Outcome assessment period	Adherence data	Findings
Amaddeo et al. [184]	31	8.9 (range 0.8–17.5y)	P	32	Median number of hours of CPAP use/night with CPAP ≥4 hrs/night	2 months	8h21m/night (5h45m -12 h 20 m)	PAP initiation is affected by: Developmental delay Behavioral problems Excellent compliance likely related to: Routine CPAP educational program Close collaboration with home care providers
Brooks et al. [97]	10	10.2 ± 3.9	P	100	NR	13 ± 6.6 months	NR	PAP initiation is affected by: Inattention
DiFeo et al. [162]	56	NR	P	66	Mean number of nights PAP was used/month Hours of usage on nights used	1 and 3 months	*Month 1:* 22 ± 8nights/month 3 ± 3 h/night *Month 3:* 19 ± 9 nights/month 2.8 ± 2.7 h/night	Strongest predictor for PAP adherence: Maternal education Poor adherence: Older typically developing youth African American youth Lower levels of social support No age-related difference in adherence among children with developmental delay
Dudoignon et al. [93]	19	7 ± 7 (range 0.4–23 y)	R	100	Mean number of nights with NIV use Number of nights NIV used for >4 h	2 ± 1 years	8h46m ± 3h59m/night	Poor PAP tolerance in patients with major behavioral disorders and family dysfunction Good adherence related to pediatric NIV team with expertise in therapeutic education and NIV
Kang et al. [169]	DD: n = 103 TD: n = 137	DD:7.9(3.2–13.1 TD: 11.0 (5.5–16.)	R	75	Percentage of nights Hours of usage on nights used, at 3 and 6 months	3 and 6 months	*Month 3:* DD Cohort 86.7% of nights used 5.0 (1.4–7.9) hrs/night TD Cohort 62.9% of nights used 4.6 (1.9–7.2) hrs/night *Month 6:* DD Cohort 90% of nights used 6.4 (18.-8.3) hrs/night TD Cohort 70.7% of nights used 5.7 (2.5–7.3) hrs/night	In children with DD: Better PAP adherence compared to TD children Increasing adherence overtime over six month period. Predictors of usage in both groups Higher median neighborhood income Higher PAP pressures
Mendoza-Ruiz-et al [131, 178]	15	Nonadherent: 5±5 Adherent: 5±3	P	33	>3 h/night at day 8 after initiation	1 month	Prior to use of table: 1 h00 ± 0h33m After use of table: 4h13m ± 1h12m	Use of a table completed by child (identified to be nonadherent to therapy) based on token economy is effective in improving CPAP adherence at one month
Nathan et al. [126]	51	11 (range 8–13)	R	73	Use of NIV ≥ 4 days/week	7 months	21/51 (42%) used NIV ≥ 4 days/week	Good adherence: Female gender Presence of comorbid conditions (asthma and genetic disease) Use of BPAP Monetary assistance Patient refusal and side effects

Author	N	Age	Design	% SHCN	Adherence measure	Duration	Results	Findings
Nixon et al. [150]	30	9.1 ± 5.5	R	73	>1 hour/night during >6 nights/week		83% were adherent for 1 hour or more on more than 50% of the nights; 72.9 nights/child; 4.7 hours/night	Consistent attempts to use CPAP after initial education session predicted longer term use; Skip CPAP nights (using CPAP for less than 1 hour) was strongly correlated with duration of use on nights used
O'Donell et al. [153]	50	9.7 ± 5.3	R	78	Days nCPAP used; % of days nCPAP used; Mean daily use; Mean daily use on days nCPAP used	46 months	76% used nCPAP for at least half the days; 52% used nCPAP for at least 75% of days; Mean daily use 4.7 hrs (IQR1.4–7.0)	Poorer compliance was associated with: Lower age; Full face mask; PAP acceptance was greatest in: Children 6–12 yo
Perriol et al. [193]	78	10.4 ± 3.2	P	72.7	Mean nightly duration of CPAP use	24 months	7.0 ± 2.7 hours/night	Higher CPAP adherence (hours per night) was associated with: Younger age; High AHI at diagnosis; Primary vs middle/high school attendance; Neurocognitive disorders at baseline
Puri et al. [167]	56	13.2 ± 3.7	R	32% w/ DD 25% w/ GS	% of nights used; % of nights used for >4 hours; Average nightly hours of use for all nights; Avg nightly hours of use for the nights used	3 months	57% of nights used; 2.8 ± 2.4 h/night	Family member on PAP therapy was associated with better PAP adherence by the child; Gender, obesity status, or OSA severity were not associated with adherence
Pascoe et al. [187]	42	12.2 ± 1.9	P	100	% days used; Days used ≥4 h/night	NR	56.1% of days used; 46.2% of days used ≥4 days; Average usage of 5.61 h on days used	Adherence barriers: Mask discomfort; Behavioral issues (refusing to use); Predictors of NIV adherence: Total number of adherence barriers; Internalizing behaviors
Trucco et al. [186]	25	2.4 (IQR 0.7–6)	R	100	Usage of overnight treatment for more than 4 h/night for >50% of the nights examined	1.9 years	Good adherence in: 7/18 CPAP patients; 4/6 bilevel NIV	Better adherence at the time of NIV initiation is related to better long-term adherence; CPAP slightly less tolerated than BPAP and oxygen supplementation
Marcus et al. [125]	56	CPAP: 12 ± 4 Bi-Flex: 12 ± 4	RCT	NR	Mean number of minutes used/night; Mean number of nights used/month	1 month and 3 months	*# of nights used:* CPAP month 1: 24 ± 6; Bi-Flex month 1: 22 ± 9; CPAP month 3: 18 ± 10; Bi-Flex Month 3: 19 ± 9; *# of minutes used:* CPAP month 1: 201 ± 135; Bi-Flex month 1: 185 ± 165; CPAP month 3: 125 ± 147; Bi-Flex month 3: 183 ± 169	Suboptimal adherence with both CPAP and Bi-Flex; Both CPAP and Bi-Flex are efficacious in treating children and adolescents with sleep disordered breathing

NR Not reported, P Prospective, Q Qualitative, R retrospective, RCT Randomized controlled trial, DD developmental delay, GS Genetic syndrome, TD typically developing

26.3 Specific PAP Adherence Factors in Children with Special Health-Care Needs

Several studies show that adherence to PAP in CSHCN is similar if not better to that seen in children without special health-care needs [106, 150, 162, 168, 169, 183], data summarized in Table 26.3. The use of PAP in CSHCN may be fraught with similar challenges to implementation as seen in children with typical development. The incorporation of PAP use into their schedule, getting accustomed to the device, and the requirement for caregiver support are examples of similar challenges [169].

In the largest study assessing adherence to PAP in children with developmental disabilities to date, Kang and colleagues found that among 103 children with DD, percentage of nights of PAP was used at 3 (86.7% in DD and 62.9% in TD, $p = 0.01$) and 6 months (90% in DD, 70.7% in TD, $p = 0.003$) was higher than in children with DD. Adherence was expressed as percentage nights used and hours of usage on nights used. The spectrum of developmental disabilities (DD) ranged from genetic syndromes ($n = 48$), CNS abnormalities ($n = 24$), autism spectrum disorder ($n = 12$), and a variety of other conditions such as idiopathic/global DD, epilepsy, craniosynostosis, mucolipidosis type II, neurofibromatosis type I, Renpenning syndrome, and unspecified intellectual disability ($n = 19$). The hours of usage between groups were similar. Both measures of adherence improved with time. Predictors of PAP usage in both groups included higher median neighborhood income and higher PAP pressures. There were 55 patients that dropped out of the study with a missing rate that was similar between groups [169].

The initial acceptance of PAP therapy in the CSHCN population may be challenging. In a successful outpatient PAP initiation program in children with complex OSA at the Hôpital Necker-Enfants Maldes in France, there was an 90% success rate for PAP acceptance and adherence, 4 of the 31 children did not accept PAP. These four children all had some degree behavioral problems and three of them were adolescents with DS [184]. The cohort of children with complex OSA in this study had medical conditions that included DS (most common diagnosis with $n = 7$), achondroplasia, crouzon syndrome, PWS, chiari malformation type 2, PRS, and MPS type II [184]. Twenty-seven participants achieved excellent adherence after 2 months with a median use of 8h21min (range 05h45min-12 h20 min) per night. CPAP was used a median of 25 nights per month (range 18–30) and 4 h/night during a median of 82 ± 17% of nights. The authors credit the high adherence rate in their program to the integrated, age-adapted education program and strict follow-up as well as close collaboration with home care providers that perform regular home visits and transmit adherence data to the team allowing for prompt adjustments in the first weeks of treatment [184] similar to observations in other studies [97]. The authors suspect that of the patients that did not accept PAP, lack of a supportive family structure as well as deficient adaptive behavior, visual-motor integration and academic achievement could be potential factors. However these were hard to elucidate due to the restrospective nature of the study.

Brooks and colleagues assessed PAP therapy in 25 children with DS who underwent polysomnography, multiple sleep latency testing (MSLT), and a battery of neuropsychological tests. The patients who were not able to tolerate PAP were deficient in tests of adaptive behavior (Vineland $p < 0.05$) visual–motor integration (Beery $p < 0.01$) and achievement (Woodcock-Johnson $p < 0.05$) compared to those successfully treated [97]. These findings suggest that inattention may be a barrier to CPAP adherence and suggest considering the evaluation and treatment of any attention deficit disorders in children having difficulty tolerating PAP [185]. In another cohort of DS patients initiated on NIV for OSA, 9/11 patients (82%) used CPAP/BIPAP for >4 h/night with average usage >8 h/night. Similar to previous findings, five patients did not tolerate PAP treatment because of major behavioral disorders and family dysfunction [93].

Better adherence in the short term may be predictive of longer-term adherence in the CSHCN population [186]. In a group of 24 young children with DS [mean age of 2.4 years old (IQR 0.7–6)] that were initiated on NIV for OSA, 11/24 (45.8%) had good adherence as defined by 4 h/night for >50% of the nights examined with average use of 8 h/night) with early adherence predicting long-term adherence. Regular follow-up was thought to be a key factor in maintaining adherence along with a multidisciplinary effort involving parents, nurses, psychologists, doctors, and play-specialists.

In children with neuromuscular disease, initial detailed education of youth and caregivers about the benefits of PPV and rapid access to troubleshooting and support early on in treatment were found to be possible key elements to promote adherence [183]. In their qualitative assessment of BPAP adherence in children with neuromuscular disease, Ennis et al. found that adherent youth were more likely to experience symptom benefit compared to nonadherent youth who also reported more adverse side effects. Nonadherent youth were found to display elements of rebellion against authority and challenge limit setting [183]. Pascoe and colleagues found poor adherence in 41 children with DMD on PAP for OSA. These patients were maintained on glucocorticoids and had preserved lung function [187]. The mean age at the time of PAP initiation was 12.2 ± 1.9y. Patients endorsed mask discomfort and sleep disruption (which may have been related to mask discomfort, leak, or pressure intolerance) as adherence barriers.

Child internalizing symptoms such as depression and anxiety were found to be predictors of lower PAP adherence as well as more adherence barriers [187].

In CSHCN that fail PAP initiation, a guided, gradual approach in a supportive setting with anticipatory guidance for assessing and managing challenges of children with complex medical needs may be helpful [144]. The initial PAP experience starts from the introduction of the device and machine to the patient, the fitting of an appropriate interface, and wearing that interface while awake with varying pressures prior to the integration of PAP placement into the bedtime routine and PAP use while asleep. Introduction to the PAP interface and machine with relaxation or distraction techniques while the child wears the device as well as allowing the child to play with the interface are some examples of creating a positive initial experience [184]. Children with craniofacial conditions who have had multiple facial surgeries may have increased sensitivity to a mask on their face [41]. In addition, CSHCN may experience the added difficulty of sensory and behavioral concerns as well as increased reliance on caregiver support [168].

The use of a CPAP age-appropriate educational program at the time of PAP initiation, behavioral assessments prior to initiation, close follow-up for the first few months of use, prompt assessment and management of issues, and side effect of PAP use are important factors linked to successful adherence in the CSHCN population [93, 106, 184, 188]. The use of an intensive CPAP program for patients with obesity, trisomy 21, and genetic syndromes which included more frequent follow-up phone calls and follow-up clinic visits compared to standard care had favorable outcomes [184]. The follow-up rate for clinic visits and titration polysomnograms was found to be higher compared to patients in the standard CPAP program [188].

Education and behavioral strategies can yield adherence improvement [189–191]. Behavioral-based adherence programs had shown promising results in PAP adherence [106, 176, 192]. In a group of 19 children with OSA and other conditions such as DS, obesity, and DD, an individualized treatment plan was associated with improvement in their average usage. The behavioral components of the treatment plan included positive reinforcement, positive coaching, behavioral rehearsal, stimulus cues, and relaxation training [176]. In the patients that did not show improvement, poor maternal buy-in to therapy and depressive symptoms were barriers to adherence. In another study that assessed adherence in 20 children with OSA and underlying complex medical conditions, behavioral intervention improved PAP tolerance and documented hours of use [106]. In this study, behavioral intervention consisted of positive reinforcement, graduated exposure, counter conditioning, as well as escape or avoidance prevention strategies [106]. Strategies to improve adherence in children with physical and cognitive delays include follow-up phone calls to assess and remotely address adherence barriers [153]. Similar efforts may be effective if psychologists provide more intensive behavioral therapy [106].

The PAP pediatric education team plays an important role in the patient's first encounter with PAP and at follow-up visits. In most studies, this team consists of a nurse with PAP expertise and therapeutic education, pediatrician, and pulmonologist [93]. The availability of a clinic RT trained in PAP use improved adherence in patients whose adherence was <50% [181, 182].

Supportive family during the patient's initial PAP experience is an equally important factor in achieving successful adherence [162, 165]. In this regard, the use of shared decision-making tools for counseling families regarding treatment options may improve agreement on treatment plan and PAP adherence [165]. This was found in a group of children with OSA without tonsillar hypertrophy. These children had comorbidities such as DS and Pierre-Robin sequence [165]. A strong partnership between the family and patient, the health-care center, and home care provider are crucial. Family dysfunction and social issues have been important factors in poor PAP adherence among CSHCN [93, 176]. Specific parental barriers to PAP adherence are low maternal education, parental nonadherence to implementing a reward system, and encouraging PAP use [162].

In summary, acceptable adherence to PAP can be achieved in the CSHCN population with resources to support initiation and close follow-up which may need to be increased from the standard protocol for children with typical development. The availability of a PAP education team to promptly troubleshoot issues with PAP usage as well as the use of a behavioral-based adherence programs are likely important factors in successful adherence in the CSHCN population.

26.4 Approach to PAP Use in Children with Special Health-Care Needs

The introduction of long-term PAP therapy in the CSHCN population can be broken down into three phases: initiation, acclimatization, and maintenance. These steps are outlined in Fig. 26.2 and in Table 26.4. The ideal candidate for PAP therapy should be cooperative and have stable upper airway obstruction and/or chronic respiratory failure [123]. Tailoring PAP treatment as individualized to the specific patient has significant potential to improve adherence to PAP therapy in children, specifically children with special health-care needs. A personalized approach to PAP therapy would take into consideration differences in individual preferences and response to treatment leading to identification of the risk of nonadherence and prescribing individualized goals for PAP use.

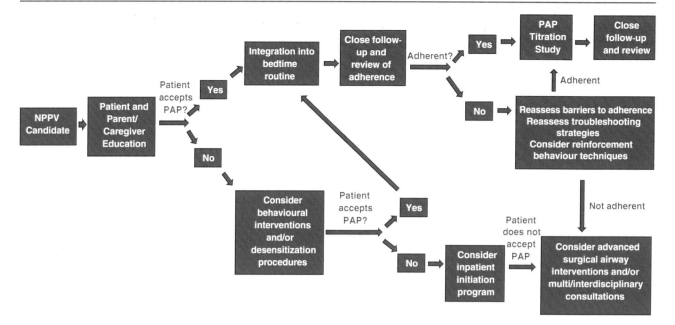

Fig. 26.2 The Approach to PAP use in CSHCN

Table 26.4 Summary of steps in the initiation, acclimatization, and maintenance phases

Initiation
1. Identify the suitability of a patient for the long-term use of NPPV
2. Discuss parental/caregiver concerns and beliefs
3. Provide education about the therapy, indication, and steps involved in NPPV therapy
4. Select appropriate interface and headgear
5. Assess the readiness and acceptance of therapy by the child
6. Use of a behavior modification-based approach; desensitization procedures; treatment of attention deficits; and/or stepwise positive reinforcement techniques as indicated

Acclimatization
1. Integration of PAP into bedtime routine
2. Positive reinforcement by family members
3. Close follow-up to identify mask and machine comfort and barriers to use
4. Promptly address specific issues that are identified
5. Plan for a titration study once the patient is using therapy regularly
6. Re-visit steps in the initiation phase as needed

Maintenance
1. Reinforcement strategy
2. Re-visit steps in the initiation and acclimatization phase as needed

26.4.1 Initiation Phase

Once a patient is identified as being a candidate for NPPV, the first step is to decide if the patient should be initiated on PAP in an inpatient or outpatient setting. Some of the considerations for inpatient initiation include failure to initiate PAP in the home or very severe sleep disordered breathing. In both cases, the first step is education of the patient and parent by the PAP team. Members of the PAP team should at minimum consist of the sleep specialist and technical personnel.

Other members of the team that have been showed to play an important role in adherence are RTs, behavioral psychologists, and nurses specialized in PAP and therapeutic education [181, 182, 184, 188]. The goal of the initiation phase is to achieve child and parent/caregiver acceptance of PAP therapy [160]. Child and parent/caregiver engagement is a crucial component in achieving this goal. To this end, maintenance of a positive and supportive approach by everyone involved is important [160]. This approach may be particularly important in the CSHCN population for whom gradual PAP exposure in a supportive setting is particularly important [144].

Patient education consists of four main categories: (1) patient and parent education; (2) review of parent/caregiver concerns and expectations; (3) goals for treatment; and (4) anticipatory guidance about common side effects, problems, and device issues and how to treat and troubleshoot them [144]. Crucial to this first step of patient and parent/caregiver education is engagement. Patient and parent education should include a review of SDB diagnosis and symptoms and the benefits of PAP. Specific age-adapted educational tools may be particularly useful and can include educational boards and cartoons, a booklet explaining PAP, and a teddy bear or doll breathing with a PAP device [184]. Healthy sleep hygiene and bedtime routine should be reviewed along with parental behavior management strategies, monitoring, and expectations. Concerns and questions by the parent should be addressed. It is particularly important to dispel inaccurate or incomplete information that the parent or caregiver may have as this can be a barrier to initial PAP acceptance [159]. It is important to identify potential limitations or barriers to incorporating PAP into the daily life of the child and address them.

Initial acceptance with first exposure is a crucial next step as an unpleasant initial first experience can lead to prolonged period of treatment rejection from both child and caregiver [159]. In children with tactile aversions, consideration should be made for a full-face mask and/or minimal nasal airflow. This is provided the child can independently dislodge the mask from the face when necessary, but this may not always be necessary specifically if there is a caregiver at the bedside to monitor the patient during sleep [159]. Desensitization procedures in addition to behavioral conditioning can be useful tools to help achieve PAP acceptance and adherence for patients in whom initial acceptance and adherence are not achieved [106]. Personalized strategies in the initiation phase of PAP use include personalizing the PAP interface to improve PAP effectiveness through reducing discomfort related to skin irritation and minimizing leak. This can be done through the use of fitting material between the mask and interface specifically in focal areas of increased pressure on the underlying skin [123]. More recently personalized three-dimensional PAP interfaces have been created 3D mask models are created with use of computed tomograpy, magnetic resonance imaging, or use of a 3D scanner. The model is then converted into a mold which is 3D printed and can then be filled with medical grade material to create the final interface [194]. These devices allow for objective measurements of the face in order to design a personalized fitting device for each patient [156]. In a pilot study assessing 3D-printed CPAP mask use in a child with Treacher Collins syndrome and severe OSA (baseline AHI = 16.4/hr), there was a 9% increase in compliance and a 24% decrease in residual AHI. There was a significant improvement in measured median mask leak from 25.2 L/min vs 6.6 L/min and leak at the 95th%tile (70.6 L/min vs 47/3 L/min). All improvements were sustained after 3 months of use. Additional patients have been enrolled, in this study and further data is pending [194].

Desensitization procedures that allow slow habituation by gradual exposure to the mask and machine may be necessary in some children with tactile aversions [160]. One example of how this would play out would be to divide procedures into daytime and nighttime practices to establish PAP as a part of routine activities for the child [195]. An example of daytime practice includes gradually introducing the mask (placing the mask in the position of the child's face) with the air turned on for increasing periods of time over a few days to wearing the mask with airflow, while the child lies down for increasing periods over a few days. Nighttime use starts with turning on the PAP machine at night without attaching it to the child so that they can get used to the noise to placing on and having the child fall asleep with the mask on. If the child is not able to fall asleep, 15 minutes of practice can be done, and the PAP can be placed after the child falls asleep. The goal is to have the child fall asleep with PAP on and use

it for the majority of the night. Daytime and bedtime practice should be continued until that goal is achieved [195]. Individually tailored behavioral interventions should be considered for children having challenges with acclimatizing to therapy and/or those with poor adherence during the maintenance phase such as inpatient admission and/or a short 2–4 week intervention with home nursing [160]. These approaches have been shown to be successful and demonstrate to the family that the child can tolerate the therapy. In addition, successful acclimatization to PAP therapy through in-patient admission or in-home intervention tends to break the cycle of patient refusal to use PAP and parental annoyance and apprehension related to lack of PAP use [160]. Treatment of attention deficits in children prior to the initiation of PAP may improve their adherence [97].

In children without tactile aversions, the interface can be tried first without the PAP device, and training can be provided for putting on and taking off the interface. If the patient is accepting of this first step, CPAP can be started at a minimal pressure and progressively increased to the highest tolerated level [184]. The patient should be encouraged to try different interfaces before determining which is most comfortable. The suitability of the interface and headgear should be assessed with pressure turned on to assess leak and comfort. During this time, the patient should be lying down calmly, and the pressure can be kept for a specified period like 30 minutes. Relaxation or distraction can be offered according to the age and preference of the child, while this is being done. Introducing the mask to the child can be made enticing with the use of stickers, videos, and picture books and allowing the child to play with the mask. Personalized books to follow the child's PAP journey can also be used. If the patient can tolerate the mask on for the period during which the machine is turned on and a pressure is applied and/or varied, this implies acceptance by the child. The final step of the initiation phase is deciding on a set pressure or a range of pressures (AutoPAP) and setting the patient up with the therapy in the home. The parent/caregiver should be provided with available resources for problem solving [144, 196].

26.4.2 Acclimatization Phase

This phase of PAP use begins after PAP acceptance and typically starts once the patient has taken home the device and starts to use it. Early follow-up and follow-up that occurs frequently is important during this phase [159]. Close follow-up with the team is important for the identification and prompt treatment of specific side effects of PAP use such as dryness, skin irritation, interface discomfort, and nasal congestion. Clinical follow-up within the first 4–6 weeks is ideal [184]. PAP should be integrated into bedtime routine to allow the patient to get accustomed to sleeping with PAP therapy which may take weeks to months. If the child is unwilling to wear PAP at night, using the mask and machine can be integrated into play time during the day with the child and parent, allowing stuffed animals, dolls, and parent to wear the mask [160]. It is crucial for regular positive reinforcement by the family during this phase. Adherence should be evaluated weekly during this phase. Home care providers trained in pediatric PAP that can perform regular home visits and transmit adherence data to the home team to allow for prompt adjustment during the first weeks of treatment and can be an important component of excellent CPAP adherence [184]. The same can be achieved with remote monitoring of data like Airview which has made data easily and readily accessible for download. If there is poor adherence, the barriers to use should be reassessed and managed by the team with regular follow-up. In children with good and excellent adherence, the progress should be rewarded and encouraged. Once the patient is using PAP regularly, consider planning for a PAP titration study with simultaneous PSG in a sleep laboratory. With the growth of telemonitoring and telemedicine, timely ongoing monitoring of PAP use is both viable and necessary. The frequency of follow-up should be personalized to the needs of the individual patient particularly in the CSHCN. Intensive initial inpatient support for PAP initiation may positively influence long-term adherence [150]. This protocol may include play therapy, cognitive behavioral therapy for older children, as well as further education and support of parents [150]. These strategies but may not be feasible and generalizable to all comers because of the high cost and limited resources of inpatient care [197]. However, this may be a consideration in specific circumstances and can be employed in specific scenarios.

26.4.3 Maintenance Phase

During this phase of PAP use, reinforcement of PAP use is the focus. The reinforcement strategies include ongoing encouragement and rewarding of good adherence and continued frequent follow-up and availability of the supportive network of the sleep physician and technical personnel to address challenges and issues.

26.5   Future Directions

PAP is an important therapy for the treatment of sleep disordered breathing in the CSHCN population. However, there is a paucity of higher level and quality studies that are adequately powered to assess factors that affect PAP adherence in this population as well as in children in general. Important parameters that still need to be defined for further large-scale

studies are the optimal adherence for positive clinical outcomes in children. This definition is crucial in setting a target for PAP usage and allow for more comprehensive assessment of facilitators and barriers to PAP use and adherence. These findings will ultimately help with designing studies to test for the efficacy of PAP adherence interventions.

Additional data on protocols outlining the introduction of PAP therapy and surveillance of PAP use in the pediatric population will help to tailor and personalize PAP initiation and use in children. Specifically, the impact of desensitization protocols, behavioral interventions, PAP education programs, and ideal follow-up times in each phase of PAP introduction are needed. Among adolescents, some of the gaps in knowledge as it pertains to PAP adherence include the inclusion of peer support groups in the promotion of adherence, understanding the influence of parenting style, family dynamics and communication, and lastly the benefit of health education and family involvement in PAP adherence strategies [170].

Future research is needed to assess the contributions of socioeconomic factors such as maternal education, race and socioeconomic status, and cultural and personal beliefs to PAP use. These findings may allow for a more targeted and customized emphasis on education of families around the use of PAP. Other specific tailored or targeted interventions for nonadherers and specific age groups of children within the group of CSHCN are important areas to understand.

Despite the technological advances in PAP interfaces, there is still limited availability of interfaces for children, specifically for CSHCN. Functional interfaces such as 3D-personalized masks may increase PAP therapy effectiveness and are a promising first step in the creation of more personalized therapy to increase PAP adherence through the improvement in patient comfort.

Acknowledgements The authors would like to acknowledge respiratory therapist, Melissa Trinh for her contribution of the photographs displayed in this chapter

References

1. McPherson M, Arango P, Fox H, Lauver C, McManus M, Newacheck PW, et al. A new definition of children with special health care needs. Pediatrics. 1998;102(1 Pt 1):137–40.
2. van Dyck PC, Kogan MD, McPherson MG, Weissman GR, Newacheck PW. Prevalence and characteristics of children with special health care needs. Arch Pediatr Adolesc Med. 2004;158(9):884–90.
3. Strickland BB, Jones JR, Newacheck PW, Bethell CD, Blumberg SJ, Kogan MD. Assessing systems quality in a changing health care environment: the 2009-10 national survey of children with special health care needs. Matern Child Health J. 2015;19(2):353–61.
4. UNICEF. Disabilities 2020. Available from: https://www.unicef.org/disabilities/.

5. U.S. Department of Health and Human Services HRaSA, Maternal and Child Health Bureau. The National Survey of Children with Special Healthcare Needs Chartbook 2005–2006 Maryland2008 [.

6. Dewan T, Cohen E. Children with medical complexity in Canada. Paediatr Child Health. 2013;18(10):518–22.

7. Pankewicz A, Davis RK, Kim J, Antonelli R, Rosenberg H, Berhane Z, et al. Children with special needs: social determinants of health and care coordination. Clin Pediatr (Phila). 2020;59(13):1161–8.

8. Tomkies A, Johnson RF, Shah G, Caraballo M, Evans P, Mitchell RB. Obstructive sleep apnea in children with autism. J Clin Sleep Med. 2019;15(10):1469–76.

9. Harris J, Malow B, Werkhaven J. Descriptive epidemiology of obstructive sleep apnea in children with autism spectrum disorder. 32nd Annual Meeting of the Associated-Professional-Sleep-Societies-LLC; Baltimore, MD2018. p. A292-A3.

10. Sivertsen B, Posserud MB, Gillberg C, Lundervold AJ, Hysing M. Sleep problems in children with autism spectrum problems: a longitudinal population-based study. Autism. 2012;16(2):139–50.

11. Johnson KP, Giannotti F, Cortesi F. Sleep patterns in autism spectrum disorders. Child Adolesc Psychiatr Clin N Am. 2009;18(4):917–28.

12. Newman CJ, O'Regan M, Hensey O. Sleep disorders in children with cerebral palsy. Dev Med Child Neurol. 2006;48(7):564–8.

13. Waters KA, Everett F, Sillence DO, Fagan ER, Sullivan CE. Treatment of obstructive sleep apnea in achondroplasia: evaluation of sleep, breathing, and somatosensory-evoked potentials. Am J Med Genet. 1995;59(4):460–6.

14. Tasker RC, Dundas I, Laverty A, Fletcher M, Lane R, Stocks J. Distinct patterns of respiratory difficulty in young children with achondroplasia: a clinical, sleep, and lung function study. Arch Dis Child. 1998;79(2):99–108.

15. Mogayzel PJ Jr, Carroll JL, Loughlin GM, Hurko O, Francomano CA, Marcus CL. Sleep-disordered breathing in children with achondroplasia. J Pediatr. 1998;132(4):667–71.

16. Tenconi R, Khirani S, Amaddeo A, Michot C, Baujat G, Couloigner V, et al. Sleep-disordered breathing and its management in children with achondroplasia. Am J Med Genet A. 2017;173(4):868–78.

17. Sisk EA, Heatley DG, Borowski BJ, Leverson GE, Pauli RM. Obstructive sleep apnea in children with achondroplasia: surgical and anesthetic considerations. Otolaryngol Head Neck Surg. 1999;120(2):248–54.

18. Collins WO, Choi SS. Otolaryngologic manifestations of achondroplasia. Arch Otolaryngol Head Neck Surg. 2007;133(3):237–44.

19. Afsharpaiman S, Sillence DO, Sheikhvatan M, Ault JE, Waters K. Respiratory events and obstructive sleep apnea in children with achondroplasia: investigation and treatment outcomes. Sleep Breath. 2011;15(4):755–61.

20. Schluter B, De Sousa G, Trowitzsch E, Andler W. Diagnostics and management of sleep-related respiratory disturbances in children with skeletal dysplasia caused by FGFR3 mutations (achondroplasia and hypochondroplasia). Georgian Med News. 2011;196-197:63–72.

21. Julliand S, Boule M, Baujat G, Ramirez A, Couloigner V, Beydon N, et al. Lung function, diagnosis, and treatment of sleep-disordered breathing in children with achondroplasia. Am J Med Genet A. 2012;158a(8):1987–93.

22. Miano S, Bruni O, Elia M, Musumeci SA, Verrillo E, Ferri R. Sleep breathing and periodic leg movement pattern in Angelman syndrome: a polysomnographic study. Clin Neurophysiol. 2005;116(11):2685–92.

23. Dosier LBM, Vaughn BV, Fan Z. Sleep Disorders in Childhood Neurogenetic Disorders. Children (Basel). 2017;4(9):82.

24. Sedky K, Bennett DS, Pumariega A. Prader Willi syndrome and obstructive sleep apnea: co-occurrence in the pediatric population. J Clin Sleep Med. 2014;10(4):403–9.

25. Nixon GM, Brouillette RT. Sleep and breathing in Prader-Willi syndrome. Pediatr Pulmonol. 2002;34(3):209–17.

26. Pavone M, Caldarelli V, Khirani S, Colella M, Ramirez A, Aubertin G, et al. Sleep disordered breathing in patients with Prader-Willi syndrome: a multicenter study. Pediatr Pulmonol. 2015;50(12):1354–9.

27. Gönüldaş B, Yılmaz T, Sivri HS, Güçer K, Kılınç K, Genç GA, et al. Mucopolysaccharidosis: Otolaryngologic findings, obstructive sleep apnea and accumulation of glucosaminoglycans in lymphatic tissue of the upper airway. Int J Pediatr Otorhinolaryngol. 2014;78(6):944–9.

28. Moreira GA, Kyosen SO, Patti CL, Martins AM, Tufik S. Prevalence of obstructive sleep apnea in patients with mucopolysaccharidosis types I, II, and VI in a reference center. Sleep Breath. 2014;18(4):791–7.

29. Hagebeuk EE, Bijlmer RP, Koelman JH, Poll-The BT. Respiratory disturbances in rett syndrome: don't forget to evaluate upper airway obstruction. J Child Neurol. 2012;27(7):888–92.

30. Sarber KM, Howard JJM, Dye TJ, Pascoe JE, Simakajornboon N. Sleep-disordered breathing in pediatric patients with Rett syndrome. J Clin Sleep Med. 2019;15(10):1451–7.

31. Akre H, Øverland B, Åsten P, Skogedal N, Heimdal K. Obstructive sleep apnea in Treacher Collins syndrome. Eur Arch Otorhinolaryngol. 2012;269(1):331–7.

32. Plomp RG, Bredero-Boelhouwer HH, Joosten KF, Wolvius EB, Hoeve HL, Poublon RM, et al. Obstructive sleep apnoea in Treacher Collins syndrome: prevalence, severity and cause. Int J Oral Maxillofac Surg. 2012;41(6):696–701.

33. Anderson IC, Sedaghat AR, McGinley BM, Redett RJ, Boss EF, Ishman SL. Prevalence and severity of obstructive sleep apnea and snoring in infants with Pierre Robin sequence. Cleft Palate Craniofac J. 2011;48(5):614–8.

34. Lee JJ, Thottam PJ, Ford MD, Jabbour N. Characteristics of sleep apnea in infants with Pierre-Robin sequence: is there improvement with advancing age? Int J Pediatr Otorhinolaryngol. 2015;79(12):2059–67.

35. Inverso G, Brustowicz KA, Katz E, Padwa BL. The prevalence of obstructive sleep apnea in symptomatic patients with syndromic craniosynostosis. Int J Oral Maxillofac Surg. 2016;45(2):167–9.

36. Suresh S, Wales P, Dakin C, Harris MA, Cooper DG. Sleep-related breathing disorder in Duchenne muscular dystrophy: disease spectrum in the paediatric population. J Paediatr Child Health. 2005;41(9–10):500–3.

37. Sawnani H, Thampratankul L, Szczesniak RD, Fenchel MC, Simakajornboon N. Sleep disordered breathing in young boys with Duchenne muscular dystrophy. J Pediatr. 2015;166(3):640–5.e1.

38. Pincherle A, Patruno V, Raimondi P, Moretti S, Dominese A, Martinelli-Boneschi F, et al. Sleep breathing disorders in 40 Italian patients with myotonic dystrophy type 1. Neuromuscul Disord. 2012;22(3):219–24.

39. Pinard JM, Azabou E, Essid N, Quijano-Roy S, Haddad S, Cheliout-Héraut F. Sleep-disordered breathing in children with congenital muscular dystrophies. Eur J Paediatr Neurol. 2012;16(6):619–24.

40. Mellies U, Ragette R, Schwake C, Baethmann M, Voit T, Teschler H. Sleep-disordered breathing and respiratory failure in acid maltase deficiency. Neurology. 2001;57(7):1290–5.

41. Cielo CM, Marcus CL. Obstructive sleep apnoea in children with craniofacial syndromes. Paediatr Respir Rev. 2015;16(3):189–96.

42. Lowe AA, Fleetham JA, Adachi S, Ryan CF. Cephalometric and computed tomographic predictors of obstructive sleep apnea severity. Am J Orthod Dentofac Orthop. 1995;107(6):589–95.

43. Miles PG, Vig PS, Weyant RJ, Forrest TD, Rockette HE Jr. Craniofacial structure and obstructive sleep apnea syndrome-a qualitative analysis and meta-analysis of the literature. Am J Orthod Dentofac Orthop. 1996;109(2):163–72.

44. Guilleminault C, Riley R, Powell N. Obstructive sleep apnea and abnormal cephalometric measurements. Implications for treatment. Chest. 1984;86(5):793–4.

45. Riha RL, Brander P, Vennelle M, Douglas NJ. A cephalometric comparison of patients with the sleep apnea/hypopnea syndrome and their siblings. Sleep. 2005;28(3):315–20.

46. Lyberg T, Krogstad O, Djupesland G. Cephalometric analysis in patients with obstructive sleep apnoea syndrome: II. Soft tissue morphology. J Laryngol Otol. 1989;103(3):293–7.

47. Sforza E, Bacon W, Weiss T, Thibault A, Petiau C, Krieger J. Upper airway collapsibility and cephalometric variables in patients with obstructive sleep apnea. Am J Respir Crit Care Med. 2000;161(2 Pt 1):347–52.

48. Nagaoka K, Tanne K. Activities of the muscles involved in swallowing in patients with cleft lip and palate. Dysphagia. 2007;22(2):140–4.

49. Aboussouan LS. Sleep-disordered breathing in neuromuscular disease. Am J Respir Crit Care Med. 2015;191(9):979–89.

50. Cohen SR, Lefaivre JF, Burstein FD, Simms C, Kattos AV, Scott PH, et al. Surgical treatment of obstructive sleep apnea in neurologically compromised patients. Plast Reconstr Surg. 1997;99(3):638–46.

51. Kerschner JE, Lynch JB, Kleiner H, Flanary VA, Rice TB. Uvulopalatopharyngoplasty with tonsillectomy and adenoidectomy as a treatment for obstructive sleep apnea in neurologically impaired children. Int J Pediatr Otorhinolaryngol. 2002;62(3):229–35.

52. Kirk V, Kahn A, Brouillette RT. Diagnostic approach to obstructive sleep apnea in children. Sleep Med Rev. 1998;2(4):255–69.

53. Worley G, Witsell DL, Hulka GF. Laryngeal dystonia causing inspiratory stridor in children with cerebral palsy. Laryngoscope. 2003;113(12):2192–5.

54. Wilkinson DJ, Baikie G, Berkowitz RG, Reddihough DS. Awake upper airway obstruction in children with spastic quadriplegic cerebral palsy. J Paediatr Child Health. 2006;42(1–2):44–8.

55. Fitzgerald DA, Follett J, Asperen V. Assessing and managing lung disease and sleep disordered breathing in children with cerebral palsy. Paediatr Respir Rev. 2009;10(1):18–24.

56. Garcia J, Wical B, Wical W, Schaffer L, Wical T, Wendorf H, et al. Obstructive sleep apnea in children with cerebral palsy and epilepsy. Dev Med Child Neurol. 2016;58(10):1057–62.

57. Prevention CfDCa. Disability and Health Promotion 2019. Available from: https://www.cdc.gov/ncbddd/disabilityand-health/obesity.html#:~:text=20%25%20of%20children%20 10%20through,without%20special%20health%20care%20 needs.&text=Annual%20health%20care%20costs%20 of,estimated%20at%20approximately%20%2444%20billion.

58. Rimmer JH, Yamaki K, Lowry BM, Wang E, Vogel LC. Obesity and obesity-related secondary conditions in adolescents with intellectual/developmental disabilities. J Intellect Disabil Res. 2010;54(9):787–94.

59. Rao DP, Kropac E, Do MT, Roberts KC, Jayaraman GC. Childhood overweight and obesity trends in Canada. Health Promot Chronic Dis Prev Can. 2016;36(9):194–8.

60. Daar G, Sarı K, Gencer ZK, Ede H, Aydın R, Saydam L. The relation between childhood obesity and adenotonsillar hypertrophy. Eur Arch Otorhinolaryngol. 2016;273(2):505–9.

61. Schwab RJ, Kim C, Bagchi S, Keenan BT, Comyn FL, Wang S, et al. Understanding the anatomic basis for obstructive sleep apnea syndrome in adolescents. Am J Respir Crit Care Med. 2015;191(11):1295–309.

62. Hsu WC, Kang KT, Weng WC, Lee PL. Impacts of body weight after surgery for obstructive sleep apnea in children. Int J Obes. 2013;37(4):527–31.

63. Kohler MJ, van den Heuvel CJ. Is there a clear link between overweight/obesity and sleep disordered breathing in children? Sleep Med Rev. 2008;12(5):347–61; discussion 63-4.

64. Horner RL, Mohiaddin RH, Lowell DG, Shea SA, Burman ED, Longmore DB, et al. Sites and sizes of fat deposits around the pharynx in obese patients with obstructive sleep apnoea and weight matched controls. Eur Respir J. 1989;2(7):613–22.

65. Schwab RJ, Gupta KB, Gefter WB, Metzger LJ, Hoffman EA, Pack AI. Upper airway and soft tissue anatomy in normal subjects and patients with sleep-disordered breathing. Significance of the lateral pharyngeal walls. Am J Respir Crit Care Med. 1995;152(5 Pt 1):1673–89.

66. Shelton KE, Woodson H, Gay S, Suratt PM. Pharyngeal fat in obstructive sleep apnea. Am Rev Respir Dis. 1993;148(2):462–6.

67. Schwab RJ, Pasirstein M, Pierson R, Mackley A, Hachadoorian R, Arens R, et al. Identification of upper airway anatomic risk factors for obstructive sleep apnea with volumetric magnetic resonance imaging. Am J Respir Crit Care Med. 2003;168(5):522–30.

68. Gleadhill IC, Schwartz AR, Schubert N, Wise RA, Permutt S, Smith PL. Upper airway collapsibility in snorers and in patients with obstructive hypopnea and apnea. Am Rev Respir Dis. 1991;143(6):1300–3.

69. Traeger N, Schultz B, Pollock AN, Mason T, Marcus CL, Arens R. Polysomnographic values in children 2-9 years old: additional data and review of the literature. Pediatr Pulmonol. 2005;40(1):22–30.

70. Arens R, Marcus CL. Pathophysiology of upper airway obstruction: a developmental perspective. Sleep. 2004;27(5):997–1019.

71. Imayama I, Prasad B. Role of leptin in obstructive sleep apnea. Ann Am Thorac Soc. 2017;14(11):1607–21.

72. Deal CL, Tony M, Höybye C, Allen DB, Tauber M, Christiansen JS. GrowthHormone Research Society workshop summary: consensus guidelines for recombinant human growth hormone therapy in Prader-Willi syndrome. J Clin Endocrinol Metab. 2013;98(6):E1072–87.

73. Bakker B, Maneatis T, Lippe B. Sudden death in Prader-Willi syndrome: brief review of five additional cases. Concerning the article by U. Eiholzer et al.: deaths in children with Prader-Willi syndrome. A contribution to the debate about the safety of growth hormone treatment in children with PWS (Horm Res 2005;63:33-39). Horm Res. 2007;67. Switzerland:203–4.

74. Eiholzer U, Nordmann Y, L'Allemand D. Fatal outcome of sleep apnoea in PWS during the initial phase of growth hormone treatment. A case report. Horm Res. 2002;58(Suppl 3):24–6.

75. Grugni G, Livieri C, Corrias A, Sartorio A, Crinò A. Death during GH therapy in children with Prader-Willi syndrome: description of two new cases. J Endocrinol Investig. 2005;28(6):554–7.

76. Miller J, Silverstein J, Shuster J, Driscoll DJ, Wagner M. Short-term effects of growth hormone on sleep abnormalities in Prader-Willi syndrome. J Clin Endocrinol Metab. 2006;91(2):413–7.

77. Riedl S, Blümel P, Zwiauer K, Frisch H. Death in two female Prader-Willi syndrome patients during the early phase of growth hormone treatment. Acta Paediatr. 2005;94(7):974–7.

78. Van Vliet G, Deal CL, Crock PA, Robitaille Y, Oligny LL. Sudden death in growth hormone-treated children with Prader-Willi syndrome. J Pediatr. 2004;144(1):129–31.

79. Widger JA, Davey MJ, Nixon GM. Sleep studies in children on long-term non-invasive respiratory support. Sleep Breath. 2014;18(4):885–9.

80. Pauli RM, Scott CI, Wassman ER Jr, Gilbert EF, Leavitt LA, Ver Hoeve J, et al. Apnea and sudden unexpected death in infants with achondroplasia. J Pediatr. 1984;104(3):342–8.

81. Helbing WA, van der Blij JF, ten Houten R, Broere G, Oorthuys JW. Attacks of apnea in an infant with achondroplasia. Tijdschr Kindergeneeskd. 1991;59(3):81–5.

82. Loughlin GM, Wynne JW, Victorica BE. Sleep apnea as a possible cause of pulmonary hypertension in Down syndrome. J Pediatr. 1981;98(3):435–7.

83. Levine OR, Simpser M. Alveolar hypoventilation and cor pulmonale associated with chronic airway obstruction in infants with Down syndrome. Clin Pediatr (Phila). 1982;21(1):25–9.

84. Kasian GF, Duncan WJ, Tyrrell MJ, Oman-Ganes LA. Elective oro-tracheal intubation to diagnose sleep apnea syndrome in children with Down's syndrome and ventricular septal defect. Can J Cardiol. 1987;3(1):2–5.

85. Bloch K, Witztum A, Wieser HG, Schmid S, Russi E. Obstructive sleep apnea syndrome in a child with trisomy 21. Monatsschr Kinderheilkd. 1990;138(12):817–22.

86. Hultcrantz E, Svanholm H. Down syndrome and sleep apnea--a therapeutic challenge. Int J Pediatr Otorhinolaryngol. 1991;21(3):263–8.

87. Eipe N, Lai L, Doherty DR. Severe pulmonary hypertension and adenotonsillectomy in a child with Trisomy-21 and obstructive sleep apnea. Paediatr Anaesth. 2009;19. France:548–9.

88. Konstantinopoulou S, Tapia IE, Kim JY, Xanthopoulos MS, Radcliffe J, Cohen MS, et al. Relationship between obstructive sleep apnea cardiac complications and sleepiness in children with Down syndrome. Sleep Med. 2016;17:18–24.

89. Chan D, Li AM, Yam MC, Li CK, Fok TF. Hurler's syndrome with cor pulmonale secondary to obstructive sleep apnoea treated by continuous positive airway pressure. J Paediatr Child Health. 2003;39(7):558–9.

90. Kasapkara ÇS, Tümer L, Aslan AT, Hasanoğlu A, Ezgü FS, Küçükçongar A, et al. Home sleep study characteristics in patients with mucopolysaccharidosis. Sleep Breath. 2014;18(1):143–9.

91. Deschildre A, Martinot A, Fourier C, Nguyen-Quang JM, Hue V, Derambure P, et al. Effects of hypocaloric diet on respiratory manifestations in Willi-Prader syndrome. Arch Pediatr. 1995;2(11):1075–9.

92. Yildirim SV, Durmaz C, Pourbagher MA, Erkan AN. A case of achondroplasia with severe pulmonary hypertension due to obstructive sleep apnea. Eur Arch Otorhinolaryngol. 2006;263(8):775–7.

93. Dudoignon B, Amaddeo A, Frapin A, Thierry B, de Sanctis L, Arroyo JO, et al. Obstructive sleep apnea in Down syndrome: benefits of surgery and noninvasive respiratory support. Am J Med Genet A. 2017;173(8):2074–80.

94. Breslin J, Spanò G, Bootzin R, Anand P, Nadel L, Edgin J. Obstructive sleep apnea syndrome and cognition in down syndrome. Dev Med Child Neurol. 2014;56(7):657–64.

95. McConnell EJ, Hill EA, Celmiņa M, Kotoulas SC, Riha RL. Behavioural and emotional disturbances associated with sleep-disordered breathing symptomatology in children with Down's syndrome. J Intellect Disabil Res. 2020;

96. Joyce A, Elphick H, Farquhar M, Gringras P, Evans H, Bucks RS, et al. Obstructive sleep Apnoea contributes to executive function impairment in young children with Down syndrome. Behav Sleep Med. 2020;18(5):611–21.

97. Brooks LJ, Olsen MN, Bacevice AM, Beebe A, Konstantinopoulou S, Taylor HG. Relationship between sleep, sleep apnea, and neuropsychological function in children with Down syndrome. Sleep Breath. 2015;19(1):197–204.

98. Edgin JO, Tooley U, Demara B, Nyhuis C, Anand P, Spanò G. Sleep disturbance and expressive language development in preschool-age children with Down syndrome. Child Dev. 2015;86(6):1984–98.

99. Combs D, Edgin JO, Klewer S, Barber BJ, Morgan WJ, Hsu CH, et al. OSA and neurocognitive impairment in children with congenital heart disease. Chest. 2020;158(3):1208–17.

100. Murata E, Mohri I, Kato-Nishimura K, Iimura J, Ogawa M, Tachibana M, et al. Evaluation of behavioral change after adeno-tonsillectomy for obstructive sleep apnea in children with autism spectrum disorder. Res Dev Disabil. 2017;65:127–39.

101. Malow BA, McGrew SG, Harvey M, Henderson LM, Stone WL. Impact of treating sleep apnea in a child with autism spectrum disorder. Pediatr Neurol. 2006;34(4):325–8.

102. Perfect MM, Archbold K, Goodwin JL, Levine-Donnerstein D, Quan SF. Risk of behavioral and adaptive functioning difficulties in youth with previous and current sleep disordered breathing. Sleep. 2013;36(4):517–25b.

103. Churchill SS, Kieckhefer GM, Bjornson KF, Herting JR. Relationship between sleep disturbance and functional outcomes in daily life habits of children with Down syndrome. Sleep. 2015;38(1):61–71.

104. Choi EK, Jung E, Van Riper M, Lee YJ. Sleep problems in Korean children with Down syndrome and parental quality of life. J Intellect Disabil Res. 2019;63(11):1346–58.

105. Bergeron M, Duggins AL, Cohen AP, Leader BA, Ishman SL. The impact of persistent pediatric obstructive sleep apnea on the Quality of Life of Patients' families. Int J Pediatr Otorhinolaryngol. 2020;129:109723.

106. Koontz KL, Slifer KJ, Cataldo MD, Marcus CL. Improving pediatric compliance with positive airway pressure therapy: the impact of behavioral intervention. Sleep. 2003;26(8):1010–5.

107. Hsiao KH, Nixon GM. The effect of treatment of obstructive sleep apnea on quality of life in children with cerebral palsy. Res Dev Disabil. 2008;29(2):133–40.

108. Kosko JR, Derkay CS. Uvulopalatopharyngoplasty: treatment of obstructive sleep apnea in neurologically impaired pediatric patients. Int J Pediatr Otorhinolaryngol. 1995;32(3):241–6.

109. Sung V, Beebe DW, Vandyke R, Fenchel MC, Crimmins NA, Kirk S, et al. Does sleep duration predict metabolic risk in obese adolescents attending tertiary services? A cross-sectional study. Sleep. 2011;34(7):891–8.

110. Tauman R, Serpero LD, Capdevila OS, O'Brien LM, Goldbart AD, Kheirandish-Gozal L, et al. Adipokines in children with sleep disordered breathing. Sleep. 2007;30(4):443–9.

111. Redline S, Storfer-Isser A, Rosen CL, Johnson NL, Kirchner HL, Emancipator J, et al. Association between metabolic syndrome and sleep-disordered breathing in adolescents. Am J Respir Crit Care Med. 2007;176(4):401–8.

112. Kheirandish-Gozal L, Sans Capdevila O, Kheirandish E, Gozal D. Elevated serum aminotransferase levels in children at risk for obstructive sleep apnea. Chest. 2008;133(1):92–9.

113. Section on Pediatric Pulmonology SboOSASAAoP. Clinical practice guideline: diagnosis and management of childhood obstructive sleep apnea syndrome. Pediatrics. 2002;109(4):704–12.

114. Lee CH, Hsu WC, Ko JY, Yeh TH, Lin MT, Kang KT. Adenotonsillectomy for the treatment of obstructive sleep apnea in children with Prader-Willi syndrome: a meta-analysis. Otolaryngol Head Neck Surg. 2020;162(2):168–76.

115. Alves RS, Resende MB, Skomro RP, Souza FJ, Reed UC. Sleep and neuromuscular disorders in children. Sleep Med Rev. 2009;13(2):133–48.

116. Villa MP, Bernkopf E, Pagani J, Broia V, Montesano M, Ronchetti R. Randomized controlled study of an oral jaw-positioning appliance for the treatment of obstructive sleep apnea in children with malocclusion. Am J Respir Crit Care Med. 2002;165(1):123–7.

117. Carvalho FR, Lentini-Oliveira DA, Prado LB, Prado GF, Carvalho LB. Oral appliances and functional orthopaedic appliances for obstructive sleep apnoea in children. Cochrane Database Syst Rev. 2016;10(10):Cd005520.

118. Julliand S, Boulé M, Baujat G, Ramirez A, Couloigner V, Beydon N, et al. Lung function, diagnosis, and treatment of sleep-disordered breathing in children with achondroplasia. Am J Med Genet A. 2012;158a(8):1987–93.

119. Howard JJM, Sarber KM, Yu W, Smith DF, Tikhtman RO, Simakajornboon N, et al. Outcomes in children with down syndrome and mild obstructive sleep apnea treated non-surgically. Laryngoscope. 2020;130(7):1828–35.

120. Maris M, Verhulst S, Wojciechowski M, Van de Heyning P, Boudewyns A. Outcome of adenotonsillectomy in children with Down syndrome and obstructive sleep apnoea. Arch Dis Child. 2017;102(4):331–6.

121. da Rocha M, Ferraz RCM, Guo Chen V, Antonio Moreira G, Raimundo FR. Clinical variables determining the success of adenotonsillectomy in children with Down syndrome. Int J Pediatr Otorhinolaryngol. 2017;102:148–53.

122. Castro-Codesal ML, Dehaan K, Featherstone R, Bedi PK, Martinez Carrasco C, Katz SL, et al. Long-term non-invasive ventilation therapies in children: a scoping review. Sleep Med Rev. 2018;37:148–58.

123. Amin R, Al-Saleh S, Narang I. Domiciliary noninvasive positive airway pressure therapy in children. Pediatr Pulmonol. 2016;51(4):335–48.

124. Marcus CL, Rosen G, Ward SL, Halbower AC, Sterni L, Lutz J, et al. Adherence to and effectiveness of positive airway pressure therapy in children with obstructive sleep apnea. Pediatrics. 2006;117(3):e442–51.

125. Marcus CL, Beck SE, Traylor J, Cornaglia MA, Meltzer LJ, DiFeo N, et al. Randomized, double-blind clinical trial of two different modes of positive airway pressure therapy on adherence and efficacy in children. J Clin Sleep Med. 2012;8(1):37–42.

126. Nathan AM, Tang JP, Goh A, Teoh OH, Chay OM. Compliance with noninvasive home ventilation in children with obstructive sleep apnoea. Singap Med J. 2013;54(12):678–82.

127. Uong EC, Epperson M, Bathon SA, Jeffe DB. Adherence to nasal positive airway pressure therapy among school-aged children and adolescents with obstructive sleep apnea syndrome. Pediatrics. 2007;120(5):e1203–11.

128. Beebe DW, Byars KC. Adolescents with obstructive sleep apnea adhere poorly to positive airway pressure (PAP), but PAP users show improved attention and school performance. PLoS One. 2011;6(3):e16924.

129. Schmidt-Nowara WW. Continuous positive airway pressure for long-term treatment of sleep apnea. Am J Dis Child. 1984;138(1):82–4.

130. Marcus CL, Radcliffe J, Konstantinopoulou S, Beck SE, Cornaglia MA, Traylor J, et al. Effects of positive airway pressure therapy on neurobehavioral outcomes in children with obstructive sleep apnea. Am J Respir Crit Care Med. 2012;185(9):998–1003.

131. Massa F, Gonzalez S, Laverty A, Wallis C, Lane R. The use of nasal continuous positive airway pressure to treat obstructive sleep apnoea. Arch Dis Child. 2002;87(5):438–43.

132. Marcus CL, Ward SL, Mallory GB, Rosen CL, Beckerman RC, Weese-Mayer DE, et al. Use of nasal continuous positive airway pressure as treatment of childhood obstructive sleep apnea. J Pediatr. 1995;127(1):88–94.

133. Waters KA, Everett FM, Bruderer JW, Sullivan CE. Obstructive sleep apnea: the use of nasal CPAP in 80 children. Am J Respir Crit Care Med. 1995;152(2):780–5.

134. Guilleminault C, Nino-Murcia G, Heldt G, Baldwin R, Hutchinson D. Alternative treatment to tracheostomy in obstructive sleep apnea syndrome: nasal continuous positive airway pressure in young children. Pediatrics. 1986;78(5):797–802.

135. Castro-Codesal ML, Dehaan K, Bedi PK, Bendiak GN, Schmalz L, Katz SL, et al. Longitudinal changes in clinical characteristics and outcomes for children using long-term non-invasive ventilation. PLoS One. 2018;13(1):e0192111.

136. Lynch MK, Elliott LC, Avis KT, Schwebel DC, Goodin BR. Quality of life in youth with Obstructive Sleep Apnea Syndrome (OSAS) treated with Continuous Positive Airway Pressure (CPAP) therapy. Behav Sleep Med. 2019;17(3):238–45.

137. Parmar A, Baker A, Narang I. Positive airway pressure in pediatric obstructive sleep apnea. Paediatr Respir Rev. 2019;31:43–51.

138. Fedor KL. Noninvasive respiratory support in infants and children. Respir Care. 2017;62(6):699–717.

139. Boldrini R, Fasano L, Nava S. Noninvasive mechanical ventilation. Curr Opin Crit Care. 2012;18(1):48–53.

140. Mehta S, Hill NS. Noninvasive ventilation. Am J Respir Crit Care Med. 2001;163(2):540–77.

141. Non-invasive ventilation in acute respiratory failure. Thorax. 2002;57(3):192–211.

142. Ramirez A, Khirani S, Aloui S, Delord V, Borel JC, Pépin JL, et al. Continuous positive airway pressure and noninvasive ventilation adherence in children. Sleep Med. 2013;14(12):1290–4.

143. Simon SL, Duncan CL, Janicke DM, Wagner MH. Barriers to treatment of paediatric obstructive sleep apnoea: development of the adherence barriers to continuous positive airway pressure (CPAP) questionnaire. Sleep Med. 2012;13(2):172–7.

144. Sawyer AM, Gooneratne NS, Marcus CL, Ofer D, Richards KC, Weaver TE. A systematic review of CPAP adherence across age groups: clinical and empiric insights for developing CPAP adherence interventions. Sleep Med Rev. 2011;15(6):343–56.

145. Kribbs NB, Pack AI, Kline LR, Smith PL, Schwartz AR, Schubert NM, et al. Objective measurement of patterns of nasal CPAP use by patients with obstructive sleep apnea. Am Rev Respir Dis. 1993;147(4):887–95.

146. Reeves-Hoche MK, Meck R, Zwillich CW. Nasal CPAP: an objective evaluation of patient compliance. Am J Respir Crit Care Med. 1994;149(1):149–54.

147. Engleman HM, Martin SE, Douglas NJ. Compliance with CPAP therapy in patients with the sleep apnoea/hypopnoea syndrome. Thorax. 1994;49(3):263–6.

148. Watach AJ, Xanthopoulos MS, Afolabi-Brown O, Saconi B, Fox KA, Qiu M, et al. Positive airway pressure adherence in pediatric obstructive sleep apnea: a systematic scoping review. Sleep Med Rev. 2020;51:101273.

149. Bhattacharjee R, Benjafield A, Armisteas J, Cistulli P, Nunez C, Pepin J-L, et al. Adherence in children using positive airway pressure therapy: a big-data analysis. Lancet Digital Health. 2020;2(2):E94–E101.

150. Nixon GM, Mihai R, Verginis N, Davey MJ. Patterns of continuous positive airway pressure adherence during the first 3 months of treatment in children. J Pediatr. 2011;159(5):802–7.

151. Aloo P, Bhattacharjee R, Benjafield A, Armisteas J, Cistulli P, Nunez C, et al. Adherence in children using positive airway pressure therapy: a big-data analysis. Lancet Digital Health. 2020;2(2):E94–E101.

152. Iglowstein I, Jenni OG, Molinari L, Largo RH. Sleep duration from infancy to adolescence: reference values and generational trends. Pediatrics. 2003;111(2):302–7.

153. O'Donnell AR, Bjornson CL, Bohn SG, Kirk VG. Compliance rates in children using noninvasive continuous positive airway pressure. Sleep. 2006;29(5):651–8.

154. Kushida CA, Halbower AC, Kryger MH, Pelayo R, Assalone V, Cardell CY, et al. Evaluation of a new pediatric positive airway pressure mask. J Clin Sleep Med. 2014;10(9):979–84.

155. Castro-Codesal ML, Olmstead DL, MacLean JE. Mask interfaces for home non-invasive ventilation in infants and children. Paediatr Respir Rev. 2019;32:66–72.

156. Shikama M, Nakagami G, Noguchi H, Mori T, Sanada H. Development of personalized fitting device with 3-dimensional solution for prevention of NIV Oronasal mask-related pressure ulcers. Respir Care. 2018;63(8):1024–32.

157. Ramirez A, Delord V, Khirani S, Leroux K, Cassier S, Kadlub N, et al. Interfaces for long-term noninvasive positive pressure ventilation in children. Intensive Care Med. 2012;38(4):655–62.

158. Teague WG. Non-invasive positive pressure ventilation: current status in paediatric patients. Paediatr Respir Rev. 2005;6(1):52–60.

159. Kirk VG, O'Donnell AR. Continuous positive airway pressure for children: a discussion on how to maximize compliance. Sleep Med Rev. 2006;10(2):119–27.

160. King MS, Xanthopoulos MS, Marcus CL. Improving positive airway pressure adherence in children. Sleep Med Clin. 2014;9(2):219–34.

161. Delord V, Khirani S, Ramirez A, Joseph EL, Gambier C, Belson M, et al. Medical hypnosis as a tool to acclimatize children to noninvasive positive pressure ventilation: a pilot study. Chest. 2013;144(1):87–91.

162. DiFeo N, Meltzer LJ, Beck SE, Karamessinis LR, Cornaglia MA, Traylor J, et al. Predictors of positive airway pressure therapy adherence in children: a prospective study. J Clin Sleep Med. 2012;8(3):279–86.

163. Roberts SD, Kapadia H, Greenlee G, Chen ML. Midfacial and dental changes associated with nasal positive airway pressure in children with obstructive sleep apnea and craniofacial conditions. J Clin Sleep Med. 2016;12(4):469–75.

164. Li KK, Riley RW, Guilleminault C. An unreported risk in the use of home nasal continuous positive airway pressure and home nasal ventilation in children: mid-face hypoplasia. Chest. 2000;117(3):916–8.

165. Bergeron M, Duggins A, Chini B, Ishman SL. Clinical outcomes after shared decision-making tools with families of children with obstructive sleep apnea without tonsillar hypertrophy. Laryngoscope. 2019;129(11):2646–51.

166. Avis KT, Gamble KL, Schwebel DC. Effect of positive airway pressure therapy in children with obstructive sleep apnea syndrome: does positive airway pressure use reduce pedestrian injury risk? Sleep Health. 2019;5(2):161–5.

167. Puri P, Ross KR, Mehra R, Spilsbury JC, Li H, Levers-Landis CE, et al. Pediatric positive airway pressure adherence in obstructive sleep apnea enhanced by family member positive airway pressure usage. J Clin Sleep Med. 2016;12(7):959–63.

168. Hawkins SM, Jensen EL, Simon SL, Friedman NR. Correlates of pediatric CPAP adherence. J Clin Sleep Med. 2016;12(6):879–84.

169. Kang EK, Xanthopoulos MS, Kim JY, Arevalo C, Shults J, Beck SE, et al. Adherence to positive airway pressure for the treatment of obstructive sleep apnea in children with developmental disabilities. J Clin Sleep Med. 2019;15(6):915–21.

170. Prashad PS, Marcus CL, Maggs J, Stettler N, Cornaglia MA, Costa P, et al. Investigating reasons for CPAP adherence in adolescents: a qualitative approach. J Clin Sleep Med. 2013;9(12):1303–13.

171. Archbold KH, Parthasarathy S. Adherence to positive airway pressure therapy in adults and children. Curr Opin Pulm Med. 2009;15(6):585–90.

172. Alebraheem Z, Toulany A, Baker A, Christian J, Narang I. Facilitators and barriers to positive airway pressure adherence for adolescents. A qualitative study. Ann Am Thorac Soc. 2018;15(1):83–8.

173. Machaalani R, Evans CA, Waters KA. Objective adherence to positive airway pressure therapy in an Australian paediatric cohort. Sleep Breath. 2016;20(4):1327–36.

174. Katz SL, Kirk VG, MacLean JE, Bendiak GN, Harrison MA, Barrowman N, et al. Factors related to positive airway pressure therapy adherence in children with obesity and sleep-disordered breathing. J Clin Sleep Med. 2020;16(5):733–41.

175. Bhattacharjee R, Benjafield A, Armistead JP, Cistulli PA, Nunez C, Pepin, J-L, Woehrle H, et al., editors. Patient engagement technology in sleep apnea to optimize PAP adherence in children. American Thoracic Society 2020 International Conference; 2020.

176. Harford KL, Jambhekar S, Com G, Pruss K, Kabour M, Jones K, et al. Behaviorally based adherence program for pediatric patients treated with positive airway pressure. Clin Child Psychol Psychiatry. 2013;18(1):151–63.

177. Weaver TE, Grunstein RR. Adherence to continuous positive airway pressure therapy: the challenge to effective treatment. Proc Am Thorac Soc. 2008;5(2):173–8.

178. Mendoza-Ruiz A, Dylgjeri S, Bour F, Damagnez F, Leroux K, Khirani S. Evaluation of the efficacy of a dedicated table to improve CPAP adherence in children: a pilot study. Sleep Med. 2019;53:60–4.

179. Amaddeo A, Caldarelli V, Fernandez-Bolanos M, Moreau J, Ramirez A, Khirani S, et al. Polygraphic respiratory events during sleep in children treated with home continuous positive airway pressure: description and clinical consequences. Sleep Med. 2015;16(1):107–12.

180. Caldarelli V, Borel JC, Khirani S, Ramirez A, Cutrera R, Pépin JL, et al. Polygraphic respiratory events during sleep with noninvasive ventilation in children: description, prevalence, and clinical consequences. Intensive Care Med. 2013;39(4):739–46.

181. Jambhekar SK, Com G, Tang X, Pruss KK, Jackson R, Bower C, et al. Role of a respiratory therapist in improving adherence to positive airway pressure treatment in a pediatric sleep apnea clinic. Respir Care. 2013;58(12):2038–44.

182. Harford KL, Jambhekar S, Com G, Bylander L, Pruss K, Teagle J, et al. An in-patient model for positive airway pressure desensitization: a report of 2 pediatric cases. Respir Care. 2012;57(5):802–7.

183. Ennis J, Rohde K, Chaput JP, Buchholz A, Katz SL. Facilitators and barriers to noninvasive ventilation adherence in youth with nocturnal hypoventilation secondary to obesity or neuromuscular disease. J Clin Sleep Med. 2015;11(12):1409–16.

184. Amaddeo A, Frapin A, Touil S, Khirani S, Griffon L, Fauroux B. Outpatient initiation of long-term continuous positive airway pressure in children. Pediatr Pulmonol. 2018;53(10):1422–8.

185. Berry R, Brooks R, Garnaldo C, Hardig S, Lloyd R, Quan S, et al. The AASM manual for the scoring of sleep and associated events: rules, terminology and technical specifications; 2017.

186. Trucco F, Chatwin M, Semple T, Rosenthal M, Bush A, Tan HL. Sleep disordered breathing and ventilatory support in children with Down syndrome. Pediatr Pulmonol. 2018;53(10):1414–21.

187. Pascoe JE, Sawnani H, Hater B, Sketch M, Modi AC. Understanding adherence to noninvasive ventilation in youth with Duchenne muscular dystrophy. Pediatr Pulmonol. 2019;54(12):2035–43.

188. Riley EB, Fieldston ES, Xanthopoulos MS, Beck SE, Menello MK, Matthews E, et al. Financial analysis of an intensive pediatric continuous positive airway pressure program. Sleep. 2017;40(2)

189. Kahana S, Drotar D, Frazier T. Meta-analysis of psychological interventions to promote adherence to treatment in pediatric chronic health conditions. J Pediatr Psychol. 2008;33(6):590–611.

190. Graves MM, Roberts MC, Rapoff M, Boyer A. The efficacy of adherence interventions for chronically ill children: a meta-analytic review. J Pediatr Psychol. 2010;35(4):368–82.

191. Pai AL, McGrady M. Systematic review and meta-analysis of psychological interventions to promote treatment adherence in children, adolescents, and young adults with chronic illness. J Pediatr Psychol. 2014;39(8):918–31.

192. Rains JC. Treatment of obstructive sleep apnea in pediatric patients. Behavioral intervention for compliance with nasal continuous positive airway pressure. Clin Pediatr (Phila). 1995;34(10):535–41.

193. Perriol MP, Jullian-Desayes I, Joyeux-Faure M, Bailly S, Andrieux A, Ellaffi M, et al. Long-term adherence to ambulatory initiated continuous positive airway pressure in non-syndromic OSA children. Sleep Breath. 2019;23(2):575–8.

194. Jea M, editor. Personalized 3D-printed CPAP masks improve CPAP effectiveness in children with OSA and craniofacial anomalies. Combined otolaryngology spring meetings. Boston, MA; 2015.

195. (CHOP) CsHoP. Non-Invasive Ventilation for Infants and Children 2020. Available from: https://www.chop.edu/health-resources/non-invasive-ventilation-infants-and-children.

196. Mihai R, Vandeleur M, Pecoraro S, Davey MJ, Nixon GM. Autotitrating CPAP as a tool for CPAP initiation for children. J Clin Sleep Med. 2017;13(5):713–9.

197. Luijks KA, Vandenbussche NL, Pevernagie D, Overeem S, Pillen S. Adherence to continuous positive airway pressure in adults with an intellectual disability. Sleep Med. 2017;34:234–9.

Kin M. Yuen and Rafael Pelayo

While understanding PAP therapy is the "gold standard" for the treatment of obstructive sleep apnea, many patients find its use challenging. This chapter will explore possible contributing factors to PAP adherence and alternative or adjunctive treatment options.

27.1 Introduction

The "gold standard" treatment for obstructive sleep apnea is the use of positive airway pressure devices. In 1981 when Colin Sullivan and colleagues first published the successful use of this treatment in five patients, the clinical practice of sleep medicine was irrevocably changed [1]. Of note, they described the treatment as "comfortable," and none of their patients had "difficulty sleeping" with their new "vacuum-cleaner blower motor"-based device. The patients had an average apnea index of 62 events per hour in NREM sleep (not an apnea hypopnea index, which presumably would have been higher). In addition, none of the patients, which included a 13-year-old boy, needed pressures greater than 10 cm to resolve their obstruction. Despite this propitious beginning, concerns about patients' adherence to this form of therapy have been present ever since. Challenges range from patients rejecting PAP initiation, continuing its use, and discontinuing its use all together. This chapter will help summarize the current data regarding factors that influence the successful use of PAP devices, their level of efficacy, and strategies to increase adherence. We will review the literature

of PAP adherence while keeping in mind the limitations of arbitrary definitions when working with individual patients. In addition, since positive airway therapy is an evolving therapeutic modality with frequent improvements in mask design and pressure delivery systems, it is important to be cautious when applying the older literature to the current situation. If medical advances allow for PAP to be retired as a treatment for OSA, historians may look back at this current time as the golden era of PAP therapy.

27.2 Overview

Adherence to positive airwave pressure therapy has become a fundamental measurement of the success of the treatment of obstructive sleep apnea. Yet, the yardsticks used can be somewhat arbitrary. Adherence is not typically discussed nor mandated by insurance providers concerning other more expensive treatments for OSA. For example, measuring adherence does not apply to surgical interventions, though with the development of hypoglossal nerve stimulators it may be useful [2, 3]. With custom-fabricated oral appliances, there is no mandated demand for an arbitrary minimal amount of hours of use. Insurance companies have used adherence in factoring whether to pay for PAP treatment. Yet if a patient does not wear their prescription eye glasses, nobody from the optometrist offices knocks on their door to ask for the glasses back. Nor does somebody from the pharmacy refuse to refill medications because one skipped prior doses. Why is PAP, which is relatively inexpensive, compared to other OSA treatments, singled out this way? There are likely a confluence of historical reasons that are not entirely medical or evidence-based, and other technological and economic factors likely contribute [4]. For example, PAP devices can be refurbished and used by other patients, unlike the other common treatment options for OSA. This allows the devices to be reclaimed and reissued. Furthermore, unlike an automobile dealer, durable medical equipment vendors are not required to inform their patients they have

K. M. Yuen (✉)
UCSF Sleep Disorders Center, Department of UCSF Pulmonary, Critical Care, Allergy and Sleep Medicine, San Francisco, CA, USA

Stanford Sleep Disorders Clinic, Stanford University, Stanford, CA, USA
e-mail: kin.yuen@stanfordalumni.org

R. Pelayo
Stanford Sleep Disorders Clinic, Stanford University, Stanford, CA, USA

been sold a previously used CPAP device. Thus, the proper functioning of these preowned units may not be optimal.

Secondly, what does treatment success mean clinically? Certainly, for a clinician, there is value in monitoring and adjusting the therapy of patients with chronic condition to enhance his/her health. However, there is more than one way to think about whether the PAP treatment is successful. If one thinks about it from the patient's perspective, then the success of the treatment could be based on the resolution of the initially presented chief complaint. For example, if a patient says he/she is seeking medical attention because his/her snoring is disturbing the bed partner, then any measure of success would have to include elimination of the snoring. If the PAP data download shows a reduced apnea-hypopnea index, but that patient is still snoring, or the PAP's noise is still disturbing the bed partner, that patient is unlikely to be satisfied with the treatment and may in the end abandon PAP. Alternatively, if PAP is to eliminate the bed partner's complaints about snoring, then when the patient is sleeping alone, or during travel, he/she is less likely to use the PAP device. In this situation, despite the patient's data download might indicate poor adherence, the patient is fully satisfied that the PAP therapy has fully addressed the primary reason for seeking treatment.

Another way to think about the treatment adherence and ultimate success is not based on the chief complaint but on prevention of consequences of untreated obstructive sleep apnea. This is analogous to the treatment of hypertension. The patient may have little awareness that some new hypertension treatment has lowered the average blood pressure by 10 mm Hg unless measured. But this could have a positive impact on possible cardiovascular sequelae. A patient may tell you that they do not feel any different when they use PAP despite having excellent measured adherence data based on a PAP download. The motivation for that patient to continue to use the PAP treatment may be simply the peace of mind that treatment will lower the risk of OSA-related complications. This scenario is not uncommon for patients with recent cardioversion or ablation for atrial fibrillation. Some view the PAP as an insurance against arrhythmia recurrence without perceiving any other benefit. As long as patients remain in sinus rhythm, PAP treatment is a success regardless of device efficacy data.

In clinical practice, there may be more than one motivating factor for patient to use PAP and those factors may change with time, and with it how patients gauge the success of their treatment. Therefore, out of necessity, arbitrary definitions of PAP adherence success were created [5–7]. This allows for research methods and results to be more uniformly applied to various populations. The arbitrary nature of these definitions must be kept in mind when working with individual patients. For example, a common parameter for PAP adherence is using the device for at least 4 hours per night [8]. It would seem intrinsically self-evident that 4 hours on PAP for a patient that habitually sleeps only 5 and a half hours would be different from the same hours on PAP for a patient that habitually sleeps 9 hours. Yet if we apply the typical PAP adherence definitions, both patients would be viewed as being adherent.

In an older review, it was estimated that up to 15% of patients discontinue CPAP after their first-night trial but that patients receiving automated PAP devices had some small increase in usage as compared to fixed pressure PAP. In that study, the improvement in PAP use with the automated system was of unclear clinical significance [9]. A more recent review by the same group again found that automated PAP had higher nightly usage when measured at 12 and 16 weeks; both machine types reduce symptoms, but that the difference between them is unlikely to be clinically important. The studies measure relatively short-term results and may not predict long-term outcomes [10]. It is worth pointing out that even if automated PAP had the same usage as fixed pressure PAP, it would still result in a potential healthcare cost saving if the automated PAP decreased the need for sleep lab PAP titrations. Our surgical colleagues tell us that only about half the patients advised to use PAP will be adherent [11]. Yet the evidence in support of using PAP as treatment for OSA is strong as reviewed by the American Academy of Sleep Medicine [12, 13]. The evidence goes beyond the United States, and PAP is used throughout the world. An international study from Saudi Arabia reported that with support and education at follow-up, PAP was successfully used among 83% of their patients during the first 10 months of being started [14]. Problems with PAP adherence do exist, and there is much room for improvement. In one study, 46–55% of those diagnosed with OSA either refuse PAP therapy outright or do not adhere to treatment [15].

Traditionally, when discussing treatment of OSA with a patient, we may offer a range of choices such as PAP, surgery, and oral combined in an individual patient to optimize their sleep health. For properly selected patients, upper airway surgery may improve the subsequent PAP adherence. Surgical intervention may play a role even in patients who are unlikely to be fully cured of their OSA by surgery, which indicates that surgery may have an adjunctive role in the management of OSA.

To further understand the challenges patients face in the use of PAP devices, first we have to understand how patients are diagnosed, their level of psychological acceptance and barriers, their underlying anatomical morphology, other comorbid conditions and support system for PAP use, patients' symptomatology, and subsequent training and follow-up to increase efficacy and to provide feedback on PAP usage.

27.3   First Thing First: Testing

A Kaiser study published in 2018 found that their patients who presented with symptoms, such as daytime sleepiness (OR 0.86; 95% CI 0.82–0.91) and snoring/gasping/choking (OR 0.87; 95% CI 0.82–0.92), were more likely to follow through with sleep testing than those without. But, those with cognitive impairment (OR 0.74; 95% CI 0.67–0.82) and obesity (OR 0.89; 95% CI 0.85–0.93) were less likely to get tested. Patients who had visits to the emergency department (ED) during the 6-month baseline period were less likely to get tested than those without visits to the ED (OR 1.15; 95% CI 1.08–1.22). The medical specialty of provider influenced the results. Among the same set of Kaiser patients, if the ordering medical provider were pulmonologists (OR 0.72; 95% CI 0.68–0.76) or sleep specialists (OR 0.74; 95% CI 0.68–0.81), their patients were more likely to pursue testing compared to those whose tests were ordered by primary care providers [16]. How these results would apply to a different medical delivery system than Kaiser's is unclear.

27.4   Chief Complaint

When a patient first starts using CPAP, at the initial follow-up visit, it is important to have a conversation about what the patient is experiencing. At this visit, it is good to take a step back to discuss what the original reason the patients sought evaluation for their sleep in the first place was. As mentioned above, circling back to the original chief complaint will help both the patient and healthcare provider put in perspective the patient's experience with CPAP. This is especially helpful if the provider at the follow-up visit is different from the provider at the initial visit prior to starting CPAP. For example, if a patient first came in because of snoring, then it is important to know if the snoring has gone away completely.

If instead the patient came in originally with a complaint of insomnia, and their insomnia is persisting, then the CPAP may be viewed as a further hindrance to their sleep. If a patient is adapting well to CPAP, and enjoying their sleep, then continuing with CPAP is a straightforward process. However, some patients will struggle with the device at first. A good question to ask the patient at that first follow-up visit is: "what would help them continue?" Most patients will tell you that they want help to make the necessary adjustment to make the device more effective and comfortable.

However, some patients when asked will tell you that even if the device works, they do not want to use it. Even if a patient tells you the device is comfortable and effective, they will not use it. If they tell you they would rather remain symptomatic than use CPAP, then the clinic encounter must pivot to a discussion of alternative treatment modalities.

At this point in the encounter, it is worthwhile to let the patient know that even if they do not want to use CPAP at the current time, that CPAP technology has progressively improved over time and that OSA is a chronic condition that can worsen over time. Therefore, although you will review alternative treatment options, it is important that the patient stay open minded to perhaps using CPAP in the future. Most patients will agree to this contingency. At this point a discussion of alternative treatment modalities for that individual patient is also appropriate.

27.5   OSA Is Different Despite "Severity" Ranking

The definition of obstructive sleep apnea has evolved to include obstructive hypopneas and respiratory effort-related arousals, RERAs. Similarly, the severity criteria have been modified. Regardless, the severity is still dependent on the frequency of obstructive events. Often, patients with similar severity may have different composites of obstructive apneas relative to obstructive hypopneas and RERAs. Therefore, we rely on frequency and severity of hypoxemia as a further guideline: oxygen desaturation index. Clinically, a "severe" patient with an AHI of 30 events per hour of sleep that is comprised of more obstructive apneas, high degree of oxygen desaturations, and low oxygen nadirs is different from a patient who had predominantly obstructive hypopneas with little oxygen desaturations. Based on current clinical guidelines, both patients are offered automatic or continuous PAP as initial treatment. Purportedly, the efficacy of PAP use increases linearly with hours of use per night by patients. Use of PAP over 5 hours per night was reported to reduce subjective sleepiness [17]. Thus, clinicians generally encourage usage of PAP over 4–5 hours per night for their patients [18].

An international study that evaluated 24-month PAP adherence among moderate-to-severe OSA patients with cardiovascular diseases (SAVE trials) reported that early adherence at 1 month, fixed CPAP pressure, and loudness of snoring were independent predictors of subsequent continual use [19]. However, in this same SAVE trial, despite moderate-to-severe OSA (mean ODI of 28.3 per hour; SD 14.1), the study population had not reported significant daytime sleepiness before treatment (mean Epworth score was 7); they were older (mean age 61.34; SD 7.58) and overweight to obese (BMI 28.67; SD 4.46) and were predominantly male (81%) [20]. Of note, this was an open trial, and the average nightly usage was less than 4 hours per night; thus, these results can be viewed as an intention to treat study rather than a treatment efficacy study.

27.6 Automatic Mode

Not all patients tolerate the default settings with automatic PAP devices. Some patients with a strong hyperarousal response tolerate PAP better with a narrow range of pressure or "CPAP" mode during adaptation. The rise in pressure nocturnally contributes to the patient's awakenings. This can be reflected in an increased "central apnea" index as recorded in PAP devices.

27.7 Anatomical Challenges

Often patients with OSA complain of nasal congestion or blockage which predisposes them to oral breathing. Yet, the same patients who may have narrow or constricted nasal passages are offered devices that pipe in high-flow air through the same spaces that had resistance. Exacerbation of nasal congestion is not a surprising result. Medication and nasal sprays that were inadequate in controlling these symptoms to begin with are not likely to be helpful after initiating PAP therapy. Admittedly, heated humidification lessens the work of breathing in these areas. Anatomical blockages include deviated septum; sinus congestion may further reduce motivation to initiate and maintain PAP use {inoue, nasal function and CPAP compliance} [21]. Surgery may play a role in helping a patient increase PAP adherence [22, 23].

27.8 Special Population

There is limited literature regarding long-term PAP adherence for children or adolescents with developmental delays, craniofacial abnormalities, and social interaction challenges [24]. A recent report from France using outpatient PAP titration for 31 children whose median (range) age was 8.9 years (0.8–17.5), with Down syndrome ($n = 7$), achondroplasia ($n = 3$), and obesity ($n = 3$) [25]. They were followed for 12.3 months (median of 2.2 and range of 25.2). The median baseline obstructive apnea-hypopnea index (OAHI) was 12.5 events/h (range 5–100). Patients had follow-up visits 1 month after PAP initiation, then 2 months after, then every 3 months thereafter for those who remained on PAP therapy. Comparing the initial 2 months' PAP usage in 27 subjects, the median compliance was 08:21 h:min/night (05:45–12:20), and a median number of 25 was used out of 30 nights [17–30] during this follow-up visit. However, for the same time period, three adolescents with Down syndrome used PAP <4 hours per night after 2 months (a boy of 16.2 years and two girls of 16.6 and 10.2 years) [25]. The fourth subject was an 8-year-old girl with "an arteriovenous cervico-facial malformation." Psychosocial stressors were reported for these four subjects with "variable degrees of developmental delay and behavior problems." A promising consideration for CPAP non-adherent children with Down syndrome is hypoglossal nerve stimulator implant [26].

27.9 Symptomatology

Patients present to a sleep clinic with varying degree of daytime sleepiness, cognitive impairment, and discomfort. Those that present because others complain of their snoring exhibit varying degree of motivation for treatment. Some are not aware of any subjective daytime deficit and often lack comorbid conditions. If they are amenable for a trial of PAP, it is also unclear what types of improvement are expected since they were asymptomatic to begin with. Similarly, patients who are referred by their primary care providers, dentists, allergists, and cardiologists may be resistant to treatment if they have not felt any daytime function decrement.

27.10 Comorbid Conditions

In 2017, an Italian study reported that "adherence was positively associated with OSAS severity and negatively associated with cigarette smoking and previous cardiovascular events at baseline." The study extended over a median of 74.8 (24.2/110.9) months, and long-term compliance to treatment was present in less than half of the patients [27].

A French study that looked at those with cardiovascular disease compared to their peers found participants whose age <60 years and lower maximal positive airway pressure levels were less likely to be compliant with PAP after 3 years: age <60 years and diabetes were independent factors predicting low compliance [28]. Cardiovascular events were defined as myocardial infarction, stroke, coronary artery disease, and atrial fibrillation. Patients were followed with "short-term" evaluation at 5 months, and "long term" at 3 years. "There was no significant impact of the presence of CV disease on compliance at 5 months. There was no significant association between gender, mask types, 90th centile positive airway pressure level, apnea/hypopnea index and short- or long-term compliance in our population."

Among those with resistant hypertension, a Spanish study similarly reported that lower adherence at 1-month follow-up for PAP therapy decreased the likelihood of future use in a population with cardiovascular risks: poor adherence was the presence of previous stroke (hazard ratio 4.00, 95% confidence interval 1.92–8.31). Sufficient adherence at 1 month also predicted good adherence at the end of the follow-up (hazard ratio 14.4, 95% confidence interval 4.94–56). Both variables also predicted adherence at a threshold of 6 hours per night [29].

27.11 Psychological Acceptance

Psychological acceptance is a continuum. Studies have shown that the presentation of disease spectrum, how patients relate the given information to their specific circumstance, their social support structure, the availability of equipment, how instructions of the use and cleaning of PAP devices are delivered, and scheduled follow-up as well as the patients' time availability all affect the "outcome measures." The more labor-intensive programs with frequent telephone, virtual, or in-person follow-ups yield better adherence rates. However, the costs of such programs can be prohibitive to be generalizable to smaller institutions or independent sleep clinics.

The acceptance and support of family members or the absence of support is also important. For teens or young adults who may be subject to peer pressure and being social accepted by peers, the use of PAP device during sleep can lessen the appeal. Acknowledgement of a sleep disorder may also further alienate someone having daytime symptoms.

27.12 Socioeconomic Status

Accessibility of care yields another layer of challenge to those that rely on public transit to reach medical providers. The costs to travel, time off from work, and childcare responsibility may interfere with motivation to go to a PAP care follow-up or compliance check. The process of appealing for medical insurance coverage for office visits, medical sleep apnea testing, and subsequent treatment may be daunting and exhausting for some patients.

Depending on the supply chain for PAP equipment, in the United States, the reliability and timeliness of receiving PAP devices and correctly sized mask interface from durable medical equipment companies can be highly variable. While those with private medical insurance may have an entire spectrum of PAP machines, mask types, and climate-controlled hoses available, those with limited resources or governmental support may have a small selection.

27.13 Gender Differences

Post-menopausal women may see a steady rise in risk of OSA [30]. Onset of events may be confined to REM sleep. The use of PAP during other stages of sleep when there is no or only mild obstructive event may awaken them more often than usual. Despite exhalation relief, and improved sensitiv-

ity to air flow obstruction, the physical act of being connected to a long hose that is attached to a fixed machine presents challenges [31–33].

Women tend to present with symptoms of insomnia more than men. In some, the hyperarousal response is stronger [34]. Wearing the mask, regardless of improvements in its construction, is still disruptive to the sleep of women with hyperarousal responses.

27.14 Environmental Factors

Some patients worry that the air blows directly onto their bed partners while using PAP devices. Others may co-sleep with their children, grandchildren, or pets. Disapproval of wearing masks from their family or significant others, discomfort of the masks, air leaks from mask displacements, noise from the machine or air leaks, dry eyes from errant air flow, and patient's unconscious mask removal in sleep may further reduce the efficacy of PAP devices. Newer and lighter PAP mask designs have been introduced to divert the air away from the bed partner, and these also make less noise. These would be expected to improve adherence.

27.15 Patient Acceptance

Whether from claustrophobia or perception of being less appealing bed partner, physical discomfort of being entangled with the hose, difficulty during travel with their home devices, and recurring expenses of refurbishments of PAP supplies, patients express various objections to PAP use. Often education and setting expectations and prompt response to patients' concerns help reduce non-adherence. Nonetheless, there is a population with a low hyperarousal threshold for whom PAP therapy is not possible despite best efforts. Newer PAP mask designs have been introduced to be less confining and to lower claustrophobic feelings. There is also short and effective psychological treatments (exposure therapy and cognitive behavioral therapy) for claustrophobia; see Chap. 6. These measures are expected to improve adherence as well.

27.16 Education

By involving family members early, this will help build a supportive environment through the treatment phase. To properly gauge patients' expectations and explain possible problems along the way often will ease transition to more successful outcomes. If there is one or two dedicated staff members (rather than rotating staffs) in the clinic responsible to help patient navigate the paperwork to qualify for PAP use, coordinate transfer of report data and prescriptions, troubleshoot questions about PAP use, obtain masks and/or return PAP equipment, assist with PAP setting changes, obtain replacement parts including distilled water, and provide feedback data to medical insurances, then patients usually report a more positive experience.

27.17 What Is Acceptable Adherence Level?

Traditionally, obtaining a follow-up appointment in a sleep clinic could take at least 1 month. Often, this is scheduled as an appointment for "adherence check" or efficacy assessment. Clinicians may help change settings of PAP machines, comfort features, or mask types during these appointments. Patients may report any improvements, air leaks, aerophagia, or other experiences to the clinicians. An artificial benchmark of 70% usage of 4 or more hours with a low apnea-hypopnea index is considered an acceptable adherence rate [35–37]. While it may be important for medical insurance to decide whether to further financially support patients for the continual use of PAP devices, studies have shown that further monitoring and encouragement from clinicians is needed beyond the first 30 days. "Drop-out" after the initial 30 days has been reported to be significant [13].

While some patients achieve 100% compliance, others could have sporadic use. Yet others may present years later to inquire for alternatives or when new equipment or technology for treatment becomes available. Follow-up frequency is also highly variable. Medicare criteria in the United States require that patient visits their sleep providers annually in order to obtain prescriptions for CPAP supplies. Private medical insurances may have different requirements. Commercial operators often have a set requirement for work allowance. Independent sleep centers may have different schedules from academic or tertiary medical centers in availability for follow-up appointments as well. Often, the frequency of follow-up rests on the patients. Those that can afford to purchase the device out of pocket may not have any follow-up at all.

27.18 What Is Acceptable Apnea-Hypopnea Index?

With the latest automatic positive airway pressure devices, an AHI of below 5 is realistically achievable provided these are predominantly obstructive in nature. Small numbers of central apneas may co-occur due to sleep instability or arousals during PAP use. Often, an even lower AHI is possible. Ultimately, patient's perception of improvement of symptoms, reduction of comorbid conditions, and lessening of observed snoring and apneas in sleep by family would be determinant whether the patient would continue its use.

27.19 CPAP Versus Bilevel PAP

In a study published in BMJ in collaboration with ResMed Science Center, of the 1496 patients with non-compliant OSA subjects identified, "30.3% used CPAP, 62.3% APAP, and 7.4% both APAP and CPAP before switching to a bilevel mode; 47.8% patients switched to Spontaneous mode and 52.2% to VAuto mode. PAP usage significantly improved by 0.9 h/day ($p < 0.001$) and all other device metrics (residual apnea–hypopnea index and unintentional mask leak) also improved after the switch. No patients had achieved US CMS criteria for compliance before the switch, and 56.8% did after" [38].

Another study of obese Asian patients who required higher PAP pressures benefitted from the use of bilevel PAP (BPAP) therapy with higher adherence [39]. The mean was AHI: 51.1/hour; CPAP needs were >15 cm H_2O and were non-adherent to CPAP therapy. When changed to bilevel, 75.7% of the cohort showed nightly adherence of >4 hours per night versus 42.9% with CPAP.

An editorial comment stated that the patient cohort that benefitted had characteristics that would make them more likely candidates for BPAP use such as: "higher BMI, comorbid congestive heart failure, higher blood CO_2, greater OSA severity and lower oxygen nadirs." However, due to higher cost of BPAP machines, that BPAP should not be considered as first-line therapy over CPAP devices [40].

27.20 Adaptive Servo Ventilation (ASV)

For patients with central sleep apnea, either as treatment emergent or complex in origin, adaptive servo ventilation may be considered if their left ventricular ejection fractions are above 45% [41].

Central apnea affects about 0.9% of patients with congestive heart failure [42]. Loop gain mechanism delays contribute to the mismatch of ventilator drive and apneic events. Javaheri et al. reported the prevalence of patients who developed PAP treatment-emergent CSA was about 8% (range 3.5–19.8%) often resolving spontaneously in 4–5 weeks to 28 weeks [43]. However, about one third will have treatment-persistent CSA: "0.9%–3.2% of all patients treated with PAP therapy for OSA will exhibit treatment persistent CSA on a long-term basis. They represent 14.3%–46.2% of treatment emergent CSA patients, who continue to experience PAP therapy-related central sleep apnea over a protracted period" [43].

Patients that exhibit central sleep apnea index of >/−5 events per hour or Cheyne-Stokes breathing pattern during polysomnography may be considered candidates for bilevel PAP treatment or ASV if they do not respond well with CPAP therapy and correction of the underlying etiology. In a recent analysis, prevalence of treatment-emergent CSA was between 0.7% and 4.2% of patients undergoing PAP treatment after 1 month or longer. Those exhibiting treatment-emergent CSA that had a higher AHI and CAI at baseline, and a higher residual AHI at their titration study, may be associated with increased likelihood of conversion to treatment-persistent CSA in the long run. However, the authors reported a statistically significant increase in compliance and improvements in daytime sleepiness among those that were transitioned from CPAP to ASV in an Australian study [44].

Regardless of etiology for CSR, the AHI was reduced from baseline AHI of 52.0 ± 29.3 vs. CPAP use at 21.3 ± 14.8* and ASV use 9.7 ± 8.5 with ASV events per hour. Epworth values also decreased from ESS baseline values of 12.2 ± 6.2 to CPAP use of 9.6 ± 5.6 and ASV use of 7.9 ± 4.6. Length of ASV use varied from 28 [16–56] days. Usage per night increased from CPAP time of 4.8 ± 2.4 to ASV time of 5.4 ± 2.2 hours [44].

Whether to change a patient with treatment-emergent or treatment-persistent central sleep apnea will depend on the patient's daytime symptoms and underlying cause. If there is persistent daytime sleepiness, elevated AHI/CAI, and hypoxemia, it is worth consideration to switch to a trial with an ASV device.

27.21   When to Refer to Dental/Oral Appliance?

Dental or oral appliances (OA) are indicated for mild-to-moderate cases of OSA as per AASM guidelines [46]. For those patients who either would not use or unable to use PAP devices, one study reported compliance rates of 83% of oral appliance usage over 4 hours per night 70% of the time in 1 year [47]. A prospective study of 21 subjects with compliance monitoring showed that the mean usage time was 5.49 hours/night, with nightly compliance (defined as >4 hours per night for 70% the nights per week) at 33%. Furthermore, compliance increased from 26% to 50% from week 1 to week 4 [48].

Patients that have some degree of bruxism but no acute temporomandibular joint pain and can increase the size of their oral airway by protruding their tongues/mandible forward may be potential candidates for mandibular advancement devices (MAD) custom manufactured by our dental colleagues. A thorough examination is recommended to exclude anatomical protrusions such as torus/tori palatini,

mandibulari, gum diseases, or TMJ abnormalities [46]. Tori will make physically fitting of dental appliances onto the gums or hard palate difficult. Exiting gingivitis or receding gums may need the mouth to be closed for proper healing or risk loss of dentition. Qualification and experience of the dental provider in manufacturing such devices also factor into the success of these patients. In some cases, expertise in TMJ pain is needed for determined patients that have ongoing issues but wish to proceed with this form of treatment. Frequency of follow-up and titration studies are best addressed elsewhere.

27.22   When to Refer to Surgery?

Despite positive airway pressure being the gold standard or first-line treatment for obstructive sleep apnea, it is important to remember that the first effective treatment for OSA was surgery. Tracheostomy was the standard until it was supplanted by CPAP. Thankfully, we no longer need to rely on tracheostomy for the vast majority of OSA patients. But just as CPAP has improved over time, so have our surgical options. CPAP technology and surgical technique improvements have perhaps spurred each other on to the benefit of our patients. It is beyond the scope of this text to review the surgical advances of OSA and excellent reviews are available [24, 45]. We will briefly discuss the role of hypoglossal nerve stimulators since PAP non-adherence is a prerequisite to their application.

When patients are unable or unwilling to continue PAP therapy, and when there are anatomical challenges to breathing, surgical intervention may be considered. A review of all the current surgical techniques is beyond the scope of this chapter [45] (Verse and de Vries, Current Concepts of Sleep Apnea Surgery (ISBN 978-3-13-240119-8), Some of the common approaches include nasal turbinate reduction, nasal valve repair, upper airway radiofrequency reduction, tonsillectomy, and uvulopalatopharyngoplasty (UPPP) as part of upper airway surgery (UAS) [23].

Surgery typically does not "cure" OSA altogether. If there is reduction of OSA by 50% with an overall AHI below 20, or the elimination of the need for CPAP, then it is considered successful. The aforementioned meta-analysis of 10/11 studies suggested UAS reduced the need to use CPAP. However, due to the heterogeneous site procedure, ranging from single UAS to multiple levels, it was difficult to report conclusively the individual procedure's success rate.

Two newer techniques worth mentioning include distraction osteogenesis maxillary expansion (DOME) or endoscopically-assisted surgical expansion (EASE) performed by different surgeons in the San Francisco Bay Area. The basis of each is to help expand the width of the maxilla [49–53].

Anatomical corrections to improve nasal congestion will improve daytime function as well as tolerance of PAP use nocturnally. Those patients that have consistently maximized nasal irrigations; inhaled nasal steroid sprays [45], nasal antihistamine sprays, or daily use oral montelukast to help control rhinitis; and continued to exhibit nasal congestion are likely candidates for an evaluation by an otolaryngologist. Furthermore, those that experience recurrent sinusitis and nasal polyps despite optimum medical treatment can similarly benefit from ENT consultation. Some patients are more risk averse compared to others. Some patients do not have adequate recovery time available after a surgical procedure to ensure complete recovery. Some patients may not have the social support to monitor eating needs for 2–4 weeks postoperatively. The ability to have a reliable transport to appointments for follow-up can also be a source of concern.

27.23 Bariatric Surgery

For patients that have been unsuccessful with PAP therapy, are not candidates for UAS, and have comorbid conditions such as morbid obesity (BMI $\geq$ 40 kg/m^2) or cardiovascular risk factors such as type 2 diabetes and hypertension, then bariatric surgery may be indicated [54].

The National Institutes of Health consensus in 1991 that detailed guideline requires that patients should have attempted to lose weight by "nonoperative means, including self-directed dieting, nutritional counseling, and commercial and hospital-based weight loss programs [55]." Additionally, there not ought to be any psychological diseases [55]. Although the surgical literature is mixed in whether preoperative weight loss helps post-operative weight loss, medical insurances often mandate pre-op weight loss before approval for bariatric surgery [56].The most commonly performed techniques include Roux-en-Y and sleeve gastrectomy. Of those undergoing bariatric surgery, mean excess weight loss was around 70% with the target BMI as 25 kg/m^2. Apnea-hypopnea index reduced from 66 to 25/hour in the severe OSA group, from 21 to 9/hour in the moderate OSA group, and from 10 to 5/hour in the mild OSA group. At least 75% of moderately severe OSA patients achieve AHI levels below 15/hour after surgery [57–59].

27.24 Surgery

27.24.1 The Road to Inspire…

A newer intervention is the use of a pacemaker-type device being implanted into the right side of the chest; one of its electrodes is attached to the hypoglossal nerve on the right to stimulate the genioglossus muscle activity, and the other electrode to intercostal area to synchronize with breathing during sleep.

What is known as the STAR (Stimulation Therapy for Apnea Reduction) trial reported reduction of AH, in 126 OSA patients with CPAP intolerance, from 29.3 to 9.0 events an hour at the end of 1 year. Sixty-six percent of subjects achieved a reduction of at least 50% and an AHI of less than 20 events an hour. The AHI reduction was accompanied by improvements in daytime sleepiness and functional outcomes of sleep. The rate of serious adverse events was less than 2 percent. Furthermore, "90% of bed partners reported soft or no snoring for their partner, as compared to only 17% of bed partners at baseline" [60].

The Inspire website indicates that patients who may qualify include those that have "moderate to severe obstructive sleep apnea (AHI 15-65), are unable to use or get consistent benefit from CPAP, are not significantly obese, are age 22 or above" (https://www.inspiresleep.com/am-i-eligible/) [61–64].

Higher success rates were found with a body mass index (BMI) generally <35 kg·m^{-2} and an absence of complete concentric collapse at the level of the velopharynx during drug-induced sleep endoscopy (DISE) examination [65, 66]. Exclusion of neuromuscular disease, hypoglossal nerve palsy, severe cardiopulmonary disease, active psychiatric disease, grade 3–4 tonsils, and anterior-posterior predominant retropalatal collapse on drug-induced sleep endoscopy was recommended to increase success and to lower risk of complications.

27.25 Conclusion

Finally, despite the many challenges a patient may face from the initiation presentation to following through with sleep testing, then beginning the journey with PAP therapy, many succeed with improved quality of life and lessened daytime symptoms and snoring.

References

1. Sullivan CE, Issa FG, Berthon-Jones M, Eves L. Reversal of obstructive sleep apnoea by continuous positive airway pressure applied through the nares. Lancet. 1981;1(8225):862–5.
2. Eisele DW, Smith PL, Alam DS, Schwartz AR. Direct hypoglossal nerve stimulation in obstructive sleep apnea. Arch Otolaryngol Head Neck Surg. 1997;123(1):57–61.
3. Eastwood PR, Barnes M, Walsh JH, Maddison KJ, Hee G, Schwartz AR, et al. Treating obstructive sleep apnea with hypoglossal nerve stimulation. Sleep. 2011;34(11):1479–86.
4. Loube DI. Technologic advances in the treatment of obstructive sleep apnea syndrome. Chest. 1999;116(5):1426–33.
5. Sanders MH, Gruendl CA, Rogers RM. Patient compliance with nasal CPAP therapy for sleep apnea. Chest. 1986;90(3):330–3.

6. Krieger J. Long-term compliance with nasal continuous positive airway pressure (CPAP) in obstructive sleep apnea patients and nonapneic snorers. Sleep. 1992;15(6 Suppl):S42–6.

7. Rauscher H, Formanek D, Popp W, Zwick H. Self-reported vs measured compliance with nasal CPAP for obstructive sleep apnea. Chest. 1993;103(6):1675–80.

8. Wickwire EM, Jobe SL, Oldstone LM, Scharf SM, Johnson AM, Albrecht JS. Lower socioeconomic status and co-morbid conditions are associated with reduced CPAP adherence use among older adult medicare beneficiaries with obstructive sleep apnea. Sleep. 2020;43(12):zsaa122.

9. Smith I, Lasserson TJ. Pressure modification for improving usage of continuous positive airway pressure machines in adults with obstructive sleep apnoea. Cochrane Database Syst Rev. 2009;(4):CD003531.

10. Kennedy B, Lasserson TJ, Wozniak DR, Smith I. Pressure modification or humidification for improving usage of continuous positive airway pressure machines in adults with obstructive sleep apnoea. Cochrane Database Syst Rev. 2019;12:CD003531.

11. Russell JO, Gales J, Bae C, Kominsky A. Referral patterns and positive airway pressure adherence upon diagnosis of obstructive sleep apnea. Otolaryngol Head Neck Surg. 2015;153(5):881–7.

12. Patil SP, Ayappa IA, Caples SM, Kimoff RJ, Patel SR, Harrod CG. Treatment of adult obstructive sleep apnea with positive airway pressure: an American Academy of Sleep Medicine systematic review, meta-analysis, and GRADE assessment. J Clin Sleep Med. 2019;15(2):301–34.

13. Patil SP, Ayappa IA, Caples SM, Kimoff RJ, Patel SR, Harrod CG. Treatment of adult obstructive sleep apnea with positive airway pressure: an American Academy of Sleep Medicine clinical practice guideline. J Clin Sleep Med. 2019;15(2):335–43.

14. BaHammam AS, Alassiri SS, Al-Adab AH, Alsadhan IM, Altheyab AM, Alrayes AH, et al. Long-term compliance with continuous positive airway pressure in Saudi patients with obstructive sleep apnea. A prospective cohort study. Saudi Med J. 2015;36(8):911–9.

15. Furukawa T, Suzuki M, Ochiai M, Kawashima H, Yokoyama N, Isshiki T. Long-term adherence to nasal continuous positive airway pressure therapy by hypertensive patients with preexisting sleep apnea. J Cardiol. 2014;63(4):281–5.

16. Gordon A, Wu SJ, Munns N, DeVries A, Power T. Untreated sleep apnea: an analysis of administrative data to identify risk factors for early nonadherence. J Clin Sleep Med. 2018;14(8):1303–13.

17. Antic NA, Catcheside P, Buchan C, Hensley M, Naughton MT, Rowland S, et al. The effect of CPAP in normalizing daytime sleepiness, quality of life, and neurocognitive function in patients with moderate to severe OSA. Sleep. 2011;34(1):111–9.

18. He J, Kryger MH, Zorick FJ, Conway W, Roth T. Mortality and apnea index in obstructive sleep apnea. Experience in 385 male patients. Chest. 1988;94(1):9–14.

19. Van Ryswyk E, Anderson CS, Antic NA, Barbe F, Bittencourt L, Freed R, et al. Predictors of long-term adherence to continuous positive airway pressure in patients with obstructive sleep apnea and cardiovascular disease. Sleep. 2019;42(10):zsz152.

20. McEvoy RD, Antic NA, Heeley E, Luo Y, Ou Q, Zhang X, et al. CPAP for prevention of cardiovascular events in obstructive sleep apnea. N Engl J Med. 2016;375(10):919–31.

21. Inoue A, Chiba S, Matsuura K, Osafune H, Capasso R, Wada K. Nasal function and CPAP compliance. Auris Nasus Larynx. 2019;46(4):548–58. https://doi.org/10.1016/j.anl.2018.11.006. Epub 2018 Dec 8. PMID: 30538069.

22. Wong JK, Rodriguez EM, Wee-Tom B, Lejano M, Kushida CA, Howard SK, et al. A multidisciplinary perioperative intervention to improve positive airway pressure adherence in patients with obstructive sleep apnea: a case series. A A Pract. 2020;14(4):119–22.

23. Ayers CM, Lohia S, Nguyen SA, Gillespie MB. The effect of upper airway surgery on continuous positive airway pressure levels and adherence: a systematic review and meta-analysis. ORL J Otorhinolaryngol Relat Spec. 2016;78(3):119–25.

24. Liu SY, Awad M, Riley R, Capasso R. The role of the revised Stanford protocol in today's precision medicine. Sleep Med Clin. 2019;14(1):99–107.

25. Amaddeo A, Frapin A, Touil S, Khirani S, Griffon L, Fauroux B. Outpatient initiation of long-term continuous positive airway pressure in children. Pediatr Pulmonol. 2018;53(10):1422–8. https://doi.org/10.1002/ppul.24138. Epub 2018 Aug 1. PMID: 30070059.

26. Caloway CL, Diercks GR, Keamy D, de Guzman V, Soose R, Raol N, et al. Update on hypoglossal nerve stimulation in children with down syndrome and obstructive sleep apnea. Laryngoscope. 2020;130(4):E263–E7.

27. Baratta F, Pastori D, Bucci T, Fabiani M, Fabiani V, Brunori M, et al. Long-term prediction of adherence to continuous positive air pressure therapy for the treatment of moderate/severe obstructive sleep apnea syndrome. Sleep Med. 2018;43:66–70.

28. Nsair A, Hupin D, Chomette S, Barthelemy JC, Roche F. Factors influencing adherence to auto-CPAP: an observational monocentric study comparing patients with and without cardiovascular diseases. Front Neurol. 2019;10:801.

29. Campos-Rodriguez F, Navarro-Soriano C, Reyes-Nunez N, Torres G, Caballero-Eraso C, Lloberes P, et al. Good long-term adherence to continuous positive airway pressure therapy in patients with resistant hypertension and sleep apnea. J Sleep Res. 2019;28(5):e12805.

30. Heinzer R, Marti-Soler H, Marques-Vidal P, Tobback N, Andries D, Waeber G, et al. Impact of sex and menopausal status on the prevalence, clinical presentation, and comorbidities of sleep-disordered breathing. Sleep Med. 2018;51:29–36.

31. Polo-Kantola P, Rauhala E, Helenius H, Erkkola R, Irjala K, Polo O. Breathing during sleep in menopause: a randomized, controlled, crossover trial with estrogen therapy. Obstet Gynecol. 2003;102(1):68–75.

32. Eichling PS, Sahni J. Menopause related sleep disorders. J Clin Sleep Med. 2005;1(3):291–300.

33. Mirer AG, Young T, Palta M, Benca RM, Rasmuson A, Peppard PE. Sleep-disordered breathing and the menopausal transition among participants in the Sleep in Midlife Women Study. Menopause. 2017;24(2):157–62.

34. Baker FC, Lampio L, Saaresranta T, Polo-Kantola P. Sleep and sleep disorders in the menopausal transition. Sleep Med Clin. 2018;13(3):443–56.

35. Chhatre S, Chang YHA, Gooneratne NS, Kuna S, Strollo P, Jayadevappa R. Association between adherence to continuous positive airway pressure treatment and cost among medicare enrollees. Sleep. 2020;43(1):zsz188.

36. Naik S, Al-Halawani M, Kreinin I, Kryger M. Centers for Medicare and Medicaid Services positive airway pressure adherence criteria may limit treatment to many Medicare beneficiaries. J Clin Sleep Med. 2019;15(2):245–51.

37. Aloia MS, Knoepke CE, Lee-Chiong T. The new local coverage determination criteria for adherence to positive airway pressure treatment: testing the limits? Chest. 2010;138(4):875–9.

38. Benjafield AV, Pepin JL, Valentine K, Cistulli PA, Woehrle H, Nunez CM, et al. Compliance after switching from CPAP to bilevel for patients with non-compliant OSA: big data analysis. BMJ Open Respir Res. 2019;6(1):e000380.

39. Ishak A, Ramsay M, Hart N, Steier J. BPAP is an effective second-line therapy for obese patients with OSA failing regular CPAP: a prospective observational cohort study. Respirology. 2020;25(4):443–8.

40. Omobomi O, Quan SF. BPAP for CPAP failures: for the many or the few. Respirology. 2020;25(4):358–9.

41. Piccini JP, Pokorney SD, Anstrom KJ, Oldenburg O, Punjabi NM, Fiuzat M, et al. Adaptive servo-ventilation reduces atrial fibrillation burden in patients with heart failure and sleep apnea. Heart Rhythm. 2019;16(1):91–7.

42. Donovan LM, Kapur VK. Prevalence and characteristics of central compared to obstructive sleep apnea: analyses from the sleep heart health study cohort. Sleep. 2016;39(7):1353–9.

43. Nigam G, Riaz M, Chang ET, Camacho M. Natural history of treatment-emergent central sleep apnea on positive airway pressure: a systematic review. Ann Thorac Med. 2018;13(2):86–91.

44. Huseini T, McArdle N, Jasper E, Kurmagadda S, Douglas J, King S, et al. The use and effectiveness of adaptive servo ventilation in central sleep apnea: a study of consecutive sleep clinic patients. J Sleep Res. 2020; 29:e13016.

45. Awad M, Capasso R. Skeletal surgery for obstructive sleep apnea. Otolaryngol Clin N Am. 2020;53(3):459–68.

46. Ramar K, Dort LC, Katz SG, Lettieri CJ, Harrod CG, Thomas SM, et al. Clinical practice guideline for the treatment of obstructive sleep apnea and snoring with oral appliance therapy: an update for 2015. J Clin Sleep Med. 2015;11(7):773–827.

47. Dieltjens M, Braem MJ, Vroegop A, Wouters K, Verbraecken JA, De Backer WA, et al. Objectively measured vs self-reported compliance during oral appliance therapy for sleep-disordered breathing. Chest. 2013;144(5):1495–502.

48. Mullane S, Loke W. Influence of short-term side effects on oral sleep appliance compliance among CPAP-intolerant patients: an objective monitoring of compliance. J Oral Rehabil. 2019;46(8):715–22.

49. Li KK, Powell NB, Riley RW, Guilleminault C. Distraction osteogenesis in adult obstructive sleep apnea surgery: a preliminary report. J Oral Maxillofac Surg. 2002;60(1):6–10.

50. Abdelwahab M, Yoon A, Okland T, Poomkonsarn S, Gouveia C, Liu SY. Impact of distraction osteogenesis maxillary expansion on the internal nasal valve in obstructive sleep apnea. Otolaryngol Head Neck Surg. 2019;161(2):362–7.

51. Iwasaki T, Yoon A, Guilleminault C, Yamasaki Y, Liu SY. How does distraction osteogenesis maxillary expansion (DOME) reduce severity of obstructive sleep apnea? Sleep Breath. 2020;24(1):287–96.

52. Yoon A, Guilleminault C, Zaghi S, Liu SY. Distraction Osteogenesis Maxillary Expansion (DOME) for adult obstructive sleep apnea patients with narrow maxilla and nasal floor. Sleep Med. 2020;65:172–6.

53. Li K, Quo S, Guilleminault C. Endoscopically-assisted surgical expansion (EASE) for the treatment of obstructive sleep apnea. Sleep Med. 2019;60:53–9.

54. Noshiro H, Tanaka M. Evaluating obesity before surgery. Ann Surg. 2005;241(2):383.

55. NIH conference. Gastrointestinal surgery for severe obesity. Consensus Development Conference Panel. Ann Intern Med. 1991;115(12):956–61. PMID: 1952493.

56. Tewksbury C, Williams NN, Dumon KR, Sarwer DB. Preoperative medical weight management in bariatric surgery: a review and reconsideration. Obes Surg. 2017;27(1):208–14.

57. de Raaff CAL, Gorter-Stam MAW, de Vries N, Sinha AC, Jaap Bonjer H, Chung F, et al. Perioperative management of obstructive sleep apnea in bariatric surgery: a consensus guideline. Surg Obes Relat Dis. 2017;13(7):1095–109.

58. de Raaff CAL, de Vries N, van Wagensveld BA. Obstructive sleep apnea and bariatric surgical guidelines: summary and update. Curr Opin Anaesthesiol. 2018;31(1):104–9.

59. Verse T, de Vries N. Current concepts of sleep apnea surgery. Stuttgart/New York: Thieme; 2019. xvi, 287 p.

60. Strollo PJ Jr, Soose RJ, Maurer JT, de Vries N, Cornelius J, Froymovich O, et al. Upper-airway stimulation for obstructive sleep apnea. N Engl J Med. 2014;370(2):139–49.

61. Dedhia RC, Woodson BT. Standardized reporting for hypoglossal nerve stimulation outcomes. J Clin Sleep Med. 2018;14(11):1835–6.

62. Woodson BT, Strohl KP, Soose RJ, Gillespie MB, Maurer JT, de Vries N, et al. Upper airway stimulation for obstructive sleep apnea: 5-year outcomes. Otolaryngol Head Neck Surg. 2018;159(1):194–202.

63. Boon M, Huntley C, Steffen A, Maurer JT, Sommer JU, Schwab R, et al. Upper airway stimulation for obstructive sleep apnea: results from the ADHERE registry. Otolaryngol Head Neck Surg. 2018;159(2):379–85.

64. Thaler E, Schwab R, Maurer J, Soose R, Larsen C, Stevens S, et al. Results of the ADHERE upper airway stimulation registry and predictors of therapy efficacy. Laryngoscope. 2020;130(5):1333–8.

65. Heiser C, Hofauer B. Predictive success factors in selective upper airway stimulation. ORL J Otorhinolaryngol Relat Spec. 2017;79(1–2):121–8.

66. Steffen A, Sommer JU, Hofauer B, Maurer JT, Hasselbacher K, Heiser C. Outcome after one year of upper airway stimulation for obstructive sleep apnea in a multicenter German post-market study. Laryngoscope. 2018;128(2):509–15.

Questionnaires Evaluating Sleep Apnea and CPAP Adherence

28

Sohaib Ahmed Shamim

28.1 IF SLEEPY

The IF SLEEPY questionnaire is used to screen for obstructive sleep apnea in children. There is a parents'/guardian's version and a child version of the questionnaire, both having the same set of questions.

The parents'/guardian's version is shown in the (Fig. 28.1).

The questionnaire includes some of the most common features of sleep apnea in children, i.e., enlarged tonsils and/or adenoids, and the most commonly experienced symptoms of obstructive sleep apnea such as breathing difficulties, hyperactivity, irritability, and excessive daytime sleepiness. A score of 3 out of 8 indicates a 70% risk of having obstructive sleep apnea and the risk increases by 5% for every increase in score.

During the validation study, a total of 150 children referred to a children's sleep clinic and their parents completed the IF SLEEPY questionnaire and had a sleep study [1]. The sensitivity was 78% for the parents' version and 45% for the child's version [1]. The IF SLEEPY, although not widely used, is a simple and sensitive screening tool for detecting obstructive sleep apnea in children [1] and performs better than most alternatives (Fig. 28.1).

28.2 STOP BANG

The STOP BANG questionnaire screens for obstructive sleep apnea in adults. It is being widely used at sleep clinics, CPAP clinics, and hospitals to screen for obstructive sleep apnea. STOP BANG is particularly useful in ruling out the anesthetic risk for patients before the surgery [2] (Fig. 28.2).

The questionnaire focuses on the main symptoms of obstructive sleep apnea such as snoring, breathing pauses, and excessive daytime sleepiness and also includes some of the common risk factors including hypertension, obesity, neck circumference, and male sex. The validation process involved surgical patients with a mean age of 57 ± 16 [2]. When only the first four items of STOP BANG are used, a total of two or more indicates significant risk for obstructive sleep apnea [2, 3]. When using the complete 8-item STOP BANG, a score of 3 out of 8 indicates a 70% risk of having obstructive sleep apnea and the risk increases by 5% for every increase in score. STOP BANG has both excellent sensitivity and specificity of more than 90% in screening patients with moderate-to-severe obstructive sleep apnea [2]. STOP BANG has less validity in some clinical populations for sleep apnea screening, including individuals with glaucoma [4]. To date there are over 450 citations relating to STOP BANG.

28.3 Epworth Sleepiness Scale (ESS)

ESS is an eight-item self-assessing questionnaire that evaluates the degree of subjective daytime sleepiness [5]. In the original validation study ESS scores were noted to be on par with the readings recorded during the multiple sleep latency test (MSLT) [5]. ESS scores also correlate with the apnea-hypopnea index (AHI) and improvement in ESS scores correlates with CPAP adherence [5, 6]. However, when evaluated in traumatic brain injury (TBI) population, the ESS failed to provide a strong correlation with the readings on the MSLT [7]. Further studies are needed to test its relevance in the TBI population.

The questionnaire assesses how likely a person is to "fall asleep" in eight different situations as opposed to feeling "just tired." The total score ranges from 0 to 24 with higher scores indicating more significant daytime sleepiness as compared to lower scores [5]. A score of 10 and above is considered significant for daytime sleepiness.

S. A. Shamim (✉)
Dow Medical College, Karachi, Pakistan

Youthdale Child and Adolescent Sleep Centre,
Toronto, ON, Canada
e-mail: Sohaib@youthdalesleepcenter.ca

© The Author(s), under exclusive license to Springer Nature Switzerland AG 2022
C. M. Shapiro et al. (eds.), *CPAP Adherence*, https://doi.org/10.1007/978-3-030-93146-9_28

Fig. 28.1 The IFSLEEPY/
IMSLEEPY are two versions
of the same questionnaire. In
older children, the
IMSLEEPY is more
appropriate, so the M [body
mass index] replaces the F
[fidget] [1]. In younger
children, the IFSLEEPY is
more appropriate, so the F
[fidget] replaces the M [body
mass index] Copyright ©
Kadmon et al. [1] Reprinted
with permission

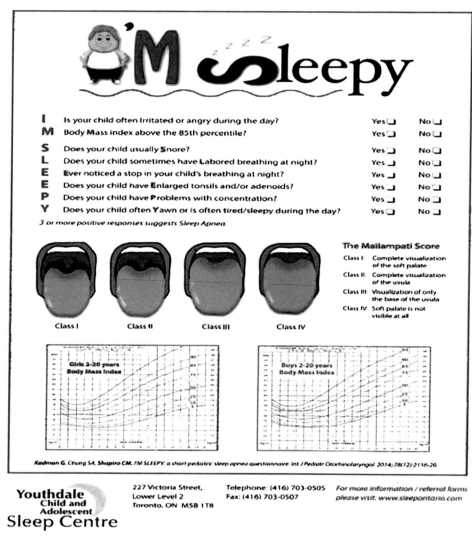

The ESS has vast utility in clinical medicine and research. The ESS has been used to assess daytime sleepiness in diverse age groups, occupations, and health conditions including military personnel [8], children and adolescents [9], commercial drivers [10], and patients with Down syndrome [11]. Choi et al. (2006) showed that a higher score on the ESS in sleep apnea patients was independently associated with impaired cardiac function [12]. The eight questions of ESS are shown in the Table 28.1.

28.4   Fatigue Severity Scale (FSS)

FSS is a nine-item self-administered questionnaire that measures tiredness or fatigue in contrast to excessive daytime sleepiness. The scale was developed and validated by Krupp et al. in 1989 [13]. The process involved completion of the FSS by 25 patients with multiple sclerosis (MS), 29 patients with systemic lupus erythematosus (SLE), and 20 healthy adults [13]. The results showed that FSS was reliable and accurate in differentiating healthy adults from patients with MS and SLE [13]. The scores of FSS in patients with SLE and MS were substantially higher (usually > 4) than healthy adults, indicating that it can be used to detect fatigue in patients with comorbid conditions [13]. The questionnaire evaluates fatigue by assessing the impact of fatigue on daily life activities such as exercise, sustained physical functioning, social life, and work life. It is particularly useful in differentiating excessive daytime sleepiness as measured by ESS from fatigue in people who describe themselves as "sleepy and tired." Learmonth et al. (2013) used FSS in their study and established that FSS has adequate reliability to assess fatigue in patients with multiple sclerosis for a 6-month period [14]. FSS has also been used in the evalua-

Fig. 28.2 The STOP BANG questionnaire screens for obstructive sleep apnea in adults. A score of 3 out of 8 indicates a 70% risk of having obstructive sleep apnea and the risk increases by 5% for every increase in score

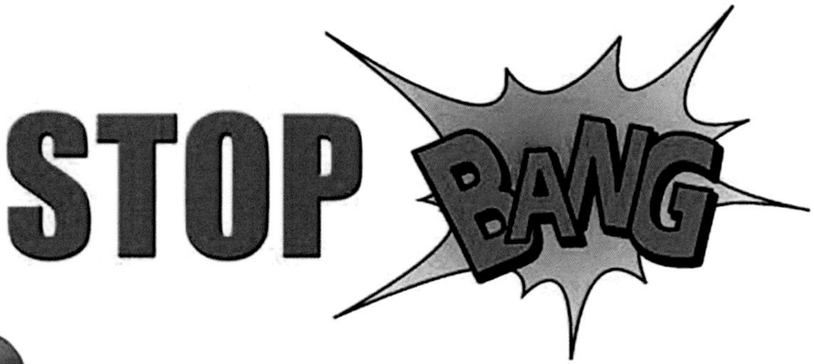

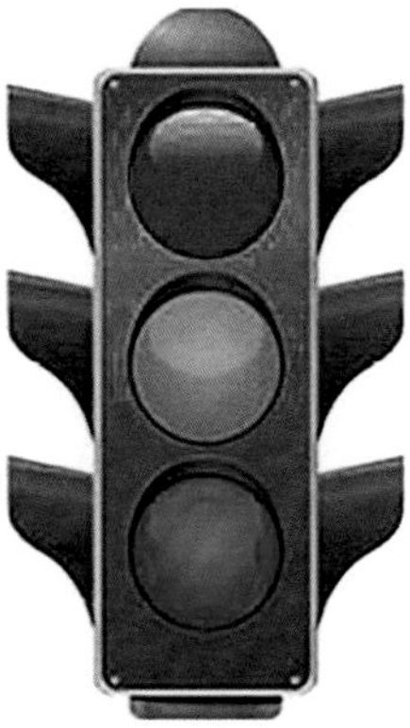

Do you **S**nore?   Yes ☐   No ☐

Do you feel **T**ired, fatigued or sleepy during the day?   Yes ☐   No ☐

Has anyone **O**bserved you stop breathing in your sleep?   Yes ☐   No ☐

Do you have high blood **P**ressure?   Yes ☐   No ☐

Please count the number of "Yes" responses and put the number in this box ☐
There is a good chance that you have Sleep Apnea if you have two 'yes' responses out of four.

My neck size is   _____cms_____inches

My height is   _____cms_____inches

My weight is   _____kgs_____lbs

B	**A**	**N**	**G**
BMI > 35	Age > 50	Neck Size > 40cm > 15.7"	Gender - Male

If height is in ft & weight in lbs is >	4'11" 167	5'0" 179	5'2" 191	5'4" 204	5'6" 216	5'8" 230	5'10" 250	6'0" 258	6'2" 272	
If height is m & weight in kgs is >	1.47 75	1.52 81	1.58 86	1.63 92	1.68 97	1.73 104	1.78 113	1.83 116	1.88 122	1.93 129

Then BMI is > 35

If you count positive responses in STOP and BANG and three out of eight factors are applicable then you should have a sleep assessment.

tion of fatigue in patients with other comorbid conditions such as cirrhosis [15], myasthenia gravis [16], and lung disease [17]. Fatigue presented a strong correlation with depressive symptomatology and quality of life. The complete FSS questionnaire is shown in the Table 28.2.

Table 28.1 The Epworth sleepiness scale (ESS)

Situation	Chance of dozing			
Sitting and reading	0	1	2	3
Watching TV	0	1	2	3
Sitting inactive in a public place (e.g., theater or a meeting)	0	1	2	3
As a passenger in a car for an hour without a break	0	1	2	3
Lying down to rest in the afternoon when circumstances permit	0	1	2	3
Sitting and talking to someone	0	1	2	3
Sitting quietly after a lunch without alcohol	0	1	2	3
In a car, while stopped for a few minutes in the traffic	0	1	2	3

Copyright © Murray Johns. Reprinted with permission from Murray Johns
0 = would *never* doze, 1 = *slight* chance of dozing, 2 = *moderate* chance of dozing, 3 = *high* chance of dozing

Table 28.2 Fatigue severity scale (FSS)

During the past week, I have found that:	Completely disagree		Neither agree nor disagree		Completely agree		
1. My motivation is lower when I am fatigued	1	2 3	4	5 6	7		
2. Exercise brings on my fatigue	1	2 3	4	5 6	7		
3. I am easily fatigued	1	2 3	4	5 6	7		
4. Fatigue interferes with my physical functioning	1	2 3	4	5 6	7		
5. Fatigue causes frequent problems for me	1	2 3	4	5 6	7		
6. My fatigue prevents sustained physical functioning	1	2 3	4	5 6	7		
7. Fatigue interferes with carrying out certain duties and responsibilities	1	2 3	4	5 6	7		
8. Fatigue is among my three most disabling symptoms	1	2 3	4	5 6	7		
9. Fatigue interferes with my work, family, or social life	1	2 3	4	5 6	7		

Copyright © Krupp et al. [13]. Reprinted with permission

28.5 Toronto Hospital Alertness Test (THAT)

THAT is a ten-item self-administered questionnaire that helps to measure alertness over the past 1 week [18]. The questionnaire uses a 6-point Likert type scale and assesses for psychological features of alertness, including the ability to feel alert, refreshed, energetic, concentrate, think of new ideas, and focus on the task at hand [18]. A score of <20 indicates poor subjective alertness and higher numbers indicate greater levels of alertness [18]. Shapiro et al. showed that THAT has an internal consistency of 0.96 and a test-retest reliability of 0.82 [19] (Table 28.3).

The clinical utility of THAT has been shown in different studies. Moller et al. (2006) used the THAT questionnaire and evaluated variances in subjective states of alertness and sleep-

Table 28.3 Toronto Hospital Alertness Test (THAT)

During the last week I felt:	Not at all	Less than ¼ of the time	¼ to ½ of the time	½ to ¾ of the time	More than ¾ of the time	All the time I was awake
	0	1	2	3	4	5
1. Able to concentrate						
2. Alert						
3. Fresh						
4. Energetic						
5. Able to think of new ideas						
6. Vision was clear noting all details (e.g., driving)						
7. Able to focus on the task at hand						
8. Mental facilities were operating at peak level						
9. Extra effort was needed to maintain alertness						
10. In a boring situation, I would find my mind wandering						

Reprinted from Shapiro et al. [19]. Copyright 2006, with permission from Elsevier

iness in patients with different sleep disorders and showed that alertness is more the opposite of fatigue than is sleepiness [20]. Shapiro et al. (2017) used THAT questionnaire and identified that different levels of alertness exist for self-described anxious and non-anxious individuals [21]. The Chinese version of THAT has been validated as well [22].

28.6 Adherence Barriers to CPAP Questionnaire (ABCQ)

The ABCQ is a unique questionnaire that illustrates the causes of CPAP noncompliance in children and adolescents in contrast to adults [23]. It is a lengthy questionnaire (31 items scored on a 5-point Likert scale) and has both child's/ youth's and parents' version that assesses a wide variety of barriers to CPAP adherence [23]. It was validated by Simon et al. (2012) [24]. The questionnaire was administered to a sample of 51 youth (age 8–17 years) at their regular appointments and compared with the usage data downloaded from the CPAP machine in a 90-day period of CPAP use [24]. The ABCQ scores had sufficient accuracy and the higher numbers of "barriers" on the questionnaire were associated with poorer compliance [24].

According to Simon et al. (2012), overall, three biggest reasons for CPAP non-adherence were:

1. Does not use when away from home
2. Child not feeling well
3. Just want to forget about obstructive sleep apnea (children in particular had more prominent psychological barriers about CPAP treatment with 43% of them scoring positive on this item) [24]

The ABCQ can be used as an effective screening questionnaire to recognize patient-specific reasons for CPAP non-adherence in children and adolescents diagnosed with obstructive sleep apnea [24]. Carmody et al. (2020) also studied the ABCQ on a sample of 181 children and determined that the ABCQ has robust psychometric properties and can be used to assess and predict non-adherence in pediatric population [25]. The full questionnaire is not reproduced but some of the items of the parents' version [24] include:

1. The CPAP makes my child's nose stuffed up (congested).
2. My child forgets to use their CPAP.
3. My child is embarrassed that they have to use their CPAP.
4. I don't understand why my child has to use their CPAP.
5. The CPAP makes my child feel sick (e.g., headache, dry mouth, stomachache).
6. My child is worried their friends will find out about their sleep apnea.

7. My child just wants to forget about their sleep apnea.
8. My child can stay healthy without using their CPAP.

28.7 Self-Efficacy Measure for Sleep Apnea (SEMSA)

The SEMSA is a 26-item self-administered questionnaire that assesses three elements: perceived risk of obstructive sleep apnea, advantages and outcome expectancy of CPAP use, and self-efficacy (the trust to take part in CPAP use) [26, 27]. Weaver et al. (2003) determined that SEMSA has an internal consistency of 0.92 and test-retest reliability between 0.68 and 0.77 [26, 28].

The questionnaire uses a 4-point Likert scale to assess patients' agreement with items in regard to perceived risks of obstructive sleep apnea, outcome expectancy of CPAP use, and self-efficacy of using CPAP [28]. Higher scores are consistent with better risk awareness, better treatment expectancy, and improved confidence to use CPAP [26, 27]. The SEMSA can be utilized to assess health awareness about obstructive sleep apnea and CPAP to improve CPAP adherence [26, 27]. The questionnaire has been cited in another Springer book *STOP, THAT and One Hundred Other Sleep Scales*, published in 2012 [28]. The French and Chinese versions of the SEMSA have been validated as well [27, 29]. The complete questionnaire could not be reproduced here but a few questions of the SEMSA are shown below.

Self-Efficacy Measure for Sleep Apnea (SEMSA)

My chances of having high blood pressure compared to people my own age and sex who do not have sleep apnea are:

Very low	Low	High	Very high

My chances of falling asleep while driving compared to people my own age and sex who do not have sleep apnea are:

Very low	Low	High	Very high

If I use CPAP, then I will not snore.

Not at all true	Barely true	Somewhat true	Very true

If I do not use CPAP, I will be less alert during the day.

Not at all true	Barely true	Somewhat true	Very true

I would use CPAP, even if I have to wear a tight mask on my face at night.

Not at all true   Barely true   Somewhat true   Very true

I would use CPAP, even if it made my nose stuffy.

Not at all true   Barely true   Somewhat true   Very true

Copyright © Terri Weaver et al. [26, 28]. Reprinted with permission

28.8 Index for Non-adherence to Positive Airway Pressure (I-NAP)

The I-Nap is a 19-item screening questionnaire that helps to measure the CPAP non-adherence risk prospectively among patients diagnosed with obstructive sleep apnea [30]. This detailed questionnaire includes a combination of other questionnaires and information such as Health Literacy Screening (HLS) questionnaire, Social Cognitive Theory Questionnaire in obstructive sleep apnea (SCT), the SEMSA, body mass index (BMI), marital status, and presenting complaints [30] to address the different risk factors that affect CPAP compliance. The questionnaire assesses risk factors such as risk awareness, daytime functioning, health literacy, and outcome expectancy to CPAP treatment [30]. Sawyer et al. (2014) conducted a study that tested I-NAP in patients newly diagnosed with obstructive sleep apnea (after CPAP titration study) and determined that I-NAP successfully identifies patients at risk of non-compliance at 1 month after CPAP initiation [30]. A cutoff point of > −4.8 for I-NAP gives a sensitivity (87%), specificity (63%), positive predictive value (60%), and negative predictive value (88%) for detecting non-adherers to CPAP (<4 hours of CPAP use) [30]. The questionnaire helps detect non-compliant patients early during CPAP treatment and can be used to plan and implement strategies to improve CPAP adherence [30]. However, there is a scarcity of the use of this questionnaire in other studies, and further validation in a more heterogeneous sample is needed to prove the clinical efficacy of I-NAP [30].

The questionnaire is shown in the Table 28.4.

28.9 CPAP Perception Questionnaire

The CPAP Perception Questionnaire is a six-item questionnaire that predicts CPAP adherence 1 month after CPAP initiation when administered in the morning after a CPAP

Table 28.4 INAP items and subscales [30]

Item or subscale	Format and number of items included	Source
Self-Efficacy Measure for Sleep Apnea (SEMSA) – outcome expectancies subscale	4-point Likert scale; 9 items	Available with permission from the author[a]
Social Cognitive Theory Questionnaire in sleep apnea – self-efficacy subscale	5-point Likert scale; 5 items	Publicly available[b]
Health Literacy Questionnaire How often do you have problems learning about your medical condition because of difficulty understanding written information?	5-point Likert scale; 1 item	Publicly available[c]
BMI	1 item	–
Marital status Married Not married		
Presenting symptoms for seeking care at sleep center Restless sleep Snoring Breathing stops in sleep Sleepiness during day Other		–
Gender Male Female		–

Copyright © Sawyer et al. [30]. Reprinted with permission
[a]Weaver et al. [26]
[b]Stepnowsky et al. [34]
[c]Chew et al. [35]

titration sleep study [31]. The complete questionnaire is shown below:

1. *How much difficulty did you have tolerating CPAP?*

No difficulty   Some difficulty   Great difficulty

1   2   3   4   5   6   7   8   9   10

2. *How uncomfortable was the mask?*

Not comfortable   Somewhat comfortable   Very comfortable

1   2   3   4   5   6   7   8   9   10

3. *How uncomfortable was the CPAP pressure?*

Not comfortable   Somewhat comfortable   Very comfortable

1   2   3   4   5   6   7   8   9   10

4. *What is the likelihood of you wearing the equipment at night almost every night?*

Very likely   Likely   Highly unlikely

1   2   3   4   5   6   7   8   9   10

5. *How beneficial do you think CPAP is going to be for your health and sleep?*

Very beneficial   Somewhat beneficial   Not beneficial

1   2   3   4   5   6   7   8   9   10

6. *What is your attitude toward CPAP therapy?*

Greatly like CPAP   Somewhat like CPAP   Intensely dislike CPAP

1   2   3   4   5   6   7   8   9   10

The retrospective study done by Balachandran et al. (2013) included 403 patients who completed the CPAP perception questionnaire after the overnight CPAP titration study and had nightly reports (downloaded from the machine) for the first 30 days of CPAP use [31].

Balachandran et al. (2013) determined that four out of six questions (questions 1, 3, 4, and 5) were better at predicting CPAP adherence post-30 days than the other two questions [31]. The questions were scored on a 10-point Likert-type scale. A score of 16 and higher was associated with difficulty tolerating CPAP and higher rates of non-adherence ($p < 0.001$) [31].

The questionnaire is unique in that it is very short, validated in a study that includes a substantial number of women and members of the African American population (groups that are often underrepresented in other CPAP adherence studies) [31]. It accurately predicts CPAP adherence after 1 month of CPAP use [31]. This makes it a very useful and handy tool to screen for patients who likely will have difficulties with adhering to CPAP treatment at the very beginning and to organize strategies to improve CPAP adherence in these patients [31]. However, this questionnaire has not been put into test in other studies and further studies are required to establish its clinical utility.

28.10 Motivation to Use CPAP Scale (MUC-S)

The MUC-S is a brief questionnaire with strong psychometric properties that assesses the behavioral aspects of motivation to use CPAP [32]. It is the first tool in its category that measures perceived motivation in patients who are prescribed CPAP [32]. The questionnaire has a total of nine items; the first six items are under the category of "Autonomous motivation" – regarding self-motivating reasons to use CPAP such as improvement in apnea, alertness, and overall health [32]. The next three items are grouped

under "Controlled motivation" which screens for people who would want to use CPAP not due to their personal preference but rather due to other people's concerns such as spouse or personnel [32]. The score ranges from 9 to 45 and elevated scores are associated with higher motivating force to use CPAP [32].

Broström et al. (2020) included 193 newly diagnosed patients with obstructive sleep apnea in their validation study [32]. The Cronbach's alpha values of 0.88 and 0.86 for both autonomous and controlled motivation factors indicated good internal consistency of the MUC-S [32]. The study indicates that physicians can utilize the MUC-S as a psychometric tool to assess motivation to use CPAP and improvement with CPAP treatment. However, further studies are needed to prove its clinical utility (Table 28.5).

28.11 Attitudes to CPAP Treatment Inventory (ACTI)

The attitudes to CPAP treatment inventory (ACTI) is a five-item self-administered scale developed and validated by Broström et al. (2011) that assesses the beliefs and attitudes to CPAP treatment [33]. The questions assess five different types of attitudes to CPAP treatment (analyzed on a 5-point Likert scale) – regarding the beliefs about the effectiveness of CPAP for problems caused by sleep apnea, improvement in overall health, improvement in quality of life, perception of CPAP as being the best treatment, and patient self-expectation of using CPAP [33] (Table 28.6). The ACTI was made by conducting detailed interviews with 23 patients, analyzing relevant research literature, and consensus of a multidisciplinary team [33]. The ACTI has been used in the validation study for the Motivation to Use CPAP Scale (MUC-S) described above.

The total sample size used in the validation process was 289 although the complete data was available for only 142 participants after 6 months [33]. The cutoff of 10 showed a high sensitivity (93%) but comparatively lower specificity (44%) at detecting CPAP use at 2 weeks and non-adherence after 6 months [33]. Unfortunately, there have not been other studies validating the clinical use of this questionnaire and further research is necessary.

CPAP adherence remains a challenge despite the recent advancements in screening and treatment strategies. From our evaluation of different questionnaires that predict CPAP adherence, we conclude that there are a variety of reasons contributing to non-adherence including behavioral factors, psychological factors, perceived health risk, outcome expectancy, and subjective factors such as degree of sleepiness, health literacy, and marital status. Sleep clinics, CPAP vendors, and clinicians who work with patients with sleep apnea can use these screening questionnaires for early identifica-

Table 28.5 The MUC-S questionnaire

Items	Response alternatives				
1. I use the CPAP treatment because it makes me feel good	Strongly agree 5	Agree 4	Undecided 3	Disagree 2	Strongly disagree 1
2. I use the CPAP treatment because it makes me feel good	Strongly agree 5	Agree 4	Undecided 3	Disagree 2	Strongly disagree 1
3. I use the CPAP treatment because I want to feel more alert	Strongly agree 5	Agree 4	Undecided 3	Disagree 2	Strongly disagree 1
4. I use the CPAP treatment because it feels important to use the CPAP	Strongly agree 5	Agree 4	Undecided 3	Disagree 2	Strongly disagree 1
5. I use the CPAP treatment because my health is important to me	Strongly agree 5	Agree 4	Undecided 3	Disagree 2	Strongly disagree 1
6. I use the CPAP treatment because it feels good to use CPAP	Strongly agree 5	Agree 4	Undecided 3	Disagree 2	Strongly disagree 1
7. I use the CPAP treatment because other people say I have to	Strongly agree 5	Agree 4	Undecided 3	Disagree 2	Strongly disagree 1
8. I use the CPAP treatment because the personnel say I have to	Strongly agree 5	Agree 4	Undecided 3	Disagree 2	Strongly disagree 1
9. I use the CPAP treatment because I have to	Strongly agree 5	Agree 4	Undecided 3	Disagree 2	Strongly disagree 1

Copyright © Broström et al. [32]. Reprinted with permission

Table 28.6 A description of the attitudes to CPAP treatment inventory (ACTI)

1. The CPAP treatment reduces the problems caused by my sleep apnea	Strongly agree 1	Agree 2	Undecided 3	Disagree 4	Strongly disagree 5
2. The CPAP treatment improves my health	Strongly agree 1	Agree 2	Undecided 3	Disagree 4	Strongly disagree 5
3. The CPAP treatment improves my quality of life	Strongly agree 1	Agree 2	Undecided 3	Disagree 4	Strongly disagree 5
4. The CPAP treatment is the best treatment for my sleep apnea	Strongly agree 1	Agree 2	Undecided 3	Disagree 4	Strongly disagree 5
5. I can use the CPAP as expected of me	Strongly agree 1	Agree 2	Undecided 3	Disagree 4	Strongly disagree 5

Copyright © Broström et al. [33]. Reprinted with permission

tion of patients who will have difficulties with adhering to a CPAP treatment plan. It opens the opportunity to strategically devise targeted strategies to help patients with CPAP adherence.

References

1. Kadmon G, Chung SA, Shapiro CM. I'M SLEEPY: a short pediatric sleep apnea questionnaire. Int J Pediatr Otorhinolaryngol. 2014;78(12):2116–20. https://doi.org/10.1016/j.ijporl.2014.09.018. Epub 2014 Oct 8. PMID: 25305064.
2. Shahid A, et al. STOP-Bang questionnaire. In: Shahid A, et al., editors. STOP, THAT and one hundred other sleep scales. New York: Springer; 2012. https://doi.org/10.1007/978-1-4419-9893-4_92.
3. Chung F, Yegneswaran B, Liao P, Chung SA, Vairavanathan S, Islam S, Khajehdehi A, Shapiro CM. STOP questionnaire: a tool to screen patients for obstructive sleep apnea. Anesthesiology. 2008;108(5):812–21. https://doi.org/10.1097/ALN.0b013e31816d83e4. PMID: 18431116.
4. Cabrera M, Benavides AM, Hallaji NAE, Chung SA, Shapiro CM, Trope GE, Buys YM. Risk of obstructive sleep apnea in open-angle glaucoma versus controls using the STOP-Bang questionnaire. Can J Ophthalmol. 2018;53(1):76–80. https://doi.org/10.1016/j.jcjo.2017.07.008. Epub 2017 Sept 27. PMID: 29426446.
5. Johns MW. A new method for measuring daytime sleepiness: the Epworth sleepiness scale. Sleep. 1991;14(6):540–5. https://doi.org/10.1093/sleep/14.6.540. PMID: 1798888.
6. Salepci B, Caglayan B, Kiral N, Parmaksiz ET, Comert SS, Sarac G, Fidan A, Gungor GA. CPAP adherence of patients with obstructive sleep apnea. Respir Care. 2013;58(9):1467–73. https://doi.org/10.4187/respcare.02139. Epub 2013 Feb 19. PMID: 23431305.
7. Mollayeva T, Kendzerska T, Colantonio A. Self-report instruments for assessing sleep dysfunction in an adult traumatic brain injury population: a systematic review. Sleep Med Rev. 2013;17(6):411–23. https://doi.org/10.1016/j.smrv.2013.02.001. Epub 2013 May 23. PMID: 23706309.

8. Hurlston A, Foster SN, Creamer J, Brock MS, Matsangas P, Moore BA, Mysliwiec V. The Epworth sleepiness scale in service members with sleep disorders. Mil Med. 2019;184(11–12):e701–7. https://doi.org/10.1093/milmed/usz066. PMID: 30951176.

9. Janssen KC, Phillipson S, O'Connor J, Johns MW. Validation of the Epworth sleepiness scale for children and adolescents using Rasch analysis. Sleep Med. 2017;33:30–5. https://doi.org/10.1016/j.sleep.2017.01.014. Epub 2017 Feb 12. PMID: 28449902.

10. Baiardi S, La Morgia C, Sciamanna L, Gerosa A, Cirignotta F, Mondini S. Is the Epworth sleepiness scale a useful tool for screening excessive daytime sleepiness in commercial drivers? Accid Anal Prev. 2018;110:187–9. https://doi.org/10.1016/j.aap.2017.10.008. Epub 2017 Nov 1. PMID: 29074223.

11. Hill EA, Fairley DM, McConnell E, Morrison I, Celmina M, Kotoulas SC, Riha RL. Utility of the pictorial Epworth sleepiness scale in the adult down syndrome population. Sleep Med. 2020;66:165–7. https://doi.org/10.1016/j.sleep.2019.10.003. Epub 2019 Oct 25. PMID: 31877508.

12. Choi JB, Nelesen R, Loredo JS, Mills PJ, Ancoli-Israel S, Ziegler MG, Dimsdale JE. Sleepiness in obstructive sleep apnea: a harbinger of impaired cardiac function? Sleep. 2006;29(12):1531–6. https://doi.org/10.1093/sleep/29.12.1531. PMID: 17252883.

13. Krupp LB, LaRocca NG, Muir-Nash J, Steinberg AD. The fatigue severity scale. Application to patients with multiple sclerosis and systemic lupus erythematosus. Arch Neurol. 1989t;46(10):1121–3. https://doi.org/10.1001/archneur.1989.00520460115022. PMID: 2803071.

14. Learmonth YC, Dlugonski D, Pilutti LA, Sandroff BM, Klaren R, Motl RW. Psychometric properties of the fatigue severity scale and the modified fatigue impact scale. J Neurol Sci. 2013;331(1–2):102–7. https://doi.org/10.1016/j.jns.2013.05.023. Epub 2013 Jun 20. PMID: 23791482.

15. Rossi D, Galant LH, Marroni CA. Psychometric property of fatigue severity scale and correlation with depression and quality of life in cirrhotics. Arq Gastroenterol. 2017;54(4):344–8. https://doi.org/10.1590/S0004-2803.201700000-85. Epub 2017 Oct 2. PMID: 28977117.

16. Alekseeva TM, Gavrilov YV, Kreis OA, Valko PO, Weber KP, Valko Y. Fatigue in patients with myasthenia gravis. J Neurol. 2018;265(10):2312–21. https://doi.org/10.1007/s00415-018-8995-4. Epub 2018 Aug 11. PMID: 30099585.

17. Talwar A, Sahni S, John S, Verma S, Cárdenas-Garcia J, Kohn N. Effects of pulmonary rehabilitation on fatigue severity scale in patients with lung disease. Pneumonol Alergol Pol. 2014;82(6):534–40. https://doi.org/10.5603/PiAP.2014.0070. PMID: 25339563.

18. Shahid A, et al. Toronto Hospital Alertness Test (THAT). In: Shahid A, et al., editors. STOP, THAT and one hundred other sleep scales. New York: Springer; 2012. https://doi.org/10.1007/978-1-4419-9893-4_96.

19. Shapiro CM, Auch C, Reimer M, Kayumov L, Heslegrave R, Huterer N, Driver H, Devins GM. A new approach to the construct of alertness. J Psychosom Res. 2006;60(6):595–603. https://doi.org/10.1016/j.jpsychores.2006.04.012. PMID: 16731234.

20. Moller HJ, Devins GM, Shen J, et al. Sleepiness is not the inverse of alertness: evidence from four sleep disorder patient groups. Exp Brain Res. 2006;173:258–66. https://doi.org/10.1007/s00221-006-0436-4.

21. Shapiro C, Truffaut L, Matharan S, Olivier V. Discriminating between anxious and non-anxious subjects using the Toronto Hospital Alertness Test. Front Psychiatry. 2017;8:5. https://doi.org/10.3389/fpsyt.2017.00005. PMID: 28210228; PMCID: PMC5288356.

22. Li S, Fong DYT, Wong JYH, Wilkinson K, Shapiro C, Choi EPH, McPherson B, Lam CLK, Ip MSM. Psychometric evaluation of the Chinese version of the Toronto Hospital Alertness Test. J Patient Rep Outcomes. 2020;4(1):32. https://doi.org/10.1186/s41687-020-00197-7. PMID: 32372244; PMCID: PMC7200959.

23. Apnea B. Barriers and correlates of adherence in pediatric obstructive sleep apnea [Internet]. Ufdc.ufl.edu. 2021 [cited 14 March 2021]. Available from: https://ufdc.ufl.edu/UFE0042668/00001.

24. Simon SL, Duncan CL, Janicke DM, Wagner MH. Barriers to treatment of paediatric obstructive sleep apnoea: development of the adherence barriers to continuous positive airway pressure (CPAP) questionnaire. Sleep Med. 2012;13(2):172–7. https://doi.org/10.1016/j.sleep.2011.10.026. Epub 2011 Dec 14. PMID: 22172967.

25. Carmody JK, Simon SL, Mara CA, Byars KC. Validation and confirmatory factor analysis of the pediatric Adherence Barriers to Continuous Positive Airway Pressure Questionnaire. Sleep Med. 2020;74:1–8. https://doi.org/10.1016/j.sleep.2020.05.025. Epub 2020 May 23. PMID: 32828897; PMCID: PMC7541536.

26. Weaver TE, Maislin G, Dinges DF, Younger J, Cantor C, McCloskey S, Pack AI. Self-efficacy in sleep apnea: instrument development and patient perceptions of obstructive sleep apnea risk, treatment benefit, and volition to use continuous positive airway pressure. Sleep. 2003;26(6):727–32.

27. Micoulaud-Franchi JA, Coste O, Bioulac S, Guichard K, Monteyrol PJ, Ghorayeb I, Weaver TE, Weibel S, Philip P. A French update on the Self-Efficacy Measure for Sleep Apnea (SEMSA) to assess continuous positive airway pressure (CPAP) use. Sleep Breath. 2019;23(1):217–26. https://doi.org/10.1007/s11325-018-1686-7. Epub 2018 Jun 26. PMID: 29946945.

28. Shahid A, et al. Self-Efficacy Measure for Sleep Apnea (SEMSA). In: Shahid A, et al., editors. STOP, THAT and one hundred other sleep scales. New York: Springer; 2012. https://doi.org/10.1007/978-1-4419-9893-4_75.

29. Lai AY, Fong DY, Lam JC, Weaver TE, Ip MS. Linguistic and psychometric validation of the Chinese version of the self-efficacy measures for sleep apnea questionnaire. Sleep Med. 2013;14(11):1192–8. https://doi.org/10.1016/j.sleep.2013.04.023. Epub 2013 Sept 16. PMID: 24051110.

30. Sawyer AM, King TS, Hanlon A, et al. Risk assessment for CPAP nonadherence in adults with newly diagnosed obstructive sleep apnea: preliminary testing of the Index for Nonadherence to PAP (I-NAP). Sleep Breath. 2014;18(4):875–83. https://doi.org/10.1007/s11325-014-0959-z.

31. Balachandran JS, Yu X, Wroblewski K, Mokhlesi B. A brief survey of patients' first impression after CPAP titration predicts future CPAP adherence: a pilot study. J Clin Sleep Med. 2013;9(3):199–205. https://doi.org/10.5664/jcsm.2476.

32. Broström A, Ulander M, Nilsen P, Lin CY, Pakpour AH. Development and psychometric evaluation of the Motivation to Use CPAP Scale (MUC-S) using factorial structure and Rasch analysis among patients with obstructive sleep apnea before CPAP treatment is initiated. Sleep Breath. 2021;25(2):627–37. https://doi.org/10.1007/s11325-020-02143-9. Epub ahead of print. PMID: 32705529.

33. Broström A, Ulander M, Nilsen P, Svanborg E, Arestedt KF. The attitudes to CPAP treatment inventory: development and initial validation of a new tool for measuring attitudes to CPAP treatment. J Sleep Res. 2011;20(3):460–71. https://doi.org/10.1111/j.1365-2869.2010.00885.x. Epub 2010 Aug 31. PMID: 20819143.

34. Stepnowsky CJ, Marler MR, Ancoli-Israel S. Determinants of nasal CPAP compliance. Sleep Med. 2002;3:239–47.

35. Chew LD, Bradley KA, Boyko EJ. Brief questions to identify patients with inadequate health literacy. Fam Med. 2004;36:588–94.

Suggested Reading

Lewinsohn PM, Seeley JR, Roberts RE, Allen NB. Center for Epidemiologic Studies Depression Scale (CES-D) as a screening instrument for depression among community-residing older adults. Psychol Aging. 1997;12(2):277–87. https://doi.org/10.1037//0882-7974.12.2.277. PMID: 9189988.

Wilkinson K, Shapiro C. Development and validation of the Nonrestorative Sleep Scale (NRSS). J Clin Sleep Med. 2013;9(9):929–37. https://doi.org/10.5664/jcsm.2996.

Shahid A, Chung SA, Maresky L, et al. The Toronto Hospital Alertness Test scale: relationship to daytime sleepiness, fatigue, and symptoms of depression and anxiety. Nat Sci Sleep. 2016;8:41–5. https://doi.org/10.2147/NSS.S91928.

Shahid A, et al. Dysfunctional beliefs and attitudes about sleep scale (DBAS). In: Shahid A, et al., editors. STOP, THAT and one hundred other sleep scales. New York: Springer; 2012. https://doi.org/10.1007/978-1-4419-9893-4_28.

Shahid A, et al., editors. STOP, THAT and one hundred other sleep scales. New York: Springer; 2012.

Compliance and Oral Appliance Use for Sleep-Related Breathing Disorders

Michael Simmons

29.1 Compliance vs. Adherence vs. Concordance (CAC)

The terms compliance and adherence are often used interchangeably in the *SRBD literature, so discussion is warranted as to whether "compliance" or "adherence" is the best terminology to describe a patient's behavior in following a prescribed therapy. Each word provides a different emphasis when it comes to the agency of the patient in the said treatment. *Compliance* is considered to be the degree to which the patient follows the therapy as prescribed by the clinician; *adherence* is thought to be more appropriate when the patient participates in concert with their healthcare provider in the choice of therapy out of a number of viable alternatives. Accordingly, if a patient does not agree to try a prescribed therapy, then compliance is zero, since the prescribed therapy was never used by the patient; in this same instance, adherence is not applicable, as the patient never agreed to the therapy. "*Concordance*" is a further element of terminology which, according to Chakrabarti [1], "emphasizes a therapeutic relationship, which facilitates clinicians' and patients' views on treatment, and supports an informed choice of treatment by patients." This speaks to the patient arriving at their choice of therapy after adequate opportunity to reflect upon unbiased information. Concordance ultimately assumes that the patient knows themselves best, including which of the potential therapies they could and would follow.

When it comes to therapy for *SRBD, there is a drop-off in compliance at each stage following diagnosis and sometimes earlier on (e.g., if the patient refuses to accept a recommended diagnostic test that might lead to an unwanted diagnosis). A large amount of the *SRBD literature reports on adherence, as the patient has often agreed, through a formal informed consent procedure in a clinical study, often overseen by an institutional review board, to use the therapy. Published reports on adherence rates do not typically address the subjects who did not agree to the proposed therapeutic trial and therefore do not reflect compliance measures. In reality the measure of compliance may be a better indicator of how effective a therapy is, since a patient unwilling to explore or try a therapy is a treatment failure in of itself. Whether the reason for non-use of a therapy is social stigma, perceived difficulty, or any other rational or other choice, it ultimately undermines the overall effectiveness of that specific therapy. Put another way, if an effective therapy is refused by a patient, its overall efficacy rate goes down. While the nuanced differences between compliance, adherence, and concordance should be acknowledged as they shape approaches to treatment, the abbreviation CAC will be used as a helpful abbreviation for the reader.

The goal of achieving better treatment outcomes in addressing *SRBD has received more attention, especially in terms of better CAC through a focus on individualized patient care approaches. One example of trying to achieve better outcomes uses a P4 model in healthcare [2, 3], which takes into consideration the four Ps: (i) *predicting* whether an illness is likely to exist, (ii) *prevention* of an illness when possible, (iii) *personalizing* the care to that individual patient, and (iv) *participation* of the patients as the most important stakeholder. The latter two Ps speak to an interest in higher patient engagement and improved treatment CAC. The P4 model in sleep medicine described by Pack [4] appears to be specifically consistent with the tenets of patient concordance in that the patient chooses their therapy from a list of viable alternatives, and this emphasis of patient choice potentially leads to better engagement in the therapy.

In the context of improving CAC, it should be acknowledged that prescribed or offered therapies are not only influenced by the unique circumstances of the patient but often depend upon the healthcare provider's specialty. Hypothetically, a patient consulting a surgeon has a surgical remedy expectation, especially since a surgeon is more likely to provide a surgical intervention. In the same context, a

M. Simmons (✉)
Encino Center for Sleep and TMJ Disorders, Encino, CA, USA

UCLA School of Dentistry 1987–2018, Los Angeles, CA, USA
e-mail: msimmons@g.ucla.edu

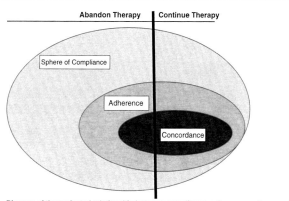

Diagram of the projected relationship between compliance, adherence and concordance and ongoing use of therapy

Fig. 29.1 Impact of CAC spheres on continuing therapy

psychologist consult would likely result in the recommendation for behavioral treatment interventions. If the problem at hand is not readily addressed by the consulted healthcare provider, the patient is potentially referred to providers skilled in other areas of sleep healthcare. In this way, the patient self-selects care as they must agree either to move in the recommended direction or self-seek alternative therapies. Helping patients make informed decisions and overcome obstacles to care may be more important than the therapy itself since the informed decision process includes patient engagement, responsibility, and ownership in their own care. In this regard, reconciling simpler therapy, which is more likely to be followed, with more efficacious therapy, which possesses better outcomes when followed, is a difficult balance to strike (see Fig. 29.1).

A public health perspective of care often utilizes a compliance model where all individuals are expected to follow the directives such as vaccination schedules and health safety regulations. In these domains there is little to no individual discussion or alternate choice of acceptable options, and compliance at a high percentage of the time is necessary for survival of the individual and population. An overlap between public health and individual *SRBD care approaches is demonstrated in specific populations such as commercial aircraft pilots or truck drivers that are obliged to fulfill specific *SRBD hours of therapy, rest, and sleep time, and their compliance is monitored as part of job requirements. Compliance in the public health sector is more of a requirement than a choice especially since there are potential penalties in noncompliance.

While the overall contention is that compliance is the most accurate measure of outcome efficacy of a single therapeutic option, there is seldom only one successful approach to a problem – indeed, the more viable treatment options available to manage a problem, the better from a CAC perspective. In treating *SRBD conditions such as obstructive sleep apnea (OSA), sleep academies have historically advo-

cated strongly for positive airway pressure (PAP) therapy as a favored first-line treatment [5] consistent with a compliance model. This privileging comes at the expense of other possible treatments, such as oral appliance therapies (OATs) and positional and surgical treatment options. It is a reasonable argument that patients may not have sufficient depth of understanding, even with informed consent and its intrinsic biases, to make the best choice of therapy. Nevertheless, every reasonable attempt should be made to satisfy an unbiased consent process allowing for treatment choices, in an effort to reach concordance. Presumably the outcome of therapy chosen by the patient results in more consistent use of the therapy but not necessarily the best efficacy of therapy.

One final but important consideration is how to define CAC in terms of various therapies for *SRBD. Notably the threshold for CAC sufficiency in PAP use is arbitrarily set very low at 4 hours per night for 5 nights per week (70% of nights) for civilians. This adds up to 20 hours of protected sleep time using PAP out of a recommended 49–56 sleep hours per week for adults, i.e., less than 50% (35.7–40.8%) of normal adult sleep time use. From a public health perspective, this would be similar to wearing a seat belt less than half the time when driving in a car. In an ideal situation, every time the patient sleeps, whether during their main sleep cycle or naps, they should have protected sleep. If the bar for PAP use were at 6 hours per 24-hour period or at 75% of sleep time usage, the CAC values reported for PAP would be dramatically less. The arbitrary benchmark choice of 4 hours per night of PAP usage [6, 7] makes little sense, is poorly validated, and completely ignores PAP's dose-dependent therapeutic impact on important health measures such as cardiovascular, metabolic, mood, and cognitive function [8, 9] as well as all-cause mortality [10]. Since the greatest reduction in mortality rates is associated with >6 hours of daily PAP use, the 6-hour minimum use standard for PAP would be at least somewhat substantiated [10]. Even with its privileged status, limited use requirement, and extensive list of improvements over the past 40 years, PAP has not proven to be the magic bullet answer to *SRBD conditions for most patients. Due consideration for alternative therapies, especially those favored by patients, must therefore be explored and OAT has the existing infrastructure and potential providers to dramatically augment PAP options to improve population-level CAC for *SRBD care.

In this chapter, the focus is on the many ways to improve CAC for *SRBD, but the overall theme is how to improve population-level care as this speaks to the largest improvement outcome. There is elaboration on improving CAC in the following ways:

A. *Reducing barriers to care*
B. *Bridging bias in therapeutic options*

C. *Increased efficiency in providing effective therapy*

D. *Reducing bias in restrictive definition of OAT*

E. *Continued OA evolution as monotherapy and combination therapy*

29.2   Improving CAC by Reducing Barriers to Care

There are many barriers to *SRBD care, but they are readily split into diagnostic barriers and treatment barriers. The current gold standard system of diagnosing and treating those with obstructive sleep apnea (OSA), according to the American Academy of Sleep Medicine (AASM), may have been beneficial at the individual patient care level but appears poorly effective at the population level. While improving CAC is critical for the "20% diagnosed" with OSA as determined by the AASM Frost and Sullivan report (F&S) [11], it would also be prudent to engage the other 80% as yet undiagnosed into therapies with the aim of improving the CAC for *SRBD at the population level. More diagnostic pathways through more primary sleep health providers allow for increased population impact and increased diversity in treatment options. This would include overall success in diagnosis and treatment of milder *SRBD conditions such as primary snoring and upper airway resistance syndrome, which are often overlooked by the medical community as not clinically significant. Current AASM guidelines for more medically troubling *SRBD conditions such as OSA also utilize an inefficient trial-and-error approach that is biased toward a poorly validated gold standard. This standard of care limits diagnosis only through physicians, and perhaps their advanced practice surrogates, with the medical communities, predetermined preference for PAP as a universal all-purpose first-line therapy. The current treatment journey for OSA can be unduly restrictive in options, costly, frustrating, time consuming, and lacking in personalized care; as a result, many patients are untreated, undertreated, dropped from care, or lost to follow-up [12]. Reliance on one preferred treatment option PAP for *SRBD is like reliance on one approach or medication class to manage all patients with one disorder such as hypertension. The consequences of such an approach are potentially deadly.

29.3   Improving CAC by Bridging Bias in Therapeutic Options

If the goal were to improve population-level care of *SRBD and especially OSA, then more treatment options would be routinely prescribed and provided to patients. If CAC were evaluated for the condition being treated as opposed to reliance on a single treatment option for a condition, we would

see much better CAC measures. Additionally, by focusing on a single objective efficacy measure of success to determine which is the gold standard therapy, we overlook additional and equally important success measures that might be provided by other "non-gold standard" therapies.

For OSA, treatment outcome improvements using the apnea hypopnea index (AHI) show PAP possesses the highest treatment efficacy per hour of use among nonsurgical therapies. Consequently, over the past 40 years the most prescribed treatment for OSA is PAP which is reflected in the F&S report [11] as 85% of OSA therapy with PAP, 10% with oral appliance therapy (OAT), and 5% with surgical therapy (Fig. 29.2). Unfortunately, the over-reliance on PAP may prove to be a poor choice since PAP may only be effective on specific subgroups with OSA and not at a general population level for those with an AHI at or above five events per hour.

If "efficacy per hour" were the only and most important measure of a therapy, and AHI the most relevant measure of efficacy, there might be some justification for the overwhelming therapy recommendation of PAP. However, efficacy per hour is by no means the only or most useful metric. Clearly "overall efficacy" is a more valid measure of treatment effect as it takes into consideration both efficacy per hour and hours of use. In addition, several other important factors which impact CAC ought to be considered:

Current *SRBD Therapy Apportionment

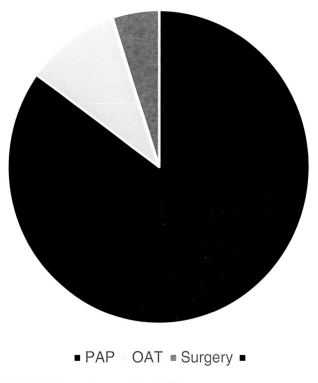

■ PAP   OAT ■ Surgery ■

Fig. 29.2 Current therapy pie for *SRBD

(i) *Willingness to try a therapy*: *PAP therapy* is not readily accepted, tolerated, or chosen by patients, in part because of its intrusive nature of tethering, bulkiness, and cumbersome interface with the human anatomy; *surgical options* may have low CAC in that patients are likely to opt out from an invasive versus conservative therapy due to surgical risk and recovery issues.

(ii) *Untoward side effects from the therapy (short and long term)*: *OAT* is limited to patients that do not have a high gag reflex; it contributes to dentition changes that are cumulative over time [8], and it may not be consistently effective in a number of OSA cases; *upper airway surgeries* in particular take time to heal where swelling during recovery can aggravate airway patency for months, leaving the patient in a transitionally worse situation than their pre-treatment status.

(iii) *Time to adapt to therapy and for therapy to be effective*: the minimum time necessary for the patient to incorporate the intervention into their daily routines and titrate to reach an effective outcome can be delayed in *PAP and OAT*; *weight loss* may be an effective therapy in a subpopulation of *SRBD patients who range from overweight to superobese, but the time to reach an effective outcome is likely prolonged, even if supplemented by bariatric surgery and for many the weight loss goal is hardly ever maintained.

Therefore, in any discussion of CAC for *SRBD, all potential therapies, including surgical, nonsurgical, combination, and observation/no therapy, must be included and compared as part of a standardized informed consent process. The disproportionate use of PAP relative to other effective therapies for *SRBD should be revisited in light of CAC levels, proof of effect for specific patient presentations, scientific developments, and patient preference. While there is more research literature supporting PAP as the highest efficacy of therapies per hour of use, other developing nonsurgical therapies for patients should be considered, including the following:

- Oral appliance therapy
- Positional therapy
- Medication management
- Nasal expiratory positive airway pressure devices
- Oropharyngeal exercises
- Non-ablative laser tightening of oropharyngeal tissues
- Orthodontic tooth and/or skeletal expansion of the tongue space
- Negative air pressure devices pulling tongue/adjacent upper airway tissues anteriorly

There has been limited discussion on specific criteria for selecting these various treatment options. For instance, Camacho et al. reported on a meta-analysis of 35 non-PAP options to address *SRBD which were subdivided by ana-

tomical subsites: nose, palate and oropharynx, tongue, skeletal surgery and jaw repositioning, and other surgical and medical interventions [9]. Each approach has various levels of proof of effect, CAC data, individual efficacy per hour of use, and overall efficacy at various *SRBD severities for various population subtypes. Others looking to improve individual CAC suggest more targeted therapies based upon phenotyping since OSA is a heterogeneous disorder [13]. However, from a cost perspective the targeted approach would be challenging and certainly is not an easy solution to address at the population level, especially since each targeted therapy would still be subject to the same CAC issues found in therapy trials.

Consideration for the body of scientific support for any therapy is not only critical in the therapeutic decision tree, but using targeted/personalized approaches where that therapy has higher impact is also a critically important aspect of future care [13, 14]. Currently a progression of PAP followed by OAT has the most substantial scientific validation of overall treatment efficacy for all severities of *SRBD. There are many reasons to choose PAP therapy, such as its high effectiveness, remote monitoring capability, customized pressure ramping, heating, humidification, ability to auto-titrate intra- and internight, and potential feedback to patients on a daily basis. Despite enormous technical advances over 40 years of use, including reduced noise and more options in interface designs, there has been little improvement in the percentage of patients able to use PAP devices in the long term. Even behavioral and support programs have not proven dramatically effective in increasing PAP CAC.

Thus, other therapies must become readily available as alternative first- and second-line options. There should also be more focus on using PAP as part of combined therapies. In addition, alternative rescue therapies should be immediately available to patients should their PAP therapy be interrupted for any reason. Interruptions are always an issue with PAP since they include the many unpredictable vagaries of life such as power or equipment failure, airway congestion, otalgia, facial trauma or procedures, transient insomnia, claustrophobia, disenchantment with the therapy, equipment noise disruption to bed partner, napping, or sleeping away from home. Since no specific therapy for *SRBD has proven itself vastly superior in overall efficacy, more consideration to the CAC potential for each viable therapy is necessary to achieve population and cost containment solutions. When viewed from this perspective, OAT stands as a tried-and-true alternative.

29.4 Why Consider OAT

There are two generally accepted reasons to consider conventional OAT for *SRBD – the treatment's overall efficacy and its preference as a therapy by patients.

1. OAs have demonstrated their clinical validity and in many cases match PAP health outcomes. Since the first case series publication, their acceptability in medical circles has increased: they began in 1982 [15] as an unvalidated, unaccepted treatment for *SRBD; by 1995 they were an acceptable treatment for primary snoring [16]; by 2005 they were a potential second-line treatment for mild-to-moderate OSA should the patient fail or refuse PAP [17]; and by 2015 they were a viable alternative for severe OSA should the patient refuse PAP [18]. The future is likely to include more evolved options for OAT as first-line optional treatment for all levels of obstructive *SRBD, including first-line treatment for severe OSA, based upon success rates of about 40–61% with severe OSA cases using a mandibular advancement design (MAD) OA [19–22]. In one PAP-OAT comparison study, success with severe OSA cases was 50% for OA versus 74.1% PAP [21]. Haviv et al. studied 52 severe OSA patients (AHI > 40) that had failed PAP with a trial of OAT. While many PAP failures with severe OSA were successful with OAT, 17.3% of the 52 users of OAT reverted back to using PAP therapy; of these, one-third would still use their OA when sleeping away from home [23]. The success of a significant portion of patients using OAT for severe OSA demonstrates that OAT should no longer be considered the rescue therapy for those who are intolerant to PAP, but as another first-line therapy option for all severities of OSA.

With this perspective, PAP would act as rescue therapy for failed or non-adherent OAT just as much as the reverse. One study showed that patients would also ideally have both of these options and potentially other conservative therapies during transient periods, during which one therapy cannot be used and alternate therapies would be available as a rescue [24]. As stated above, having multiple therapies increases the potential for adherence to overall therapeutic efficacy, independent of therapeutic choice for that specific patient and their circumstance during that sleep cycle. Treatment parameters that dictate patients must fail one therapy (e.g., PAP) in order to try another therapy (e.g., OAT) push a compliance monotherapy model of care and hinder patient choice and self-efficacy.

The overall success rates of OAT in addressing comorbidities of *SRBD are also similar to PAP. Proof includes high-level evidence, such as randomized controlled trials, systematic reviews, and meta-analyses [25–37]. Studies have shown that OAT improves cardiovascular function [38, 39] and hypertension [40–43], with one study showing this benefit in severe OSA patients at 1 year follow-up [37]. Another study showed statistically greater improvement in cardiac function by OAT relative to PAP therapy [44]. Both OAT and PAP have been shown to be equally effective in reducing cardiac event fatality with severe OSA when compared to non-treatment groups [45], and reducing AHI to below 15, which might favor PAP therapy, is not necessary to achieve significant cardiovascular improvement [21]. Improvements from OAT in addressing *SRBD also include improved quality of life, reduced sleepiness (i.e., a lower score in the Epworth Sleepiness Scale), and improvement in neuro-behavioral measures [45–52]. Moreover, the effects of OAT have been shown to be long term [53, 54]—for instance, a recent study showed good and stable treatment effects by both PAP and OAT after a 10-year follow-up period, confirming both therapies provide similar health benefit at 10 years (albeit slightly better for CPAP), and therefore both therapies are appropriate for long-term management of OSA [55].

2. OAT is less cumbersome, more portable, easier to use, better tolerated, and consistently reported in comparison studies as the preferred therapy for *SRBD over PAP by most patients. The evidence supporting this includes over 20 years' worth of publications showing higher CAC rates with OAT [24, 56]. OAT is chosen by more patients who tried both therapies and were given either option [21, 57, 58]. Adherence to OAT is over 80% at the end of 1 year [59] which is better than PAP's overly optimistic adherence values of 60% by F&S [11]. One well-controlled study included 108 treatment naïve/newly diagnosed moderate-to-severe obstructive sleep apnea participants, who completed both OAT and PAP arms of the study with a washout period. Study findings indicated nonsignificant difference in overall efficacy with both therapies, which included objective and subjective outcome measures (arterial blood pressure, sleepiness, quality of life, and driving simulator performance), but 51% of participants preferred OAT versus 23% who preferred PAP therapy [46].

This preference for OAT occurs despite a more involved titration process than that required for PAP. In general, it can take from a few days to a few months to arrive at the most effective mandibular position for those using OAT, although noticeable effects can be present on the first night. In most cases, delays in achieving best effect occur because OA benefit potentially increases through advancing the mandible gradually to determine the best effect. The best mandibular target position is typically not known or predictable for each individual although there is some evidence that there is a dose-dependent effect with more effect as the mandible is advanced further anteriorly [60, 61]. Tan et al. [58] found 17 out of the 21 mild-to-severe OSA subjects who completed both arms of their CPAP and OAT crossover study preferred the OAT. Both therapies had statistically similar improvements in the AHI and Epworth Sleepiness Scale. Another study by Yamamoto et al. [57], which included 40 moderate-to-severe OSA participants who finished both CPAP and OA arms of therapy, showed similar cardiovascular and symp-

Table 29.1 Some factors to consider in Mandibular Advancement Device (MAD) oral appliance options to manage *SRBD

Pre-conceived beliefs	Perceived benefits	Realized benefits
Candidacy for therapy	Ease of use	Overall efficacy
Time to achieve effectiveness	Maintenance	Repairability
Problem-solving adaptation	Patient expectations of benefits	Getting physician prescription for OAT (in the USA)
Access to care	Offered as treatment option	Design choices
Adaptability to dentition change	Adjustability	Side effects
Past experience with OAs	Co-treating sleep bruxism	Bed partner expectation
Combination with PAP therapy	Combination positional therapy	Other combination therapy
Hypoallergenic material options	Durability	Cost
Objective feedback on effectiveness	Independent compliance monitoring	Temporary failure contingency planning

tom improvement, but the OAT was preferred by participants on all 9 subjective measures with 8 of the 9 measures statistically significant. These subjective preference measures included: simplicity in setting and removal, comfortability, stability, time needed to get used to the device, simplicity of maintenance, appearance of the device, bed partner's acceptance, and overall satisfaction.

If the reader accepts that compliance with therapy is king, then OAT should be used more often than the 10% reported by F&S [11] and closer to double the rate that PAP is used for OSA. Like any therapy for *SRBDs, OAT has pros and cons to consider in addition to the patient's informed comparisons to other potential interventions. Some of the many areas to consider for OAT are shown in Table 29.1; they include ease of use, time to reach efficacy, overall efficacy, cost, durability, and maintenance. In addition, for any determination of success involving therapy such as OAT, there must be clarity as to the valid measures of success, both on a subjective and objective basis, short term and long term. For example, using AHI measures as the metric of success with therapy is increasingly suspect; there is evidence that the time under 90% oxygen saturation or oxygen desaturation index improvement may be more reflective of health benefits [62].

29.5 Improving CAC Through Efficiency in Providing Effective Therapy

Better efficiency in arriving at effective therapy is likely to result in more use of that therapy but not necessarily improved overall efficacy. For example, a recent Cochrane study found positional therapy had better adherence than CPAP with immediate effects but still had less overall efficacy [63]. In order to speed up attaining an effective therapeutic dose, both PAP and OAT can be titrated over a single night in a lab setting. Such titration can help to solve some of the adaptation issues and initial barriers to use. In the case of OAT, a lab titration can result in increased normalization of breathing parameters in about 30% of subjects who were otherwise considered OA failures [64].

The concept of a home-based, self-, or auto-adjusting PAP or OAT has been explored. This process requires feedback on objective successful sleep parameters through connection to a home-based sleep testing device. Such a device has a feedback loop which automatically adjusts or gives the user information on how to self-adjust the device. This can be accomplished using an OA over multiple nights with feedback guidance from a sleep testing device as simple as a snoring app on a smart phone, a pulse oximeter, or a more sophisticated sleep monitor. Waking the patient within single sleep cycles to adjust an OA leads to sleep fragmentation and a more difficult process, but the OA protrusion can readily be adjusted on a night-by-night basis without this additional sleep disruption. By comparison, an auto-PAP can change air pressure within a single night automatically without waking the patient, which has a distinct advantage over any current OA titration. There has been one home-based auto-OAT on the market for use as an auto-adjusting theragnostic device over several nights. This system, called the home MATRx, had a small motor connected to an adjustable temporary oral appliance, which was moved in tiny 0.2 mm increments during the sleep cycle to determine the best mandibular protrusion to manage *SRBD events without causing awakenings [65].

The temporary MATRx OA used to determine the best mandibular advancement was bulky with associated lip seal issues and the process was not tolerated by all patients; nevertheless, it allowed for hundreds of incremental 0.2 mm machine-driven titrations during one night, designed to be so small as to not fragment the patient's sleep. Independent testing showed good predictability of this device in determining the effective mandibular protrusion, although about 8 out of 33 (24%) participants had inconclusive results in predicting response [66]. The MATRx auto-titrating OA could also test effectiveness with no mandibular protrusion before advancing the mandible. This should be compared to the standard recommended titration process of OAT, which typically starts at 50–70% of maximum mandibular protrusion. Starting the mandibular protrusion at a minimum of 50% of maximum protrusive range may overshoot the needed protrusive position of the mandible in managing *SRBD, putting more strain on the patient's stomatognathic system than necessary and potentially leading to reduced CAC. This is of interest since at least one study showed some patients may need 25% or less protrusion [67] to be effective; and in another study, 10 out of 26 patients had a greater than 50% reduction in AHI without any mandibular protrusion, speaking to an effect from preventing mandibular retrusion as the mechanisms of action [68].

No system of titration or calibration is perfect, but the auto-titrating process of auto-PAP remains superior as an ongoing therapeutic remedy in instances where increased PAP pressure is indicated. This would be of potential benefit intranight during specific sleep architecture and/or body position, or over time due to severity progression of the *SRBD and specifically to overcome internight variability. However beneficial this auto-PAP technology may appear in effectiveness, it is not associated with statistically significant increased PAP adherence compared to conventional CPAP [69]. It is also important to recognize that while efficacy and overall sophistication of PAP may be higher than OAT per hour of use, the overall mean disease alleviation of PAP and OAT has been determined to be similar [21, 70, 71]. The mean disease alleviation is a combination of efficacy per hour of use and the number of hours used per night. More efficacy per hour by PAP is matched by more hours of use with OAT [21]. Despite the limits of OA titration, most OA adaptation problems can be mitigated and ultimately result in a high percentage of OAT hours of use during sleep.

29.6 Increased CAC by Reducing Bias in Restrictive Definition of OAT

Although OAs are evolving at a fast pace, the definition of an OA is overly restrictive, which limits the OA treatment options supported by medical reimbursement and consequently reduces CAC. The definition of an OA has been addressed by the American Academy of Dental Sleep Medicine (AADSM) several times since 2014 and updated most recently in March 2019 [72, 73]. As currently defined:

> An oral appliance is custom fabricated using digital or physical impressions and models of an individual patient's oral structures and physical needs. A custom-fabricated oral appliance

may include a prefabricated component; however, it is not a primarily prefabricated item that is subsequently trimmed, bent, relined, or otherwise modified. It is made of biocompatible materials and engages both the maxillary and mandibular arches. The oral appliance has a mechanism that advances the mandible in increments of 1 mm or less with a protrusive adjustment range of at least 5 mm. This mechanism may or may not include fixed mechanical hinges or metallic materials. In addition, reversal of the advancement must be possible. The protrusive setting must be verifiable. The appliance is suitable for placement and removal by the patient or caregiver. It maintains a stable retentive relationship to the teeth, implants, or edentulous ridge, prevents dislodging, and retains the prescribed setting during use.

OAT for *SRBD is clearly much larger than this narrow definition, which was probably developed for insurance standardization and reimbursement purposes. The narrow OA definition by the AADSM limited to mandibular advancement devices (MAD) was attributed to insufficient high-quality evidence to support other OATs such as tongue retaining/guiding devices (TRDs) and non-adjustable appliances, such as monobloc and single arch OAs [18]. MAD devices can be divided into customized versus prefabricated OAs. Prefabricated OAs can be provided and adjusted by dentists as a temporary or trial OA but other prefabricated OAs include designs are available over the counter (OTC) and are used as self-treatment by patients. Customized appliances have been shown to be superior to prefabricated OAs in efficacy due to better retention (fit and comfort) and range of protrusion available [74, 75]. Although the AADSM rejected OA designs, such as TRDs, monoblocs, single arch designs, trial appliances, and even OTC models, these options have a place in care, and consideration should be given as to which patient population would benefit most from each type (Tables 29.2 and 29.3).

A completely different consideration design in OA therapy is incorporating active orthodontic approaches to increase the size of the upper airway. This approach would include orthodontic tooth and skeletal expansion devices that may include pediatric growth and development of both the maxillary and mandibular dental arches, in an anterior poste-

Table 29.2 Some of the many options with MAD-type OA designs

Type	OTC	Premade	Custom	Others
Base material	Acrylic	Nylon	Metal	Others
Retention	Soft or hard liner	Metal clasps	Distal tooth wrap	Others
Adjustability	Infinite	0.5–1 mm	Unilateral	Others
Action	Push	Pull	Lock	Others
Connector	Metal bar or hook	Nylon/acrylic	Rubber/elastic	Others
Coloration	Clear	White	Single color	Others
Interarch movement	Horizontal or vertical only	Vertical and horizontal	No movement	Others
Durability	Up to 1 year	Up to 3 years	3–5 years	>5 years
Modify/repair	None	In office	In lab	Others
Add-ons	Anterior disclusion vertical height	Tongue lifts/nares spreaders	Elastic bands/air tubes	Others
Component parts	One	Two	Three	> three

Table 29.3 Some of the many options in a broader definition of OAT

Type of OAT	Option A	Option B	Option C	Option D	Option E
Trial	*OTC MAD*	*Prefab MAD*	*TRD*	*MATRx*	*No protrusion*
Monobloc	*Maxillary*	*Mandibular*	*Fused/locked Max/ Mand*	*Variable lock of Max/ Mand*	*Increased vertical mouth opening, tongue space*
Bibloc	*Connected push*	*Connected pull*	*Separate*	*Multiple connectors*	*Ability to protrude into passive range*
Combination OA therapy	*Connect PAP to oral airway*	*Connect PAP to nasal airway*	*Connect to PAP oronasal airway*	*MAD/TRD combination*	*Tongue lift, nares spread, air suction*
More OAT combinations	*OAT/EPAP*	*OAT/body positional*	*OAT/soft tissue surgical*	*OAT/oral exercise*	*OAT/non-ablative laser*
Orthodontic OAT	*Growth in children*	*Development in adults*	*Surgical assist*	*Use of temp anchorage devices*	*With orthognathic surgery*

rior as well as transverse aspect [76, 77]. The dental arches can also be potentially addressed in adult upper airway enlargement using midface skeletal expanders, sometimes using temporary anchorage devices or removable orthodontic devices [78–80]. This is a long-term therapy but may be potentially curative or preventive as opposed to the *SRBD management-type approach utilized in MAD therapy. Expanding dental arches may require surgical assistance in addition to temporary anchorage devices.

One final aspect to OAT that is not often discussed is the ability of OAs to increase the CAC of PAP therapy; in this way, OAT functions as part of a combination therapy. There are three situations in which this is helpful:

(i) A strapless interface of PAP therapy, by using an oral appliance to securely hold the nasal or oronasal PAP interface, allows for less irritation of PAP straps and less leaking from positional changes that that may break the mask interface seal. This designation would also include the OPAP or Oventus designs of blowing PAP air through the oral appliance or an OA air channel allowing inspired air to bypass the tongue [81, 82].

(ii) Concurrent use of an oral appliance which holds the mandible forward to help partially open the airway and can result in lower and potentially more tolerable PAP pressure by about 30% up to 45%, resulting in easier adherence to PAP therapy [82, 83].

(iii) Stabilizing the mandible during sleep with an oral appliance allows the facial contours to remain more stable during all sleep stages, which contributes to a more consistent PAP interface air seal.

Sadly, the narrow AADSM definition of OAT is restricting the many options within this OA therapeutic group that can be effective as stand-alone and combination therapy. This limitation detracts from the ultimate goal of improved *SRBD outcomes.

29.7 Increased CAC Through Continued OA Evolution

While evolution of PAP therapy has been the main thrust of research for *SRBD, there have been significant but less robust inroads with surgical interventions (e.g., multilevel approaches) [84] and if considering OAT's broader definition. While PAP appears to be nearing its zenith of treatment acceptance, other alternative therapies continue to develop.

OAT started many years before the first published use of CPAP by Sullivan et al. in 1981 [85]; Pierre Robin is credited with first using oral appliances in treating breathing issues in 1923 [86]. However, OAT in its broader definition still remains in its infancy in regard to impact on upper airway function and development. Future improvements are possible through modifying old OA designs, tweaking current designs, adding new designs, and development of new paradigms of OA therapy in the upper airway growth and development arena.

Even TRDs, which fell out of favor in part because they are less reliable and not adjustable, still continue to be used today for a small number of patients such as the edentulous, those with limited range of mandibular protrusion or with significant temporomandibular joint disorders. Chang et al. reported results of a systemic review and meta-analysis of conventional TRDs effects as decreasing the AHI by 53% and decreasing the Epworth Sleepiness Scale scores by 2.8 points [87]. High-tech companies have tried to emulate and improve the effects of a passive TRD in tongue protrusion during sleep, using an active negative suction to pull oral soft tissues away from blocking the upper airway. One product named Winx was reported to be 30–40% effective [88], but the company is no longer in business. A more recently published device specifically addressing anterior suctioning of the tongue showed positive clinical effects while still in the development stage [89] and a newer intraoral negative air pressure therapy is currently commercially available by prescription.

When comparing various types of OA designs for insights into improved CAC, Deane et al. found treatment success (AHI < 5) with TRDs to be about 45% in a cohort of 22 OSA patients (5 mild, 11 moderate, and 6 severe OSA; 16 male) and 68% of subjects with a MAD [90]. Compliance was relatively poor with the tongue retention device, and 91% of subjects preferred the MAD design OA. Johal et al. [75] compared custom-made OAs to OTC designs, which are a subset of pre-fabricated OAs, and found that the custom designs had greater patient preference. The advantages of the custom OA include patient comfort, smaller size, greater range of mandibular protrusion, more precise adjustment, as well as overall better fit and retention. Custom OAs were also more effective. A treatment outcome of AHI < 5 was found in 64% of patients with mild OSA using custom OA as compared to 24% with the premade OAs. In addition, the custom OAs were worn more than their premade counterparts (on average 7 versus 3 nights/week; 5 versus 3 hours/night) and were preferred at a rate of 21 to 1.

In some cases, an OA may have its design tweaked for improvement by addition of tongue guidance straps/buttons/prongs, nares spreaders under the upper lip, changing vertical height of the oral appliance and adding tubing to attach oxygen or PAP. Several designs of OAs have been used as carriers to specifically attach PAP, or as novel strapless and stable PAP interfaces in multiple head positions that may deliver air through the mouth, the nose, or both. These combination approaches, while useful, are more the exception than rule and often require more advanced training to deliver this level of therapy. There is also scant evidence to support any notion that they impact CAC or overall efficacy beyond the individual patient.

To address specific patient preferences and achieve high CAC levels, mechanisms to advance the mandible provided by dentists have been developed to include adjustable screws or guiding ramps with infinite settings, advancement bars, or straps providing 0.5–1 mm increments of change. Each of the many designs speaks to ease of use, durability, size, comfort, and calibration/titration. Some devices are better adjusted by the dentist, others by the patient. For example, an oral appliance may be "monobloc" in design, where the maxillary and mandibular arch components are joined together, whereas others are "bibloc," so that the maxillary and mandibular arches have readily adjustable connection systems. While the simpler options involving less adjustment are preferred by some patients, one recent design of OA, took an opposite approach that allows for different types of adjustment systems that can be attached to the same maxillary and mandibular arch components. These variable adjustment systems allow for changes in the flexibility and range of motion of the interarch connectors to address unwanted side effects, such as temporary TMJ arthralgia, which might otherwise reduce ongoing OA usage (Photo 29.1).

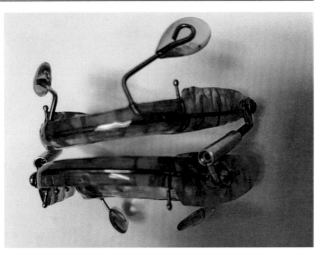

Photo 29.1 Image of an OA (MAD) with added ball clasps for rubber bands, nares spreaders, and tongue lifts. Rubber bands may be used to help keep the upper and lower components together and encourage a mouth closed position. Rubber bands may cover over the body of the tongue to restrict tongue movement

To increase the number of people that can be successfully treated with OAT, various OAs have different attributes: ranges in and ease of titration of the mandible anteriorly and vertically, ease of repair, types of materials used to account for allergies (e.g., acrylic or metal), and ease of adaptation to a changing dentition should the patient have dental work. Nevertheless, there are some patients for whom OAT is not the most easy or effective option. For patients with poor dexterity or hand strength, some OAs may not be usable without help. For patients with exaggerated gag responses or orofacial pain conditions, there may be intermittent OA use and limited range of adjustment, and, in some cases, no OA may be tolerable. For patients that are edentulous, or have very few remaining sound teeth, there may be inadequate retention to keep an OA in place, requiring use of dental adhesives or supplementation of OA anchorage by dental implants. For patients with cognitive challenges, dementia, or motor dyskinesias, support by a caregiver may be required for any chance of success. In some of these challenging cases, the OAT is an easier therapy than CPAP, but no conservative therapy is consistently successful. At this time, most OA modifications are made by trial and error and utilized by dentists with more experience in applying OAT as there are insufficient studies demonstrating clear advantages for specific subtypes of OSA or specific populations.

29.8 Increasing CAC with OAT

Reasons that patients will not start or try OAT once it is introduced through an impartial informed consent process can range from lack of insurance approval for this therapy, out-of-pocket costs, access to care, barriers in getting US physician approval and prescription for OAT, pre-conceived biases from patients and physicians against OAT, recent orthodontic or planned dental work, heightened gag response, dental disease or orofacial pain, or dysfunction conditions. There is no currently published research that addresses the percentage of drop-off in trying OAT for the various reasons, once recommended, but this aspect is important to identify and address in increasing CAC.

Once OAT is started the two main reasons for patients to stop using their OA are lack of efficacy, often subjectively determined by the continued presence of snoring, and untoward side effects, which can be short- or long-term and range from mild to severe. OATs can fail to meet a patient's expectations of efficacy through subjective and/or objective findings, such as an insufficiency of effect, otherwise termed a partial effect. This could mean there is a normalized AHI, but snoring is still disruptive to the bed partner or snoring is normalized and the AHI with OAT is not acceptable to the care provider. In this instance, the uninformed patient may proverbially throw in the towel rather than supplement the partial effect by modifying the OA or combining OAT with another therapy. Even in the case of highly validated MAD devices, it is still difficult to predict the OAT's overall efficacy and CAC, as it requires a multidimensional assessment of both anatomy and physiology, together with ample time to address potential side effects and resolve adaptation problems [66, 91].

Best predictions of OA effect are by actual use of an OA during sleep, with measures of outcome over a period of days to weeks. Pre-emptive OA trials can be performed with drug-induced endoscopy using midazolam or propofol, which mimics non-REM sleep [92] or a home or sleep lab based testing of various mandibular protrusions while using a temporary OA. While these best predictions of efficacy indicate a high likelihood of effect, they do not predict the patient will continue to wear the OA, as side effects may not have revealed themselves until several months of use. Additionally, discontinued use due to lack of objective measures of improvement may only reflect a single night's poor performance effect and not the average improvement noted over a week or longer. Therefore, over-reliance on limited objective data can result in abandoning an otherwise helpful therapy.

Untoward side effects that reduce CAC may be divided into short term (up to 2 months) and long term, as well as be separated by mild to severe impact. Side effects that impact CAC should be addressed as early into treatment as possible and especially during the titration period, when patients may be naïve to potential untoward outcomes of using an OA during sleep. Some side effects are frequent and occur early into treatment, such as excess salivation, but these are considered mild and usually they dwindle over time. A salivary response is expected with initial placement of an oral appliance, as the brain perceives the OA as something to be digested. With

time, this autonomic response wanes; thus, excess salivation is not a typical reason reported in the literature to discontinue use of the OA. Severe side effects, such as headaches, jaw pain, temporomandibular joint dysfunction symptoms (e.g., jaw joint noises), arthralgia, or myalgia, can greatly impact use and may be acute enough to warrant discontinuation of use for weeks to months or indefinitely. However, once resolved, even the more severe side effects may permit the patient to return to OA use. This type of treatment "holiday" can be alternated with another *SRBD therapy should the patient have multiple options of care.

Some commonly expected side effects in addition to hypersalivation include dry mouth, especially if lip incompetency is present or aggravated by the OA, chewing difficulties for a short time after removal of the OA, and temporary bite challenges in bringing the posterior teeth into the normal bite. These typically resolve within a few hours following use and often reduce in frequency and severity with tine and frequency of use of the OA. A morning mandibular repositioning device, tooth index matrix, or exercise routine can mitigate short- and long-term bite changes accompanying OA use.

Mullane and Loke [93] reported on short-term side effects on 21 non-PAP-compliant OSA subjects who subsequently used OAT for 4 weeks. The first 4 weeks are typically a titration period in which the OA has increased mandibular protrusion and the time when side effects would be more frequently expected. The study goal was to determine which side effects impact OA use and also if there was a discrepancy between subjective and objective reports of length of time of OA use per night. Subjects were therefore blinded as to the OA having a use compliance chip and were told the attached sensor in the OA was a "pressure sensor" to detect tooth movement. Subjective and objective measures of OA hours of use were not statistically different. This outcome, while different to the significant discrepancies in PAP subjective and objective use, has been confirmed by several other studies that used covert OA compliance measurement for varying periods of time [94, 95]. Mullane and Loke also noted that usage time of the OA almost doubled over the 4 weeks once the untoward side effects were addressed. They reported reduced compliance hours of use with OAs with moderate-to-severe side effects, such as jaw discomfort and noises or soft tissue (gum) discomfort. More frequent side effects of excess salivation, xerostomia, or tooth discomfort had less impact on OA hours of use. In this regard, more than 50% of their subjects endorsed some level of discomfort with: 67% excess salivation, 62% xerostomia, 61% tooth discomfort, 56% chewing difficulties in the morning, 55% jaw discomfort, and 51% jaw joint noises. Tooth movement and bite changes were never reported as severe by any of the subjects.

In terms of compliance and specific hours of therapy use, there is literature on both PAP and OAT that may be compared. Dieltjens et al. [96] evaluated 51 subjects after OA use for a year finding objective average daily OA use of 6.4+/−1.7 hours, which was subjectively overestimated by participants by 30 minutes. The regular use rate of the OA was 83% and the discontinuation rate at the 1-year follow-up was 9.8%. Other research of covert measuring of OA use allowing comparison of objective to subjective OA use has shown no significant time difference of subjective versus objective hours of OA use per night and no anthropometric or polysomnographic parameters correlated with compliance. There was also no correlation found between objective compliance and reports of excessive daytime sleepiness, suggesting that improved sleepiness is not a strong enough subjective improvement to continue using an OA. Snoring, however, showed increased objective compliance with a larger decrease in socially disturbing snoring. Dry mouth was the only adverse effect that correlated with less objective compliance at the 3-month follow-up. Newer compliance methods for OAT are being clinically proven as effective should the need arise to validate hours of OA usage [97]. By comparison Kribbs et al. [98] covertly monitored PAP use in 35 patients for an average of 106 days finding average use for 66% of the days with a mean duration of use of 4.88 hours. Subjectively, these same patients over-reported PAP use by 69 mins. The researchers noted that the more regular PAP users had significantly more years of education.

As well as the general advantages and disadvantages of OAT already discussed, there are specific OAT advantages and disadvantages as listed in Table 29.4.

Table 29.4 Advantages and disadvantages to the various types of OAT

Type of OAT	Advantages	Disadvantages
OTC	Cost, availability, self-help remedy. Helpful for benign conditions	Often lacks professional diagnosis and misses pathology. Poor: fit, retention, comfort, efficacy, durability
Pre-fabricated	Cost, trial device	Poor: comfort, durability
TRD	Cost, trial device, may help with compromised TMJ/teeth	Lacks adjustability, less efficacy and comfort
MAD	Highest efficacy, options of design, materials, add-ons	Relatively high cost, lack of clarity as to the best design for individual patients
Combination	More improvement in greater range of severity	High cost, often requires multiple providers, not patient-friendly
Orthodontic	Potentially curative in specific populations: children or narrow or retruded dental arches. May need surgical assistance for effect	Most: costly, invasive, required time to complete, time to reach efficacy. May not resolve *SRBD requiring management with PAP or other OAT

29.9 Comparing OAT and PAP Therapy for Future Overall *SRBD CAC

Comparing OAT to CPAP has been done by various authors and the conclusions are consistent in showing CPAP is more efficacious per hour of use and has a broader reach in the range of OSA severities that it brings back into the normal range when used (Tables 29.5 and 29.6). Other positive attributes of PAP include adherence monitoring which may be seamlessly uploaded to healthcare providers. In addition to immediate machine algorithm-driven feedback on the effectiveness of therapy, time of use, air leakage, apnea hypopnea index during each sleep cycle, PAP measured objective outcomes may also be shared with the end user (see Table 29.1) which can help the end use patient stay engaged in treatment. Of course, there is also a litany of negative attributes associated with PAP usage as listed in Table 29.3, any and all of which can impact CAC. A 20-year review of PAP shows a persistently low adherence despite efforts toward behavioral intervention and patient coaching [99]. Other authors have opined that "new PAP modes do not appear to be the "magic bullet" to improve "suboptimal adherence to PAP" [100]. This addresses the question whether CPAP should continue to be considered the gold standard of therapy for OSA [99].

Using the phenotypic conceptual framework of targeted OSA therapy, the authors estimate that >50% of all OSA patients could be treated with one or more non-PAP interventions [101, 102]. Since multiple authors report fewer than 50% of patients adequately tolerate the first-line therapy of PAP, there should be other first-line treatments [103, 104]. For instance, an OSA patient can nap in a semi-recliner chair and otherwise provide positional therapy if they are positional apnics or use an OA if camping or backpacking and needing to travel light. One single first line therapy for *SRBD neither fits all patients for a single circumstance nor fits all circumstances for any one patient. The ability to have multiple optional therapies to choose between, depending on circumstances, would help overall CAC especially as a short-term alternative [105]. The improved therapeutic outcomes would be based upon the reasonable assumption that more options of effective therapy will be associated with higher overall efficacy and treatment CAC as opposed to a specific doctor dictated therapy CAC.

While little has been reported on barriers to the various alternative treatment options for *SRBD in the USA, the F&S report [11] illustrates the deficit in use of OAT. In France, low socioeconomic status (SES) constitutes a barrier to access to OAT that speaks to inequalities in healthcare access [106]. According to the authors, even though the cost of the OA is reimbursed by the national health insurance, OAs are not prescribed as they should be due to a requirement for adequate oral health of candidate patients that pre-

Table 29.5 Positive attributes of PAP and OAT

Positive attributes of PAP	*Positive attributes of OAT*
Highest efficacy/hour of use	Highest compliance/hours of use per 24 hours
Off the shelf – premade	Requires no power source for use
Broader range of severities that it brings back to normal	Pt. preference over PAP, surgery, and positional therapy
Objective daily feedback information for the patient	Highly portable and self-contained
Remote objective feedback for health provider	Easy maintenance
Can self-adjust according to need – intra- and inter-night	Can only be worn by the patient it was prescribed for
Adjustable controls for heat, humidification, ramping, etc.	Can collect compliance data
Effective starting on first night of use	Many designs and adjustment mechanisms
	Ability for bed partner to adjust during sleep
	Components can deliver other therapies (topical medications)
	Works with nasal congestion
	Works with prone sleeping
	Can concurrently treat temporomandibular disorders
	Can mitigate some headaches
	Can act as a stable strapless PAP interface connector
	Eliminates tooth wear and fractures from sleep bruxism
	Can stabilize mandible for better full face PAP seal
	Readily monitored objectively by patient-driven self-testing

Table 29.6 Negative Attributes of PAP and OAT

Negative attributes of PAP	*Negative attributes of OAT*
Lowest adherence in hours of use per 24 hours	Ineffective in 15–60% related to severity and individuality
May be worn by someone other than the patient	Can move teeth – crowd maxillary and splay mandibular
Claustrophobia in some	Can stress teeth, restorations, and aggravate soft tissues
May dislodge with movements during sleep	Can contribute to temporomandibular dysfunction
Not compatible with prone sleep position	May need refitting/remake after new dental restorations
High maintenance	Will not work in those with heightened gag reflex
Requires periodic filter and interface replacement	Usually requires sufficient number of stable teeth or implants
Noise of equipment can disturb bed partner	Usually requires sufficient ability to protrude mandible
Aerophagia in some	Outcome dependent on provider skill level
Tethering to face is required	Mandible may stay mildly protruded after use for hours
Power source is required	Self-treatment options confound proper use
Not readily portable (e.g., difficult to use in airplane travel)	Lacks self-adjustment intra-night
Unflattering cosmetics	Lacks real-time remote monitoring of use or efficacy
Leaves temporary facial marks from straps	
Long-term intrusion of mid face from mask retention straps	
Difficulty in maintaining air seal	

cludes many with low SES [106]. In a 2014 paper, the barriers to more use of OAT were identified as related to organizational issues, industrial development, different effectiveness, contraindications, side effects, and both dental and medical professional organizational issues [107]. These issues have all been addressed to some degree in this chapter and it is clear that the public will benefit from elimination of these barriers.

Given that the F&S report [11] indicates management of OSA in the best light and finds that 80% of those with OSA are undiagnosed and that PAP adherence for those that accept this therapy is 60%, it follows that the current gold standard protocols of diagnosis and management miss not only the undiagnosed 80% but also a substantial proportion of the remaining 20% who try therapy. According to F&S [11], this would be about another 7% of the population with OSA (40% non-adherent × 85% receiving PAP therapy × 20% diag-

nosed = approx. 7%). Therefore, current gold standards of treatment of OSA using PAP as first-line gold standard therapy are not providing care for a minimum of 87% of the population with OSA. In reality, even the 87% with OSA not getting care is a conservative figure; since PAP is not 100% effective when used, PAP use adherence values are set at 4 hours when at least 6 hours/night is indicated, resulting in CAC values for PAP usage closer to 25% as a long-term measure. Most importantly, the F&S estimate of 12% of the US adult population with OSA dramatically underestimates epidemiologists' assessment that over 25% of US adults have OSA [11, 108] and countries such as Switzerland show over 35% of adults with OSA [109]. In effect it would appear that only a few percent (<5%) of the population with OSA are managed long-term with current gold standards and better solutions are indicated.

Another sad reflection of the CAC failure to treat the public health problem of *SRBD was revealed by Russel et al.

[110], who reviewed the outcomes of a cohort of 616 participants receiving treatment in an academic hospital that met OSA inclusion criteria. While 42% of patients had documented adherence to PAP, about 50% of the non-adherent group did not have continued treatment or even referral for alternative care, and only 35% of the non-adherent group were referred for further attempts at management of the diagnosed OSA. This points to an enormous gap in the continuity of care for those patients that are non-adherent to PAP therapy, indicating a knowledge gap in viable alternative therapies, over reliance on PAP therapy when other therapies are available and increasingly chosen and/or a lack of follow-up and resources for those that cannot tolerate PAP (Fig. 29.3).

Despite positive attributes both PAP and OAT have significant limitations and side effects that reduce compliance. See Table 29.6.

Overall, OAT is a much simpler therapy and has very limited features in comparison to CPAP. OAs can be adjusted internight but not easily intranight without typically waking the patient and contributing to fragmented sleep. Although OAs have options for compliance monitoring, there is no immediate feedback or remote short-range wireless communication technology as to the OA effectiveness and hours of use. Patients are currently required to bring their OA to the dentist to upload compliance data, if tracked, although such data may be stored for a month or more. Furthermore, there is no auto-adjusting of OAT as needed, such as during REM sleep, after drinking alcohol, smoking, or when the sleeper is in a supine position. Night-to-night variability in sleep breathing parameters cannot be automatically addressed, since no "smart oral appliance" is currently marketed. The closest contemporary oral appliance to a self-adjusting design would be by using the MATRx system for an off-label indication. In June 2021 the MATRx home system was discontinued by the developers/manufacturers.

Table 29.2 compares the differences between PAP and OAT. The obvious differences include less untoward side effects of OA, less tethering, less reliance upon a power source, and less background equipment noise to nearby sleepers. Additionally, an OA provides fringe benefits to the user such as protection of the teeth from sleep bruxism wear patterns and some tooth splinting as well as some effects as a tooth retainer. For both OAT and PAP there are a litany of side effects which patients may state prevents them from using therapy more frequently. In both therapies, a period of adaptation is normal and the need for support by the healthcare provider is essential to enable ongoing utilization of therapy (Table 29.7).

29.10 Improving CAC for *SRBD

After discussion of the two most frequently prescribed conservative *SRBD therapies with highest overall efficacy, the question remains as to why choose one therapy over the other. If cost containment principles allowed for both of these and other treatment options to be used, with the end goals of higher CAC and lower overall healthcare costs associated with treated *SRBD, then consideration should be given for multiple primary, backup, and rescue therapies. Certainly, OAT has many options available within this category of therapy when considering both management and potentially preventive/curative OA approaches along with the possibilities of combination therapy with other *SRBD therapies.

*SRBD Projected Future Therapy Apportionment

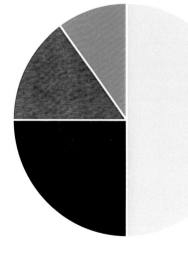

OAT ■ PAP ■ Surgery ■ Other

Fig. 29.3 Future therapy pie for *SRBD

Table 29.7 Comparative advantages of PAP vs. OAT

Measure	PAP – advantage	OAT – advantage
Compliance/adherence		+
Patient preference		+
Durability of components		+
Maintenance		+
Portability		+
Power requirement		+
Ease of use		+
Intrinsic noise		+
Tethering		+
Only fits intended user		+
Mean disease alleviation	+	+
Cost	+	+
Funding and research	+	
Efficacy	+	
Success with all severities	+	
Data connectivity to provider	+	
Direct user feedback	+	
Auto-adjusting option	+	
Compliance monitoring	+	

While there has been a great deal of attention to discovering the predictors of OAT success, including morphometric features, cephalometric measures, BMI, symptoms, behaviors, comorbidities, and sleep index severities, no concrete predictors have been found. Even if a high positive predictive value of OA effectiveness were determined for an individual, there would still be the challenge of CAC with that OA design over time. While there are patterns for prediction, success with OAT is best determined from a therapeutic trial. This OA trial can be self-assessed by the patient using an OA and getting feedback from a bed partner or monitoring device over multiple nights or with an intranight trial at various mandibular protrusive positions in an auto-titrating or lab setting. This is akin to a medication trial for other chronic health conditions. Trials may result in early termination of a medication just as for an OA due to side effects or lack of efficacy, or only found effective if used in combination with other medications or therapies.

29.11 Improving CAC for OAT (Top 10 Approaches)

1. Overcome SES barriers to receiving OAT including the elimination of the requirement for physician prescription for OAT.
2. Increase the number of therapeutic options for patients including multiple primary therapies, backup, and rescue therapies.
3. Application of health behavior models and behavioral techniques such as motivational interviewing to enable success with OAT and more development of concordance in care.
4. Educate healthcare providers on an impartial list of effective *SRBD therapy options with pros and cons for each therapy. Update the gold standard of care to include both personalized care at the individual level and at the population level by attention to population and disease phenotypes.
5. Increase the number of primary sleep healthcare providers from neuroscience, dentistry, and pharmacy able to manage SRBD using a stepped care model and develop better measures of success with therapy.
6. Enable trial, OTC, and auto testing OA design options to overcome resistance to trying OA along with pre-testing to determine nonresponders to OAT.
7. Increase medical insurance reimbursement for OAT both MAD and non-MAD alternatives along with encouraging a wider definition of OAT to include more interest in both management and curative approaches to *SRBD.
8. Increase patient self-testing options to support objective as well as subjective changes when using OAT.
9. Frequent coaching, remotely or in-person, to overcome adaptation hurdles along with increasing patient self-efficacy in OAT by providing up-front solutions to common side effects.
10. Address night-to-night variability with formalized adjustment protocols of the OA and supportive alternate therapies.

29.12 Conclusion

There are large gaps in current protocols to diagnose and treat those with *SRBD. There is a need for population-based solutions involving many different portals of entry into diagnosis and flow of care with staged care. The simple cases may be managed entirely by primary care sleep providers, including those in family medicine, neuroscience, pharmacy, and dentistry, whereas the more complicated *SRBD cases may require care coordinated by a sleep specialist. Better population-level solutions for *SRBD are needed that reflect a sensitivity to CAC measures, and coordinated therapies to increase overall effectiveness. The solution is not a better CAC single therapy outcome but a coordination of all therapies for better *SRBD disorder outcome. OAT has an increasingly important future role in *SRBD care.

References

1. Chakrabarti S. What's in a name? Compliance, adherence and concordance in chronic psychiatric disorders. World J Psychiatry. 2014;4(2):30–6. https://doi.org/10.5498/wjp.v4.i2.30.
2. Hood L, Heath JR, Phelps ME, Lin B. Systems biology and new technologies enable predictive and preventative medicine. Science. 2004;306(5696):640–3.
3. Weston AD, Hood L. Systems biology, proteomics, and the future of healthcare: toward predictive, preventative, and personalized medicine. J Proteome Res. 2004;3(2):179–96.
4. Pack A. Further development of P4 approach to OSA. Sleep Med Clin. 2019;14:379–89.
5. Epstein LJ, Kristo D, Strollo PJ Jr, Friedman N, Malhotra A, Patil SP, Ramar K, Rogers R, Schwab RJ, Weaver EM, Weinstein MD; Adult Obstructive Sleep Apnea Task Force of the American Academy of Sleep Medicine. Clinical guideline for the evaluation, management and long-term care of obstructive sleep apnea in adults. J Clin Sleep Med. 2009;5(3):263–76. PMID: 19960649; PMCID: PMC2699173
6. Bakker JP, Weaver TE, Parthasarathy S, Aloia MS. Adherence to CPAP: what should we be aiming for, and how can we get there? Chest. 2019;155(6):1272–87. https://doi.org/10.1016/j.chest.2019.01.012. Epub 2019 Jan 23. PMID: 30684472
7. Sawyer AM, Gooneratne NS, Marcus CL, Ofer D, Richards KC, Weaver TE. A systematic review of CPAP adherence across age groups: clinical and empiric insights for developing CPAP adherence interventions. Sleep Med Rev. 2011;15(6):343–56. https://doi.org/10.1016/j.smrv.2011.01.003. Epub 2011 Jun 8. PMID: 21652236; PMCID: PMC3202028
8. Antic NA, Catcheside P, Buchan C, et al. The effect of CPAP in normalizing daytime sleepiness, quality of life, and neurocog-

nitive function in patients with moderate to severe OSA. Sleep. 2011;34:111–9.

9. Weaver TE, Maislin G, Dinges DF, et al. Relationship between hours of CPAP use and achieving normal levels of sleepiness and daily functioning. Sleep. 2007;30:711–9.

10. Campos-Rodriguez F, Pena-Grinan N, Reyes-Nunez N, et al. Mortality in obstructive sleep apnea-hypopnea patients treated with positive airway pressure. Chest. 2005;128:624–33.

11. https://aasm.org/resources/pdf/sleep-apnea-economic-crisis.pdf.

12. Carberry JC, Amatoury J, Eckert DJ. Personalized management approach for OSA. Chest. 2018;153(3):744–55. https://doi.org/10.1016/j.chest.2017.06.011. Epub 2017 Jun 16. PMID: 28629917

13. Osman AM, Carter SG, Carberry JC, Eckert DJ. Obstructive sleep apnea: current perspectives. Nat Sci Sleep. 2018;10:21–34. Published 2018 Jan 23. https://doi.org/10.2147/NSS.S124657. Paredes N, Colak O, Gargoum A, Miguez M, Mayoral P, Lagravère Vich M. Anteroposterior and vertical effects of mandibular advancement devices in sleep-disordered patients: a systematic review. J Dent Sleep Med. 2021;8(2).

14. Camacho M, Chang ET, Neighbors CLP, Noller MW, Mack D, Capasso R, Kushida CA. Thirty-five alternatives to positive airway pressure therapy for obstructive sleep apnea: an overview of meta-analyses. Expert Rev Respir Med. 2018;12(11):919–29. https://doi.org/10.1080/17476348.2018.1522253. Epub 2018 Oct 3. PMID: 30204000

15. Cartwright RD, Samelson CF. The effects of a nonsurgical treatment for obstructive sleep apnea. The tongue-retaining device. JAMA. 1982;248:705–9.

16. Schmidt-Nowara W, Lowe A, Wiegand L, Cartwright R, Perez-Guerra F, Menn S. Oral appliances for the treatment of snoring and obstructive sleep apnea: a review. Sleep. 1995;18(6):501–10.

17. Kushida CA, Morgenthaler TI, Littner MR, et al. Practice parameters for the treatment of snoring and Obstructive Sleep Apnea with oral appliances: an update for 2005. Sleep. 2006;29(2):240–3. https://doi.org/10.1093/sleep/29.2.240.

18. Ramar K, Dort LC, Katz SG, Lettieri CJ, Harrod CG, Thomas SM, Chervin RD. Clinical practice guideline for the treatment of obstructive sleep apnea and snoring with oral appliance therapy: an update for 2015. J Clin Sleep Med. 2015;11(7):773–827.

19. Holley AB, Lettieri CJ, Shah AA. Efficacy of an adjustable oral appliance and comparison with continuous positive airway pressure for the treatment of obstructive sleep apnea syndrome. Chest. 2011;140:1511–6.

20. Byun JI, Kim D, Ahn SJ, Yang KI, Cho YW, Cistulli PA, Shin WC. Efficacy of Oral appliance therapy as a first-line treatment for moderate or severe obstructive sleep apnea: a Korean Prospective Multicenter Observational Study. J Clin Neurol. 2020;16(2):215–21. https://doi.org/10.3988/jcn.2020.16.2.215. PMID: 32319237

21. Lam B, Sam K, Lam JC, Lai AY, Lam CL, Ip MS. The efficacy of oral appliances in the treatment of severe obstructive sleep apnea. Sleep Breath. 2011;15(2):195–201. https://doi.org/10.1007/s11325-011-0496-y.

22. Doff MHJ, Hoekema A, Wijkstra PJ, van der Hoven JH, Slater JJRH, de Bont LGM, Stegenga B. Oral appliance versus continuous positive airway pressure in obstructive sleep apnea syndrome: a 2-year follow-up. Sleep. 2013;36(9):1289–96.

23. Haviv Y, Zini A, Almoznino G, Keshet N, Sharav Y, Aframian DJ. Assessment of interfering factors in non-adherence to oral appliance therapy in severe sleep apnea. Oral Dis. 2017;23(5):629–35. https://doi.org/10.1111/odi.12633.

24. Lorenzi-Filho G, Almeida FR, Strollo PJ. Treating OSA: current and emerging therapies beyond CPAP. Respirology. 2017;22(8):1500–7. https://doi.org/10.1111/resp.13144.

25. Ferguson KA, Ono T, Lowe AA, Keenan SP, Fleetham JA. A randomized crossover study of an oral appliance vs nasal-continuous

positive airway pressure in the treatment of mild-moderate obstructive sleep apnea. Chest. 1996;109:1269–75.

26. Oral appliances for obstructive sleep apnea: an evidence-based analysis. Ontario health technology assessment series 2009;9:1–51.

27. Oral appliances for treatment of snoring and obstructive sleep apnea: a review of clinical effectiveness. CADTH technology overviews 2010;1:e0107.

28. Aarab G, Lobbezoo F, Hamburger HL, Naeije M. Oral appliance therapy versus nasal continuous positive airway pressure in obstructive sleep apnea: a randomized, placebo-controlled trial. Respiration. 2011;81:411–9.

29. Bennett LS, Davies RJ, Stradling JR. Oral appliances for the management of snoring and obstructive sleep apnoea. Thorax. 1998;53(Suppl 2):S58–64.

30. Ferguson KA, Cartwright R, Rogers R, Schmidt-Nowara W. Oral appliances for snoring and obstructive sleep apnea: a review. Sleep 2006;29:244–262. Giles TL, Lasserson TJ, Smith BJ, White J, Wright J, Cates CJ. Continuous positive airways pressure for obstructive sleep apnoea in adults. Cochrane Database Syst Rev 2006:CD001106.

31. Hensley M, Ray C. Sleep apnoea. Clin Evid. 2009;2009:2301.

32. Hoekema A. Efficacy and comorbidity of oral appliances in the treatment of obstructive sleep apnea-hypopnea: a systematic review and preliminary results of a randomized trial. Sleep Breath. 2006;10:102–3.

33. Lettieri CJ, Paolino N, Eliasson AH, Shah AA, Holley AB. Comparison of adjustable and fixed oral appliances for the treatment of obstructive sleep apnea. J Clin Sleep Med. 2011;7:439–45.

34. Lim J, Lasserson TJ, Fleetham J, Wright J. Oral appliances for obstructive sleep apnoea. Cochrane Database Syst Rev. 2006:CD004435.

35. Marklund M, Verbraecken J, Randerath W. Non-CPAP therapies in obstructive sleep apnoea: mandibular advancement device therapy. Eur Respir J. 2012;39:1241–7.

36. Mehta A, Qian J, Petocz P, Darendeliler MA, Cistulli PA. A randomized, controlled study of a mandibular advancement splint for obstructive sleep apnea. Am J Respir Crit Care Med. 2001;163:1457.

37. Hoekema A, Voors AA, Wijkstra PJ, et al. Effects of oral appliances and CPAP on the left ventricle and natriuretic peptides. Int J Cardiol. 2008;128:232–9.

38. Itzhaki S, Dorchin H, Clark G, Lavie L, Lavie P, Pillar G. The effects of 1-year treatment with a herbst mandibular advancement splint on obstructive sleep apnea, oxidative stress, and endothelial function. Chest. 2007;131:740–9.

39. Barnes M, McEvoy RD, Banks S, et al. Efficacy of positive airway pressure and oral appliance in mild to moderate obstructive sleep apnea. Am J Respir Crit Care Med. 2004;170:656–64.

40. Gotsopoulos H, Kelly JJ, Cistulli PA. Oral appliance therapy reduces blood pressure in obstructive sleep apnea: a randomized, controlled trial. Sleep. 2004;27:934–41.

41. Iftikhar IH, Hays ER, Iverson MA, Magalang UJ, Maas AK. Effect of oral appliances on blood pressure in obstructive sleep apnea: a systematic review and meta-analysis. J Clin Sleep Med. 2013;9:165–74.

42. Otsuka R, Ribeiro de Almeida F, Lowe AA, Linden W, Ryan F. The effect of oral appliance therapy on blood pressure in patients with obstructive sleep apnea. Sleep Breath. 2006;10(29–36):8.

43. Yoshida K. Effect on blood pressure of oral appliance therapy for sleep apnea syndrome. Int J Prosthodont. 2006;19:61–6.

44. Anandam A, Patil M, Akinnusi M, Jaoude P, El Solh AA. Cardiovascular mortality in obstructive sleep apnea treated with continuous positive airway pressure or oral appliance: an observational study. Respirology. 2013;18:1184–90.

45. Hoekema A, Stegenga B, Wijkstra PJ, van der Hoeven JH, Meinesz AF, de Bont LG. Obstructive sleep apnea therapy. J Dent Res. 2008;87:882–7.

46. Phillips CL, Grunstein RR, Darendeliler MA, Mihailidou AS, Srinivasan VK, Yee BJ, Marks GB, Cistulli PA. Health outcomes of continuous positive airway pressure versus oral appliance treatment for obstructive sleep apnea: a randomized controlled trial. Am J Respir Crit Care Med. 2013;187(8):879–87. https://doi.org/10.1164/rccm.201212-2223OC. PMID: 23413266

47. Levendowski DJ, Morgan TD, Patrickus JE, et al. In-home evaluation of efficacy and titration of a mandibular advancement device for obstructive sleep apnea. Sleep Breath. 2007;11:139–47.

48. Machado MA, Prado LB, Carvalho LB, et al. Quality of life of patients with obstructive sleep apnea syndrome treated with an intraoral mandibular repositioner. Arq Neuropsiquiatr. 2004;62:222–5.

49. Naismith SL, Winter VR, Hickie IB, Cistulli PA. Effect of oral appliance therapy on neurobehavioral functioning in obstructive sleep apnea: a randomized controlled trial. J Clin Sleep Med. 2005;1:374–80.

50. Rose EC, Barthlen GM, Staats R, Jonas IE. Therapeutic efficacy of an oral appliance in the treatment of obstructive sleep apnea: a 2-year follow-up. Am J Orthod Dentofac Orthop. 2002;121:273–9.

51. Saletu A, Anderer P, Parapatics S, Matthai C, Matejka M, Saletu B. Effects of a mandibular repositioning appliance on sleep structure, morning behavior and clinical symptomatology in patients with snoring and sleep disordered breathing. Neuropsychobiology. 2007;55:184–93.

52. Walker-Engstrom ML, Wilhelmsson B, Tegelberg A, Dimenas E, Ringqvist I. Quality of life assessment of treatment with dental appliance or UPPP in patients with mild to moderate obstructive sleep apnoea. A prospective randomized 1-year follow-up study. J Sleep Res. 2000;9:303–8.

53. Marklund M, Franklin KA. Long-term effects of mandibular repositioning appliances on symptoms of sleep apnoea. J Sleep Res. 2007;16:414–20.

54. Walker-Engstrom ML, Tegelberg A, Wilhelmsson B, Ringqvist I. 4-year follow-up of treatment with dental appliance or uvulopalatopharyngoplasty in patients with obstructive sleep apnea: a randomized study. Chest. 2002;121:739.

55. Uniken Venema JAM, Doff MHJ, Joffe-Sokolova D, Wijkstra PJ, van der Hoeven JH, Stegenga B, Hoekema A. Long-term obstructive sleep apnea therapy: a 10-year follow-up of mandibular advancement device and continuous positive airway pressure. J Clin Sleep Med. 2020;16(3):353–9. https://doi.org/10.5664/jcsm.8204. Epub 2020 Jan 14.PMID: 31992403

56. Sutherland K, Phillips CL, Cistulli PA. Efficacy versus effectiveness in the treatment of obstructive sleep apnea: CPAP and oral appliances. J Dental Sleep Med. 2015;2(4):175–81.

57. Yamamoto U, Nishizaka M, Tsuda H, Tsutsui H, Ando SI. Crossover comparison between CPAP and mandibular advancement device with adherence monitor about the effects on endothelial function, blood pressure and symptoms in patients with obstructive sleep apnea. Heart Vessel. 2019;34(10):1692–702. https://doi.org/10.1007/s00380-019-01392-3. Epub 2019 Mar 29. PMID: 30927057

58. Tan YK, L'Estrange PR, Luo YM, Smith C, Grant HR, Simonds AK, Spiro SG, Battagel JM. Mandibular advancement splints and continuous positive airway pressure in patients with obstructive sleep apnoea: a randomized crossover trial. Eur J Orthod. 2002;24:239–49.

59. Sutherland K, Dalci O, Cistulli PA. What do we know about adherence to oral appliances? Sleep Med Clin. 2021;16(1):145–54. https://doi.org/10.1016/j.jsmc.2020.10.004. Epub 2020 Dec 7. PMID: 33485526

60. Kato J, Isono S, Tanaka A, et al. Dose-dependent effects of mandibular advancement on pharyngeal mechanics and nocturnal oxygenation in patients with sleep-disordered breathing. Chest. 2000;117:1065–72.

61. Bamagoos AA, Cistulli PA, Sutherland K, et al. Dose-dependent effects of mandibular advancement on upper airway collapsibility and muscle function in obstructive sleep apnea. Sleep. 2019:pii: zsz049. https://doi.org/10.1093/sleep/zsz049.

62. Azarbarzin A, Sands SA, Stone KL, Taranto-Montemurro L, Messineo L, Terrill PI, Ancoli-Israel S, Ensrud K, Purcell S, White DP, Redline S, Wellman A. The hypoxic burden of sleep apnoea predicts cardiovascular disease-related mortality: the osteoporotic fractures in men study and the sleep heart health study. Eur Heart J. 2019;40(14):1149–57. https://doi.org/10.1093/eurheartj/ehy624. Erratum in: Eur Heart J. 2019 Apr 7;40(14):1157. PMID: 30376054; PMCID: PMC6451769

63. Srijithesh PR, Aghoram R, Goel A, Dhanya J. Positional therapy for obstructive sleep apnoea. Cochrane Database Syst Rev. 2019;5(5):CD010990. https://doi.org/10.1002/14651858.CD010990.pub2. PMID: 31041813; PMCID: PMC6491901

64. Almeida FR, Parker JA, Hodges JS, Lowe AA, Ferguson KA. Effect of a titration Polysomnogram on treatment success with a mandibular repositioning appliance. J Clin Sleep Med. 2009;5(3):198–20.

65. Remmers JE, Topor Z, Grosse J, Vranjes N, Mosca EV, Brant R, Bruehlmann S, Charkhandeh S. Jahromi SA.A feedback-controlled mandibular positioner identifies individuals with sleep apnea who will respond to oral appliance therapy. J Clin Sleep Med. 2017;13(7):871–80.

66. Sutherland K, Ngiam J, Cistulli PA. Performance of remotely controlled mandibular protrusion sleep studies for prediction of oral appliance treatment response. J Clin Sleep Med. 2017;13(3):411–7.

67. Aarab G, Lobbezoo F, Hamburger HL, Naeije M. Effects of an oral appliance with different mandibular protrusion positions at a constant vertical dimension on obstructive sleep apnea. Clin Oral Investig. 2010;14:339–45. https://doi.org/10.1007/s00784-009-0298-9. Epub 2009 Jun 18. PMID: 19536571

68. Anitua E, Durán-Cantolla J, Almeida GZ, Alkhraisat MH. Minimizing the mandibular advancement in an oral appliance for the treatment of obstructive sleep apnea. Sleep Med. 2017;34:226–31. https://doi.org/10.1016/j.sleep.2016.12.019. Epub 2017 Jan 29. PMID: 28228337

69. Powell ED, Gay PC, Ojile JM, Litinski M, Malhotra A. A pilot study assessing adherence to auto-bilevel following a poor initial encounter with CPAP. J Clin Sleep Med. 2012;8(1):43–7. https://doi.org/10.5664/jcsm.1658. PMID: 22334808; PMCID: PMC3266339

70. Vanderveken OM, Dieltjens M, Wouters K, De Backer WA, Van de Heyning PH, Braem MJ. Objective measurement of compliance during oral appliance therapy for sleep-disordered breathing. Thorax. 2013;68(1):91–6. https://doi.org/10.1136/thoraxjnl-2012-201900. Epub 2012 Sep 19. PMID: 22993169; PMCID: PMC3534260. [see 41,67,68 ref below all refs}

71. Dieltjens M, Vanderveken O. Oral appliances in obstructive sleep apnea. Healthcare (Basel). 2019;7(4):141. https://doi.org/10.3390/healthcare7040141.

72. Scherr SC, Dort LC, Almeida FR, Bennett KM, Blumenstock NT, Demko BG, Essick GK, Katz SG, McLornan PM, Phillips KS, Prehn RS, Rogers RR, Schell TG, Sheats RD, Sreshta FP. Definition of an effective oral appliance for the treatment of obstructive sleep apnea and snoring. J Dental Sleep Med. 2014;1(1):51.

73. Mogell K, Blumenstock N, Mason E, Rohatgi R, Shah S, Schwartz D. Definition of an effective oral appliance for the treat-

ment of obstructive sleep apnea and snoring: an update for 2019. J Dent Sleep Med. 2019;6(3)45. Barnes M, McEvoy RD, Banks S, Tarquinio N, Murray CG, Vowles N, Pierce RJ. Efficacy of positive airway pressure and oral appliance in mild to moderate obstructive sleep apnea. Am J Respir Crit Care Med. 2004;170:656–64.

74. Vanderveken OM, Devolder A, Marklund M, et al. Comparison of a custom-made and a thermoplastic oral appliance for the treatment of mild sleep apnea. Am J Respir Critical Care Med. 2008;178:197–202.

75. Johal A, Haria P, Manek S, Joury E, Riha R. Ready-made versus custom-made mandibular repositioning devices in sleep apnea: a randomized clinical trial. J Clin Sleep Med. 2017;13(2):175–82.

76. Colak O, Paredes NA, Elkenawy I, Torres M, Bui J, Jahangiri S, Moon W. Tomographic assessment of palatal suture opening pattern and pterygopalatine suture disarticulation in the axial plane after midfacial skeletal expansion. Prog Orthod. 2020;21(1):21. https://doi.org/10.1186/s40510-020-00321-9. PMID: 32686018; PMCID: PMC7370251

77. Bahammam SA. Rapid maxillary expansion for obstructive sleep apnea among children - systematic review and meta-analysis. Sleep Sci. 2020;13(1):70–7. https://doi.org/10.5935/1984-0063.20190123.

78. Abdullatif J, Certal V, Zaghi S, Song SA, Chang ET, Gillespie MB, Camacho M. Maxillary expansion and maxillomandibular expansion for adult OSA: a systematic review and meta-analysis. J Craniomaxillofac Surg. 2016;44(5):574–8. https://doi.org/10.1016/j.jcms.2016.02.001. Epub 2016 Feb 6. PMID: 26948172

79. Singh GD, Griffin T, Cress SE. Biomimetic oral appliance therapy in adults with severe obstructive sleep apnea. J Sleep Disord Ther. 2016;5(227):2167–277

80. Chamberland S. Consideration of Maxillary Skeletal Expansion (MSE) and Mandibular Symphyseal Distraction Osteogenesis (MSDO) for the treatment of sleep apnea and snoring. J Dent Sleep Med. 2020;7(2)

81. Moore RW, Hart WT. OPAP--a new approach to the management of obstructive sleep apnea. Funct Orthod. 2000;17(1):29–30.

82. Tong BK, Tran C, Ricciardiello A, Donegan M, Chiang AKI, Szollosi I, Amatoury J, Carberry JC, Eckert DJ. CPAP combined with oral appliance therapy reduces CPAP requirements and pharyngeal pressure swings in obstructive sleep apnea. J Appl Physiol (1985). 2020;129(5):1085–91. https://doi.org/10.1152/japplphysiol.00393.2020. Epub 2020 Sep 10. PMID: 32909921

83. El-Solh AA, Moitheennazima B, Akinnusi ME, Churder PM, Lafornara AM. Combined oral appliance and positive airway pressure therapy for obstructive sleep apnea: a pilot study. Sleep Breath. 2011;15(2):203–8.

84. Pang KP, Montevecchi F, Vicini C, Carrasco-Llatas M, Baptista PM, Olszewska E, Braverman I, Kishore S, Chandra S, Yang HC, Chan YH, Pang SB, Pang KA, Pang EB, Rotenberg B. Does nasal surgery improve multilevel surgical outcome in obstructive sleep apnea: a multicenter study on 735 patients. Laryngoscope Investig Otolaryngol. 2020;5(6):1233–9. https://doi.org/10.1002/lio2.452. PMID: 33364416; PMCID: PMC7752065

85. Sullivan CE, Issa FG, Berthon-Jones M, Eves L. Reversal of obstructive sleep apnoea by continuous positive airway pressure applied through the nares. Lancet. 1981;1(8225):862–5. https://doi.org/10.1016/s0140-6736(81)92140-1.

86. Robin P. La chute de la base de la langue considérée comme une nouvelle cause de gans la respiration naso-pharyngienne. Bull Acad Natl Med. 1923;89:37–41.

87. Chang ET, Fernandez-Salvador C, Giambo J, Nesbitt B, Liu SY, Capasso R, Kushida CA, Camacho M. Tongue retaining devices for obstructive sleep apnea: a systematic review and meta-analysis. Am J Otolaryngol. 2017;38(3):272–8. https://doi.org/10.1016/j.amjoto.2017.01.006. Epub 2017

88. Schwab RJ, Kim C, Siegel L, et al. Examining the mechanism of action of a new device using oral pressure therapy for the treatment of obstructive sleep apnea. Sleep. 2014;37(7):1237–47. Published 2014 Jul 1. https://doi.org/10.5665/sleep.3846.

89. Fukuda T, Takei Y, Nakayama H, Inoue Y, Tsuiki S. Continuous tongue suction as a potential therapy for obstructive sleep apnea: a feasibility study. J Dent Sleep Med. 2020;7(3)

90. Deane SA, Cistulli PA, Ng AT, Zeng B, Petocz P, Darendeliler MA. Comparison of mandibular advancement splint and tongue stabilizing device in obstructive sleep apnea: a randomized controlled trial [published correction appears in Sleep. 2009;32(8):table of contents.

91. Sutherland K, Takaya H, Qian J, Petocz P, Ng AT, Cistulli PA. Oral appliance treatment response and polysomnographic phenotypes of obstructive sleep apnea. J Clin Sleep Med. 2015;11(8):861–8.

92. Huntley C, Cooper J, Stiles M, Grewal R, Boon M. Predicting success of oral appliance therapy in treating obstructive sleep apnea using drug-induced sleep endoscopy. J Clin Sleep Med. 2018;14(8):1333–7. https://doi.org/10.5664/jcsm.7266. PMID: 30092884; PMCID: PMC6086966

93. Mullane S, Loke W. Influence of short-term side effects on oral sleep appliance compliance among CPAP-intolerant patients: an objective monitoring of compliance. J Oral Rehabil. 2019;46(8):715–22. https://doi.org/10.1111/joor.12802.

94. Smith YK, Verrett RG. Evaluation of a novel device for measuring patient compliance with oral appliances in the treatment of obstructive sleep apnea. J Prosthodont. 2014;23(1):31–8.

95. Lowe AA, Sjoholm TT, Ryan CF, Fleetham JA, Ferguson KA, Remmers JR. Treatment, airway and compliance effects of a titratable oral appliance. Sleep. 2000;23(Suppl 4):S172–8.

96. Dieltjens M, Verbruggen AE, Braem MJ, et al. Determinants of objective compliance during oral appliance therapy in patients with sleep-disordered breathing: a prospective clinical trial. JAMA. Otolaryngol Head Neck Surg. 2015;141(10):894–900. https://doi.org/10.1001/jamaoto.2015.1756.

97. J Prosthodont. 2014;23(1):31–38. Smith YK, Verrett RG. Evaluation of a novel device for measuring patient compliance with oral appliances in the treatment of obstructive sleep apnea. J Prosthodont. 2014;23(1):31–8. https://doi.org/10.1111/jopr.12076. Epub 2013 Jul 25. PMID: 23889695.

98. Kribbs NB, Pack AI, Kline LR, et al. Objective measurement of patterns of nasal CPAP use by patients with obstructive sleep apnea. Am Rev Respir Dis. 1993;147(4):887–95. https://doi.org/10.1164/ajrccm/147.4.887.

99. Rotenberg BW, Murariu D, Pang KP. Trends in CPAP adherence over twenty years of data collection: a flattened curve. J Otolaryngol Head Neck Surg. 2016;45(1):43. https://doi.org/10.1186/s40463-016-0156-0. PMID: 27542595; PMCID: PMC4992257

100. Quan SF, Awad KM, Budhiraja R, Parthasarathy S. The quest to improve CPAP adherence—PAP potpourri is not the answer. J Clin Sleep Med. 2012;8(1):49–50.

101. Eckert DJ, White DP, Jordan AS, Malhotra A, Wellman A. Defining phenotypic causes of obstructive sleep apnea. Identification of novel therapeutic targets. Am J Resp Crit Care Med. 2013;188(8):996–1004.

102. Eckert DJ. Phenotypic approaches to obstructive sleep apnoea - new pathways for targeted therapy. Sleep Med Rev. 2018;37:45–59. https://doi.org/10.1016/j.smrv.2016.12.003. Epub 2016 Dec 18. PMID: 28110857

103. Weaver TE, Grunstein RR. Adherence to continuous positive airway pressure therapy: the challenge to effective treatment. Proc Am Thor Soc. 2008;5(2):173–8.

104. Wozniak DR, Lasserson TJ, Smith I. Educational, supportive and behavioural interventions to improve usage of continuous positive airway pressure machines in adults with obstructive sleep apnoea.

Cochrane Database Syst Rev. 2014;(1):CD007736. Published 2014 Jan 8

105. Almeida FR, Mulgrew A, Ayas N, et al. Mandibular advancement splint as short-term alternative treatment in patients with obstructive sleep apnea already effectively treated with continuous positive airway pressure. J Clin Sleep Med. 2013;9(4):319–24.

106. Fleury M, Le Vaillant M, Pelletier-Fleury N. IRSR sleep cohort group. Socio-economic status: a barrier to access to mandibular advancement device therapy for patients with obstructive sleep apnea syndrome in France. PLoS One. 2015;10(9):e0138689. https://doi.org/10.1371/journal.pone.0138689. PMID: 26402443; PMCID: PMC4581831

107. Fleury B, Lowe AA. ORal Appliance Network for Global Effectiveness Group. Current barriers and study needs for oral appliance therapy: the personal perspective of a physician and dentist. J Dental Sleep Med. 2014;1(3):123–7.

108. Peppard PE, Young T, Barnet JH, Palta M, Hagen EW, Hla KM. Increased prevalence of sleep-disordered breathing in adults. Am J Epidemiol. 2013;177(9):1006–14. https://doi.org/10.1093/aje/kws342. Epub 2013 Apr 14

109. Heinzer R, Vat S, Marques-Vidal P, et al. Prevalence of sleep-disordered breathing in the general population: the HypnoLaus study. Lancet Respir Med. 2015;3(4):310–8. https://doi.org/10.1016/S2213-2600(15)00043-0.

110. Russell JO, Gales J, Bae C, Kominsky A. Referral patterns and positive airway pressure adherence upon diagnosis of obstructive sleep apnea. Otolaryngol Head Neck Surg. 2015;153(5):881–7. https://doi.org/10.1177/0194599815596169.

Utilization of Wake-Promoting Drugs in Patients on CPAP Therapy

Russell Rosenberg

30.1 Introduction

30.1.1 Prevalence of Excessive Daytime Sleepiness in Obstructive Sleep Apnea

The prevalence of obstructive sleep apnea (OSA) has continued to increase over the last few decades, likely in part due to the growing obesity and diabetes epidemics, with recent estimates suggesting that nearly 1 billion adults worldwide have OSA [1–3]. Excessive daytime sleepiness (EDS) is a key symptom of OSA, but estimations of its prevalence have been inconsistent, and due to its multidimensional nature, it is difficult to establish sleepiness accurately [4]. Some reports approximate that 50–80% of patients with OSA report EDS prior to initiating therapy [5, 6], whereas others claim that 60–70% do not report EDS [7]. These discrepancies could be due to a number of reasons, such as under-recognition in the clinic due to ambiguity in patient reporting of symptoms, prevalence overlap with other comorbid etiologies of EDS, insufficient screening questionnaires, and low agreement among various EDS assessment tools. Alternatively, there is increasing recognition that OSA is a heterogenous disorder with different patterns of clinical presentation.

Among those who do report EDS, studies have shown that the severity of EDS does not correlate with the severity of OSA (as determined by apnea hypopnea index [AHI]), suggesting that factors other than respiratory events and arousal contribute to EDS in this population [8–11]. Indeed, EDS has been shown to persist in some patients despite normalization of breathing, oxygenation, and sleep quality with continuous positive airway pressure (CPAP) therapy (the gold standard treatment for OSA) [12, 13] Population- based studies have estimated that 9–22% of CPAP-treated patients continue to experience EDS, even when other potential causes of sleepiness, such as medications, comorbidities, and inadequate sleep duration, are controlled [14, 15]. There is a dose- response relationship between objectively measured CPAP adherence and persistence of sleepiness on treatment.

To complicate matters, prevalence rates of EDS based on self-report measures are often inconsistent with rates based on objective measures. Prospective studies have suggested that 22–34% of patients self-report EDS after CPAP use; however, objective measures of EDS indicate that, within those populations, up to 65% of patients may experience residual EDS [16–18]. This discrepancy suggests that some patients may not be aware of their sleepiness.

30.1.2 Consequences Associated with EDS in OSA

The adverse effects of EDS are multifactorial and extend beyond the individual patient, also impacting the patient's family, workplace, and society. At the individual level, EDS diminishes mood, quality of life, and cognitive functioning [19–21]. In the workplace, EDS debilitates daily functioning, productivity, and social interactions [19, 22]. Specifically, individuals with EDS have been shown to have impairments in work productivity and activity, such as difficulties with time management, work quantity and quality, and on- the-job social interactions [19, 22]. At the societal level, impairments in cognitive functioning can lead to increased risk of motor vehicle and occupational accidents, thereby posing a safety risk to patients and the community. It has been estimated that individuals with OSA have a 2.5- and 1.8-fold increased risk of getting into a motor vehicle and workplace accident, respectively, when compared to those without OSA [23, 24]. This is particularly concerning considering some patients may be unaware of their sleepiness [16–18]. Indeed, recent evidence demonstrated that OSA was associated with increased motor vehicle crash risk even among those without self-reported EDS, indicating that these individuals failed to recognize the presence or severity of their cognitive impairments [25].

R. Rosenberg (✉)
Neurotrials Research, Atlanta, GA, USA
e-mail: rrosenberg@neurotrials.com

© The Author(s), under exclusive license to Springer Nature Switzerland AG 2022
C. M. Shapiro et al. (eds.), *CPAP Adherence*, https://doi.org/10.1007/978-3-030-93146-9_30

30.1.3 Unmet Need and Objective

Despite emphasis on EDS as a key feature of OSA and the accompanying physical and mental burdens, EDS is often overlooked and underdiscussed in the primary care setting [26]. Given the potential deleterious consequences that EDS may have on patient and public safety, it is critical for physicians to recognize EDS in order to give patients the opportunity to access to diagnosis and receive treatment. Furthermore, the high prevalence of OSA may exceed the capacity of tertiary sleep centers, and with advances in assessment and treatment technologies, it is being advocated that primary care may need to manage simpler cases, reserving referrals to sleep specialists for more complex cases [27]. Thus, it is vital that HCPs be informed on how to manage EDS along the clinical pathway, including how to appropriately screen for and diagnose EDS, when to intervene to enhance adherence to primary OSA treatment, when to use pharmacotherapy, how to choose a suitable agent, and when to refer to a sleep specialist.

Recent reviews have provided thorough reports of the definition, prevalence, pathophysiology, assessment tools, and treatment options associated with EDS in patients with OSA [28, 29]; however, there is a need for step-by-step guidance for practice procedures to help HCPs and respiratory/sleep specialists appropriately evaluate and manage EDS in the OSA population. This review aims to provide suggestions for procedures that can be implemented into routine clinical practice to screen for, identify, and manage EDS in patients with OSA.

30.2 Screening for EDS

30.2.1 Risk Factors for EDS in OSA

Risk factors for EDS in patients with OSA are not well defined, but some have been identified (Table 30.1) [6, 7, 18]. Among patients who have already been diagnosed with and treated for OSA, those with severe EDS at diagnosis are more likely to experience residual EDS after CPAP treatment [6, 14, 15, 18]. Other possible risk factors include younger age and depression [14, 15]. Interestingly, baseline severity of OSA, based on AHI, and body mass index (BMI) do not appear to be risk factors for residual EDS in patients who are adherent to CPAP therapy [6, 14, 15, 18]. It is inconclusive whether comorbid diabetes and hypertension influence the risk of residual EDS, as some [6], but not all [14, 15, 18] studies have reported an association.

Table 30.1 Risk factors for EDS in patients with OSA based on a combination of available studies

Risk factor	Odds ratio
Diabetes [6]	6.9
Baseline[a] EDS [6, 18]	1.3–5.1[b]
Not getting enough sleep [7]	4.6
Heart disease [6]	2.9
Awaken with leg cramps [7]	2.4
Chronic pain [18]	2.3
COPD [7]	2.0
Wake up too early [7]	1.8
Wake up during night [7]	1.8
Respiratory disease [7]	1.8
Depression [18]	1.8
Habitual snorer [7]	1.6
Trouble falling asleep [7]	1.5
Asthma [7]	1.2
Lower respiratory disturbance index [6]	1.0

COPD chronic obstructive pulmonary disease, *CPAP* continuous positive airway pressure, *EDS* excessive daytime sleepiness, *OSA* obstructive sleep apnea
[a]Pre-CPAP treatment
[b]Odds of experiencing residual EDS after CPAP treatment

30.2.2 Subjective Symptoms of EDS

In theory, the easiest way for a HCP to identify whether a patient with OSA has EDS is through recognition of subjective symptoms. Unfortunately, patients' complaints are not always straightforward and illuminating. A patient may use terms other than EDS to express their sleepiness or they may describe associated consequences, such as feeling tired, unrefreshed awakening, lack of energy, feeling fatigued, napping, morning headaches, irritability, or difficulty concentrating [1, 30, 31]. In fact, patients are more likely to report fatigue, tiredness, and lack of energy than sleepiness [30]. Furthermore, they tend to consider lack of energy to be a bigger problem than sleepiness per se [30]. As previously discussed, some patients may simply be unaware of their sleepiness or may not perceive their sleepiness to be troublesome [16–18, 25]. In these cases, symptomatic indications of EDS may be even more subtle. To reduce ambiguity, initial screening for EDS should begin with a clinical consultation, during which the clinician can obtain a thorough past medical history and physical examination. However, the most effective way to ensure EDS is not missed is to use specific screening tools. Patients suspected of having OSA should be assessed for EDS. In addition, since EDS can persist in some patients despite treatment with CPAP therapy, all patients diagnosed with OSA and treated should be assessed for EDS as well.

30.2.3 Self-Report Assessments of EDS

Self-report questionnaires are brief, inexpensive tools, making them convenient for routine clinical practice to screen for EDS (Table 30.2).

The Epworth Sleepiness Scale (ESS) is the most commonly used self-administered assessment for EDS. The ESS is a validated, patient-reported questionnaire for EDS that assesses the propensity to fall asleep in real-world situations [32]. Specifically, patients are asked to rate, on a scale of 0–3 with higher numbers indicating more sleepiness, how likely they would be to doze off or fall asleep in various situations, such as while sitting and reading, watching television, or riding as a passenger in a car. The questionnaire consists of eight items and can be self-administered, making it convenient for use in the clinic. Instructions while administering the ESS can be tailored depending on the time period of interest. For example, patients can be asked to answer the questions based on their level of sleepiness over the last few days, week, or month.

Total scores can range from 0 to 24, with higher scores representing greater levels of sleepiness. To identify a patient with EDS, scores ≤10 are considered within the normal range, whereas scores >10 indicate EDS [32, 33].

Advantages of the ESS include its brevity, accessibility, and widespread use in clinical and research studies. The eight-item questionnaire takes ~2–3 minutes to complete and has been translated, tested, and validated in many languages, making it convenient and accessible to clinicians and researchers around the world [34]. In addition, the ESS has been shown to have high internal consistency in measuring EDS in patients with OSA [11, 35]. Some [11, 36], but not all [37–39], studies have found the ESS to have good test–retest reliability in controlled clinical trial settings or when administered in similar clinical settings, with less reliability when administered across different primary and secondary care settings (e.g., between a PCP and sleep specialist visit). Finally, the widespread use of the ESS has produced extensive evidence for normative scores in clinical and nonclinical samples, facilitating interpretation of results. The main disadvantage of the ESS is its reliance on self-report, making it susceptible to patient's self-awareness of their sleepiness.

The Stanford Sleepiness Scale (SSS) is another self-report assessment tool that can be used to quantify EDS. In contrast

Table 30.2 Tools for evaluating EDS

Tools	Characteristics assessed	Findings suggestive of EDS	Utility	Administrator
Self-report measures				
Epworth Sleepiness Scale (ESS)	Sleep propensity in daily situations (trait sleepiness)	Score >10	To screen for and/or diagnose EDS	Any HCP
Stanford Sleepiness Scale (SSS)	Degree of sleepiness at point in time (state sleepiness)	Score >3	Not ideal for clinical purposes	Any HCP
Karolinska Sleepiness Scale (KSS)	Degree of sleepiness at point in time (state sleepiness)	Score ≥7	Not ideal for clinical purposes	Any HCP
Objective measures				
Multiple Sleep Latency Test (MSLT)	Ability to fall asleep	Mean sleep latency <8 minutes	To make a differential diagnosis (e.g., rule out EDS associated with narcolepsy) To confirm severity of EDS to justify pharmacotherapy	Sleep specialist
Maintenance of Wakefulness Test (MWT)	Ability to stay awake	Mean sleep latency ≤19 minutes	To characterize response to wake-promoting treatment To evaluate functional severity of EDS (i.e., if patient's ability to remain awake is a safety risk)	Sleep specialist
Oxford Sleep Resistance (OSLER) Test	Ability to stay awake	N/A[a]	Simplified behavioral-based version of the MWT	Sleep specialist
Psychomotor Vigilance Test (PVT)	Sustained vigilance (reaction time; lapses in attention)	N/A[b]	To evaluate functional severity of EDS (i.e., if patient's ability to remain awake is a safety risk)	Any HCP
Actigraphy	Graphical summary of sleep and wakefulness patterns; estimates of sleep parameters (e.g., sleep latency, TST, WASO, SE)	N/A	To improve diagnostic accuracy (e.g., rule out insufficient sleep as cause of EDS)	Sleep specialist

EDS excessive daytime sleepiness, *HCP* healthcare provider, *SE* sleep efficiency, *TST* total sleep time, *WASO* wake after sleep onset
[a]No standard cutoff; however, OSLER test mean sleep latency has been shown to be consistent with MWT mean sleep latency
[b]No standard cutoff; however, patients with EDS have been shown to have lower reaction times, greater variability in reaction times across a task, and longer and more frequent lapses

to the ESS, which measures trait EDS over a period of time (e.g., the previous weeks), the SSS measures state EDS at a specific point in time. The SSS asks patients to rate, on a Likert-type scale of 1–7, their level of sleepiness at the current moment. Patients are asked to select the statement that best describes their current perceived state, ranging from [1] feeling active, vital, alert, or wide awake to [7] no longer fighting sleep, sleep onset soon, and having dream-like thoughts [40, 41]. Since the SSS measures situational EDS, it can be administered repeatedly (e.g., every 15 minutes) to observe changes in sleepiness across the day. As such, the SSS is more often used in research settings and is for the most part impractical for clinic settings. Experimentally induced chronic sleep restriction and total sleep deprivation have been shown to increase SSS scores; however, widely available normative data are sparse [41–43]. As a result, the SSS is not well suited for making clinical judgments regarding EDS, especially if administered at a single clinic visit only.

Similar to the SSS, the Karolinska Sleepiness Scale (KSS) is another state focused self- report questionnaire that measures EDS. Patients are asked to rate their sleepiness on a 9-point Likert-type scale by selecting the statement that best reflects their current psycho-physical state (within the prior 10 minutes). Statements range from [1] extremely alert to [9] extremely sleepy – fighting sleep. Scores ≥ 7 correspond to physiologic signs of sleepiness, such as increased alpha and theta activity or difficulty keeping one's eyes open as determined by electroencephalography (EEG) and electrooculography (EOG), respectively [44]. Similar to the SSS, the KSS is sensitive to fluctuations in prior sleep and time of day and typically is not used for clinical purposes [45].

30.2.4 Choosing a Screening Tool

To summarize, self-report questionnaires place little burden on time, cost, and other resources and can be administered in conjunction with the clinical interview, making them convenient for routine clinical practice. The ESS is the best option available for PCPs to realistically implement into day-to-day practice to assess for EDS, although it is limited by a patient's perception of their sleepiness and the potential for lower test– retest reliability along a clinical pathway from primary care to specialist settings, a consideration that warrants further research. Some of these limitations can be overcome if the ESS is filled in separately by the partner of the patient.

30.3   Evaluation

If a patient with OSA is suspected of having EDS, several additional steps should be considered prior to making a diagnosis. Firstly, the HCP should confirm the nocturnal upper airway obstruction is being optimally treated. If the patient continues to experience EDS despite adherence to primary OSA therapy, the HCP should rule out other potential causes of EDS, including lifestyle factors and other competing etiologies. Only after the completion of these evaluation steps should a diagnosis of residual EDS be made.

30.3.1 Optimization of OSA Therapy

The first step in managing a patient with OSA who appears to have EDS is to determine whether the underlying airway obstruction and associated sleep fragmentation is being optimally treated. To start, the clinician should assess whether the patient is adherent to his/her primary OSA therapy, such as CPAP or a mandibular advancement device (MAD). Although some patients who are adherent to CPAP continue to experience EDS, residual EDS has been shown to significantly improve with increased CPAP use, signifying that residual EDS is not completely resistant to CPAP treatment [14]. However, an estimated 30–40% of patients with OSA do not use CPAP as recommended (i.e., are nonadherent) [46]. Data from randomized controlled trials (RCTs) suggest that this prevalence may be even higher, with 50% and 75% of patients being classified as nonadherent after 1 and 5 years of treatment, respectively. Patient adherence to CPAP may depend on several factors, such as demographic characteristics (e.g., age, sex, marital status, socioeconomic status), disease characteristics (e.g., AHI, nocturnal hypoxemia, EDS), technologic factors, patient experience of diagnostic procedures and initial CPAP exposure, psychosocial factors (e.g., risk perception, treatment outcome expectations, self-efficacy), and patient perception of response to CPAP (e.g., symptom improvement) [47].

To determine whether a patient is using their device as recommended, the clinician should ask the patient (and, when available, their bed partner) how many hours per night and nights per week the device is used. For those using CPAP, telemonitoring devices are available that can provide clinicians with objective data on usage [27]. A variety of interventions are available to help improve adherence, such as troubleshooting technical issues (e.g., airway leaks, pressure adjustments, humidity settings), improving side effects (e.g., mask discomfort, dry mouth), and cognitive- behavior therapies such as framing. Detailed approaches to implementing these interventions have been published and are beyond the scope of this review [48–51]; however, establishing whether the HCP or sleep specialist is responsible for optimizing adherence is relevant. Studies have shown that clinical management of patients with OSA, including adherence to CPAP, tends to be better when the patient is treated by a board-certified sleep specialist rather than a HCP [52, 53]. For example, some patients may not be sufficiently adherent to CPAP, despite the best efforts by both patient and HCP. In these cases, referral to a sleep specialist may be appropriate.

30.3.2 Differential Diagnosis

If the patient is still experiencing EDS after optimal adherence to primary OSA therapy has been confirmed, the next course of action is to rule out other potential causes of EDS, beginning with lifestyle factors. The most common cause of EDS in the general population is insufficient sleep, with more than one third of American adults sleeping less than is recommended to prevent cognitive, health, and safety-related impairments [54, 55]. Indeed, patients with OSA who do not get enough sleep have a 4.6-fold increased risk of having EDS (Table 30.1) [6, 7, 18]. HCPs should advise patients to get at least 7 hours of sleep each night [55], maintain a consistent sleep/wake, create a comfortable sleep environment (e.g., dark, quiet bedroom with a cooler temperature; electronics, including cell phones, turned off or silenced), and practice good sleep hygiene (e.g., avoid electronics and arousing/stressful activities, such as social media, email, finances, or an action movie, prior to bed). In addition to optimizing sleep, HCPs should evaluate a patient's diet (e.g., caffeine consumption) and exercise habits.

In addition to lifestyle factors, EDS can have many other etiologies, such as medications, substance abuse, other sleep disorders, psychiatric disorders, or medical disorders (Table 30.3). For instance, OSA and depression can both cause EDS and have many other overlapping symptoms, such as poor concentration, irritability, psychomotor impairments, and weight gain; also see Chap. 19 [56]. If the HCP assumes EDS is due to OSA before making a differential diagnosis, the patient may miss an opportunity to receive treatment for depression. In most cases, a differential diagnosis can be made based on a clinical interview (health history and physical examination); however, further testing with questionnaires, laboratory tests, or objective assessments may be needed in other cases.

30.3.3 Objective Assessments for EDS

Several objective assessments are available to evaluate EDS (Table 30.2). Unfortunately, most objective assessments are time consuming, expensive, and complex to administer (i.e., require an experienced technologist and/or sleep laboratory). For these reasons, it is not feasible to use these assessments to assess EDS in routine practice; however, they may be helpful when attempting to make a differential diagnosis (e.g., rule out narcolepsy as the cause of EDS) [57, 58], justify use of pharmacotherapy, or evaluate response to treatment.

Table 30.3 Differential diagnosis of EDS

Lifestyle factors
Insufficient sleep
Diet
Exercise
Sleep disorders
Narcolepsy (type 1 or 2)
Idiopathic hypersomnia
Kleine–Levin syndrome
Circadian rhythm sleep–wake disorders
Restless legs syndrome
Periodic limb movement disorder
Psychiatric disorders
Depression
Anxiety
Substance use
Medical disorders
Diabetes
Hypothyroidism
Renal disease
Hepatic encephalopathy
Medications
Antihistamines
Anxiolytics
Antidepressants
Anticonvulsants
Beta blockers
Mood stabilizers
Antipsychotics
Opioids
Sedative–hypnotics

EDS excessive daytime sleepiness

The Multiple Sleep Latency Test (MSLT) and Maintenance of Wakefulness Test (MWT) are the most commonly used objective assessments for characterizing an individual's ability to fall asleep or stay awake, respectively. Prior to undergoing the MSLT, a full polysomnogram is required. The clinical MSLT protocol consists of five 20-minute nap opportunities, performed at 2-hour intervals with the first nap opportunity occurring 1.5–3 hours after awakening from the nocturnal sleep episode (recorded by in-laboratory polysomnography). During each nap opportunity, the patient is asked to try to fall asleep in a sleep-inducing environment (i.e., lying down in a dark, quiet bedroom). When using the MSLT to diagnose EDS, the outcome of interest is mean sleep onset latency, or the average amount of time it takes the patient to fall asleep, as determined by EEG and EOG. A mean sleep latency <8 minutes is considered indicative of EDS [57, 59]. When using the MSLT to determine whether narcolepsy is a potential cause of EDS, the presence of sleep onset rapid eye movement periods (SOREMPs) is considered in combination with mean sleep onset latency [57].

A PSG is not required prior to an MWT. The MWT is similar to the MSLT; however, rather than assessing a patient's ability to fall asleep, it assesses a patient's ability to stay awake [58]. To do so, the patient is instructed to remain awake for as long as possible while seated in a dark, quiet environment. A variety of MWT protocols have been used, but a four-trial 40-minute test is recommended for clinical purposes [58]. Similar to the MSLT, the trials are performed at 2-hour intervals, with the first beginning 1.5–3 hours after awakening, and the outcome of interest is mean sleep onset latency. A mean sleep latency ≤19 minutes on the 40-minute MWT has been suggested to indicate EDS [60]; however, the American Academy of Sleep Medicine (AASM) advises that the MWT should not be used for diagnostic purposes [57]. Instead, it may be useful to evaluate response to treatment or assess whether an individual's ability to remain awake poses a public or personal safety risk, such as those employed in public transportation [58]. It is important to note that MSLT reflects sleepiness and MWT reflects wakefulness on a single day. As such, they are most informative when performed while the patient is well rested (i.e., has adhered to his/her typical sleep/wake schedule for at least a week and has obtained optimal sleep the night prior to the test) and compliant with primary OSA therapy [58].

The use of EEG to determine sleep latency renders the MSLT and MWT burdensome, labor intensive, and complex for settings other than a sleep laboratory. Although less standardized, there are tests that use methods other than EEG to objectively quantify EDS. The Oxford Sleep Resistance (OSLER) Test and Psychomotor Vigilance Task (PVT) use simple behavioral-based methods to measure sleep latency and sustained vigilance, respectively. Similar to the MWT, the OSLER test measures a patient's ability to stay awake in a non-stimulating environment during four 40-minute trials [61, 62]. Instead of using EEG to determine sleep onset, the OSLER instructs patients to press a button each time a flash of dim light appears on a device; sleep onset is determined by failure to respond after 21 seconds. Studies have shown that the OSLER test can estimate mean sleep latency and discriminate patients with EDS associated with OSA from healthy participants as accurately as the MWT [61]. Although still time consuming, this method is less expensive and requires less training for administration and interpretation than the MWT.

The PVT is a simple behavioral task that assesses a patient's ability to sustain attention by measuring reaction time. Participants are instructed to attend to a focal point and press a button as quickly as possible in response to a randomly reoccurring visual stimulus over a period of 10 minutes, although variations of the test have been used (e.g., auditory or tactile stimuli and durations other than 10 minutes) [63–65]. Various outcomes can be assessed, such as median reaction time or lapses in attention (defined as reaction times >500 ms). Studies have shown that patients with OSA have impaired PVT performance compared with healthy controls [66], and patients with more severe EDS (i.e., higher ESS scores) have significantly longer reaction times and more

lapses in attention than those with less severe EDS [67]. Although slowed reaction time and lapses in attention can be applicable to real-world outcomes, such as driving off the road or going through a red light [68], thresholds indicative of EDS have not been established, making it difficult for HCPs to use PVT results to make clinical decisions.

One advantage of the PVT is that it is available on a portable device and, more recently, as an app for mobile devices [63, 69]. In theory, this accessibility would be convenient for routine clinical care; however, to date, the PVT has had limited utility outside research and clinical trial settings.

Finally, home-based wearables, such as actigraph watches, can provide insight into sleep and wakefulness patterns in the home environment. Sleep diaries are often used to estimate at-home sleep/wake schedules, but they are susceptible to bias, cumbersome to complete, and impractical for patients with impaired cognition, literacy, or motivation. Actigraphy estimates sleep parameters based on activity and light exposure levels, providing an objective alternative to sleep diaries [70]. Actigraphy is less obtrusive and less expensive and requires less expertise to administer and analyze than the MSLT or MWT. In addition, actigraphy can capture 24-hour sleep habits over long periods (weeks or months) in the real world, as opposed to a single day in the laboratory. Typically, actigraphy is used to improve diagnostic accuracy of the MSLT or MWT (i.e., to ensure the patient has obtained sufficient sleep prior to test day), rather than as a diagnostic test in and of itself [57, 70, 71]. However, a recent meta-analysis conducted by an AASM task force determined that actigraphy-based sleep latency estimates are reliable enough to be used for clinical decision-making, including assessment of treatment-related changes, in patients with insomnia [70]. However, its reliability in estimating sleep latency in patients with OSA has not been examined and few studies have directly compared the diagnostic reliability of actigraphy with polysomnography-based assessments, especially in regard to EDS. Nonetheless, actigraphy may serve as a useful tool when attempting to make a differential diagnosis (e.g., to rule out insufficient sleep as a cause for EDS).

30.3.4 Correlation Between Subjective Symptoms, Self-Report Assessments, and Objective Assessments

Subjective symptoms and self-report measures of EDS often do not correlate with objective measures of EDS. In patients with OSA, complaints of sleepiness, tiredness, lack of energy, and fatigue have been found to have no association with MSLT mean sleep latency [30]. In addition, a systematic review concluded that there was only a moderate association between the ESS and MWT and a weak association between the ESS and MSLT [11]. There are several possible explanations for the low agreements between self-report and objective measures of EDS. As previously discussed, patients may simply be unaware of the severity of their sleepiness, especially if their baseline reference for feeling "normal" has gradually shifted. On the other hand, patients may be reluctant to report negative feelings associated with disease, for fear of work- or driving- related implications. Indeed, research has shown that close relatives often describe the patient as having more severe levels of sleepiness than the patient themself reports [72]. Another potential reason may be that these assessments measure different dimensions of EDS. For example, objective PVT performance has been shown to be associated with ESS scores, but not with MSLT sleep latency [73]. The authors postulated that the PVT and ESS may predict impaired performance, whereas the MSLT may predict physiologic sleep propensity [73].

30.3.5 Choosing an Evaluation Method

To summarize, objective assessments can be useful when attempting to make a differential diagnosis. EEG-based objective assessments of EDS are not practical options for primary care settings. If the HCP suspects their use is necessary, the HCP should refer the patient to a sleep specialist for further evaluation; the sleep specialist will determine what additional testing is appropriate. Behavioral-based objective assessments show promise for use in routine care as they are less influenced by patient perception than self-report assessments and are more accessible than EEG-based assessments; however, to date, their clinical utility has been limited and additional research is needed to establish cutoff values indic-

ative of EDS. Once the clinician has confirmed that the patient's symptoms are indeed residual EDS associated with OSA, the severity of EDS should be evaluated with the ESS or objective assessments.

Characterizing the severity of the residual EDS will be helpful for making treatment decisions.

30.4 Treatment

Only after a diagnosis of residual EDS and altered quality of life associated with OSA has been confirmed and other contributing conditions have been ruled out should pharmacologic treatment with a wake-promoting agent or stimulant be considered. The decision to prescribe a trial of pharmacotherapy can be based upon EDS severity. In general, ESS scores ≥ 10 indicate that the patient's EDS is burdensome and interfering with daily life; however, this threshold is not absolute. Clinical judgment should be made on an individual basis, especially for patients whose occupations may pose a personal and/or public safety risk (e.g., those working in public transportation, healthcare, or childcare). As previously discussed, several objective assessments are available to help evaluate the functional severity of EDS. If pharmacologic treatment is determined to be appropriate, it is important to note that pharmacotherapy for EDS should not replace primary treatment of the underlying airway obstruction. Moreover, there is the risk for pharmacotherapy to decrease CPAP use. Clinicians should monitor patients' CPAP use after initiating pharmacologic treatment to confirm adherence. Key information for the treatment options discussed below is summarized in Table 30.4.

Table 30.4 Pharmacotherapy options for EDS in OSA

Agent	Dosing	Side effects	Drug interactions/contraindications
FDA-approved			
Modafinil (Provigil®) [74]	200 mg/day Initiate at 100 or 200 mg/day Administer once daily in morning	Serious rash, including Stevens–Johnson syndrome Headache Nausea Nervousness Rhinitis Diarrhea Back pain Anxiety Insomnia Dizziness Dyspepsia	Steroidal contraceptive Cyclosporine CYP2C19 substrates (e.g., omeprazole, phenytoin, diazepam)
Armodafinil (Nuvigil®) [75]	150 or 250 mg/day Initiate at 150 mg/day Administer once daily in morning	Serious rash, including Stevens–Johnson syndrome Headache Nausea Dizziness Insomnia	Steroidal contraceptive Cyclosporine CYP2C19 substrates (e.g., omeprazole, phenytoin, diazepam)

(continued)

Table 30.4 (continued)

Agent	Dosing	Side effects	Drug interactions/contraindications
Solriamfetol (Sunosi™) [85]	37.5, 75, or 150 mg/day Initiate at 37.5 mg/day Administer once daily on waking	Headache Nausea Decreased appetite Insomnia Anxiety	Monoamine oxidase inhibitors Drugs that increase blood pressure and/or heart rate Dopaminergic drugs
Off-label			
Pitolisant (Wakix®) [90]	17.8–35.6 mg/day Initiate at 8.9 mg/day Administer once daily in morning	Insomnia Nausea Anxiety QT interval prolongation	Patients with severe hepatic impairment CYP2D6 inducers CYP3A4 substrates, including hormonal contraceptives
Methylphenidate (Ritalin®) [96]	5, 10, or 20 mg/day Administer 20–30 mg 2 or 3 times daily, preferably 30–45 minutes before meals (maximum dose of 60 mg/day)	Tachycardia Palpitations Headache Insomnia Anxiety Hyperhidrosis Weight loss Decreased appetite Dry mouth Nausea Abdominal pain	Monoamine oxidase inhibitors Antihypertensive drugs Halogenated anesthetics
Amphetamines (e.g., Adderall® [97] and Dexedrine® [98])	5–60 mg/day Initiate at 10 mg/day Administer at the lowest effective dose and adjust on an individual patient basis Administer in divided doses; first dose upon awakening with subsequent doses at intervals of 4–6 hours Avoid late evening doses due to resulting insomnia	Palpitations Tachycardia Blood pressure increased Sudden death Cardiomyopathy Overstimulation Restlessness Dizziness Irritability Insomnia Euphoria Dyskinesia Dysphoria Depression Tremor Headache Exacerbation of motor and phonic tics and Tourette's syndrome Aggression Anger Logorrhea Dermatillomania Vision blurred Mydriasis Dry mouth Unpleasant taste Diarrhea Constipation Anorexia/weight loss Urticaria Hypersensitivity reactions (angioedema and anaphylaxis) Serious skin rash, including Stevens–Johnson syndrome and toxic epidermal necrolysis Impotence Changes in libido Frequent/prolonged erections Alopecia Rhabdomyolysis	Patients with advanced arteriosclerosis, symptomatic cardiovascular disease, moderate-to-severe hypertension, hyperthyroidism, known hypersensitivity or idiosyncrasy to the sympathomimetic amines, glaucoma, or agitated states Patients with history of drug abuse Monoamine oxidase inhibitors Acidifying agents, adrenergic blockers, alkalinizing agents, tricyclic antidepressants, CYP2D6 inhibitors, serotonergic drugs, antihistamines, antihypertensives, chlorpromazine, ethosuximide, haloperidol, lithium carbonate, meperidine, methenamine therapy, norepinephrine, phenobarbital, phenytoin, propoxyphene, proton pump inhibitors, veratrum alkaloids

30.4.1 Modafinil and Armodafinil

Modafinil (Provigil®; Teva Pharmaceuticals, North Wales, PA) and armodafinil (Nuvigil®; Teva Pharmaceuticals) are approved in the United States to improve wakefulness in adults with EDS associated with narcolepsy, OSA, or shift work disorder [74, 75]. Both agents have demonstrated efficacy in reducing EDS and improving wakefulness in patients with OSA in short-term RCTs [76–79] and long-term open-label extension trials, improving ESS scores by ~2 points and MWT sleep latency by ~3 minutes compared with placebo [80–82]. Modafinil had previously been approved for this indication in the European Union; however, in 2011, the European Medicines Agency (EMA) withdrew the indication for OSA from the marketing authorization due to a poor benefit/risk profile [83]. Specifically, the EMA concluded that risk of serious cardiovascular disorders, neuropsychiatric disorders, and skin and hypersensitivity disorders outweighed any potential benefit for EDS in patients with OSA [83].

In terms of dosing, modafinil can be initiated at 100 or 200 mg/day (maximum recommended dose of 200 mg/day), taken as a single dose in the morning. Doses up to 400 mg/day have been well tolerated; however, evidence does not suggest additional benefit with doses higher than 200 mg/day [74]. Similarly, armodafinil can be initiated at 150 or 250 mg/day (maximum recommended dose of 250 mg/day), taken as a single dose in the morning. Although 250 mg/day is a Food and Drug Administration (FDA)- approved dose, there is limited evidence suggesting additional benefit beyond 150 mg/day [75].

The most common side effect experienced with both agents is headache, although armodafinil tends to be associated with a lower rate of headache than modafinil [84]. Other common side effects include nausea, dizziness, insomnia, upper respiratory tract infection, and anxiety [84]. In addition, serious skin rashes, such as Stevens–Johnson syndrome and toxic epidermal necrolysis, and hypersensitivity, including angioedema and anaphylactoid reaction, have been reported. Therefore, the EMA withdrew approval due to potential adverse cardiovascular effects, and the FDA issued a warning for use in patients with known cardiovascular disease [74, 75]. A recent meta-analysis concluded that modafinil and armodafinil may slightly increase blood pressure, but not by a clinically significant amount [82]. Regardless, clinicians should monitor patients' blood pressure prior to initiating and routinely during treatment with modafinil or armodafinil. Particularly relevant to a large number of patients is modafinil and armodafinil's interaction with hormonal contraceptives. These agents can reduce the effectiveness of birth control; therefore, if prescribed to premenopausal women, alternative methods of contraception are recommended and should be discussed.

30.4.2 Solriamfetol

Solriamfetol (Sunosi™; Jazz Pharmaceuticals, Inc., Palo Alto, CA) is a dopamine/norepinephrine reuptake inhibitor approved in the United States and European Union to improve wakefulness in adults with EDS associated with narcolepsy or OSA [85, 86]. Solriamfetol has demonstrated efficacy in reducing EDS and improving wakefulness in patients with OSA in short-term RCTs [87, 88] and a long-term open-label extension trial, improving ESS scores by ~2–5 points and MWT sleep latency by ~5–13 minutes compared with placebo [89].

In terms of dosing, solriamfetol can be initiated at 37.5 mg/day and then titrated up 1 dose level every 3 days to 75 mg/day or a maximum dose of 150 mg/day [85]. Solriamfetol should be administered once daily upon awakening, and administration within 9 hours of scheduled bedtime should be avoided due to its potential to interfere with sleep.

The most common side effects with solriamfetol treatment include headache, nausea, decreased appetite, insomnia, and anxiety [85]. In addition, solriamfetol treatment has been associated with small mean increases in heart rate and blood pressure in patients with OSA, although increases were greatest for the 300 mg/day dose, which is not FDA-approved [87]. Regardless, patients' hypertension should be controlled prior to initiating solriamfetol, and heart rate and blood pressure should be monitored periodically during treatment. The FDA advises that use in patients with unstable cardiovascular disease, serious heart arrhythmias, or other serious heart problems should be avoided.

Solriamfetol is contraindicated with monoamine oxidase inhibitors; therefore, clinicians should avoid prescribing solriamfetol with this antidepressant.

30.4.3 Pitolisant (Off-Label)

Pitolisant (Wakix®; Harmony Biosciences, LLC, Plymouth Meeting, PA) is a histamine-3 receptor antagonist approved in the United States to improve wakefulness in adults with EDS associated with narcolepsy [90]. Although not currently FDA-approved for EDS associated with OSA, a recent phase 3 RCT demonstrated the efficacy of pitolisant in reducing EDS in patients with OSA who refused CPAP therapy, improving ESS scores by ~3 points relative to placebo [91]. In contrast to modafinil, armodafinil, and solriamfetol, pitolisant was not effective in improving objective wakefulness.

In terms of dosing, pitolisant has been tested in Europe at doses of 5, 10, and 20 mg/day in patients with OSA, with administration occurring once daily upon awakening. Treatment was initiated at 5 mg/day, followed by a 2-week titration period [91]. These doses are lower than those FDA-approved for patients with narcolepsy, which consists of a recommended 8.9 mg initiation dose followed by stable doses of 17.8–35.6 mg/day [90].

The most common side effect associated with pitolisant is headache. Other common side effects include insomnia, nausea, and vertigo [91]. In patients with narcolepsy, pitolisant is contraindicated in patients with severe hepatic impairment. Additionally, the FDA issued a warning for use with drugs that increase the QT interval and in patients with risk factors for prolonged QT interval, as pitolisant has been associated with QT interval prolongation [90]. Similar to modafinil and armodafinil, pitolisant can reduce the effectiveness of hormonal contraceptives.

30.4.4 Stimulants (Off-Label)

Stimulants, such as methylphenidate (Ritalin®; Novartis Pharmaceuticals Corporation, East Hanover, NJ) and amphetamines (Adderall® [Teva Select Brands, Horsham, PA] or Dexedrine® [Teva Pharmaceuticals]), have also been used off-label to treat EDS associated with OSA. Importantly, no RCTs or published data exist to support their use in the OSA population. In addition, stimulants are associated with extensive side-effect profiles that limit their use. Furthermore, there is a high potential for abuse and addiction with stimulants. As such, most are classified as schedule II controlled substances.

30.4.5 Follow-Up

After initiating a trial of pharmacotherapy, the clinician should follow up with the patient to evaluate efficacy, side effects, and adherence to primary OSA therapy. To determine efficacy, the HCP can re-administer the ESS. Determining whether a patient has responded to treatment based on ESS scores can be considered based on the absolute score or the degree of change. In the first case, ESS scores may have decreased within the normal range ($\leq$10); however, significant improvement may not be observable until after many weeks of stable treatment [77, 91, 92]. In the second case, the clinician can assess the percent reduction (improvement) in ESS scores relative to baseline, using a reduction in ESS score $\geq$25% from baseline as a threshold for a clinically meaningful response to treatment [93, 94]. Alternatively, some data suggest that a 2- to 3-point reduction in ESS score, corresponding to an effect size of 0.5, represents the minimal clinically important difference [91].

In addition to evaluating efficacy, the HCP should monitor for adverse events, particularly cardiovascular side effects (e.g., hypertension). Heart rate and blood pressure should be monitored prior to initiating and periodically

throughout treatment with any wake-promoting agent or stimulant. With modafinil and armodafinil, some side effects, such as rashes, may occur weeks after initiation. With solriamfetol, the most common early-onset side effects (those that occur during the first week of treatment) are short-lived (~10 days in duration) [95].

Finally, the HCP should monitor changes in the use of primary OSA therapy to ensure the underlying airway obstruction continues to be treated. Adherence can be assessed through self-report or, in the case of CPAP devices, digital recordings of usage data.

30.4.6 Choosing an Agent

To summarize, choosing a pharmacologic agent to treat residual EDS in a patient with OSA should be individualized to the patient, taking into account the evidence available regarding an agent's efficacy and safety profile, cost, and patient characteristics (e.g., cardiovascular conditions, childbearing potential, or other comorbid conditions). Among the pharmacotherapies available, modafinil, armodafinil, and solriamfetol have the most evidence from RCTs to support their use in patients with OSA. Pitolisant may be an alternative, but, to date, data are limited. While stimulants can be used, no clinical trials demonstrating their efficacy exist and they are associated with more side effects than the other agents. For these reasons, wake-promoting agents are likely a better treatment option for patients with known cardiovascular disorders, such as hypertension. For women of childbearing potential, solriamfetol may provide a better treatment option than modafinil, armodafinil, or pitolisant as it does not interact with hormonal contraceptives. Regardless of which agent is chosen, the HCP should assess a patient's response to treatment during follow-up visits. Efficacy should be evaluated with the ESS and tolerability by assessing adverse events. In addition, the HCP should periodically monitor blood pressure (6-monthly) and heart rate, consider a 12-lead ECG annually, and monitor adherence to primary OSA therapy.

Whether to treat patients who struggle with adherence to primary OSA therapy with a pharmacologic agent warrants discussion. First and foremost, treatment of EDS with a wake-promoting agent or stimulant is not a replacement for treatment of the underlying airway obstruction. For every patient, best efforts should be made to optimize adherence to CPAP or other airway therapies. Even in patients who are adherent, pharmacologic treatment has the potential to reduce motivation to use CPAP. This has been demonstrated with modafinil and armodafinil, although data suggest that adherence to primary OSA therapy remains stable during treatment with solriamfetol [84, 87]. Pitolisant has only been evaluated in patients with OSA who refused CPAP treatment; therefore, it is unknown whether pitolisant impacts on primary OSA therapy adherence [91]. Sometimes, despite the best efforts by clinician and patient, patients remain nonadherent to primary OSA therapy. In these cases, investigation of the potential causes for nonadherence is warranted and interventions such as changing masks, evaluating pressure, and CBT may be considered.****.

30.5 When to Refer to a Sleep Specialist

In cases when the HCP may be unable to evaluate or manage a patient's EDS, a referral to a sleep specialist for further evaluation and/or testing (e.g., an MSLT, MWT, or overnight polysomnography) may be necessary. This could be, for example, when a HCP may want to confirm that OSA is being optimally treated before prescribing wake- promoting pharmacotherapy for residual EDS, or a HCP may have uncertainty about the cause of EDS, especially in cases that may have multiple sources.

30.6 Conclusions

EDS negatively impacts patients' ability to function in daily life and is a risk factor for patient and public health. As such, it is important for any physician to be able to recognize, evaluate, and manage EDS in patients with OSA in order to provide patients with the opportunity to receive treatment. Due to the high prevalence, it falls to the HCPs to assess patients diagnosed with OSA for EDS with the ESS. If a patient is suspected of having EDS, the HCP should first confirm the nocturnal apneas and hypopneas are being optimally treated. If the patient continues to experience EDS despite adherence to CPAP or other OSA therapies, the patient should be reviewed in clinic, and, when appropriate, questionnaires, physical examination, laboratory tests, or objective assessments to rule out other potential causes of EDS should be considered. After a differential diagnosis of residual EDS associated with OSA has been confirmed, pharmacologic treatment using a wake-promoting agent may be considered. Consistent use of this proposed approach to screening and management can help PCPs identify patients with EDS, improve diagnostic accuracy, and enhance management strategies in the primary care setting and make optimal use of secondary and tertiary resources in specialist centers.

References

1. Young T, Palta M, Dempsey J, Skatrud J, Weber S, Badr S. The occurrence of sleep-disordered breathing among middle-aged adults. N Engl J Med. 1993;328(17):1230–5.

2. Peppard PE, Young T, Barnet JH, Palta M, Hagen EW, Hla KM. Increased prevalence of sleep-disordered breathing in adults. Am J Epidemiol. 2013;177(9):1006–14.
3. Benjafield AV, Ayas NT, Eastwood PR, et al. Estimation of the global prevalence and burden of obstructive sleep apnoea: a literature-based analysis. Lancet Respir Med. 2019;7(8):687–98.
4. American Academy of Sleep Medicine. Obstructive sleep apnea, adult. International Classification of Sleep Disorders. 3rd ed. Darien, IL: American Academy of Sleep Medicine; 2014. p. 53–62.
5. Bailly S, Destors M, Grillet Y, et al. Obstructive sleep apnea: a cluster analysis at time of diagnosis. PLoS One. 2016;11(6):e0157318.
6. Koutsourelakis I, Perraki E, Economou NT, et al. Predictors of residual sleepiness in adequately treated obstructive sleep apnoea patients. Eur Respir J. 2009;34(3):687–93.
7. Kapur VK, Baldwin CM, Resnick HE, Gottlieb DJ, Nieto FJ. Sleepiness in patients with moderate to severe sleep-disordered breathing. Sleep. 2005;28(4):472–7.
8. Macey PM, Woo MA, Kumar R, Cross RL, Harper RM. Relationship between obstructive sleep apnea severity and sleep, depression and anxiety symptoms in newly-diagnosed patients. PLoS One. 2010;5(4):e10211.
9. Lipford MC, Wahner-Roedler DL, Welsh GA, Mandrekar J, Thapa P, Olson EJ. Correlation of the Epworth sleepiness scale and sleep-disordered breathing in men and women. J Clin Sleep Med. 2019;15(1):33–8.
10. Gabryelska A, Białasiewicz P. Association between excessive daytime sleepiness, REM phenotype and severity of obstructive sleep apnea. Sci Rep. 2020;10(1):34.
11. Kendzerska TB, Smith PM, Brignardello-Petersen R, Leung RS, Tomlinson GA. Evaluation of the measurement properties of the Epworth Sleepiness Scale: a systematic review. Sleep Med Rev. 2014;18(4):321–31.
12. Patil SP, Ayappa IA, Caples SM, Kimoff RJ, Patel SR, Harrod CG. Treatment of adult obstructive sleep apnea with positive airway pressure: an American Academy of sleep medicine systematic review, meta-analysis, and GRADE assessment. J Clin Sleep Med. 2019;15(2):335–43.
13. Epstein LJ, Kristo D, Strollo PJ Jr, et al. Clinical guideline for the evaluation, management and long-term care of obstructive sleep apnea in adults. J Clin Sleep Med. 2009;5(3):263–76.
14. Gasa M, Tamisier R, Launois SH, et al. Residual sleepiness in sleep apnea patients treated by continuous positive airway pressure. J Sleep Res. 2013;22(4):389–97.
15. Pepin JL, Viot-Blanc V, Escourrou P, et al. Prevalence of residual excessive sleepiness in CPAP-treated sleep apnoea patients: the French multicentre study. Eur Respir J. 2009;33(5):1062–7.
16. Antic NA, Catcheside P, Buchan C, et al. The effect of CPAP in normalizing daytime sleepiness, quality of life, and neurocognitive function in patients with moderate to severe OSA. Sleep. 2011;34(1):111–9.
17. Weaver TE, Maislin G, Dinges DF, et al. Relationship between hours of CPAP use and achieving normal levels of sleepiness and daily functioning. Sleep. 2007;30(6):711–9.
18. Budhiraja R, Kushida CA, Nichols DA, et al. Predictors of sleepiness in obstructive sleep apnoea at baseline and after 6 months of continuous positive airway pressure therapy. Eur Respir J. 2017;50(5):1700348.
19. Stepnowsky C, Sarmiento KF, Bujanover S, Villa KF, Li VW, Flores NM. Comorbidities, health-related quality of life, and work productivity among people with obstructive sleep apnea with excessive sleepiness: findings from the 2016 US National Health and Wellness Survey. J Clin Sleep Med. 2019;15(2):235–43.
20. Lal C, Strange C, Bachman D. Neurocognitive impairment in obstructive sleep apnea. Chest. 2012;141(6):1601–10.
21. Werli KS, Otuyama LJ, Bertolucci PH, et al. Neurocognitive function in patients with residual excessive sleepiness from obstruc-

tive sleep apnea: a prospective, controlled study. Sleep Med. 2016;26:6–11.

22. Mulgrew AT, Ryan CF, Fleetham JA, et al. The impact of obstructive sleep apnea and daytime sleepiness on work limitation. Sleep Med. 2007;9(1):42–53.

23. Tregear S, Reston J, Schoelles K, Phillips B. Obstructive sleep apnea and risk of motor vehicle crash: systematic review and meta-analysis. J Clin Sleep Med. 2009;5(6):573–81.

24. Garbarino S, Guglielmi O, Sanna A, Mancardi GL, Magnavita N. Risk of occupational accidents in workers with obstructive sleep apnea: systematic review and meta-analysis. Sleep. 2016;39(6):1211–8.

25. Gottlieb DJ, Ellenbogen JM, Bianchi MT, Czeisler CA. Sleep deficiency and motor vehicle crash risk in the general population: a prospective cohort study. BMC Med. 2018;16(1):44.

26. Won CH, Bogan RK, Doghramji K, et al. Assessing communication between physicians and patients with excessive daytime sleepiness associated with treated obstructive sleep apnea: insights from an ethnographic study of in-office visits [abstract]. Am J Respir Crit Care Med. 2019;199:A1390.

27. Pépin JL, Tamisier R, Hwang D, Mereddy S, Parthasarathy S. Does remote monitoring change OSA management and CPAP adherence? Respirology. 2017;22(8):1508–17.

28. He K, Kapur VK. Sleep-disordered breathing and excessive daytime sleepiness. Sleep Med Clin. 2017;12(3):369–82.

29. Javaheri S, Javaheri S. Update on persistent excessive daytime sleepiness in obstructive sleep apnea. Chest. 2020;158:776–86.

30. Chervin RD. Sleepiness, fatigue, tiredness, and lack of energy in obstructive sleep apnea. Chest. 2000;118(2):372–9.

31. Vernet C, Redolfi S, Attali V, et al. Residual sleepiness in obstructive sleep apnoea: phenotype and related symptoms. Eur Respir J. 2011;38(1):98–105.

32. Johns MW. A new method for measuring daytime sleepiness: the Epworth Sleepiness Scale. Sleep. 1991;14(6):540–5.

33. Johns M, Hocking B. Daytime sleepiness and sleep habits of Australian workers. Sleep. 1997;20(10):844–9.

34. About the Epworth Sleepiness Scale. 2020. Available at: https://epworthsleepinessscale.com/about-the-ess/. Accessed 16 Oct 2020.

35. Lapin BR, Bena JF, Walia HK, Moul DE. The Epworth Sleepiness Scale: validation of one-dimensional factor structure in a large clinical sample. J Clin Sleep Med. 2018;14(8):1293–301.

36. Rosenberg R, Babson K, Menno D, et al. Epworth Sleepiness Scale Test-Retest reliability analysis in solriamfetol studies [abstract]. Sleep. 2020;43(Suppl 1):A285–6.

37. Taylor E, Zeng I, O'Dochartaigh C. The reliability of the Epworth Sleepiness Score in a sleep clinic population. J Sleep Res. 2019;28(2):e12687.

38. Campbell AJ, Neill AM, Scott DAR. Clinical reproducibility of the Epworth Sleepiness Scale for patients with suspected sleep apnea. J Clin Sleep Med. 2018;14(5):791–5.

39. Nguyen AT, Baltzan MA, Small D, Wolkove N, Guillon S, Palayew M. Clinical reproducibility of the Epworth Sleepiness Scale. J Clin Sleep Med. 2006;2(2):170–4.

40. Hoddes E, Dement W, Zarcone V. The development and use of the Stanford sleepiness scale (SSS) [abstract]. Psychophysiology. 1972;9:150.

41. Hoddes E, Zarcone V, Smythe H, Phillips R, Dement WC. Quantification of sleepiness: a new approach. Psychophysiology. 1973;10(4):431–6.

42. Carskadon MA, Dement WC. Cumulative effects of sleep restriction on daytime sleepiness. Psychophysiology. 1981;18(2):107–13.

43. Herscovitch J, Broughton R. Sensitivity of the Stanford sleepiness scale to the effects of cumulative partial sleep deprivation and recovery oversleeping. Sleep. 1981;4(1):83–91.

44. Akerstedt T, Gillberg M. Subjective and objective sleepiness in the active individual. Int J Neurosci. 1990;52(1–2):29–37.

45. Shahid A, Wilkinson K, Marcu S, Shapiro CM, Karolinska Sleepiness Scale (KSS). STOP, THAT and one hundred other sleep scales. New York: Springer; 2012. p. 209–10.

46. Rotenberg BW, Murariu D, Pang KP. Trends in CPAP adherence over twenty years of data collection: a flattened curve. J Otolaryngol Head Neck Surg. 2016;45(1):43.

47. Weaver TE, Sawyer AM. Adherence to continuous positive airway pressure treatment for obstructive sleep apnoea: implications for future interventions. Indian J Med Res. 2010;131:245–58.

48. Weaver TE. Novel aspects of CPAP treatment and interventions to improve CPAP adherence. J Clin Med. 2019;8(12):2220.

49. Weaver TE, Grunstein RR. Adherence to continuous positive airway pressure therapy: the challenge to effective treatment. Proc Am Thorac Soc. 2008;5(2):173–8.

50. Sawyer AM, Gooneratne NS, Marcus CL, Ofer D, Richards KC, Weaver TE. A systematic review of CPAP adherence across age groups: clinical and empiric insights for developing CPAP adherence interventions. Sleep Med Rev. 2011;15(6):343–56.

51. Pengo MF, Czaban M, Berry MP, et al. The effect of positive and negative message framing on short term continuous positive airway pressure compliance in patients with obstructive sleep apnea. J Thorac Dis. 2018;10(Suppl 1):S160–s169.

52. Parthasarathy S, Haynes PL, Budhiraja R, Habib MP, Quan SF. A national survey of the effect of sleep medicine specialists and American Academy of Sleep Medicine Accreditation on management of obstructive sleep apnea. J Clin Sleep Med. 2006;2(2):133–42.

53. Parthasarathy S, Subramanian S, Quan SF. A multicenter prospective comparative effectiveness study of the effect of physician certification and center accreditation on patient-centered outcomes in obstructive sleep apnea. J Clin Sleep Med. 2014;10(3):243–9.

54. Sleep and sleep disorders data and statistics. 2017. Available at: https://www.cdc.gov/sleep/data_statistics.html. Accessed 16 Oct 2020.

55. Watson NF, Badr MS, Belenky G, et al. Recommended amount of sleep for a healthy adult: a joint consensus statement of the American Academy of Sleep Medicine and Sleep Research Society. Sleep. 2015;38(6):843–4.

56. Ejaz SM, Khawaja IS, Bhatia S, Hurwitz TD. Obstructive sleep apnea and depression: a review. Innov Clin Neurosci. 2011;8(8):17–25.

57. American Academy of Sleep Medicine. International classification of sleep disorders. 3rd ed. Darien, IL: American Academy of Sleep Medicine; 2014.

58. Littner MR, Kushida C, Wise M, et al. Practice parameters for clinical use of the multiple sleep latency test and the maintenance of wakefulness test. Sleep. 2005;28(1):113–21.

59. Sateia MJ. International classification of sleep disorders-third edition: highlights and modifications. Chest. 2014;146(5):1387–94.

60. Doghramji K, Mitler MM, Sangal RB, et al. A normative study of the maintenance of wakefulness test (MWT). Electroencephalogr Clin Neurophysiol. 1997;103(5):554–62.

61. Bennett LS, Stradling JR, Davies RJ. A behavioural test to assess daytime sleepiness in obstructive sleep apnoea. J Sleep Res. 1997;6(2):142–5.

62. Priest B, Brichard C, Aubert G, Liistro G, Rodenstein DO. Microsleep during a simplified maintenance of wakefulness test. A validation study of the OSLER test. Am J Respir Crit Care Med. 2001;163(7):1619–25.

63. Dinges DF, Powell JW. Microcomputer analyses of performance on a portable, simple visual RT task during sustained operations. Behav Res Methods Instrum Comput. 1985;17(6):652–5.

64. Naito E, Kinomura S, Geyer S, Kawashima R, Roland PE, Zilles K. Fast reaction to different sensory modalities activates common fields in the motor areas, but the anterior cingulate cortex is involved in the speed of reaction. J Neurophysiol. 2000;83(3):1701–9.

65. Jung CM, Ronda JM, Czeisler CA, Wright KP Jr. Comparison of sustained attention assessed by auditory and visual psychomotor vigilance tasks prior to and during sleep deprivation. J Sleep Res. 2011;20(2):348–55.

66. D'Rozario AL, Field CJ, Hoyos CM, et al. Impaired neurobehavioural performance in untreated obstructive sleep apnea patients using a novel standardised test battery. Front Surg. 2018;5:35.

67. Batool-Anwar S, Kales SN, Patel SR, Varvarigou V, DeYoung PN, Malhotra A. Obstructive sleep apnea and psychomotor vigilance task performance. Nat Sci Sleep. 2014;6:65–71.

68. Thomann J, Baumann CR, Landolt HP, Werth E. Psychomotor vigilance task demonstrates impaired vigilance in disorders with excessive daytime sleepiness. J Clin Sleep Med. 2014;10(9):1019–24.

69. Deering S, Amdur A, Borelli J, Headapohl W, Stepnowsky CJ. A three-minute mobile version of the psychomotor vigilance task [abstract 1053]. Sleep. 2018;41(Suppl 1):A391–2.

70. Smith MT, McCrae CS, Cheung J, et al. Use of actigraphy for the evaluation of sleep disorders and circadian rhythm sleep-wake disorders: an American Academy of Sleep Medicine systematic review, meta-analysis, and GRADE assessment. J Clin Sleep Med. 2018;14(7):1209–30.

71. Martin JL, Hakim AD. Wrist actigraphy. Chest. 2011;139(6):1514–27.

72. Li Y, Zhang J, Lei F, Liu H, Li Z, Tang X. Self-evaluated and close relative- evaluated Epworth Sleepiness Scale vs. multiple sleep latency test in patients with obstructive sleep apnea. J Clin Sleep Med. 2014;10(2):171–6.

73. Li Y, Vgontzas A, Kritikou I, et al. Psychomotor vigilance test and its association with daytime sleepiness and inflammation in sleep apnea: clinical implications. J Clin Sleep Med. 2017;13(9):1049–56.

74. Provigil [package insert]. North Wales, PA: Teva Pharmaceuticals; 2018.

75. Nuvigil [package insert]. North Wales, PA: Teva Pharmaceuticals; 2018.

76. Pack AI, Black JE, Schwartz JR, Matheson JK. Modafinil as adjunct therapy for daytime sleepiness in obstructive sleep apnea. Am J Respir Crit Care Med. 2001;164(9):1675–81.

77. Black JE, Hirshkowitz M. Modafinil for treatment of residual excessive sleepiness in nasal continuous positive airway pressure-treated obstructive sleep apnea/hypopnea syndrome. Sleep. 2005;28(4):464–71.

78. Hirshkowitz M, Black JE, Wesnes K, Niebler G, Arora S, Roth T. Adjunct armodafinil improves wakefulness and memory in obstructive sleep apnea/hypopnea syndrome. Respir Med. 2007;101(3):616–27.

79. Roth T, White D, Schmidt-Nowara W, et al. Effects of armodafinil in the treatment of residual excessive sleepiness associated with obstructive sleep apnea/hypopnea syndrome: a 12-week, multicenter, double-blind, randomized, placebo-controlled study in nCPAP-adherent adults. Clin Ther. 2006;28(5):689–706.

80. Hirshkowitz M, Black J. Effect of adjunctive modafinil on wakefulness and quality of life in patients with excessive sleepiness-associated obstructive sleep apnoea/hypopnoea syndrome: a 12-month, open-label extension study. CNS Drugs. 2007;21(5):407–16.

81. Black JE, Hull SG, Tiller J, Yang R, Harsh JR. The long-term tolerability and efficacy of armodafinil in patients with excessive sleepi-

ness associated with treated obstructive sleep apnea, shift work disorder, or narcolepsy: an open-label extension study. J Clin Sleep Med. 2010;6(5):458–66.

82. Chapman JL, Vakulin A, Hedner J, Yee BJ, Marshall NS. Modafinil/ armodafinil in obstructive sleep apnoea: a systematic review and meta-analysis. Eur Respir J. 2016;47(5):1420–8.

83. European Medicines Agency. Modafinil - Article 31 referral - Annex I, II, III, IV. 2011. Available at: https://www.ema.europa.eu/ documents/referral/modafinil-article-31-referral-annex-i-ii-iii-iv_ en.pdf. Accessed 24 Jan 2019.

84. Sukhal S, Khalid M, Tulaimat A. Effect of wakefulness-promoting agents on sleepiness in patients with sleep apnea treated with CPAP: a meta-analysis. J Clin Sleep Med. 2015;11(10):1179–86.

85. Sunosi® (solriamfetol) tablets Prescribing Information. Palo Alto, CA: Jazz Pharmaceuticals, Inc; 2019.

86. Sunosi® (solriamfetol) tablets summary of product characteristics. Dublin, Ireland: Jazz Pharmaceuticals Ireland Ltd; 2020.

87. Schweitzer PK, Rosenberg R, Zammit GK, et al. Solriamfetol for excessive sleepiness in obstructive sleep apnea (TONES 3): a randomized controlled trial. Am J Respir Crit Care Med. 2019;199(11):1421–31.

88. Strollo PJ Jr, Hedner J, Collop N, et al. Solriamfetol for the treatment of excessive sleepiness in OSA: a placebo-controlled randomized withdrawal study. Chest. 2019;155(2):364–74.

89. Malhotra A, Shapiro C, Pepin JL, et al. Long-term study of the safety and maintenance of efficacy of solriamfetol (JZP-110) in the treatment of excessive sleepiness in participants with narcolepsy or obstructive sleep apnea. Sleep. 2020;43(2):zsz220.

90. Wakix [package insert]. Plymouth Meeting, PA: Harmony Biosciences; 2019.

91. Dauvilliers Y, Verbraecken J, Partinen M, et al. Pitolisant for daytime sleepiness in obstructive sleep apnea patients refusing CPAP: a randomized trial. Am J Respir Crit Care Med. 2020;201(9):1135–45.

92. Rosenberg R, Baladi M, Menno D, Bron M. Clinically relevant effects of solriamfetol on excessive daytime sleepiness: a post-hoc analysis of the magnitude of change in clinical trials in adults with narcolepsy or obstructive sleep apnoea [abstract]. Sleep Med. 2019;64(suppl):S325.

93. Scrima L, Emsellem HA, Becker PM, et al. Identifying clinically important difference on the Epworth Sleepiness Scale: results from a narcolepsy clinical trial of JZP-110. Sleep Med. 2017;38:108–12.

94. Lammers GJ, Bogan R, Schweitzer PK, et al. Thresholds for clinically meaningful changes on the Epworth sleepiness scale and maintenance of wakefulness test sleep latency [abstract]. Presented at: Biennial World Sleep Congress; September 20–25, 2019; Vancouver, BC, Canada.

95. Rosenberg R, Schweitzer PK, Malhotra A, et al. Incidence and duration of common adverse events in a solriamfetol (JZP-110) phase 3 study for treatment of excessive daytime sleepiness in obstructive sleep apnea [abstract 0569]. Sleep. 2019;42(suppl 1):A226–7.

96. Ritalin [package insert]. East Hanover, NJ: Novartis Pharmaceuticals Corporation; 2019.

97. Adderall [package insert]. Horsham, PA: Teva Pharmaceuticals; 2017.

98. Dextroamphetamine sulfate [package insert]. North Wales, PA: Teva Pharmaceuticals; 2016.

Improving CPAP Adherence Using Telehealth

31

Ajmal Razmy

31.1 Pathogenesis of Obstructive Sleep Apnea

Fundamentally we understand that sleep is an integral part of our daily health needs. However, what outcomes would arise if one did not get the recommended amount of sleep? Those that suffer with obstructive sleep apnea (OSA) do have to deal with the consequences of disrupted sleep. OSA is a sleep breathing disorder that blocks breathing during sleep causing sleep to be disrupted and waking up to occur [1]. Approximately 6.4% of Canadians were diagnosed with OSA in 2017. This number is most likely an underestimate of the number of people who have OSA because many people with mild OSA do not get tested and therefore are not diagnosed [2]. In normal sleep, blood pressure decreases, and the body avoids physiological stress as sympathetic activity decreases [1]. In OSA patients, [laryngeal and pharyngeal] muscles relax constricting their airway and lowering oxygen intake. The brain is able to sense breathing difficulty and the patient will awake from their sleep. Many factors ranging from genetics to lifestyle choices affect one's predisposition for developing OSA.

The most common factor that increases the risk of developing OSA is excess weight. Fat can deposit around the upper airway, narrowing the opening, and disrupt breathing, enhancing the probability of developing OSA [1]. Also, there are cases where the upper airway is narrowed by an inherited genetic predisposition. This could include having a thicker neck or having other body parts obstructing airflow such as tonsils [1]. Men are more likely to develop OSA and the risk increases as people get older [1]. Lifestyle modification such as smoking cessation, limiting alcohol use, and decreased sedative drug use may lower the risk of developing OSA. The resultant impact of OSA can be vast, ranging from

decreased performance to impairment secondary to an accident, and as such the detection and treatment of OSA is a health imperative.

31.2 Obstructive Sleep Apnea: Symptoms and Consequences

Many OSA patients do not recall their frequent disruptions in nighttime sleep as they occur very quickly. However, these constant disruptions can result in excessive daytime sleepiness [3]. OSA taxes the ability to use sleep to restore the body and minimize physiological stress. These common symptoms can negatively impact one's concentration and attention increasing the risk of injuries [1]. Excessive daytime sleepiness can also affect people's mood by increasing irritability and potentially enhance depressive emotions. OSA also contributes to oxygen levels during sleep and a rise in blood pressure. Repeated increases in blood pressure may eventually lead to heart disorders or heart disease. Therefore, OSA can negatively impact daily activity as well as long-term health and it is crucial to participate in treatments to decrease the severity of the disease.

31.3 Obstructive Sleep Apnea: Treatment

Obesity is one of the main causes of OSA development. Many clinicians will inform the patient that their top priority should be to lose weight. Weight loss has been proven to lower the risk of OSA development in vulnerable patients as well as lower the severity in already diagnosed OSA patients [2]. Additionally, surgeries are available that could either widen the upper airway or aid in weight loss. Many anatomical problems that block the upper airway can be removed to allow air to pass through the airway during sleep. Examples of anatomical structures that would need surgery to correct are enlarged tonsils, restricted nasal cavity, enlarged tongue, and more [4]. However, these surgeries are considered the

A. Razmy (✉)
Joseph Brant Hospital, Burlington, ON, Canada

Cleveland Clinic Canada, Toronto, ON, Canada

© The Author(s), under exclusive license to Springer Nature Switzerland AG 2022
C. M. Shapiro et al. (eds.), *CPAP Adherence*, https://doi.org/10.1007/978-3-030-93146-9_31

last resort and are not commonly ordered by specialists [4]. Surgeries represent an invasive treatment option for OSA; however, most prescribed treatments are used to lower the severity of the disorder. The most commonly prescribed treatment is continuous positive airway pressure (CPAP). It can be incredibly effective at improving restorative sleep and reducing OSA symptoms. CPAP is prescribed to all OSA patients, even patients who have undergone surgery to correct their OSA [4]. All of these treatments are possible, but CPAP is the most effective and the safest form.

31.4 Continuous Positive Airway Pressure (CPAP)

CPAP is a machine that aids in breathing during sleep for patients with OSA. Most CPAP machines are a mask that covers the nose and mouth with a strap that wraps around the head to keep it in place. The machine is connected to a tank of water which helps increase air pressure in the throat [5]. This will prevent apneas and allow OSA patients to obtain a restorative sleep. CPAP has been proven to reduce symptom severity of OSA. The machine can significantly reduce snoring and breathing disruptions when used properly. In a randomized control trial, patients were assigned to the conservative treatment with or without CPAP, and it was seen that after 3 and 6 months, patients who received CPAP experienced reduced OSA symptoms [6]. These include daytime fatigue, irritability, and high blood pressure [6]. As well this trial presented data that suggests CPAP aids in increasing cognitive function, such as visual memory, and vigilance, in OSA patients faster than non-CPAP-related treatment [6]. However, more research should be done on this topic. Patients who use CPAP regularly will experience reduced daytime fatigue, lower blood pressure, and a lower risk of developing heart disease. Although CPAP is the most effective noninvasive treatment for OSA, it still has potential side effects. These include dry nose, sore throat, bloating, and irritation of the face [5]. However, side effect burden typically decreases with consistent CPAP treatment. Unfortunately, for a multitude of different reasons outlined below, adherence to CPAP remains a pivotal challenge.

31.5 CPAP and Adherence

Sleep specialists will often prescribe CPAP to OSA patients knowing that it will greatly lower OSA symptoms. Despite the large amount of information on how helpful CPAP treatment is for OSA, many patients do not adhere to the treatment. In a meta-analysis about CPAP and compliance, one study determined that on average, CPAP is used for 4.6 hours a night. With the assumption that the participants were receiving 7 hours of sleep a night, the adherence rate was 34.1% [7]. Also adherence rates for CPAP treatment have not changed significantly over the last 15 years, consistently hovering around 30–40% [7]. New methods need to be explored to increase CPAP adherence. When discussing patient adherence, steps are needed to be able to improve adherence for all forms of treatment. With medication compliance, clinicians need to provide the simplest presentation of the treatment to improve adherence. Patients are less likely to comply to the medication when dosing instructions become complicated or too frequent. In addition, clinicians need to educate the patients about the treatment to increase the probability for the patient to follow treatment recommendations. As well in intervening treatments, such as CPAP, clinicians should attempt to help the patient understand the severity of the disorder and the effectiveness of the treatment [8]. These are standard steps to improve adherence that clinicians should use early on in the treatment. The first few weeks are the most important to establish the habit of using the machine regularly. If the patient does not follow the treatment recommendations in the first few months, it increases the risk of the patient to never use the treatment [9]. These new methods need to address problems and concerns that patients commonly have with CPAP. Increasing adherence to CPAP is the first step to successfully treating OSA.

There are many potential reasons for why a patient may not comply with CPAP treatment. It is important to consider the fact that wearing a new apparatus to engage in an activity that we find so integral to living will be met with apprehension. Most patients report the mask being uncomfortable while they sleep. When beginning to wear the mask, the irritation frequently wakes people from sleep and then the patients do not reapply the mask so they can fall asleep easier [10]. Unfortunately, this would render the CPAP machine ineffective as it needs to be used throughout the whole night. That is a common misconception as many patients believe they are using the machine enough and more than they actually are [10]. Even taking one night off from using the machine can result in daytime fatigue and elevated blood pressure [7]. Not only does the misconception around the treatment lead to lower compliance but there are many other social factors as well. Intuitively, the severity of OSA can play a role in how motivated patients will be to comply with the treatment. In addition, anxiety and lack of social support can reduce compliance [11]. That is why it is important to motivate patients frequently during the first few months starting the treatment to keep their compliance high. However, there are not enough sleep specialists or working hours to provide each OSA patient with frequent in-person meetings. The need for innovative measures to meet patients where they are at and help motivate and educate them regarding the use of CPAP can be met using technology to enhance the patient experience.

31.6 The Emerging Method of Telehealth

31.6.1 What Is Telehealth?

In day-to-day life, most people consider using technology a daily activity. Telehealth aims to utilize technology to provide healthcare services. Computers and other mobile devices can be used to transmit healthcare information and provide routine checkups to patients [12]. Although some participants may not feel comfortable with the thought of online appointments, telehealth can help with saving the patient's and clinician's time. Anecdotal evidence suggests that once patients become familiar with the procedural elements of telehealth, often this becomes the preferred choice with follow-up care. We have seen this fast-forwarded during the COVID-19 pandemic with transitions to work from home and clinical consultations increasingly being virtual. Smaller tasks such as prescription refills and reviewing test results can be done quickly through a virtual appointment, saving the patient's time for not having to travel and see the doctor and as well the clinician's time who can keep their practice from getting too busy with patients [12]. Telehealth also has the capability to have synchronous or asynchronous appointments . Asynchronous appointments are helpful for patients who can lose motivation to continue their treatment, such as CPAP treatment, at any point in the day [13]. The patients are able to receive the necessary support and coaching required to maintain their motivation at any point in the day [13]. With a wide range of capabilities and rapidly evolving technology, telehealth may be the new method needed to promote CPAP adherence.

Telehealth has a number of advantages over in-person appointments. Healthcare through telehealth is more accessible to people in isolated communities and for those with mobility deficiencies or lack of transportation [14]. Anyone who has tried to park in busy urban clinical settings can attest to both the financial and time costs of attending in vivo assessments. Medical specialists will be more available to patients as not every community has a large number of specialists [14]. Patients who are deaf or blind can still benefit from telehealth. Telehealth provides many benefits for patients however; clinicians and specialists also benefit from it. Telehealth greatly reduces costs and saves time which can allow clinicians to be more flexible in certain situations where a patient may need more time commitment [14]. With new technology being created, both the clinicians and patients will need to adapt to the services. This could lead to clinicians refusing to provide telehealth services and patients preferring in-person appointments as that is what they are accustomed to. However, this has not been the experience during the COVID-19 pandemic with many clinicians with limited computer know-how pivoting to telehealth. Telehealth has a great potential to solve many healthcare issues and it may be part of the solution to increase CPAP adherence in patients with OSA.

31.6.2 Telehealth and CPAP Compliance

Early adherence to CPAP treatment is the most important to lead to regular CPAP use. Telehealth services allow for regular checkups and informative appointments shortly after CPAP has been prescribed. This gives clinicians the opportunity to identify OSA patients who don't use CPAP sufficiently [3]. Educational interventions have been shown to increase CPAP compliance and telehealth offers a variety of options on how to deliver these [7]. Synchronous and asynchronous videos and phone calls are commonly used to inform patients on the importance of their treatment and answer any questions they may have. It is easy to assume that patients retain the information we provide after an assessment but it is often not the case. Educational materials via telehealth can be useful for patients as reminders of what has been discussed and time-saving for providers to use as summaries of information they have provided. OSA does not typically require in-hospital evaluation or treatment. Telehealth allows patients to get the service they need wherever and whenever it is the most convenient for them. With advanced technology, patients are more open to the idea of using online resources for their healthcare services, and clinicians see similar, if not better, CPAP compliance results when they provide telehealth services [15]. CPAP treatment can take a few days to weeks until the patient gets used to it. Patients can have facilitated access to specialists who can inform them and guide them through problems they are having as they arise. Without telehealth patients may be driven away from using CPAP before their next in-person follow-up. Telehealth has great potential to improve CPAP compliance within OSA patients as supported by many studies.

Telehealth is not only useful for patient clinician interventions, but it also has the ability to transport medical data from patients to practitioners. Information such as sleeping patterns and snoring are good indicators of whether or not a patient has developed OSA [9]. Through certain apps and other storage devices, these data can be transmitted from the patient to the clinician to make an effective decision on the patient's status. Once agreement has been established between the patient and the clinician to use in telehealth services, results show that telehealth is associated with similar compliance rates as in-person appointments [14]. This means that telehealth is a viable option to promote CPAP adherence. Telehealth also provides service to all communities, even in some where sleep specialists may not be available. Phone coaching is able to provide support to the patients and educate them on CPAP quicker, as more appointments can be completed in a shorter time frame than in-person appointments. As coaching becomes less required, patients can continue to learn about their treatment through a variety of apps and asynchronous videos.

31.6.3 Telehealth Programs

Results may show that telehealth promotes CPAP compliance, but the programs need to be properly structured to demonstrate positive results. An example of a structured program that promotes CPAP compliance is U-Sleep. This online application analyzes CPAP data such as total time in use and allows the patient to follow their progress [16]. Accountability measures such as this are highly impactful with regard to improving adherence. Also, calls can be arranged if the patient is in need of general advice from a practitioner. After the data is analyzed by the app, if the patient has met their compliance goal, they will receive a message of encouragement and congratulations. If the patient does not meet the compliance goal, clinicians will be able to easily identify that this patient needs follow-up appointments [16]. This will minimize the time necessary for clinicians to promote CPAP use. Patients who use U-Sleep demonstrate improved compliance with CPAP with resolution of severe OSA symptoms with efficient use of clinical time [16]. There are many programs available that work in a similar manner that help promote CPAP compliance. The biggest barrier to effective OSA treatment is insufficient CPAP use and it seems telehealth may be able to aid in overcoming some of the barriers of CPAP adherence. Well-structured online services that provide frequent reminders to use CPAP as well as motivational comments are likely to promote compliance. With the necessary engagement by patients and clinicians, a structured program for the patient to follow, and an availability of technology for the patients, telehealth may be one of the methods with a potential to improve CPAP adherence and to promote sleep quality for patients with OSA.

References

1. Javaheri S, Barbe F, Campos-Rodriguez F, Dempsey JA, Khayat R, Javaheri S, et al. Sleep apnea: types, mechanisms, and clinical cardiovascular consequences. JACC. 2017;69(7):841–58. Available from: https://doi.org/10.1016/j.jacc.2016.11.069

2. Sleep Apnea in Canada, 2016 and 2017. Statistics Canada; 2018 Oct. Available from: https://www150.statcan.gc.ca/n1/en/pub/82-625-x/2018001/article/54979-eng.pdf?st=0jjuVpOA.

3. Kwiatkowska M, Idzikowski A, Matthews L. Telehealth-based framework for supporting the treatment of obstructive sleep apnea. Stud Health Technol Inform. 2009;143:478–83. https://doi.org/10.3233/978-1-58603-979-0-478.

4. Carvalho B, Hsia J, Capasso R. Surgical therapy of obstructive sleep apnea: a review. Neurotherapeutics. 2012;9(4):710–6. https://doi.org/10.1007/s13311-012-0141-x.

5. Chowdhury O, Wedderburn CJ, Duffy D, Greenough A. CPAP review. Eur J Pediatr. 2012;171:1441–8. https://doi.org/10.1007/s00431-011-1648-6.

6. Monasterio C, Vidal S, Duran J, Ferrer M, Carmona C, Barbé F, et al. Effectiveness of continuous positive airway pressure in mild sleep apnea-hypopnea syndrome. Am J Respir Crit Care Med. 2001;164(6):939–43. Available from: https://doi.org/10.1164/ajrccm.164.6.2008010

7. Rotenberg BW, Murario D, Pang KP. Trends in CPAP adherence over twenty years of data collection: a flattened curve. J Otolaryngol Head Neck Surg. 2016;45(1):43. https://doi.org/10.1186/s40463-016-0156-0.

8. Winnick S, Lucas DO, Hartman AL, Toll D. How do you improve compliance? Pediatrics. 2005;115(6):e718–24. Available from: https://doi.org/10.1542/peds.2004-1133

9. Villanueva JA, Suarez MC, Garmendia O, Lugo V, Ruiz C, Montserrat JM. The role of telemedicine and mobile health in the monitoring of sleep-breathing disorders: improving patient outcomes. Smart Homecare Technol Telehealth. 2017;4:1–11. Available from: https://doi.org/10.2147/SHTT.S108048

10. Devaraj UH, Ramachandran P, Biradar P, Akkara P, D'Souza G. CPAP compliance among patients with moderate/severe OSA – Appearances are deceptive! Sleep Med. 2015;16:S356–7. Available from: https://doi.org/10.1016/j.sleep.2015.02.479

11. Broström A, Pakpour AH, Nilsen P, Gardner B, Ulander M. Promoting CPAP adherence in clinical practice: a survey of Swedish and Norwegian CPAP practitioners' beliefs and practices. J Sleep Res. 2018;27(6):e12675. https://doi.org/10.1111/jsr.12675.

12. Tuckson RV, Edmunds M, Hodgkins ML. Telehealth. N Engl J Med. 2017;377:1585–92. https://doi.org/10.1056/NEJMsr1503323.

13. Langarizadeh M, Tabatabaei MS, Tavakol K, Naghipour M, Rostami A, Moghbeli F. Telemental health care, an effective alternative to conventional mental care: a systematic review. Acta Inform Med. 2017;25(4):240–6. https://doi.org/10.5455/aim.2017.25.240-246.

14. Parikh R, Touvelle MN, Wang H, Zallek SN. Sleep telemedicine: patient satisfaction and treatment adherence. Telemed J E Health. 2011;17(8):609–14. https://doi.org/10.1089/tmj.2011.0025.

15. Zia S, Fields BG. Sleep telemedicine: an emerging field's latest frontier. Chest. 2016;149(6):1556–65. Available from: https://doi.org/10.1016/j.chest.2016.02.670

16. Munafo D, Hevener W, Crocker M, Willes L, Sridasome S, Muhsin M. A telehealth program for CPAP adherence reduces labor and yields similar adherence and efficacy when compared to standard of care. Sleep Breath. 2016;20:777–85. https://doi.org/10.1007/s11325-015-1298-4.

The CPAP Machine, Mask and Interface

32

Julia Lachowicz and Matthew T. Naughton

32.1 Historical Background

Though the modern continuous positive airway pressure (CPAP) device, known as an airflow generator, now forms the cornerstone of intervention in obstructive sleep apnoea (OSA) management, it only becomes established in recent decades. CPAP has been described in medical literature from the late 1930s, with accounts of its application in the treatment of acute pulmonary oedema [1]. This preceded the use of manually delivered intermittent positive pressure ventilation in Denmark during the polio epidemics of the early 1950s [2]. Renewed interest followed from a description by Ashbaugh et al. in 1967 [3] of a series of Vietnam War soldiers with acute respiratory distress syndrome, where benefits of CPAP were seen in relation to hypoxaemia and atelectasis.

The translation of CPAP from hospital to the domiciliary setting remained elusive until the 1980s. Professor Colin Sullivan of Sydney, Australia, published a milestone account of five patients treated with low-level overnight CPAP via a nasal mask to successfully prevent obstructive apnoeas [4]. One of the crucial steps was to have a mask with a built-in exhalation valve, rather than an under-water seal. At the request of patients who had experienced symptomatic benefit from CPAP application during the trials, machines were then produced for home use and partnerships with industry developed, with a small but substantial number of patients using home CPAP devices within 10 years of Sullivan's publication [5].

32.2 Technological Advances

Technological advances occurred simultaneously in variations of positive airway pressure therapy. Non-invasive ventilation with bilevel positive airway pressure (BPAP) became recognised during the late 1980s and early 1990s as efficacious in the management of chronic severe respiratory failure secondary to a variety of causes associated with alveolar hypoventilation, providing an alternative to tracheostomy and intermittent positive pressure ventilation [6, 7].

Inspiratory and expiratory PAP settings (IPAP and EPAP) could be made, where the difference between the two (IPAP and EPAP) was equivalent to the 'pressure support' term used in the intensive care unit (ICU). Further developments came with the introduction of a device "back-up" respiratory rate for times of prolong central apnea.

The devices were sensitive enough to detect a change in flow and thus change from inspiratory to expiratory pressures – the sensitivity being high, medium or low and dependent on the proprietary software. Devices were also able to set an inspiratory pressure duration with a minimum and maximum time in milliseconds. Another important aspect was to ensure the EPAP value be set at a least value of 4 cmH_2O to prevent rebreathing and CO_2 inhalation.

It is important to note that the BPAP is a device with set IPAP and EPAP pressures and delivers variable tidal volumes. Assuming the patient is breathing 15 breaths per minute with a tidal volume of 500 ml per breath, the minute volume of ventilation is 7.5 litres per minute (lpm). The intentional leak from most masks is about 25 lpm; thus, about 33 lpm air needs to be delivered. The PAP devices can deliver up to 200 lpm; thus, there is enormous redundancy in the pumps in the setting of excessive leak.

It is also important to differentiate the more elaborate ventilators used in ICU with intubated and mechanically ventilated patients, where the ventilators often have settings for tidal volume with peak and plateau pressures, in addition

J. Lachowicz
Alfred Hospital, Melbourne, VIC, Australia

M. T. Naughton (✉)
Alfred Hospital and Monash University, Melbourne, VIC, Australia
e-mail: m.naughton@alfred.org.au

© The Author(s), under exclusive license to Springer Nature Switzerland AG 2022
C. M. Shapiro et al. (eds.), *CPAP Adherence*, https://doi.org/10.1007/978-3-030-93146-9_32

337

to PEEP (positive end-expiratory pressure). These ICU ventilators are a closed system: there is no intentional leak at the mask.

In the late 1990s auto-setting PAP (APAP) devices were developed in the hope of improving adherence and improving the control of AHI in obstructive sleep apnoea [8, 9]. These auto-CPAP devices were developed with the aim of facilitating PAP titration outside of a sleep laboratory, with implications for the cost and convenience of CPAP initiation. Of note was that each industry producer used confidentially designed software that dictated pressure changes such that significant treatment differences occur between one device and another. The APAP technology has been incorporated into the BPAP devices as a variable EPAP.

In the 1980s, the original CPAP devices were loud and unwieldy, weighing 7 kg and adapted from pump technology used for heating swimming pools, spas and jacuzzis [10]. Across many iterations, the modern CPAP machine and mask interface have been fine-tuned to improve patient comfort and ease of use.

Cold passover humidification was initially developed but soon deemed to be relatively ineffective. Heated humidification was then developed as an additional add-on, now integrated within the device to improve the quality of life and symptoms of patients with nasopharyngeal adverse effects of conventional CPAP use [11]. Heated tubing was also developed to minimise precipitation within the tubing. Moreover, 'automatic' humidification has been developed to take into consideration external room temperatures.

Ramp functionality has been developed, delivering a lower starting pressure of CPAP that eases the transition to higher fixed pressures that may contribute to pressure intolerance [12]. Some devices can detect arousals from deep sleep during the night and thus automatically drop the pressure and begin a ramp function.

Expiratory pressure relief, sometimes referred to as C-Flex, reduces the amount of pressure during the latter stages of expiration [12].

Modern CPAP machines are significantly smaller and quieter than early designs, with options now existing for battery-powered, portable devices [13]. Most modern CPAP devices create less noise than standard background noise levels.

32.3 Mask Technology

The patient-CPAP interface is customisable with nasal, oronasal (frequently termed 'full-face mask') and nasal cushion (or 'nasal pillow') designs. Influences on the choice of mask encompass patient preference, anatomic variation, sex, the presence of chronic nasal obstruction and facial hair [12]. The quality and comfort of mask fit has implications for mask leak and patient adherence [14]. The requirement for

higher CPAP pressures, lower adherence and elevated residual apnoea-hypopnoea index has been associated with the oronasal mask design [15]. New technologies becoming integrated into mask development include computerised facial mapping translated to 3D printing to deliver bespoke fit [16], suggesting that the CPAP interface of the future will be increasingly customised to the individual. Importantly, masks are made of silicone and are latex-free, thus minimising the chance of latex allergy.

32.4 CPAP Initiation

For most adult patients, CPAP is commenced in the outpatient setting following a confirmed diagnosis of OSA. Exceptions to this include the hospitalised patient identified as being at high risk of OSA in the perioperative setting, and patients in the emergency department or ambulance receiving emergent treatment for acute pulmonary oedema.

Various methods can be used to achieve an optimal CPAP setting. An overnight in-laboratory CPAP implementation study, or split-night protocol that combines a diagnostic polysomnogram during early sleep with CPAP implementation and titration during later sleep, has traditionally been favoured [17]. During an overnight PAP titration in a sleep laboratory, following mask fitting, pressures commence at 4 cmH_2O (note to avoid rebreathing and CO_2 retention) and increase in steps of 2 cmH_2O every 5–15 minutes in response to obstructive apnoeas, and in steps of 1 cmH_2O every 5–15 minutes in response to obstructive hypopnoeas and/or snoring. Note that the 'precise' pressure to control upper airway instability (i.e., snoring or obstructive sleep-disordered breathing) will vary with body position and sleep stage. In general terms, neck flexion and supine positioning reduce airway luminal size (i.e., higher pressures are required). Moreover, 'periodic breathing' is most likely to occur in non-REM stages 1 and 2, uninterrupted snoring in slow-wave sleep and hypoxemia during REM sleep. Thus, choosing an optimal CPAP pressure should take into consideration sleep stage, body position and mask leak.

With benefits in relation to cost, timeliness and access to a sleep laboratory, an alternative method is the use the APAP machine [18]. APAP machines calculate the required pressures based on measurement of apnoeas and inspiratory flow limitation, with the 90th or 95th percentile pressure after 1–2 weeks used to guide the fixed CPAP pressure in the long term (see Fig. 32.1).

Mathematical models, whereby algorithms incorporating patient body mass index, neck circumference and AHI are used, have also been developed to establish an optimal CPAP pressure. The choice of technique used to establish CPAP pressure in moderate-to-severe OSA has not been shown to

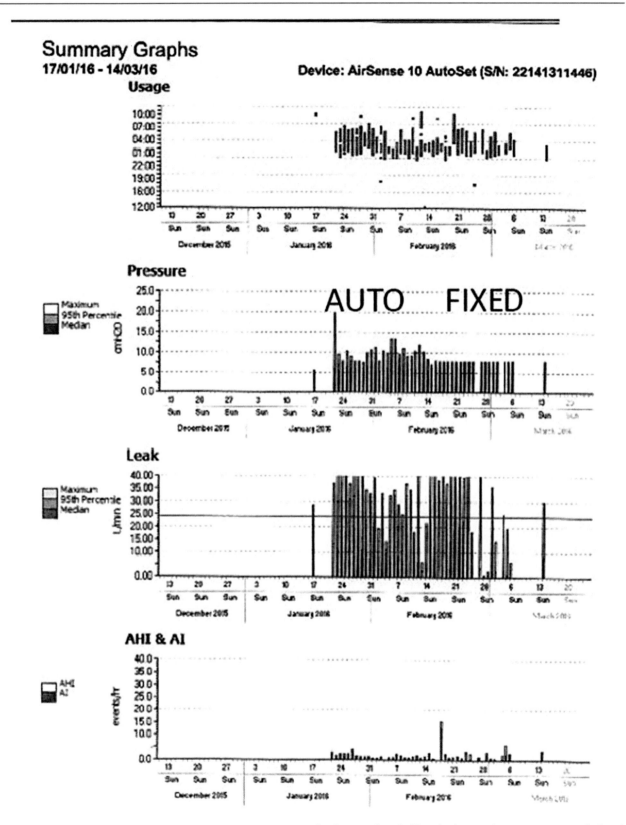

Fig. 32.1 An illustration of an APAP download over a 2-week period during which time auto-PAP was used for 1 week from which a 95th percentile pressure was derived from which a CPAP setting was made for the second week. Note the four graphs: usage, pressures, leak and residual AHI

alter clinical outcome, allowing judicious physician preference and resource availability to be equally considered [18].

Whilst it is yet to be formally validated, many sleep physicians make use of a 'ten per cent rule' as a helpful method to clinically estimate an appropriate CPAP starting pressure when a formal titration study is not immediately practicable [19]. In this method, the CPAP pressure is set based upon 10% of the patient's body weight: as such a patient who weighs 100 kg, is given 10 cmH2O CPAP. This simple approach is supported by the large SAVE [20] and RICCADSA [21] randomised controlled trials in which mean CPAP pressures were 9.6 and 9.9 cmH$_2$O, respectively, for mean body weights of 81 and 90 kg. Regardless of the initial method chosen, an overnight CPAP polysomnogram review study remains an option to fine-tune CPAP pressures over time.

32.5 Clinical Conditions

With greater knowledge of cardio-pulmonary physiology during sleep, there has been a greater precision as to which clinical groups might benefit from PAP beyond OSA.

Patients with neuromuscular weakness and chest wall diseases can respond well with BPAP; however, randomised controlled trial support is limited to motor neurone disease without bulbar disease where a survival and quality of life benefit was shown.

32.5.1 Obesity Hypoventilation Syndrome

For patients with obesity hypoventilation (PaCO$_2$ > 45 with BMI > 30 and no other cause identified), a question debated has been whether BPAP was superior to CPAP. Three randomised controlled trials have confirmed that both forms of PAP are equally effective – see Table 32.1.

Table 32.1 NIV vs CPAP for stable obesity hypoventilation syndrome

	Piper [22]	Howard [19]	Masa [23]
Comparator	CPAP vs BPAP	CPAP vs BPAP	CPAP vs BPAP
N x duration	36 × 3 months	82 × 3 months	225 × 5.4 years
Age (mean, years)	50	53	62
BMI (mean, kg/m²)	53	55	50
AHI (events/h)	16	82	68
PaCO$_2$ (mean, mmHg)	51	60 ->45	50 ->44
Settings and BURR	14 vs 16/10 spont	15 vs 19/12 and 15	11 vs 20/8 and 14
Outcomes	Change in CO$_2$	Change in CO$_2$	Hospital, survival
BPAP > CPAP?	No	No	No

Note: *BURR* back-up respiratory rate

Table 32.2 Utility of BPAP vs best medical treatment in chronic hypercapnic COPD

Author	McEvoy [24]	Struik [25]	Kohnlein [26]	Murphy [27]
Patients	Stable on LTOT	Stable COPD	Immediate post-AECOPD	2–4 weeks post-AECOPD
N and duration (months)	144 × 28	201 × 12	195 × 12	106 × 12
Age – mean	68	63	64	67
Male (%)	65	60	62	47
BMI (kg/m²)	26	24	25	22
PaCO$_2$ (mmHg)	54	59	58	59
FEV$_1$ (ml)	600	680	27%	600
LTOT (%)	100	70	65	100
Bilevel settings	13/5 and BURR = NS	19/5 and BURR =15	22/5 & BURR>14	24/4 and BURR 14
Usage (h/night)	4.5	6.5	5.9	7.6
PSG	Yes	No	No	No
CO$_2$ fall	Yes	No	Yes	No
Mortality (NIV vs others)	22 vs 31	30	12 vs 33	63% vs 80%
Improved HRQOL	No	No	Yes	Yes

32.5.2 Stable Hypercapnic COPD

For patients with stable hypercapnic COPD, the role of BPAP has been debated for 20 years. Once factors such as excessive oxygen, sedatives and other drugs that might influence CO$_2$ level are taken into account, the data suggest there is a significant role for bilevel PAP; see Table 32.2.

32.5.3 Congestive Heart Failure

Patients with heart failure due to reduced ejection fraction and OSA respond well to CPAP. Many patients however have a combination of obstructive sleep apnoea and central sleep apnoea with Cheyne-Stokes respiration (CSA-CSR), a form of periodic breathing. CPAP has been shown to be efficacious in CSA-CSR; however, adherence has been problematic. At this point it is important to understand that CSA-CSR is a condition associated with hyperventilation due to sympathetic nervous system activation, the severity of which usually parallels the severity of the heart failure. The role of CPAP in CSA-CSR was based mainly upon the observation studies in which CPAP was effective in patients with acute pulmonary oedema.

In order to improve the adherence to PAP therapy in chronic heart failure with SDB (either OSA or CSA-CSR),

Table 32.3 A comparison of the two large randomised controlled trials of adaptive servo-controlled ventilation

	SERVE-HF [29]	ADVENT-HF [30]
Commercial sponsor	ResMed	Philips Respironics
ASV trigger	Minute ventilation	Peak flow
Default pressure, cmH₂O	EPAP = 5, PSmin = 5	EPAP = 4, PSmin = 0
Mask used (FFM, nasal, NA)	76, 15, 19 (%)	Nasal > FFM
Patients × duration of follow-up	1351 × 31 months	860 × 60 months
Entry LVEF (%)	<45	<45
Entry AHI	>15	>15 (non-sleepy)
SDB type	CSA > 50%	CSA and OSA
Sleep study	Lab PSG and home PG	Lab PSG
Central reporting laboratory	No	Yes
Follow-up	Telephone and clinics	1-month PSG and clinic
Results	Negative	Not yet available

an additional form of PAP known as adaptive servo-ventilation PAP (ASV) was developed [28]. The aim was for the device to 'learn' the patients' minute volume of ventilation with minimal support, then provide some CPAP and variable amounts of pressure support, whilst aiming to maintain minute volume of ventilation at about 80% of the patients' prevailing minute ventilation.

The utility of ASV has been overshadowed in heart failure with reduced ejection fraction by an unexpected increase in all-cause and cardiovascular mortality seen with this treatment in the subsequent SERVE-HF randomised controlled trial [29]. Another industry-sponsored trial (ADVENT-HF [30]) continues with completion estimated in 2021. Importantly, the two trials (SERVE-HF and ADVENT-HF) vary in device settings, patient recruitment and study protocol (see Table 32.3).

Whether ASV will be useful in other forms of SDB, such as CSA due to narcotics, CPAP itself (see later) or unknown cause (i.e. idiopathic), remains to be determined.

32.6 Contraindications to CPAP Therapy

There remain circumstances where the use of CPAP is contraindicated or should be pursued with caution. Certain surgical procedures, which involve breaching the paranasal sinuses, pituitary fossa, skull base, retropharynx or middle ear, are at theoretical risk from post-operative CPAP delivery [31], with reports including cases of pneumoencephalus. Facial pathology, including local infection and fracture, may render the application of the CPAP mask unfeasible. CPAP use is not desirable in the context of a reduced conscious state or in patients unable to protect their own airway.

32.7 Adherence to CPAP

Critical to the success of CPAP to manage symptoms of OSA and improve patient quality of life is adequate patient adherence to therapy [13]. Adherence, a process whereby an individual chooses to act in concert with the advice of their healthcare provider, has been differentiated from the notion of compliance, which conceptualises the degree to which the individual follows the medical advice given [32]. Adherence implies joint understanding and agreement between patient and physician. Convention regards CPAP adherence to confer at least 4 hours of use per night for five or more night per week [33]. It is estimated that short-term non-adherence to CPAP in the initial 2 weeks of use is approximately 25%, comparable to that of complex management paradigms in non-OSA disease states [34]. Long-term estimates suggest non-adherence varies between 46% and 83% of patients with OSA [14].

Crawford et al. [32] have described the complex nature of adherence to CPAP, adapting the biopsychosocial model of health (Fig. 32.2). Traditional biomedical components include the age and sex of patients, symptom burden, AHI and CPAP pressure. Psychosocial factors include the patient's understanding and attitude towards their OSA and CPAP therapy, self-efficacy and social milieu which contextualise the impact of the disease on the patient. The clinician's understanding of these patient-related variables is integral to the therapeutic relationship and successful navigation of ongoing CPAP adherence and is also a basis for inter-disciplinary collaboration with behavioural sleep specialist, social workers and PAP treatment coordinators to help with non-medical factors that interfere with CPAP adherence.

On occasions when dealing with non-adherence to CPAP, one should stop and reassess the indication to trial CPAP (usually one of the following: noise of snoring, an AHI threshold, excessive sleepiness in the setting of adequate sleep duration, assumed cardiovascular risk or high pre-test probability of a post-operative complication). Is there alignment between the patients' priority of problem(s) with yours (being an experienced sleep clinician)? See also Chap. 6. It is also wise to ensure an ethical behaviour to the provision of CPAP, namely, don't simply treat the AHI, consider alternative treatments and ensure long-term follow-up with management of existent medical issues (commonly obesity and sleep deprivation). In patients that don't succeed on any treatment, our advice is to continue to follow up and maintain contact in case change occurs.

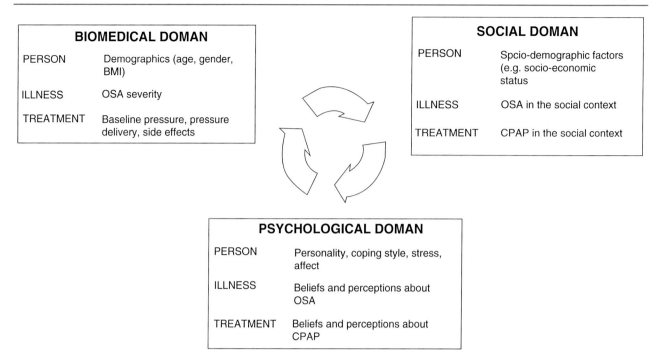

Fig. 32.2 Biopsychosocial model of CPAP adherence. (Adapted from Crawford et al. [32])

32.8 Dealing with CPAP Side Effects

Crucial to optimising adherence to CPAP is an awareness of the potential clinical side effects of therapy and the approach to their management. Side effects are encountered by up to two thirds of patients on CPAP [12]. The choice of CPAP interface has implications for air leakage and skin irritation [35]. As well as adjusting the choice of interface for fit and patient preference, adjuncts such as chin straps and different manufacturing materials for masks and mask straps can impact fit.

Imperfect mask fit can also lead to abrasions of the skin, particularly over the nasal bridge. Skin breakage over bone, similar to pretibial lacerations, can lead to significant cellulitis and potentially thrombosis of the cerebral sagittal sinus. Rarely, skin grafts and prolonged courses of antibiotics may be required. Employment of barrier creams and mask liners can assist with preventing or reversing this [12].

Nasal side effects relate to pressure intolerance and can include nasal dryness, ciliary dysfunction and impaired nasal mucociliary clearance. Nasal inflammation may manifest as rhinorrhoea [36]. Heated humidification is likely to improve the symptoms of many nasal side effects, with intranasal steroids also considered.

Pressure intolerance to CPAP can have a range of manifestations. Strategies to overcome these include reducing CPAP pressure, adopting ramping options and using APAP, which gives on average a reduction in pressure in relation to fixed PAP [12]. In the context of transsphenoidal surgery,

CSF leak has been described [37]. More commonly, aerophagy leading to eructation, abdominal discomfort or gastro-oesophageal reflux is encountered [38].

CPAP air leakage may also lead to air blowing into the eyes or being transmitted from the nasolacrimal duct to the eyes [12]. This can lead to hyperaemia of the conjunctiva, conjunctivochalasis and endophthalmitis [39]. Glaucoma has been shown to be associated with OSA; however, the effects of CPAP on glaucoma have not been established [12].

Paediatric and rare adult case reports exist of mid-facial hypoplasia postulated to be secondary to CPAP use [40]. It is suspected that nasal cushion masks may decrease the frequency of this complication. Dental complications, including movement of teeth and tooth chipping secondary to chin strap use, have been described [12]; middle ear pain can also occur.

An important potential adverse effect of CPAP therapy is the development of treatment-emergent central sleep apnoea. Mechanisms may include concomitant opioid use, changes to respiratory ventilatory control or upper airway reflexes [41]. This is commonly seen within the first month of CPAP, but usually does not persist for greater than 1 month, reflecting it is probably a result of the changing respiratory drive. On occasions, CSA can result from over-zealous CPAP levels (i.e. too high and impeding venous return) – where the 10% body weight rule can be considered. Management strategies include CPAP reduction or change to ASV therapy.

Further challenges include the noise associated with CPAP machines and a sensation of claustrophobia that some patients develop. Graded exposure therapy has been suggested for the latter [42]. Risk of infectious complications, particularly in association with humidified machines, has been theorised but not consistently demonstrated in the literature [12]. Education regarding CPAP cleaning and maintenance continues to be emphasised.

32.9 CPAP Remote Monitoring

It is well recognised that adherence to CPAP varies from 20% to 80% depending on patient symptoms, severity and type of SDB and co-existent pathology (both psychological and physical). As with the pacemaker industry, assessment of objective adherence by most devices is extremely helpful. A sophisticated digital memory of usage, leak and residual AHI (severity and type) can be downloaded directly from the device or remotely via the Internet (see Figs. 32.3 and 32.4).

It is our opinion that some patients benefit from APAP over CPAP. These patients include those with positional OSA, or where there is considerable night-to-night variability of OSA as seen in patients in whom generous levels of alcohol are consumed sporadically.

Similarly, there are a group of patients in whom APAP may be less effective in our opinion. These patients include those who have (a) had a uvulopalatoplasty and continue to have OSA, (b) periodic breathing [e.g. due to heart failure or narcotics] and (c) periodic limb movements [periodic limb movements are associated with periodic skeletal movements which can trigger additional breaths noted by the APAP device].

Moreover, remote monitoring (which can also allow changes to pressure be made remotely) can now make CPAP therapy more dynamic. For example, in a recent analysis of ~2.6 million users with one device manufacturer, the 90-day adherence to CPAP was 6 hours per night with a mean residual AHI of 3.2 events per hour [43].

During the period of analysis [43], 2.62 million patients met the inclusion criteria; 23.4% of patients were excluded for the following reasons: >1 HME (1.9%), invalid data entry (10.1%), more than one PAP modality used or data from SD card (9.2%) and age ≤18 years (0.7%). The 95th percentile pressure was 10.9 cmH$_2$O and 95th percentile leak of 23 lpm. Note however 23% of the population were excluded and the modality of therapy was variable, namely, APAP in 50%, CPAP in 41%, bilevel PAP in 8% and ASV in 1%.

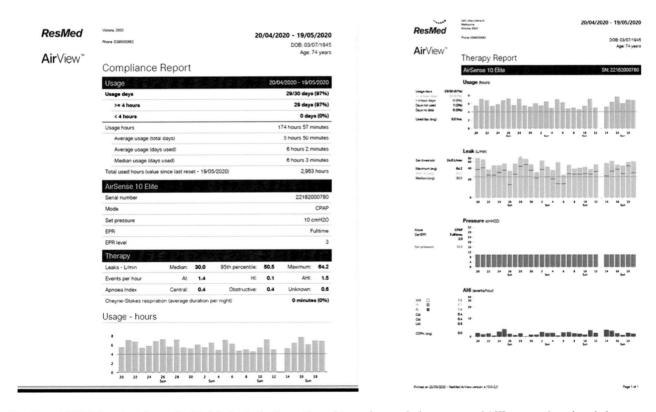

Fig. 32.3 A CPAP download from a ResMed device indicating settings, dates and usage, leak, pressure and AHI across a 4-week period

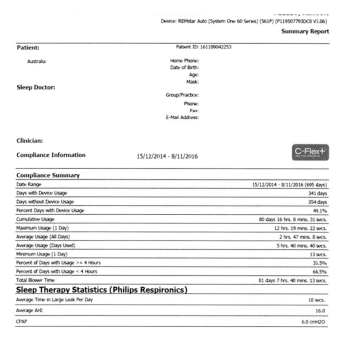
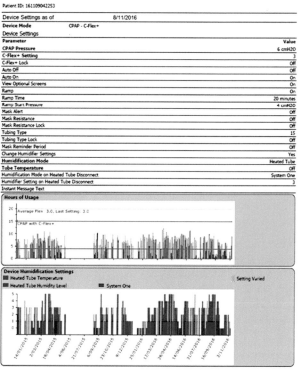

Fig. 32.4 A CPAP download from a Philips Respironics device over 695 days illustrating the settings and a graphic summary of the usage and humidification

32.10 CPAP in the COVID-19 Environment

Recent global virus pandemics including the severe acute respiratory syndrome-associated coronavirus of 2003 (SARS-CoV) and the human coronavirus pandemic of 2019 (COVID-19) have highlighted the potential role of CPAP in treating respiratory failure as well as the theoretical risk of aerosol generation and viral spread [44]. Measurement of exhaled air dispersion from patient-simulating machines receiving non-invasive ventilation has been performed to further characterise the risk of nosocomial infection to healthcare workers, demonstrating that the choice of face mask and degree of associated patient to CPAP interface leak, as well as the level of pressure used, affect the distance of aerosol dispersion [45].

In clinical practice, this has incited the use of bacterial-viral filters to be utilised in conjunction with the exhalation port of CPAP circuits, with the associated transition from vented to non-vented facemasks to reduce theoretical nosocomial spread [44]. The presence or absence of environmental factors such as sufficient room-air exchanges and negative-pressure rooms has been theorised to further augment the risk infection spread from generated aerosols. Robust prospective data to stratify the risk of infection to healthcare workers from CPAP applied to patients with acute respiratory infections remains unforthcoming, and in its absence, the use of extensive personal protective equipment by healthcare workers, including use of N95 respirators, has become commonly practised [45].

32.11 Summary

The CPAP machine has evolved into a sophisticated device for the chronic management of OSA. Best practice is facilitated by close observation of barriers to long-term adherence across biomedical, social and psychological domains, and thorough understanding and attention regarding the potential adverse effects of therapy. The future of CPAP therapy is likely to promote greater customisation of machine and interface variables to the individual patient and will be tempered by the effects of recent global viral pandemics to deliver safety and efficacy to both patients and healthcare workers.

References

1. Barach AL, Martin J, Eckman M. Positive-pressure respiration and its application for the treatment of acute pulmonary edema and respiratory obstruction. Proc Am Soc Clin Invest. 1937;16:664–80.
2. Andersen EW, Ibsen B. The anaesthetic management of patients with poliomyelitis and respiratory paralysis. Br Med J. 1954;1:786–8.

3. Ashbaugh DG, Bigelow DB, Petty TL, Levine BE. Acute respiratory distress in adults. Lancet. 1967;2(7511):319–23.

4. Sullivan CE, Berthon-Jones M, Issa FG, Eves L. Reversal of obstructive sleep apnoea by continuous positive airway pressure applied through the nares. Lancet. 1981;317(8225):862–5.

5. Kirby T. Colin Sullivan: inventive pioneer of sleep medicine. Lancet. 2011;377(9776):1485.

6. Pierson DJ. History and epidemiology of noninvasive ventilation in the acute-care setting. Respir Care. 2009;54(1):40–52.

7. Leger P, Bedcam JM, Cornette A, Reybat-Degat O, Langevin B, Polu JM, Jeannin L, Robert D. Nasal intermittent positive pressure ventilation. Long-term follow-up in patients with severe chronic respiratory insufficiency. Chest. 1994;105(1):100–5.

8. Berkani M, Lofaso F, Chouaid C, d'Ortho MP, Theret D, Grillier-Lanoir V, Harf A, Housset B. CPAP titration by an auto-CPAP device based on snoring detection: a clinical trial and economic considerations. Eur Respir J. 1998;12(4):759–63.

9. Lofaso F, Lorino AM, Duizabo D, Najafi Zadeh H, Theret D, Goldenberg F, Harf A. Evaluation of an auto-CPAP device based on snoring detection. Eur Respir J. 1996;9(9):1795–800.

10. Mansfield DR, Antic N, Rajaratnam S, Naughton M, EBSCOhost, editors. Sleep medicine. Melbourne: IP Communications; 2017.

11. Soudorn C, Muntham D, Reutrakel S, Chirakalwasan N. Effect of heated humidification on CPAP therapy adherence in subjects with obstructive sleep apnea with nasopharyngeal symptoms. Respir Care. 2016;61(9):1151–9.

12. Ghadiri M, Grunstein RR. Clinical side effects of continuous positive airway pressure in patients with obstructive sleep apnoea. Respirology. 2020;25:593–602. https://doi.org/10.1111/resp.13808.

13. Galetke W, Puzzo L, Priegnitz C, Anduleit N, Randerath WJ. Long-term therapy with continuous positive airway pressure obstructive sleep apnea: adherence, side effects and predictors of withdrawal – a 'real-life' study. Respiration. 2011;82:155–61.

14. Lebret M, Martinot JB, Arnol N, Zerillo D, Tamislier R, Pepin JL. Factors contributing to unintentional leak during CPAP treatment: a systematic review. Chest. 2017;151:707–19.

15. Deshpande S, Joosten S, Turton A, Edwards BA, Landry S, Mansfield DR, Hamilton GS. Oronasal masks require a higher pressure than nasal and nasal pillow masks for the treatment of obstructive sleep apnea. J Clin Sleep Med. 2016;12:1263–8.

16. Hsu DY, Cheng YL, Bien MY, Lee HC. Development of a method for manufacturing customised nasal mask cushion for CPAP therapy. Australas Phys Eng Sci Med. 2015;38:657–64.

17. Rosenthal L, Nykamp K, Guido P, Syron ML, Day R, Rice M, Roth T. Daytime CPAP titration: a viable alternative for patients with severe obstructive sleep apnea. Chest. 1998;114:1056–60.

18. West SD, Jones DR, Stradling JR. Comparison of three ways to determine and deliver pressure during nasal CPAP therapy for obstructive sleep apnoea. Thorax. 2006;61:226–31.

19. Howard ME, Piper AJ, Stevens B, Holland AE, Yee BJ, Dabscheck E, Mortimer D, Burge AT, Flunt D, Buchan C, Rautela L, Sheers N, Hillman D, Berlowitz DJ. A randomised controlled trial of CPAP versus non-invasive ventilation for initial treatment of obesity hypoventilation syndrome. Thorax. 2017;72(5):437–44.

20. McEvoy RD, Antic NA, Heeley E, et al. CPAP for prevention of cardiovascular events in obstructive sleep apnea. N Engl J Med. https://doi.org/10.1056/NEJMoa1606599.

21. Peker Y, Glantz H, Eulenburg C, Wegscheider K, Herlitz J, Thunström E. Effect of positive airway pressure on cardiovascular outcomes in coronary artery disease patients with non-sleepy obstructive sleep apnea: the RICCADSA randomized controlled trial. Am J Respir Crit Care Med. 2016;194(5):613–20.

22. Piper AJ, Wang D, Yee BJ, Barnes DJ, Grunstein RR. Randomised trial of CPAP vs bilevel support in the treatment of obesity hypoven-

tilation syndrome without severe nocturnal desaturation. Thorax. 2008;63:395–401.

23. Masa JF, Mokhlesi B, Benitez I, et al. Long-term clinical effectiveness of continuous positive airway pressure therapy versus non-invasive ventilation therapy in patients with obesity hypoventilation syndrome: a multicentre open label, randomised controlled trial. Lancet. 2019;393:1721–32.

24. McEvoy RD, Pierce RJ, Hillman D, et al., Australian trial of non-invasive Ventilation in Chronic Airflow Limitation (AVCAL) Study Group. Nocturnal non-invasive nasal ventilation in stable hypercapnic COPD: a randomised controlled trial. Thorax. 2009;64(7):561–6.

25. Struik FM, Sprooten RT, Kerstjens HA, et al. Nocturnal non-invasive ventilation in COPD patients with prolonged hypercapnia after ventilatory support for acute respiratory failure: a randomised, controlled, parallel-group study. Thorax. 2014;69(9):826–34.

26. Köhnlein T, Windisch W, Köhler D, et al. Non-invasive positive pressure ventilation for the treatment of severe stable chronic obstructive pulmonary disease: a prospective, multicentre, randomised, controlled clinical trial. Lancet Respir Med. 2014;2(9):698–705.

27. Murphy PJ, Rehal S, Arbane G, et al. Effect of home noninvasive ventilation with oxygen therapy vs oxygen therapy alone on hospital readmission or death after an acute COPD exacerbation. JAMA. 2017;317:2177–86.

28. Kopelovich JC, de la Garza GO, Greenlee JDW, Graham SM, Udeh CI, O'Brien EK. Pneumocephalus with BiPAP use after transsphenoidal surgery. J Clin Anaes. 2012;24(5):415–8.

29. Crawford MR, Espie CA, Bartlett DJ, Grunstein RR. Integrating psychology and medicine in CPAP adherence – new concepts? Sleep Med Rev. 2013;18:123–39.

30. Sawyer AM, Gooneratne NS, Marcus CL, Ofer D, Richards KC, Weaver TE. A systematic review of CPAP adherence across age groups: clinical and empiric insights for developing CPAP adherence interventions. Sleep Med Rev. 2011;15:343–56.

31. DiMatteo MR. Variations in patients' adherence to medical recommendations – a quantitative review of 50 years of research. Med Care. 2004;2:200–9.

32. Lebret M, Martino JB, Arnol N, Zerillo D, Tamisier R, Pepin JL, Borel JC. Factors contributing to unintentional leak during CPAP treatment: a systematic review. Chest. 2017;151:707–19.

33. AlAhmari MD, Sapsford RJ, Wezicha JA, Hurst JR. Dose response of continuous positive airway pressure on nasal symptoms, obstruction and inflammation in vivo and in vitro. Eur Respir J. 2012;40:1180–90.

34. Effect of Adaptive Servo Ventilation (ASV) on Survival and Hospital Admissions in Heart Failure (ADVENT-HF). https://clinicaltrials.gov/ct2/show/NCT01128816.

35. Teschler H, Dohring J, Wang YM, Berthon-Jones M. Adaptive pressure servo-ventilation: a novel treatment for Cheyne-stokes respiration in heart failure. Am J Respir Crit Care Med. 2001;164(4):614–9.

36. Cowie MR, Woehrle H, Wegscheider K, Angermann C, d-Ortho MP, Erdmann E, Levy P, Simonds AK, Somers VK, Zannad F, Teschler H. Adaptive servo-ventilation for central sleep apnea in systolic heart failure. N Engl J Med. 2015;373(12):1095–105.

37. Kuzniar TJ, Gruber B, Mutlu GM. Cerebrospinal fluid leak and meningitis associated with nasal continuous positive airway pressure therapy. Chest. 2005;128:1882–4.

38. Mystkowski S, Watson N. Association of CPAP related aerophagia and gastroesophageal reflux disease. Sleep. 2007;30:A325.

39. Harrison W, Pence N, Kovacich S. Anterior segment complications secondary to continuous positive airway pressure machine treatment in patients with obstructive sleep apnea. Optometry. 2007;78:352–5.

40. Roberts SD, Kapadia H, Greenlee G, Chen ML. Midfacial and dental changes associated with nasal positive airway pressure in

children with obstructive sleep apnea and craniofacial conditions. J Clin Sleep Med. 2016;12:469–75.

41. Dernaika T, Tawk M, Nazir S, Younis W, Kinasewitz GT. The significance and outcome of continuous positive airway pressure-related central sleep apnea during split-night sleep studies. Chest. 2007;132:81–7.

42. Means MK, Edinger JD. Graded exposure therapy for addressing claustrophobic reactions to continuous positive airway pressure: a case series report. Behav Sleep Med. 2007;5:105–16.

43. Cistulli P, Armitstead J, Pepin J, Woehrle H, Nunez C, Benjafield A, Malhotra A. Short-term CPAP adherence in obstructive sleep apnea: a big data analysis using real world data. Sleep Med. 2019;59:114–6.

44. Elliot M, Nava S, Schonhofer B, editors. Non-invasive ventilation and weaning: principles and practice. 2nd ed. Florida: CRC Press; 2019.

45. Hui DS, Chow BK, Lo T, Ng SS, Ko FK, Gin T, Chan MT. Exhaled air dispersion during non-invasive ventilation via helmets and a total facemask. Chest. 2015;147(5):1336–43.

How to Start Using CPAP and Benefiting From CPAP Use: The CPAP Vendor's Practical Information to Patients

33

Alex Novodvorets

Most readers already know that CPAP is the gold standard for sleep apnea treatment. There are four types of sleep apnea: obstructive sleep apnea (OSA), central sleep apnea (CSA), mixed or complex sleep apnea, and hypopnea. The severity of sleep apnea is determined by the number of times during the night that a person stops breathing for a period of over 10 seconds. This is commonly followed by a drop in their oxygen level.

Although 75% of the population are not aware of having sleep apnea[1] when they do have a condition, approximately 26% of adults have at least mild sleep apnea,[2] making it a very common but still unrecognized disorder. This means one in five people would stop breathing at least five times every hour of sleep. The prevalence of sleep apnea in the USA is similar to asthma and diabetes.[3] While everybody knows what snoring is, it is considered a social condition that does not require treatment. However, snoring (which occurs when there is an obstruction or collapsed airway) is an indicator that one might have sleep apnea – a completely collapsed airway that prevents air movement and causes oxygen deprivation with impact particularly on the heart and the brain (Fig. 33.1).

In this chapter we will bust a few *myths about CPAP*:

1. I don't need sleep apnea treatment.
2. CPAP machines are noisy and will disrupt my sleep more than snoring would.
3. A CPAP mask is bulky and not comfortable, my friend couldn't get used to it.
4. I have been snoring for decades; I'm fine.

Signs and symptoms of obstructive sleep apnea include:

- *Morning headache*
- Excessive daytime *sleepiness*
- *Loud snoring*
- Awakening with a dry mouth or sore *throat*

There is a need to treat sleep apnea even if there are no clear symptoms. If left untreated, sleep apnea can lead to:

- High blood pressure
- Diabetes
- Irregular heart rhythms
- Heart disease/stroke/heart attack
- Driving and work-related accidents

Almost 40 years ago, Dr. Colin Sullivan successfully treated sleep apnea for the first time by delivering continuous positive airway pressure through the upper airway.

CPAP is a treatment, not a cure .... It helps only as long as you use it. The night you stop using the CPAP, your symptoms and snoring will return.

33.1 CPAP or Flow Generator

A CPAP machine (Fig. 33.2) creates positive air pressure and delivers it through the mask to keep the airway open and prevent its collapse. *As a result, the snoring stops and sleep apnea disappears.* There are different types of air pressure treatments: fixed-pressure CPAP, auto-adjusting CPAP (APAP), and bi-level CPAP (VPAP).

In order to improve compliance with CPAP therapy, new CPAP machines have Bluetooth or wireless connectivity to allow remote monitoring and troubleshooting.

---

[1]Young et al. Sleep 2008

[2]Peppard et al. J Am Med Assoc 2013

[3]US Dep of Health and Human Services, Centers for Disease Control and Prevention 2008

A. Novodvorets (✉)
CPAP Clinic, Vaughan, ON, Canada
e-mail: alex@cpapclinic.ca

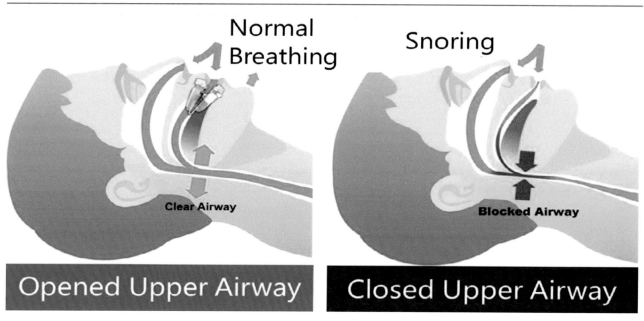

Fig. 33.1 Open and blocked airways

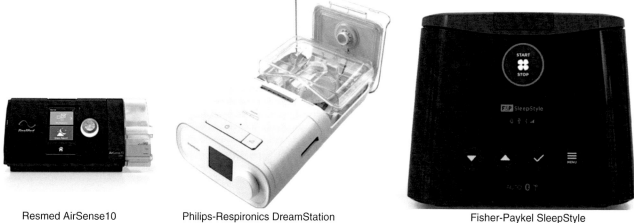

Resmed AirSense10   Philips-Respironics DreamStation   Fisher-Paykel SleepStyle

Fig. 33.2 Examples of the current PAP machine brands and models

With compliance monitoring, the provider can check the usage, leak level, and apnea index that the CPAP machine reported via the manufacturer's website. Your provider can then contact you to resolve the issue or, if required, can share the therapy report with the patient's physician, and this connectivity allows the vendor to adjust the therapy pressure or mode based on the prescription from your specialist.

33.2 CPAP Mask: The Key to a Successful CPAP Therapy

The upper airway has four compartments: the nose and mouth, the pharynx, the larynx, and the trachea. Breathing through the nose is normal and healthier because:

1. The nose purifies small particles and adjusts the air to your body's temperature.
2. The nose humidifies the air and adds resistance to the air stream.

Breathing through the mouth becomes necessary when you have nasal congestion due to allergies or a cold, a deviated septum, as well as enlarged adenoids or enlarged tonsils. For some people with sleep apnea, it may become a habit to sleep with their mouth open to accommodate their need for oxygen. However, this does not make them mouth-breathers and once they start CPAP therapy, they revert back to nasal breathing, which is healthier.

CPAP masks are constantly getting smaller, softer, lighter, and more comfortable (Fig. 33.3).

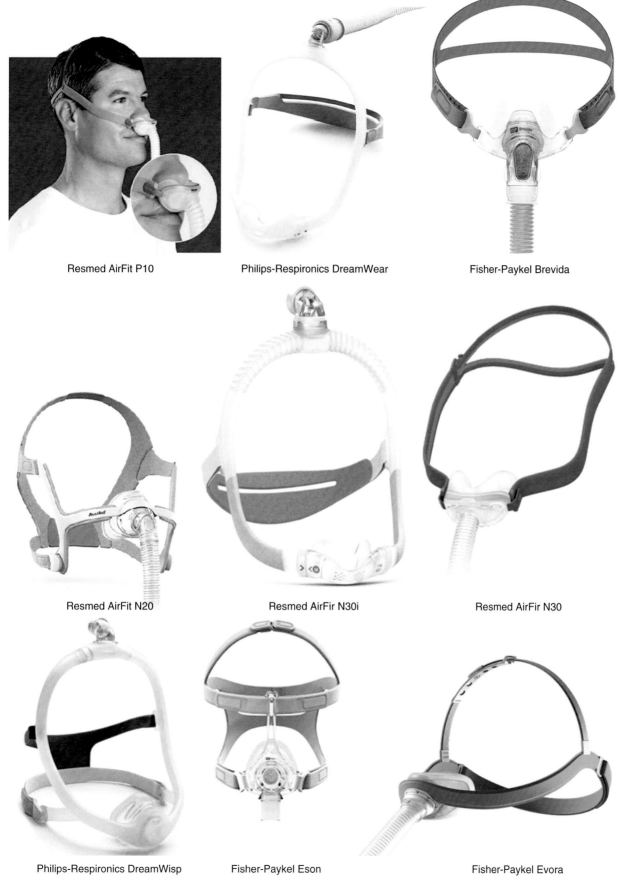

Resmed AirFit P10   Philips-Respironics DreamWear   Fisher-Paykel Brevida

Resmed AirFit N20   Resmed AirFir N30i   Resmed AirFir N30

Philips-Respironics DreamWisp   Fisher-Paykel Eson   Fisher-Paykel Evora

Fig. 33.3 PAP masks

The weight of a CPAP mask has reduced in the last decade from 300 grams to only 17 grams and has a single soft headgear strap that fits all and does not require any adjustment.

There are two types of masks: nasal and full-face masks (Fig. 33.4). While nasal masks provide air exclusively through the nose, the full-face masks need to be more by those who breathe through the mouth.

Nasal masks have three configurations (Fig. 33.5):

Another variation of the nasal mask is the hose position: this type of mask is placed on top of the head and the tube is placed behind the pillow to allow more freedom moving without pulling the mask.

The first step in finding the right CPAP mask is to determine if a nasal mask will be sufficient or if the full-face mask is required.

Nasal masks are the lightest and smallest. They tend to provide an unobstructed view, allowing the patient to watch TV or read before falling asleep. However, there are some disadvantages: they are easy to remove during sleep and if the strap is not adjustable, it needs to be replaced often because it scratches and wears out.

Full-face masks are more complex, making them harder to get used to (Fig. 33.6). They have also evolved from a large cover for the nose and mouth to going under the chin as well as drastically trimming the weight and size.

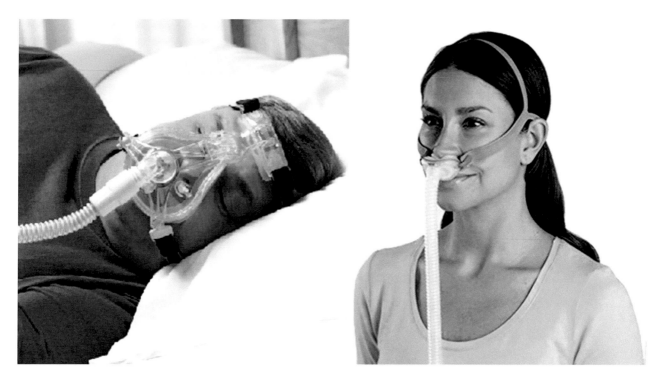

Fig. 33.4 The two main types of PAP masks

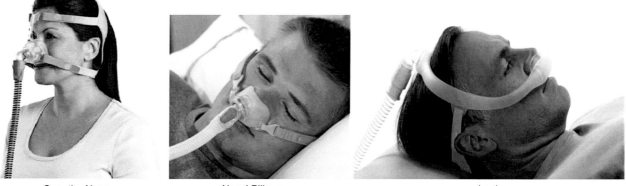

Over the Nose   Nasal Pillows   under the nose

Fig. 33.5 Nasal masks

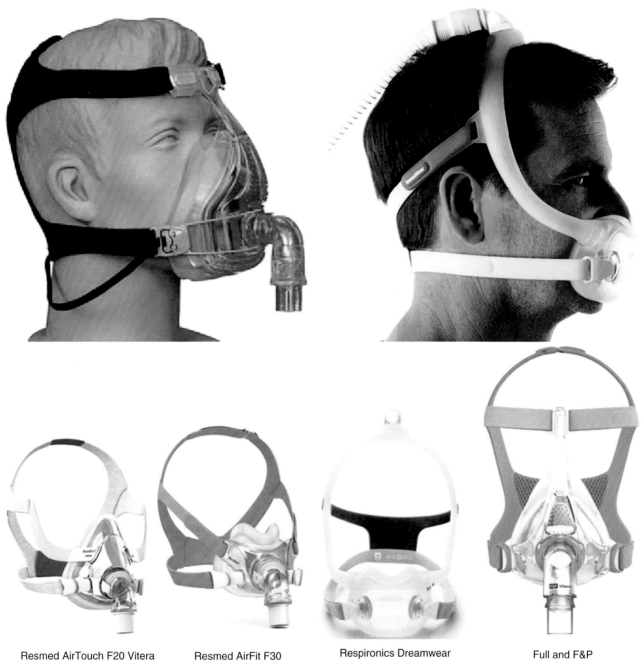

| Resmed AirTouch F20 Vitera | Resmed AirFit F30 | Respironics Dreamwear | Full and F&P |

Fig. 33.6 The most popular full-face masks

There are over 140 different masks types and sizes. This makes the fitting process challenging, but allows one to find the best fitting mask to ensure higher compliance and successful CPAP therapy.

There are endless articles and "How-to …" videos about each and every mask, but you will have the most success if you go over your options with an experienced and caring CPAP consultant who will spend as much time as you need, usually 30–60 minutes, to try on different masks and help you understand how they work and which features are important.

33.3 Common Problems and Possible Solutions

33.3.1 Dry Nose or Mouth

Humidification is not sufficient. You can increase the humidity level on your CPAP machine or even purchase a heated hose that will be able to carry more humidity without creating condensation in the tube.

33.3.2 The Pressure Is Too High

New CPAP machines have advanced ramp functionality that starts increasing the pressure only after you fall asleep and not during a set time. In addition, the majority of new PAP machines are auto-PAP; these machines deliver 30% less pressure by monitoring the airway resistance and adjusting the pressure to the level required at every moment instead of keeping a fixed pressure.

Factors that may lead to a change in pressure requirement include a, b, c, d, etc.

33.3.3 Skin Irritation or Red Areas

Although the masks are latex-free and not supposed to cause allergic reactions, many people still develop skin irritation. First, try to loosen the straps. If the skin irritation does not resolve, it is time to replace the mask or cushion. Then, rinse the mask thoroughly with running water to ensure no detergent is left on the silicone. Another option is to use cloth liners or a cloth mask.

33.3.4 Unconscious Mask Removal While Sleeping

Trying to remember and explain your behavior while sleeping tends to be a difficult task. Therefore, you can't know the exact reason why you remove the mask. Whether it's claustrophobia or the mask not fitting, you can try to prevent unconscious mask removal by addressing each factor separately. There is a very short and effective treatment for claustrophobia – if you need help, ask a referral to a psychologist who is trained in cognitive behavioral therapy (for more details in claustrophobia treatment, see Chap. 6). If the mask is not fitting, ask for a consultation with your PAP provider.

33.4 CPAP Care and Equipment Cleaning and Maintenance

Daily/weekly routines that only take 5 minutes:

1. Unplug your CPAP machine from the power source.
2. Disconnect the mask and air tubing from the CPAP machine.
3. Disassemble your mask into three parts (headgear, cushion, and frame).
4. Clean your mask cushion and headgear in a sink to remove any oils with mild soap without alcohol or antibacterial chemicals.

   Avoid using stronger cleaning products, including dish detergents, as they may damage the mask or leave harmful residue.
5. Rinse again thoroughly with warm, drinking-quality water.
6. Place the cushion and frame on a flat surface, on top of a towel, to dry. Avoid placing them in direct sunlight.

SoClean and Lumin CPAP sanitizers are additional alternatives to help keep your equipment clean (Fig. 33.7). Both options are designed for automated CPAP cleaning and sanitizing that kills 99.9% of CPAP germs and bacteria in your mask, hose, and reservoir. You don't need water or any chemicals in order to enhance your CPAP cleaning experience.

33.5 SoClean Versus Lumin

SoClean uses ozone gas to disinfect and it takes 2 hours, while Lumin uses UV-light technology and has a short (5-minute) cycle. The ozone gas can leak everywhere, while the UV light can't get through dark silicone or go inside heated hoses. Using either of those devices can give you a peace of mind, but they do not replace washing the mask regularly and periodic replacement of your CPAP supplies every 3–6 or 12 months, based on the manufacturer's recommendations.

33.6 Lifestyle and Traveling with Your CPAP

Don't let sleep apnea stop you from traveling the world. With the increase of technology in the field of sleep medicine, sleep apnea patients can now travel with ease (Fig. 33.8). CPAP shouldn't impact your travel plans any longer.

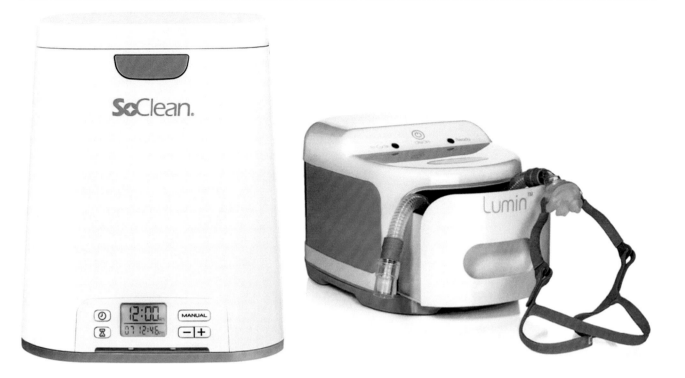

Fig. 33.7   CPAP sanitizers

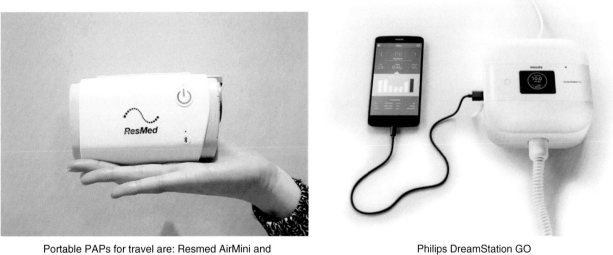

Portable PAPs for travel are: Resmed AirMini and   Philips DreamStation GO

Fig. 33.8   Potable PAP devices

33.7   Conclusion – DO NOT GIVE UP!

Treating your apnea is very important. You will experience problems getting used to your CPAP and it will take a few weeks or even months to get comfortable wearing the mask. However, once you get used to it, your life will change and the improvement and lack of fatigue will motivate you to keep using the CPAP.

Elaine Huang

As a treatment coordinator, my main role is to work along-side the treating sleep physicians and assist the clients to navigate through their treatment plan. As a team, we have been very fortunate to receive much valuable guidance from our team of supportive sleep doctors, as well as constructive feedback from clients and the different medical suppliers we frequently work with. We continue to fine-tune our methods to find the best way to effectively steer the clients through what may seem like a confusing process and to ensure each client obtain the best care for their sleep apnea treatments.

As a CPAP treatment coordinator, my first in-person meeting with a client starts after the client has received their diagnosis and treatment recommendations from their sleep physician. Although the physician has already taken the time to explain the client's diagnosis and the next steps, clients may not be able to retain all of the information provided or know where exactly to start planning and how to take the necessary action. Often clients initially appear agreeable with their treating physician's recommendations, but they may be too apprehensive to discuss their hesitation with their sleep physicians, or not to know what questions to ask before the meeting ended. Furthermore, often there is a waiting period until the client can have their next appointment with their sleep doctor, and the client would benefit from having a resolution to their concerns sooner. My role was created specifically to tend to this need and act as an additional link between the doctor, the sleep laboratory, the client, and the medical supplier, to make sure the client proceeds with and continues to receive support with their treatment plan. Having a treatment coordinator in place gives the clients an additional channel to have a more casual conversation and have someone with whom they can make a detailed treatment plan. My objective for each patient is that they walk out of the sleep clinic feeling confident with their next step and have a clear treatment plan in place.

34.1 Different Stages of Grief After Diagnosis and Coping with the Diagnosis

Once the client has finished their meeting with their treating physician, the information that has been provided by their doctors slowly starts to sink in, and often clients feel trapped and overwhelmed. The client may have seemed agreeable with the recommended actions during their meeting with the physician, as all the information logically makes sense at first. It is usually shortly after the meeting that all their questions and doubts appear. Often, once I sit down with the client, to help them plan for their next step, this is when the clients start to go through their emotions and come up with questions.

Many clients may feel as though they have been delivered with a punishment sentence that they have a sleep disorder, being pushed to decide on a major lifestyle change and purchase. Most clients may go through different stages of "grief" while coping with their new diagnosis (Table 34.1).

Clients go through some stage of "grief," and it may not be in any specific order. It's important for me as the treatment coordinator to recognize that their emotions are natural, to be patient with the clients' questions, to provide as

Table 34.1 Understanding the different post-diagnosis emotions using Elisabeth Kubler-Ross's five stages of grief

Stages of grief	Examples of expression
Denial	It is not true/it can't be/the testing must be wrong
Anger	Why me? Why is my body failing me? Why am I being forced to fix this?
Bargaining	Is there any medicine that I can take to make this go away? Can I do this after my next big work assignment/exam/family event?
Depression	I am now old and frail and need a device to get proper sleep./ My husband will never love me now that I need to wear a mask to sleep
Acceptance	I will do what needs to be done for my health

E. Huang (✉)
Sleep and Alertness Clinic, Toronto, ON, Canada
e-mail: elaine@sleepalert.ca

much emotional support as needed, and to recognize which "stages of grief" clients are in. Some clients need to be provided with statistical information to realize that immediate treatment is needed. For some others, a review of the information that their treating sleep physician has just provided is helpful. The primary focus of this initial meeting is to emphasize the positive aspects of the treatment and that multiple treatment options are available for their diagnosis. A secondary focus is to establish a solid level of rapport and trust so that the clients know they have firm support from the sleep laboratory and their doctors to get through the process of obtaining treatment. Clients need to know that they are not facing their diagnosis alone. Many clients may bargain, claiming that they will comply with the treatment once their plate is a little less full. The clients need to recognize that one's sleep and therefore health is of utmost importance. A simple "Yes, I will do it" will not be sufficient. A solid plan with timeline needs to be set in place, so the clients can visualize themselves following a treatment plan. A relatively smaller group of clients may respond positively to the diagnosis right from the start. The client may be relieved that they have an answer to what they have been suspecting for years, that their condition has finally been defined, and that a single treatment may serve to ease their other chronic illness, such as chronic headache and unexplained high blood pressure. It is important for all clients to be reminded that treatment for sleep apnea is not only in place to treat the symptoms, such as snoring or waking up to gasp for breath but also can help them to reach their long-term health goals. Treatment can be presented in a positive light as a resolution for a health concern, not as a punishment. It is not only about living longer, but to live healthier so one can stay active and enjoy life.

34.2 Treatment Options and Accessibility

A common misconception that many clients have is that any client attending a sleep clinic, who receives a sleep apnea diagnosis, will be prescribed continuous positive airway pressure (CPAP) as a method of treatment. PAP therapy involves wearing a mask through the night when going to sleep; the mask is connected to a machine with a motor that generates positive airway pressure to keep the client's airway open. PAP is certainly considered as the "golden standard" for clients who have been diagnosed with sleep apnea. However, it is not the least intrusive sleep apnea treatment method. It is most accessible, and, depending on the jurisdiction, it may be the most affordable option for most clients (e.g., if it is the only treatment that receives government financial support). PAP is usually the first recommended option, but not the only option available. To make the client better understand, I often use the analogy to compare treatment for sleep apnea with treatment for vision correction, which includes the use of glasses, lenses, or laser eye surgery. PAP therapy is a management treatment, it is not a cure, and it is only effective if it is being used. This is similar to one using glasses for vision correction. One must always use CPAP to get more quality sleep; this is akin to one who would always need to put on glasses when they want to see clearly. Some clients may consider oral appliance therapy, which is also similar to wearing contact lenses to correct one's vision. Oral appliance therapy involves wearing a dental device when going to sleep to ensure that the lower jaw protrudes forward in order to open up the airway. This line of treatment is more costly in many situations and takes slightly longer to fabricate and an additional assessment may be needed to make sure the particular patient is a good candidate before proceeding. For clients who have sleep apnea that occurs mainly in certain positions (e.g., when sleeping on their backs), their treating sleep doctor may recommend a positional device to promote sleeping on their sides as opposed to on their backs, to minimize the apneas. Some clients may discuss with their treating sleep physicians the possibility of proceeding with an ear-nose-throat (ENT) consultation before deciding on treatment options. (In children, this is a first-line treatment but it is not often applicable in adults.) Some may decide to proceed with oral and maxillofacial surgery, which is similar to having laser eye surgery, as a more permanent solution.

The client needs to be reminded that their treating sleep physician has recommended what would work best for their diagnosis and medical history. Even though the different treatment options and reasoning for focusing on one or two paths have been explained to the client during their meeting with their doctor, the client may not be able to retain all the information as there may have been a great deal of information covered. As a treatment coordinator, once I see a copy of what the client has been recommended, my role is to make sure the client have all the available information and resources to proceed to the next step. I rehearse the detailed steps needed, the approximate cost, whether additional supportive funding is available, and the time frame for obtaining the treatment. Once the client has a chance to hear the treatment information again, they may better understand that their sleep physician focuses mostly on the one treatment option that is most suitable for them and that they are ultimately in control of their treatment. This allows the clients' anxiety to abate. Lower anxiety levels certainly help clients to make better informed decisions. Although some clients may initially have doubts, once they have had time to process the information mentally, so that they can feel comfortable with making the next step, most would follow the primary recommendation advised by their treating physicians.

The majority of the clients choose to start with PAP therapy, as it is the most effective and accessible treatment for most. Some clients may choose to start with PAP while they wait to obtain their oral appliance or arrange oral and maxillofacial surgery at a later date. Some may choose to proceed with more than one treatment option before deciding which one works best for them. Clients should know that they are free to choose what would work for them and that they are never at fault and will not be criticized even if they do change their mind subsequently. As a treatment coordinator, if the client chooses to change their treatment path, I would also assist with the necessary steps. For example, if a client decides to change between PAP therapy and oral appliance therapy, then I would first go over the basic information, such as the next steps involved, the necessary correspondence, appointments, cost, and approximate time frame until they can be on the new treatment. This ensures that even if the initial treatment plan did not work out well, clients do not get lost in the process and can be directed onto an alternative treatment path that may work better for them.

To motivate clients to proceed with their treatment plan as soon as possible, an important part of my role as a treatment coordinator is to emphasize the accessibility of all the treatments. For example, clients who need an initial oral appliance therapy may consider discussing it with their dentist or see a new dentist to have their initial assessment. Some dentists do charge for the initial assessment, while others do not; or some may have shorter wait times than others. I often assist clients to establish what they would prefer and do a comparison to help them decide the best way to proceed. Many clients may choose to proceed with a MatrX sleep study before investing in the full cost of a customized oral appliance. MatrX sleep study is a laboratory sleep study involving the use of a temporary dental device; its goal is to test whether an oral appliance can indeed be effective in treating a client's sleep apnea. In some cases, given the right amount of coordination, clients can have their customized oral appliance within weeks from when they have been diagnosed, while the regular process can take 2–3 months. To give an example with PAP therapy, not all clients are aware that PAP therapy is partially funded in the province in which I am working, and additional support is available for those who are on social assistance. Most private insurance providers would also cover some or all of the remaining client costs. Most clients may not realize how common or accessible PAP therapy is until they have been prescribed to initiate the therapy. If the client is ready to proceed, they can be fitted with their equipment and ready to start on the same day as when they have been initially diagnosed. Individual clients with specific needs, such as language support, or limited mobility needs can always be accommodated. Often once the individual client's needs have been identified, I would offer a list of nearby providers to the clients for their consideration. It is the client's choice on which medical provider they would like to attend for their long-term treatment. My role as a treatment coordinator is to make sure the clients have all the support and necessary information to do so.

34.3 Medical Suppliers and Equipment Manufacturers

It is also helpful for clients to have a brief overview of what happens at the next appointment with a medical supplier. Many clients may be leery of medical suppliers, thinking that they would be pushed to purchase overpriced medical supplies that they don't need. As a treatment coordinator, my role is unique in the sense that I'm not in a position to sell any service or products, and therefore, clients often see me as an unbiased information resource who is solely there for their benefits. Clients are more inclined to attend a medical supplier if they have a general expectation of what decisions need to be made, and if they are armed with example questions they may wish to ask the medical supplier before purchasing a CPAP device. For example, finding the right mask is crucial for clients to be successful with their PAP therapy. Clients can be fitted with a nasal pillow (under the nose), nasal (over the nose), or full-face (over nose and mouth) mask based on their individual needs and comfort. All the masks do the same job, which is to deliver the positive airway pressure to the client, and it is up to the client to choose the mask at the medical supplier. Most clients would test their first mask at the medical supplier's office before taking the equipment and supplies home, but the real test is when the clients wear the mask at home on their own. Therefore, it is most beneficial for clients to choose a provider that provides a thorough demonstration on how to properly fit a mask by themselves, and has a flexible mask exchange policy, so that if the first mask being fitted is not working well, the clients can go back and exchange for a different mask size or style. It is common for clients to take 1–2 attempts before finding the right mask fit. Clients also often wonder if they should select products from one manufacturer over others. All PAP machines, regardless of manufacturer, have the same basic function, which is to generate positive airway pressure to keep the client's airway open during sleep. For the clients' ease of access, PAP masks and machines are made to be universally adaptable. There are more advanced PAP machine models that would allow the client to track their treatment progress, adjust the temperature settings on the humidifier, or have specific breathing technology that would make it more comfortable for clients to breathe out against the incoming positive airway pressure.

Some clients who travel often would seek a manufacturer that makes travel-friendly PAP units and the client may need to consider the compatibility between the unit they use at home and the unit they take when they are on the road. Some clients may seek to keep the cost low and do not have much interest in having additional features on their PAP unit. Sleep clinics should receive the latest information updates from all the main manufacturers, so they can pass on the information to clients. During my initial meeting with the client, I would give a brief overview of what typical features clients could have. This information may prompt the client to ask more questions and therefore be more prepared prior to their purchase decision. Some clients may prefer to receive all the basic information on the different models offered by different manufacturers, do their research, and then have a phone or in-person discussion with me as an unbiased resource, before they see a CPAP provider for their equipment purchase. It is up to the client to decide whether a specific feature is important to them, and how much they would like to invest in a more advanced unit. Going back to spectacles and vision analogy, this is similar to choosing a different type of glass lenses. Clients can choose basic plastic lenses that would do the job and help one see better or transition lenses that could bring more comfort or ease but at a slightly higher price point. The most important information for me to share with the client is that they need to obtain the necessary equipment to be on treatment, regardless if it is the most expensive or the most economical model. As long as treatment has been initiated, then they have already taken the most difficult step in this entire process.

34.4 Therapy Expectation and Troubleshooting

Once clients have initiated their sleep therapy of choice, as a treatment coordinator, I need to make sure the clients have a realistic expectation of their treatment outlook, and to help follow through until the client is on a steady path for their treatment plan. For example, clients proceeding with the oral appliance therapy may initially report that they find morning soreness in their teeth or jaw muscles, or that there is more drooling than before. The soreness should slowly dissipate as the client's body gets used to the mouthguard, but if the discomfort is causing distress or more disruption than they had before the treatment, then the client needs to know they should be returning to the dentist for potential adjustments, or return to see their sleep physician for a further discussion. For clients proceeding with PAP therapy, having a realistic expectation is important for clients to be adherent to the therapy. Clients should know that they may take 1–6 months to fully get used to the treatment, or the client may only be able to use the therapy between 4 and 6 hours for the first month or two. Some clients may have unrealistic expectations that once they start treatment, they should be able to sleep through the night with the treatment in place and waking up feeling fully refreshed. Starting any kind of medical treatment is a huge change for one's routine and lifestyle, and it is expected

to take time and dedication. If the client is too harsh on themselves and blames themselves for not being able to tolerate the therapy right from the start, then they are more likely to give up and jump to the conclusion that the therapy is not working at all. A step-by-step process needs to be laid out and reasonable goals set for the client. For clients who are especially nervous with initiating PAP therapy, they may benefit from generating a plan with a treatment coordinator, so they have a tangible goal set for each step, and an agreed time frame to reach such goal. Clients who have anxiety about CPAP use or stay hesitant benefit from a referral to a psychologist behavioral sleep specialist (Chap. 6) (Table 34.2).

It is important to recognize that starting PAP therapy is a major lifestyle change, and it takes a great deal of commitment. Clients should be encouraged once they have reached a milestone, such as sleeping through the night for more than 4–6 hours with the therapy for the first time. At the same time, clients need to be motivated to persevere even if they have had a slow start.

Once the client is started on PAP therapy, the first month is crucial to starting on the right track for the treatment and staying on track. If a client has not been fitted with the right mask from the start or receives the support to make the therapy more tolerable, it may lead the client into thinking the therapy is meant to be uncomfortable. Over time, the client may become frustrated and therefore will eventually refuse the treatment. In some cases, the client may refuse follow-up appointments with their doctors as well. Clients need to be encouraged and followed up regularly within the first

Table 34.2 Example of a step-by-step guide to get used to PAP therapy

Step 1	Obtain equipment and supplies; ensure mask fits comfortably on the client's face. Client can wear the mask without any tubing or therapy in place during the day while preoccupied with an active task to increase familiarity, such as when washing dishes
Step 2	Client can put on mask during the day without treatment turned on while client is relaxed and preoccupied with other tasks, such as watching television or reading
Step 3	Client to put on mask during the day with treatment turned on while occupied with other tasks, such as watching television or reading, for 10–20 minutes at a time, or for as long as they are comfortable with
Step 4	Client to put on mask and turn on therapy at night 30 minutes before bed time, and try to fall asleep with therapy in place if possible
Step 5	Client is able to fall asleep with therapy in place and tries to sleep through the night with the therapy as long as possible
Step 6	Client is able to fall asleep and maintain sleep through the night with the therapy, and nightly usage hours can slowly increase with repeat usage

Note: This process is different for clients who have claustrophobia or other CPAP-related anxiety; see Chap. 6

1–3 months to ensure initial obstacles have been tackled. For example, mask discomforts are usually discovered within the first week or so. There are certain areas that the clients can try to fix at home. The client should know that if they have attempted all the potential fixes, but the mask is still not working well to provide a therapeutic seal, they are not at fault and should not be embarrassed to reach out for help. Clients should feel comfortable speaking to their PAP home-care medical provider and explaining what the difficulty is and to find an alternative. If clients are not comfortable with connecting with their original medical supplier, they should be connecting with a different medical supplier with whom the client may have a better rapport. A treatment coordinator is helpful in this regard, to step in and bridge the gap between the client and the home-care medical provider. Often when I contact the client for follow-up, clients will express their difficulties. We would have a short communication over phone or email. Having the initial in-person meeting to establish trust and rapport makes it easier for the client to speak about their concerns. Once we run through all the basic troubleshooting over phone or email, if the client is not comfortable with doing it on their own, I would offer to relay the issues to their corresponding home-care medical provider. If the client expresses that they no longer wish to return to the same provider, whatever reason it may be, I will simply assist the client with finding a new home-care medical provider, so that they can receive the care that they need. Ongoing support is important for every client who needs treatment.

34.5 Ongoing Therapy Compliance Monitoring

For every client, there is ongoing testing or follow-ups to make sure the treatment continues to be effective. If the treating sleep physician sees that the client is doing well, they may recommend the client to return for a follow-up in a year or two for re-evaluation. During this time, clients proceeding with oral appliance therapy may be returning to their dentist for routine follow-ups to ensure comfort and therapy efficacy monitored via a home sleep test. Clients proceeding with PAP therapy can return to their home-care medical providers for ongoing follow-up and servicing, or monitor their own PAP treatment progress with the monitoring technology that is available on most PAP units. Some clients may not be comfortable with having their therapy information accessed by their home-care provider due to confidentiality concerns and may prefer to have their therapy information retained solely at their sleep laboratory and doctors' offices only. For clients with severe sleep apnea, their sleep physician may direct that the client be followed up more closely, in terms of the client having frequent in-person follow-ups with the physician, additional support for the client to initiate and stay on treatment, as well as accessing the client's compliance report on a more regular basis to ensure therapy success. A treatment coordinator can further assist with these goals, such as helping clients retrieve their therapy information, ensure relevant testing is on schedule, retaining the client's therapy information for the client's chart records, and helping the client understand the basics from their compliance information.

Most of the latest PAP units record valuable information on the client's PAP use, which is helpful for troubleshooting and routine monitoring. Clients may benefit from understanding their PAP reports, such as the system's leakage values or the overall apnea-hypopnea index (AHI) values. The system leakage value indicates whether the client's current mask is providing a sufficient seal, or whether there is any significant leakage found on the system, which may indicate mouth breathing or tubing leakage. The AHI value is an average record of breathing events per hour. By monitoring whether the AHI stays within a normal range, the client can self-monitor how well their treatment is working at the current parameters. Giving the client the access and ability to understand their therapy information often encourages the client to achieve their next "personal best" statistical record and contributes to improved therapy compliance (Fig. 34.1).

To avoid clients falling off track, every client should get a printed or emailed timeline on the next steps at the sleep clinic and doctor's office, and both hard and soft copies of the treatment coordinator's contact info. A phone call or email follow-up should be done at the 1-month mark to make sure the client is progressing well. If there are any obstacles, the earlier they are tackled, the more likely the client will be continuing to be adherent to the treatment. Additional phone calls, emails, or in-person visits can be scheduled at the client's convenience or based on their preferences. Support from a treatment coordinator should be readily available, but not too frequent that it disturbs the client's regular daily schedule or creates a nuisance. A general check on the client's chart progress should be done at around 2–3 months after initiating the treatment, to ensure that all the treating physician's instructions and recommended testing have been carried out. For clients who are progressing well, a general email follow-up at 6 months would be ideal. Clients can respond if there is an issue, or retain the clinic's contact info in their email records should a need arise in the future (Table 34.3).

Ongoing communication that occurs between the medical supplier and the doctor's office is important to make sure the client continues to do well with their therapy. Clients may benefit from knowing what happens behind the scenes so that they do not feel that they are forgotten once they leave a sleep laboratory or sleep doctor's office. Medical suppliers routinely communicate in clients' progress reports to the sleep laboratory. If there is an issue that the medical provider

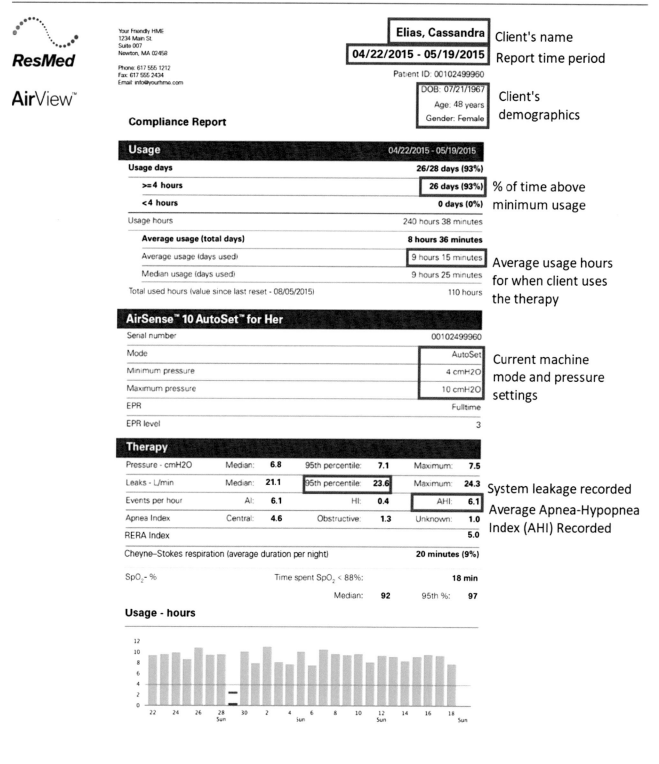

Fig. 34.1 Example of information obtained from a client's PAP unit. Client details are illustrative and not based on any real person. Source: ResMed, "AirView™ report guide", resmedwebinars.com, n.p. 2016. May 12th, 2020 < https://resmedwebinars.com/assets/uploads/ AirView_Report_Guide_1018991.pdf>

Table 34.3 Suggested general follow-up schedule

Time after recommended to initiate therapy	Action
Within 1 week	Email client with a list of next steps at the sleep clinic and contact info, including: Next sleep test date Next follow-up appointment Date with treating physician
After 2–4 weeks	Phone call or email to follow up on progress
After 2–3 months	General chart check to ensure client has proceeded with all recommended appointments
Every 6 months or as directed by sleep physician	Email to follow up on general progress and recommendation for client to stay in touch if difficulties arise in the future

cannot resolve, whether it be a PAP home-care provider or the client's dentist, then the report gets flagged for the sleep physician's attention and advice. This happens, for example, if the client has been doing well with their treatment of choice for 1–2 years, but now has been observing the same symptoms as before treatment was initiated, such as snoring, or that they are no longer waking up with refreshed sleep. The sleep physician may provide directions for the medical supplier to adjust certain settings on the client's PAP unit; the client may be scheduled to return to the sleep laboratory for further testing or an in-person assessment with the sleep physician. At this point, a treatment coordinator can provide additional values to ensure all the steps directed by the sleep physician have been communicated to and carried out by the medical supplier, a continued communication channel is opened between the sleep laboratory and the client, and most importantly, that the client does not get lost in the progress without having their concerns resolved. Once the concern is resolved, the client can once again be grouped as routinely followed up at the 6-month point for ongoing support or as directed by their sleep physicians.

While the sleep doctors, the sleep laboratory, or the medical suppliers all work in harmony to treat the clients for their sleep disorders, a treatment coordinator acts as a catalyst to give the extra boost that the clients may often need to achieve success with their treatment plan.

The Respiratory Therapist and the Vendor's Perspective on CPAP Adherence

35

Barbara Capozzolo, Marcel A. Baltzan, Kateri Champagne, and Dave Johnson

Obstructive sleep apnea (OSA) is a common sleep disorder characterized by intermittent partial or complete upper airway obstruction during sleep, associated with recurrent arousals, nocturnal intermittent hypoxia, sleep fragmentation, and poor sleep quality [1]. Continuous positive airway pressure (CPAP) is a well-established and evidence-based treatment for moderate-to-severe OSA, which significantly ameliorates the symptoms of the syndrome as well as its cardiovascular consequences [2]. However, CPAP acceptance and adherence in daily clinical practice is often problematic [2]. Long-term adherence to CPAP therapy is a major concern because diminished adherence or therapy abandonment results in diminished benefit and recurrence of OSA [3]. Non-adherence rates are reported at 50% with 20–30% of patients stopping CPAP during the first 2 weeks of therapy [3]. Factors affecting CPAP adherence include patient characteristics such as ethnicity, disease and symptom severity, increased nasal resistance, education about therapy benefits, patient perception of benefits, social support and partner interaction, and psychological and other comorbidities (insomnia) [4]. Side effects of CPAP such as aerophagia, pressure ulcerations, skin changes on the face, and a sense of claustrophobia when using the mask can also inhibit long-term use of CPAP.

Several studies show that adherence to CPAP therapy can be improved with numerous strategies: patient educational training and information at the start of therapy, timely approach to the resolution of possible causes of non-adherence to therapy, structured follow-up, and motivational support [1]. Moreover, CPAP adherence might be improved by an intensive follow-up program, including family support, management of side effects of CPAP therapy, and behavioral therapy, where problems may be addressed through a multidisciplinary team approach [2]. In addition, various methods have been proposed to increase adherence, such as achieving proper titration, using the most appropriate device, proper humidification of the upper airways, and educational and psychological programs [5]. These interventions are based on theoretical models and their aim is to remove all barriers that the patient perceives in using CPAP [5]. This suggests the need for an educational program based upon the structured models of adherence developed in the hospital setting [5]. Intervention cannot be based only on solving technical problems, but must be related to socioeconomic and psychological factors, which may affect the ability of the patient to manage their health problems and are closely linked with daily use of CPAP [5].

OSA management includes assessing the level of adherence with treatment outcomes [3]. CPAP can be a demanding therapy to undertake, and patients require a high level of input and support during the initial phase of therapy [3]. The translation of CPAP clinical assessments needs to include a review of subjective and objective use, improvement with CPAP in the outcomes with which OSA is associated, adverse effects, and any other limitations to therapy [3].

Respiratory therapists, registered nurses, and polysomnography technicians play an important role in CPAP adherence. These healthcare professionals (HCPs) are a point of reference for the patient and in some cases the only support system that they may have. HCPs with the highest adherence rates are passionate about the subject; often they or a family member wears the device and has seen the positive results from therapy. They are patient, persistent, non-judgmental, and empathetic. They take the extra time to hold the patient's hand when necessary.

B. Capozzolo (✉) · K. Champagne · D. Johnson
Institut de Médecine du Sommeil, Montréal, QC, Canada
e-mail: info@institutdemedecinedusommeil.ca

M. A. Baltzan
Institut de Médecine du Sommeil, Montréal, QC, Canada

Centre Intégré Universitaire des Soins et Services Sociaux du Nord de L'île de Montréal, Montréal, QC, Canada

Mount Sinai Hospital, Centre Intégré Universitaire des Soins et Services Sociaux du Centre-ouest de L'île de Montréal, Montréal, QC, Canada

McGill University, Faculty of Medicine, Department of Epidemiology Biostatistics and Occupational Health, Montréal, QC, Canada

A good HCP has a solid background knowledge in OSA and the consequences that can occur with non-adherence. The education a patient receives is the key to adherence. Education is the don't-pass-go step. If the patient doesn't understand sleep apnea and the purpose of wearing CPAP each night, the chances of adherence decrease. One of the greatest problems that a HCP faces is that often the patient doesn't know they have sleep apnea. They have been told by the sleep physician they wake up hundreds of times a night, but they do not recall waking up. They are skeptical that they have a sleeping problem because they can fall asleep almost anywhere. This is where the home care company and the sleep physician need to be on the same page. If the sleep physician does not convey the severity of OSA to the patient, then when the home care company is reviewing all the consequences of untreated OSA and telling the patient this condition is serious, the patient thinks the home care company is just trying to sell something. The best scenario is when the clinic is educating the patient on OSA and the home care company is on the same page and reviewing essentially the same information.

The first interaction with the patient provides an opportunity to determine what drove the patient to be evaluated and allow those working for a home care company and providing CPAP devices to understand the perception and motivation towards the therapy. Furthermore, a multidisciplinary approach permits the utilization of various tools to aid adherence to therapy. In the following, various sections will be expanded upon to permit patients to rise above the difficulty they may experience and increase their chances to adhere to their CPAP therapy.

35.1   Education and Follow-Up

The role of education in improving CPAP use in the long run has only received modest attention until now [5]. Strategies to improve CPAP adherence include providing education, follow-up, and support during the first 2 weeks of therapy when the risk of abandoning therapy is highest [3]. Educational programs need to include information on treatments of OSA, the risks and consequences of untreated OSA, dispelling myths, sleep hygiene, CPAP therapy, equipment management, acclimating to CPAP, desensitization, troubleshooting, and managing commonly encountered problems [3]. Furthermore, individuals need to know when and who to call for assistance before a decision is made to abandon therapy [3]. It has been demonstrated that therapeutic education of 2 hours every 6 months increased CPAP use by at least 1 hour per night in more than 90% of patients [5, 6]. Several different education programs have been proposed, including information sessions, telephone calls, delivery of audiovisual material, CPAP-user group meetings, and training for

patient's family members [7]. The notion of providing education using different approaches (audio, booklet, feedback, psychological) is complimentary. A comprehensive educational program to improve CPAP adherence is an important component in caring for this population [3]. Educational interventions which inform patients about CPAP benefits and consequences of non-adherence and guide a habitual routine of CPAP use may result in improved adherence [3]. Education and regular HCP follow-up appointments are essential in improving CPAP adherence especially during the first few weeks of therapy when the risks of abandoning therapy are highest. The use of patient-friendly literature allows the patient to rehearse different components [3].

Patients appear to establish their patterns of use in the first few days. The CPAP providers' goal is to make CPAP usage a habit and part of the bedtime routine. Patients receive a great deal of information at setup and sometimes they forget some of their education. A patient that forgets to put water in their humidifier chamber may struggle for the first night and after a couple hours find their nose dry or stuffy and take the mask off. If this goes uncorrected, they would try the second night, struggle for a couple of hours and take the mask off. They may try again on the third night however by about the fourth night they have decided they can't wear CPAP and the device goes into the closet or back to the home care company. Therefore, it is important that the HCP follows up with the patient in the first few nights to deal with any issues, monitor adherence, and provide support and encouragement.

As healthcare professionals, time should be spent discussing the patient's understanding of OSA – what it is that they have been told by their physician and review any questions that they may have. Educating them while reviewing that the OSA is a chronic syndrome and explaining what happens during the night while they are sleeping to the upper airway will increase their understanding of the syndrome. HCPs are encouraged to use terminology that is both easy to follow and also easy to understand. Moreover, consequences of untreated OSA as well as their current comorbidities should be reviewed with the patient. If the patient can understand what the syndrome is and how their comorbidities and their quality of life are linked to the syndrome, the chances of the patient adhering to the therapy increase. Following these discussions with the patient, the HCP will use these observations in order to establish specific goals with the client, which will then be followed up on and repeatedly be reinforced throughout the initiation of the client's CPAP therapy.

Moreover, in understanding not only their goals but also what they expect to gain from using the CPAP, one can encourage and empower the patient to attain adherence to therapy. The patient requires HCPs to be available to them when they not only have difficulty but also when they have questions. Information sheets or booklets, videos to review, step-by-step instructions on their equipment, and HCPs with expertise are useful troubleshooting tools and resources for the patient. This education and support will aid in reducing their chances in abandoning the therapy. Continuous encouragement when things may not be going well, as well as troubleshooting any issues, permits us to work as a team. This approach will hopefully enable the patient to become adherent with therapy.

An HCP needs to put the severity of OSA in perspective. An apnea hypopnea index of 20 means nothing to a patient but one can use the analogy to explain how much sleep disruption this may cause. For example, one can say to the patient that if someone rang your doorbell every 3 minutes, it wouldn't take you long to call the police. If you allowed it to go on all night, you would go to work tired, irritable, and complain to your coworkers that someone rang your doorbell every 3 minutes all night. Likewise, if your sleep is disrupted every 3 minutes by a breathing problem, you will experience consequences in your daily life.

You never get a second chance to make a first impression with CPAP. That is why the job the HCP does at the initial setup is so important. This interaction includes sleep apnea education, picking out the right device, and selecting the right mask. The setup needs to be flawless. Therefore, as HCPs, we should have at our disposal and use various tools to educate the patient about OSA. If we are able to properly educate and inform the patient on OSA as a chronic syndrome, the impact of OSA on their quality of life and the importance of their OSA being treated, the first step in management of the syndrome has been attained. Following this, education should focus on their ability to use the device and to properly manipulate their device accessories.

35.2 Psychosocial Aspects

Facilitating learning, engaging in self-care practices, and developing habitual behaviors help to promote adherence to improve health and reduce cardiovascular health in OSA patients [3]. Behavioral interventions such as patient education, systematic desensitization, and sensory awareness for claustrophobia have been shown to improve CPAP adherence [3, 8]. Findings suggest that cognitive perception of OSA and CPAP is formulated in the context of receiving patient education about the disease and treatment during early experiences on CPAP and emphasize the importance of assessing and guiding patients' formulation of accurate outcome expectancies to promote CPAP adherence [9]. Furthermore, studies suggest that patients who experience difficulties and proactively seek solutions to resolve problems (active coping) are more likely to be adherent than those who use passive coping styles [9]. In addition, beliefs (i.e., cognitive perceptions) about OSA and CPAP formed with patients' confidence in their ability to use this therapy influence adherence to CPAP [9]. Once we overcome any issues and objections, we get closer to therapy becoming a habit resulting in long-term adherence.

Patients need to not only be ready but must also accept to begin CPAP therapy. Just as is the case with any change, many thoughts may go through a patient's mind. What will others think of me having to wear a mask? Will I frighten them because of the mask? How will I travel be it for work or pleasure with a device? What will my significant other think of me and the therapy? These are all questions and concerns that should be addressed by the patient's HCP. Moreover, patients may feel embarrassed when discussing their sleep problems especially when it involves their significant other or their friends. Being told that they are disrupting their spouse', friends', or travel partners' sleep because of loud snoring, for example, can influence their decision to be tested for OSA. These same individuals can then also impact their decision to be treated with CPAP. The feeling of embarrassment of having to sleep with a mask may also influence their usage of the CPAP. Thoughts of what others may think because we are using a CPAP, facial redness from the mask in the morning, and even traveling with friends for the first time with the CPAP are all realistic preoccupations that the patient may have and will have to get through in order to properly adhere to the therapy. As HCPs, showing understanding towards what they are feeling permits us to devise tools that can aid them in overcoming them and help them to feel comfortable in these situations. A patient that is mentally prepared to make this lifestyle change will result in an increased chance in adherence to the therapy.

In addition, as HCPs, time should be invested in understanding what has motivated the patient to initially be investigated and treated for OSA. The information that we obtain from them regarding whether they have come of their own free will, or because they were pushed or encouraged by their spouse, can permit us to also understand their level of motivation (or lack thereof) for their treatment. This will in turn allow us to organize how we will proceed with our patient. The amount of encouragement, follow-up, and guidance that will be required by us to ensure that they can be adherent to the therapy long term will also depend on how motivated they are towards the therapy.

The HCP should try to understand the patient's expectations towards the therapy. What are they expecting to gain by using CPAP? They may also believe that weight loss will permit them to soon be "cured" of sleep apnea resulting in them being able to discontinue the CPAP, and believe that the therapy is temporary, influencing adherence. Helping them to understand that the therapy is generally long term eliminates any misconceptions that they will be cured of the disease after a brief period of CPAP usage. It is our job as HCPs to encourage an active lifestyle and sleep hygiene while reinforcing that this may not in fact permit them to stop the therapy. Furthermore, it is important that we continue to inform them that their OSA will not be cured or eliminated with short-term usage of the device and that in fact their OSA is being treated because of the therapy.

As HCPs, we need to ensure that realistic goals and expectations for symptom improvements are set. Although in some cases patients see improvements with the first night of therapy, some patients may take longer (3 to 6 months), and we must reinforce and continuously encourage the patient to not stop the therapy. Reviewing their initial reasons for consulting as well as their symptoms permits us to ask the appropriate questions to see if there have been any improvements.

35.3 Spousal Support

Findings are mixed in studies that have examined spousal involvement in CPAP adherence. Sharing a bed with a spouse or partner has been associated with higher adherence in two studies [10]. However, higher marital conflict and seeking treatment because of a spouse (rather than self-referral) have been associated with poorer adherence [10]. For patients living with "spouses," the spouse will likely be an integral component to any successful intervention [11]. Because of the dyadic (pairing of two individuals) nature of sleep for many adults, the impact of OSA and its treatment extend beyond merely the context of the individual patient [11]. Spousal influence has been identified as one major factor in patient self-efficacy of CPAP use, and a spouse remains the primary and foremost resource of social support [11].

Elsewhere in health literature, spousal involvement has been related to improvements in a range of health behaviors, including diet, exercise, and visiting the doctor, particularly when the involvement is viewed as positive and collaborative [10]. The most effective types of spousal involvement include providing encouragement or helping make changes to facilitate the behavior [10]. However, negative types of involvement, such as criticism, have been associated with psychological distress or ignoring the spouses' request for behavior change [10]. Thus, it is critical to understand the characteristics, role, and impact of spousal involvement in CPAP adherence before any successful interventions involving spouses can be developed to improve CPAP use [11].

Due to the multidimensional nature of CPAP adherence, one type of intervention is unlikely to meet the need of all patients [11]. For patients living with spouses, spouses can be invited to participate in educational, supportive, or behavioral programs aiming to improve CPAP adherence [11]. HCPs need to assess the burden of OSA to the spouses early in the process of disease diagnosis and educate both patients and their spouses as to the positive health benefits of using CPAP, including increased sexual function and improved marital relations [11]. If the patient knows someone who wears CPAP and it has improved their quality of life, that helps with adherence. If the person they know doesn't wear their CPAP, it's important to let them know that sometimes people struggle but the majority of patients can get used to wearing it.

The patient's initial evaluation to determine if there is OSA is often related to complaints by the spouse because of snoring or even concern with them stopping to breathe. Thus, once diagnosed, their decision to start CPAP therapy is often also related to them. The spouse's opinion, reaction, and expression towards the therapy can at times influence their CPAP adherence and decision to start the therapy. The spouse may express concern that the device may be noisy and might disrupt their sleep. In other cases, they may inform the patient that if they sleep with a CPAP they will be doing so in a separate bedroom, some may have the opposite perspective and comment that only if the spouse uses CPAP would the partner tolerate sharing a bed. Some may simply associate CPAP to extra work because of the cleaning of the equipment. These are situations that can influence the patient's decision to not only begin therapy but also their adherence should they begin CPAP therapy, hence the importance of the HCP considering the spouse's support when there is the initial interaction with the patient.

The involvement of the spouse at the first appointment is strongly encouraged so that any misconceptions towards the therapy and/or any concerns that they may have towards the therapy can be addressed. The spouse's negative feelings towards the CPAP are just as important as that of the patients as this too can cause the patient to stop. Furthermore, concerns that the patient may have such as intimacy with their spouse can negatively influence their adherence to therapy. That is, at least at the beginning of the treatment, less intimacy with partners related to CPAP can be an obstacle to embracing this therapy [12]. This suggests the need to assess the impact of CPAP on intimacy and sexual relationships and discuss with CPAP users methods to enhance this important activity, such as engaging in sexual behavior prior to applying the headgear and commencing therapy [12]. More than many other diseases and treatments, OSA and CPAP treatment affect not only the patients, but also their partners [12]. Reviewing and providing tools to overcome these negative feelings towards the therapy will permit the patient and their spouse to gradually adapt to the therapy and their new bedtime routine.

As HCPs, we need to understand that any concerns that the spouse may have can influence the patient's daily usage of the CPAP. Spending time going over any concerns as well as any questions that the spouse may have should be taken into consideration when the HCP is going through the CPAP education with the patient, hence, once again, the importance of encouraging their presence at appointments. Moreover, encouraging the spouse's participation in the therapy will aid the patient as they will have a feeling of being in it together or working as a team. The link should be made that if the OSA is being treated, there can be an improvement in their quality of life not only individually but also as a couple. CPAP therapy should be seen as a collaborative process between the two.

35.4   Motivational Enhancement

Motivational enhancement therapy (MET) for CPAP is a theory-driven approach based on the principles of motivational interviewing, which aims to elicit critical thought in the patient regarding his or her ambivalence towards treatment and highlight the patient's own motivating statements around the therapy [4]. The Motivation to Engage in Treatment (MET) model, developed by Drieschner et al. [13], can be seen as an adaptation of the SCT to explain and predict adherence to different types of treatments [14]. The model posits that adherence to a treatment is dependent on six cognitive and emotional internal determinants: problem recognition, level of suffering, external pressure, perceived cost of treatment, perceived suitability of treatment, and outcome expectancy [14]. Cognitive behavioral therapy and motivational strategies positively influence self-management of chronic disease and behavioral readiness to change [3]; also see Chap. 6.

At the beginning of the initiation to CPAP as well as throughout the first month, it is important for the HCP to evaluate and determine what stage they are in with regard to changing their behavior towards treating OSA and using CPAP. Time should be spent exploring if there are any discrepancies between their behaviors and their goals, and if so, how we can proceed to motivate them to overcome the issues they may have encountered to attain their goals. Furthermore, HCPs should avoid any arguments with the patient and accept that there may be ambivalence when patients speak with us. It is in these situations that the HCP should express empathy towards the patient and proceed with open-ended questions permitting the patient to inform us on what may be causing them to feel this way. Furthermore, positive reinforcement should be used to support the patient's perception of their ability to change.

Having the patient verbalize any discomfort with the therapy or the mask itself can give us direction on how we should proceed in order to help improve CPAP adherence. The patient may feel anxiety, fear, discomfort, pain, shame, or even embarrassment towards the idea of having to wear the mask. In some cases, patients may require longer periods to adapt, thus the importance of the HCP to spend time encouraging them to overcome these obstacles.

As HCPs, we should inform the patients we are aware that this is an adaptation period and that certain difficulties may be encountered along the way. However, it is important to stress that they shouldn't be discouraged should they not have the ability to wear the CPAP the entire night the first night. Tools to help them overcome difficulty to adapt to the therapy should be explained, for example, using the device every night with gradual increases in usage, meaning increasing the time by 15–30 minutes a night. Other tools to help adapt to the therapy may be turning on the device and using it while taking an afternoon nap, while watching TV or even reading a book. Familiarizing themselves with not only the mask interface on them but also the pressure and algorithm of the device will help them to control their breathing while using it. These are all cues that can help in reducing their stress when faced with the idea of having to sleep with the CPAP.

Furthermore, in cases where the patient is having difficulty adapting to CPAP therapy because of claustrophobia, time should be spent evaluating which mask interface will be possible without them feeling closed in (e.g., using a pillow (or direct nasal mask) or even a mask that doesn't have to be secured tightly). In addition, as HCPs, we may have to provide tools that may result in a step-by-step process which may include a desensitization period or refer the patient to a psychologist trained in cognitive behavioral therapy who can provide a short and effective claustrophobia treatment (see Chap. 6).

Asking the appropriate questions (e.g., any anxiety or fear they may have, any pain or shame they have) will help us to determine what the next course of action should be with our patient. The use of open-ended questions such as "Tell me how you are doing on CPAP so far?" may permit the patient to not only express how they are feeling, but it also permits them to feel as if they are involved, helping them value their participation in the therapy. Encouraging open communication with family and friends regarding therapy can also be an aid. Discussing the therapy with family members or friends that currently use the device can help them to see that they are not alone and that they have someone they can turn to in case they feel that they aren't being successful with CPAP. When there is a psychological factor (e.g., fear, anxiety, shame etc.) that makes CPAP use challenging for the patient, a referral to a psychologist (behavioral sleep specialist) is warranted (Chap. 1.6).

New devices with modems permit additional motivational tools to help CPAP adherence. HCPs are now able to verify how the therapy is proceeding on a day-to-day basis as opposed to only when the patient is in their office. This permits them to contact the client immediately when they see things are not going well in order to review what issues they have encountered or simply positively reinforce the importance of pushing through their problems. There are also smart phone applications or websites, which permit the patient to be more invested in their CPAP adherence as they can see how well they have been using the device, as well as how their mask adjustment is and how well their OSA is being treated. These applications provide the patient with encouragement when things are going well and tools when they see that they are having difficulty with the therapy. Receiving daily updates through these applications empowers the patient, especially when things are going well, and as such should be encouraged by the HCP.

35.5 Difficulty with the Mask Interface, CPAP Device, and Side Effects

Approximately two-thirds of CPAP users experience side effects, though these side effects have not been shown to be significantly influential on CPAP adherence [9]. Yet, the amelioration of CPAP side effects has motivated the development of comfort-related technological advances in CPAP equipment [9]. These technological advances include nasal and face mask innovations, humidified systems, and pressure relief modality add-on options [9]. Side effects from treatment, such as dry throat, nasal congestion, and mask leaks, tend to be common and are believed to reduce adherence [14]. Moreover, initial acceptance of CPAP may also be influenced by nasal resistance [9]. Various types of CPAP machines are available and can monitor the effectiveness of treatment, losses from the mask, persistence of snoring, and residual AHI [5]. This supporting system seems to be closely linked to the success of adherence with ventilation [5]. Comfort techniques and troubleshooting adverse effects such as mask fit, air leakage, and nasal congestion are important aspects of CPAP management and contribute to overall adherence [3].

As HCPs, we may encounter situations in which the patient expresses their discomfort with the mask. In general, the full-face (oronasal) mask should be used as a last resort (AASM 2019). Thus, the discussion and evaluation of the correct mask by the HCP is of great importance. Time should be spent evaluating any possible causes that would limit the use of a nasal or direct nasal mask. In some cases, a multidisciplinary approach may be necessary in order to bring the patient to using these models of masks. For example, should nasal congestion be present, regular nasal saline rinses or the opinion of an experienced physician may facilitate the use of a nasal mask by the patient. Furthermore, patients may complain of skin irritation in the area of the face that the mask is placed or even headgear marks on their face in the morning. Items such as a cloth barrier between the mask and the skin may aid in decreasing the skin irritation or marks on the face. As

HCPs, if we can reduce or eliminate this issue, chances are they will proceed with the therapy, especially if they realize the benefits of the therapy. Mask leaks may also be a source of frustration to the patient resulting in them either constantly waking up to fix the mask or simply deciding that it isn't worth it and stopping the therapy. As HCPs, fixing this problem is important. Reviewing their mask adjustment to ensure that it has a proper seal around the nose and that the headgear is securely in place will go a long way in helping your patient with the therapy. In addition, items such as CPAP pillows can also facilitate in reducing mask leaks.

Another issue that may cause the patient to have difficulty with the therapy is the pressure itself. As HCPs, we understand the concept that they are breathing against a positive pressure. However, for the patient, this sensation of having difficulty or having to actively exhale when they breathe out may cause the patient to panic and decide to stop using CPAP. Adding comfort features which will decrease the pressure as the patient goes through the expiration phase of the breathing pattern can help some patients to adapt to this new therapy. In addition, changes in modality may also be beneficial in increasing adherence to therapy. Moreover, in cases where the patient may have difficulty with the initial pressure setting, features such as a ramp may aid in CPAP usage. The ramp permits the patient to adapt to a lower pressure setting for a limited time while the device gradually increases the pressure. This will not only permit the patient to adapt to higher pressure settings but also facilitate falling asleep with the therapy. It is important to verify that the patient is getting enough air flow even at the lowest ramp pressure setting.

Dry mouth, dry throat, and even water in the mask and tube are all complaints that patients can have when using the therapy. As HCPs, listening to the patients' concerns when this happens to them is important. If we can rectify these issues, we not only increase the patients' comfort with the therapy but also help them to increase their usage of the therapy. Using the tools that are available with the new devices such as heated tubes can help to regulate the humidity required for comfortable therapy, and if all else fails, as HCPs we will have to consider the use of a chin restraint or even a full-face mask.

Spending time understanding any issues that the patient has with their therapy will in the long run help the HCP to provide the appropriate tools for patient to continue to use their CPAP. If we can help them overcome any technical difficulties that they have with the device itself, patients will feel more at ease with this new bedtime routine. Furthermore, troubleshooting mask issues, pressure issues, and humidity issues can only aid in their CPAP adherence.

35.6 Conclusion

The role of respiratory therapists, registered nurses, and polysomnography technicians in CPAP adherence is multifaceted. There is no cookie cutter model that can be used for all patients. The HCPs need to ask questions and listen to what the patients are telling them about their thoughts, feelings, and experiences of the treatment. Spending time understanding any concerns that the patients and/or their spouse may have with the therapy will aid us to provide the necessary encouragement and information to facilitate the use of the CPAP. Furthermore, providing patients with tools such as smart phone applications and/or videos will not only permit them to see how they are doing and help them if they are having difficulty with the therapy but also engage them in the therapy. Finally, spending an adequate amount of time educating the patient on not only OSA but also the therapy as well as ensuring proper follow-up at the initiation to CPAP therapy can aid CPAP adherence. Taking a multidisciplinary approach is often essential to help patients achieve consistent CPAP use.

References

1. Bue AL, Salvaggio A, Isidoro SI, Romano S, Marrone O, Insalaco G. Usefulness of reinforcing interventions on continuous positive airway pressure adherence. BMC Pulm Med. 2014;14(1):78.
2. Bouloukaki I, Giannadaki K, Mermigkis C, Tzanakis N, Mauroudi E, Moniaki V, et al. Intensive versus standard follow-up to improve continuous positive airway pressure adherence. Eur Respir J. 2014;44(5):1262–74.
3. Wellins AM, Shurpin K, Hood P, Shangold L. Impact of an obstructive sleep apneas education program on Continuous Positive Airway (CPAP) adherence a pilot study. Adv Nurs Patient Care Int J. 2018;1(2):1–15.
4. Desai U, Joshi JM. How to improve adherence to continuous positive airway pressure therapy? Indian J Sleep Med. 2019;14(4):67–9.
5. Piana GL, Scartabellati AA, Lundefined C, Lundefined R, Pundefined R, Mundefined C, et al. Long-term adherence to CPAP treatment in patients with obstructive sleep apnea: importance of educational program. Patient Prefer Adherence. 2011;5:555–62.
6. Likar LL, Panciera TM, Erickson AD, Rounds S. Group education sessions and adherence with nasal CPAP therapy. Chest. 1997;111(5):1273–7.
7. Rueda AD, Santos-Silva R, Togeiro SM, Tufik S, Bittencourt LRA. Improving adherence by a basic educational program with nurse support for obstructive sleep apneas syndrome patients. Sleep Sci. 2009;2(1):8–13.
8. Kribbs NB, Pack AI, Kline LR, Getsy JE, Schuett JS, Henry JN, et al. Effects of one night without nasal CPAP treatment on sleep and sleepiness in patients with obstructive sleep apnea. Am Rev Respir Dis. 1993;147:1162–8. https://doi.org/10.1164/ajrccm/147.5.1162.
9. Sawyer AM, Gooneratne NS, Marcus CL, Ofer D, Richards KC, Weaver TE. A systematic review of CPAP adherence across age groups: clinical and empiric insights for developing CPAP adherence interventions. Sleep Med Rev. 2011;15(6):343–56.
10. Baron KG, Gunn HE, Czajkowski LA, Smith TW, Jones CR. Spousal involvement in CPAP: does pressure help? J Clin Sleep Med. 2012;08(02):147–53.
11. Ye L, Malhotra A, Kayser K, Willis DG, Horowitz JA, Aloia MS, et al. Spousal involvement and CPAP adherence: a dyadic perspective. Sleep Med Rev. 2015;19:67–74. https://doi.org/10.1016/j.smrv.2014.04.005.
12. Ye L, Pack AI, Maislin G, Dinges D, Hurley S, McCloskey S, Weaver TE. Predictors of continuous positive airway pressure use during the first week of treatment. J Sleep Res. 2012;21:419–26.
13. Drieschner KH, Lammers SMM, van der Staak CPF. Treatment motivation: an attempt for clarification of an ambiguous concept. Clin Psych Rev. 2004;23:115–37.
14. Broström A, Nilsen P, Johansson P, Ulander M, Strömberg A, Svanborg E, et al. Putative facilitators and barriers for adherence to CPAP treatment in patients with obstructive sleep apnea syndrome: a qualitative content analysis. Sleep Med. 2010;11(2):126–30.

Part VII

Global and Historical Perspectives

Global Perspective of CPAP Adherence

Jessica Rosen, Arezu Najafi, Khosro Sadeghniiat-Haghighi,
Ravi Gupta, Slavko M. Janković, Jianhua Shen,
and Yu Jin Lee

Sleep medicine global distribution

Country	Number of people trained in sleep medicine or active within the Sleep Medicine Society	Number of sleep labs	Population (*estimate*)
Armenia	14 members of the Armenian Sleep Disorders Association	3	2,958,000
Australia New Zealand	951 members of the Australasian Sleep Association	73 accredited services (including facilities in Australia, New Zealand, and Singapore)	25,360,000 4,917,000
Austria	~200 members of the Austrian Sleep Research Association	31 ASRA-certified	8,859,000
Belgium	373 members of the Belgian Association for Sleep Research and Sleep Medicine	72 authorized to prescribe CPAP Additional 28 centers perform sleep studies without CPAP license	11,460,000
Bulgaria	45 members of the Bulgarian Society of Somnology	11 centers	7,000,000
China	3000 registered members in the Chinese Sleep Research Society	>3000	1,444,216,107
Croatia	40 members of the Society for Sleep Medicine of the Croatian Medical Association	2	4,076,000
Czech Republic	155 members of the Czech Sleep Research and Sleep Medicine Society	50	10,650,000
Denmark	68 members of the Danish Society for Sleep Medicine	4	5,806,000
Finland	201 members of the Finnish Sleep Research Society	11	5,518,000
France	400 members of the French Sleep Research and Medicine Society President	52 certified centers	67,060,000
Greece	55 members of the Hellenic Sleep Research Society	33	10,720,000
Hungary	120 members of the Hungarian Sleep Research Society	12	9,773,000
Finland	201 members of the Finnish Sleep Research Society	11	5,518,000
France	400 members of the French Sleep Research and Medicine Society President	52 certified centers	67,060,000
India	WSS international Sleep Certificate/ABSM: ~70 Trained during residency: ~400 (*"Trained" is different from those having a part of curriculum only*)	~1000	1,366,000,000

continued

J. Rosen (✉)
New York Medical College, Valhalla, NY, USA
e-mail: jrosen11@student.nymc.edu

A. Najafi · K. Sadeghniiat-Haghighi
Occupational Sleep Research Center, Baharloo Hospital, Tehran
University of Medical Sciences, Tehran, Iran

R. Gupta
Department of Psychiatry and Division of Sleep Medicine, All
India Institute of Medical Sciences, Rishikesh, Uttarakhand, India

S. M. Janković
Clinic of Neurology, Clinical Center of Serbia, Belgrade, Serbia

J. Shen
Beijing Medipertis Sleep Medicine Center, Beijing, China

Y. J. Lee
Department of Psychiatry and Center for Sleep and Chronobiology,
Seoul National University College of Medicine,
Seoul, Republic of Korea

© The Author(s), under exclusive license to Springer Nature Switzerland AG 2022
C. M. Shapiro et al. (eds.), *CPAP Adherence*, https://doi.org/10.1007/978-3-030-93146-9_36

Country	Number of people trained in sleep medicine or active within the Sleep Medicine Society	Number of sleep labs	Population (*estimate*)
Iran	43	>30	83,992,949
Israel	70 sleep doctors (estimated number due to the absence of a subspecialty)	12	9,053,000
Italy	350 members of the Italian Sleep Medicine Society	56 accredited sleep medicine centers	60,360,000
Japan	3700 registered members in the Japanese Sleep Research Society	102 approved	126,300,000
Poland	98 members of the Polish Sleep Research Society	9	37,970,000
Russia	97 members of the Russian Society of Somnologists	10–50	144,400,000
Serbia	2	2	6,945,000
Slovenia	30 members of the Slovene Sleep Society	3	2,081,000
Spain	603 members of the Spanish Sleep Society	33 accredited	46,940,000
Sweden	498 members of the Swedish Sleep Society	11 centers provide full PSG services. Additional 25 centers provide mainly diagnosis and treatment of sleep-disordered breathing	10,230,000
Switzerland	301 members of the Swiss Society for Sleep Research, Sleep Medicine and Chronobiology	6	8,545,000
Turkey	919 members of the Turkish Sleep Medicine Society	31	82,000,000
USA	7500 board certified 10,000 members of the American Academy of Sleep Medicine	>2500 accredited	328,200,000

Data has been obtained from sleep medicine professionals within the respective countries, as well as from the World Sleep Society (https://worldsleepsociety.org/) and the European Sleep Research Society: Sleep Research and Sleep Medicine Europe (https://esrs.eu/)

36.1 Iran

36.1.1 Prevalence of OSA in Iran

A nationwide study on OSA in Iran is ongoing and is yet to be released. Currently, the prevalence estimates include 59.9% high risk for OSA among train drivers [4], 8.8% in a general population study in North West of Iran [5], and 44% in a meta-analysis [6]. Despite the high reported prevalence and the fact that diagnosis and management of OSA as a disease with several metabolic and cardiovascular consequences is important, OSA in Iran is under-diagnosed and under-treated [7].

An investigation by our research center on CPAP adherence has shown that only 33% of participants undergoing titration study adhered to CPAP use for at least four hours, 70% of days of a month for a six-month period [8]. Another unpublished survey by our team followed patients advised by a physician to use CPAP. The results show that only 30% of these patients actually bought a CPAP device, highlighting the important issue of cost and education and the need for healthcare authorities to be aware of the potential consequence of untreated OSA. Several factors can be considered in Iran that influence CPAP adherence. These include patient-specific factors, as well as those related to the devices, healthcare system, and government.

36.1.2 Patient-Related Factors

Elderly patients have been shown to have higher rates of non-adherence to CPAP [8]. Among our adherent patients, weight loss is often reported. Weight loss may have influenced their psychological motivation to comply with CPAP. Reports suggest that body mass index (BMI), respiratory disturbance index (RDI), education, and marital status may influence adherence. Although 92% of adherent patients felt more refreshed and satisfied with CPAP device after treatment, educational and marital status, BMI, and RDI did not show a significant correlation with patients' adherence [8]. Additional polysomnographic characteristics such as sleep efficiency, arousal index, and mean O2 saturation were also not associated with higher CPAP adherence. Compliant patients were more likely to have poor sleep quality than non-compliant ones, indicated by sleep efficiency in their first night polysomnography; but the trend was not statistically significant.

Cultural issues in acceptance and adherence of CPAP device and insufficient education of patients prior to PAP titration study also affect PAP adherence. Before accreditation of sleep clinics by the Ministry of Health in Iran and launching training of sleep medicine specialists, the number of trained sleep physicians was limited. This had led to non-trained physicians and even companies related to PAP devices providing services to patients with OSA. Nonprofessional training and visit of patients during process of diagnosis, management, and follow-up influence adherence of patients and lead to loss of follow-up.

In Iran the price of PAP device is three to five times more than a salary of a middle-income worker per month. Although we have not published data on this issue, in our clinical practice we see that most patients who are in the low- and middle-income range do not buy a CPAP device or it takes them a long time (e.g., two–three years) to establish the necessary budget for buying a CPAP device. This issue pushes them toward other alternative treatments such as position therapy and weight loss or upper airway surgery that is much cheaper and covered by insurance companies. Although there is regulation regarding management of OSA among commercial drivers and posing restrictions in driving when they have an untreated OSA, some do not adhere to treatment as they do not need their health license after retirement or quitting their job. For this group, the problem of funding also exists and affects their compliance.

There have not been Iranian studies on the role of psychological factors in CPAP adherence. However, in a survey by Salmani et al. in our sleep clinic, about 40% of patients reported symptoms of depression, and according to the literature this may affect our patients' adherence [9].

Family and healthcare support are also important. Albeit in our survey marital status was not related to adherence, we see in our clinical practice that more adherent patients have spousal or family support.

Lack of awareness of the importance of sleep both in the health professional and in the lay community is another issue that affects the adherence of our patients. Limited native language data on sleep problems and in-attention of some health sectors to sleep problems as a cause of noncommunicable diseases have led to less informed and nonadherent patients.

36.1.3 PAP Device-Related Factors

Complications of PAP treatment, such as mask discomfort, nasal drying, nasal irritation, and intolerance of air pressure from the CPAP device and other equipment-related factors, contribute to non-adherence in our population. The most common complaints of patients were snoring and morning headache which were reported in 34 (85%) and 12 (30%) participants in our survey. Our patients also reported higher pressures of CPAP device as a cause of their non-adherence. Humidifier use and chin strap use during CPAP therapy were reported by 34 (85%) and ten (25%) compliant patients, respectively. The most common complication among CPAP users was difficulty with breathing and discomfort with full-face mask. Full-face mask was used by 30 patients (75%), while the rest of the participants used nasal mask [8].

Although not investigated yet, our patients especially younger ones mention lifestyle change and stigma especially in early years of their marital life as a cause for their non-adherence.

36.1.4 Healthcare System and Physician-Related Factors

The sleep medicine fellowship training program was launched in Iran seven years ago. Although the number of trained physicians is now above 40, the distribution and number are still limited relative to the population of the country. This inequality and disparity in access to sleep medicine professionals may result in insufficient and even wrong diagnosis and management of OSA. In addition, non-sleep medicine-trained healthcare workers and some un-authorized company practices in this field cause uncertainty for patients and in the healthcare system. Although sleep medicine physicians educate their patients well, interference of non-authorized healthcare professionals and even PAP companies lead to loss of follow-up of patients in some cases influencing their adherence.

These maleficent processes in sleep medicine are improving a lot after accreditation of sleep clinics by the Ministry of Health and the introduction of legislation of standard protocols for performing sleep tests under the supervision of sleep medicine fellowships. Auto-PAPs and home sleep tests are not popular yet, as there are still some non-authorized centers who use them inappropriately. However, the Iranian Sleep Medicine Society plans to regulate home sleep studies and auto-PAP in OSA diagnosis and management in the near future. Currently, auto-PAP devices have high price and are not affordable by low- and middle-income patients and we anticipate this will remain the situation in the near future.

Healthcare programs for follow-up of patients are very important. Although it is performed at sleep clinics at the present time, all healthcare professionals involved in the care of patients need to be involved at every step from technicians who meet with the patients in the CPAP titration night, through the ones who schedule patients to all clinicians in the patient's circle of care.

36.1.5 Governmental Issues

At the present time, we have regulations for drivers with OSA to be treated with CPAP before obtaining their health license. The numbers of those who can afford the price of PAP devices are limited and we have to prescribe alternative treatments in some cases. Another issue that exists is the price for PAP titration study and also PAP devices which are not covered by insurance companies at the present time. Several private insurance companies cover the cost; however, the main ones are not still persuaded to cover the expenses. A lot of efforts are being made to include sleep tests and modalities of treatment of OSA in the coverage plan of insurance companies.

36.1.6 Future Perspectives

We hope that by expanding our training system on sleep medicine fellowship, we can overcome disparity in distribution and availability of trained sleep medicine professionals in Iran. Additionally, by networking and increasing the awareness of public, healthcare sectors and professionals, authorities, and insurance companies, the availability and affordability of standard sleep medicine practice modalities will continue to increase.

36.2 India

Positive airway pressure (PAP) therapy is considered the first-line treatment of OSA among individuals who are not candidates for surgical management to improve daytime sleepiness and quality of life [10]. However, clinical experience suggests that a sizable number of patients with obstructive sleep apnea do not adhere to the PAP therapy. Available literature suggests that multiple issues prevent PAP adherence, e.g., comorbid disorders such as insomnia, gastroesophageal reflux, depression, poor experience with PAP during titration night, severity of OSA, no perceived improvement in clinical symptoms, severity of daytime sleepiness, issues related to interface and humidification, adverse effects arising out of PAP use, and ineffective pressure, to name a few [11, 12]. However, of importance to note is that these studies were conducted in countries where PAP devices are dispensed by the medical insurance agencies.

In India, there are a multitude of other factors that play a role in PAP adherence. The study by Suri et al. [13] was one of the first pieces of literature to report PAP adherence in India: only 25% of patients with OSA initiated the nasal continuous airway pressure (n-CPAP) therapy out of 1200 participants. This reported adherence rate has not appeared to change over the years, as two recent studies reported that out of all patients with OSA who were advised to use CPAP therapy, only 15% and 20% purchased it [14, 15]. The observed difference between these two reports is most likely to be related to the financial status of the patients visiting the two centers. A rent-free trial of CPAP device to the patients at their home could be another factor that could account for larger number of patients who initiated the therapy [13].

One of the main determinants for non-initiation of therapy in India is the cost of the device. Most of the patients need to pay for the device from their own pocket, unlike in countries like the United States and United Kingdom where the associated costs of device are taken care by way of medical insurance agencies or the state, respectively [13]. In addition, even when the cost of therapy was borne by an agency in India, delay in procurement of the device due to administrative reasons was a significant reason reported for non-initiation of treatment (Table 36.1) [14]. The question of whether financial issues, as reported by patients, are an important part of non-initiation of PAP therapy was examined by Goyal et al. [14]. They reported that total family income was more important than individual patient income when determining whether to purchase a machine [14].

Table 36.1 Factors influencing CPAP compliance in India

S.N.	Factors	Study
1.	**Non-initiation of treatment**	
A.	*Sociodemographic*	
	Cost of device, administrative delay in procurement, frequent change of place of job, irregular working shifts	Suri et al., Ninan et al., Goyal et al.
B.	*Cognitive barriers*	
	Not ready to use it lifelong; stigma related to wearing a device to sleep; obtrusive, alternate therapy to cure illness; treatment is not required; treatment ineffective; can't sleep with mask; denial of OSA; claustrophobia; socially not acceptable; not acceptable to spouse	Suri et al., Periwal et al., Goyal et al.
C.	*Concurrent medical opinion*	
	Not suggested as useful by another physician	Goyal et al.
D.	*Adverse effects of PAP*	
	Nasal discomfort	Goyal et al.
2.	**Poor adherence to PAP**	
A.	*Sociodemographic*	
	Power failure, frequent traveling, weather conditions do not suit PAP use	Suri et al., Ramachandran et al.
B.	*Medical factors*	
	Rhinitis, asthma, need for voiding at night, anxiety, depression, poor sleep maintenance, no improvement of symptoms	Suri et al., Ramachandran et al., Goyal et al.
C.	*PAP device related*	
	Maintenance of device expensive, noise	Suri et al., Ramachandran et al.
D.	*Interface related*	
	Air leak, pressure sores, skin changes, poor fitting	Suri et al., Ramachandran et al.
E.	*Cognitive barriers*	
	Claustrophobia, socially not acceptable, lifelong not acceptable, therapy ineffective, too busy to use it, OSA is not a serious disease	Suri et al., Ramachandran et al., Goyal et al.
F.	*Adverse effects of therapy*	
	Dryness in mouth and nose, nasal stuffiness, pain in nose, feeling of pressure in throat, headache, aerophagia	Suri et al., Ramachandran et al., Goyal et al.

Additional determinants that have been reported regarding non-initiation of PAP in India include cognitive barriers to the use of PAP therapy, ranging from denial of having OSA to stigma of using a device while sleeping by the patient themselves, their spouse, or society [14]. Sharing a bedroom with other members of one's family, besides a spouse, is not uncommon in Indian society due to a multitude of factors. Important to note is that this reason also independently contributes to the inability to initiate therapy [13]. Social stigma attached to PAP use was reported by 15–30% of participants for not initiating the treatment; however, it appeared to reduce over time [13, 14]. Even after the initiation of treatment, nearly half of the patients showed poor adherence due to social reasons [16]. In addition, nearly one third of patients in India are not comfortable with the fact that they have to use PAP throughout life and nearly the same proportion of patients search for alternate modes of treatment such as weight loss and surgery [13, 14]. In conjunction, this leads to both non-initiations and poor adherence to the treatment.

Lastly, it is not unusual for PAP devices to appear intrusive and cumbersome to patients in the early part of therapy; many patients take time to overcome this. Moreover, adverse effects with the use of PAP therapy are not uncommon. Some commonly reported adverse effects include mask-related skin changes, nasal stuffiness, dryness in nose and mouth, and aerophagia, to name a few. These issues have been found to act as barriers for non-initiation and poor adherence to PAP therapy in approximately one quarter of patients [13, 14]. These issues are best addressed during follow-up visits in PAP clinic. These factors are modifiable and can be dealt by choosing proper interface from the range of masks that are available these days, use of humidifier, and using telemedicine for the follow-up of the patients [17]. Similarly, issues related to poor mask fitting and leakage may also be dealt by use of customized masks [18]. However, follow-up in the PAP clinic is also poor in India. In fact, Suri et al. [13] reported that only 50% of patients visited a PAP clinic during the initial 6 months of therapy.

36.3 Serbia

The data below are unpublished and represent the professional experience and the attitude of the author who works at the (1) Department for Sleep Medicine and Epilepsy, Clinic of Neurology, Clinical Center of Serbia, School of Medicine, Belgrade, and (2) the Bel Medic Center for Sleep and epilepsy, Bel Medic General Hospital, Belgrade, Serbia.

It is estimated that the frequency of sleep apnea (SA) in the population of Serbia for the age group up to 50 years is between 6% and 7%. In older adults, the frequency of SA rises at the minimum to 15–20%. The most frequent types of apneas are obstructive and central and the conditions commonly underlying SA are obesity, chronic obstructive pulmonary disease, use of antidepressants and sedatives, alcohol overuse, and craniofacial abnormalities. In Serbia there are two accredited sleep laboratories with one neurologist-somnologist and one neurologist educated in sleep diagnostics. The most frequently used questionnaires are Epworth Sleepiness Scale, Berlin, Stop Bang, and Stanford Sleepiness Scale, and the most common daytime test used in the assessment of OSA is multiple sleep latency test (MSLT).

The dominant treatment for SA in Serbia is CPAP, with oral applicance therapy performed occasionally. Although frequently prescribed by physicians as the best therapy for

SA, the CPAP apparatus is not covered by the state health insurance. Upon medical advice, patients purchase CPAP from personal funds. Important to note as well is that professional drivers are not forced by law to pass sleep laboratory diagnostics. However, if the clinic makes the diagnosis of SA with hypersomnolence, drivers are forbidden to pursue this career route (this is also typically seen with the diagnosis of narcolepsy or epilepsy).

There is a higher adherence to CPAP in patients with SA within Serbia, most likely the consequence of patients having to acquire the CPAP from their own resources and are therefore more motivated to use it. On the other hand, the population groups who can afford CPAP typically have a higher awareness that the use of CPAP is important for their health. In these cases, the adherence to CPAP is at least from five to six hours/night sleep. On the other hand, the percentage of patients who fall within the category of having the resources to afford CPAP treatment is very small. Controls for setting the CPAP parameters are performed according to the fixed time protocol. Generally, there is no reimbursement for the prescribed CPAP in patients with SA resulting in small number being treated in relation to real needs. Supported by the institutes of occupational health, the general awareness exists that the patients not treated SA use pharmacologic treatment and medical services far more than those utilizing CPAP.

There is no internally defined cutoff point to define the adequate CPAP compliance nor the level of compliance needed to obtain the highest health benefit from the treatment and there are significant differences in CPAP use among patients. Only in rare cases does the patient with SA undergo the PSG retest to assess the efficiency of CPAP therapy. Lack of compliance is certainly present but is less than could be expected compared to countries with the established state reimbursement policy.

36.4 China

36.4.1 Introduction to OSA in China

Although traditional Chinese medicine, including acupuncture, has been used for treating sleep problems since ancient time, the development of modern sleep medicine in China has come about later than in the Western world. In 1982, Dr. Xiehe Liu, a worldwide famous professor and psychiatrist from the West China University of Medical Sciences, brought modern sleep medicine from England to China. In the same year, he established the first sleep laboratory. Since 1998, sleep medicine has been developed rapidly, and since 2002 continuous positive airway pressure (CPAP), bilevel PAP (BiPAP) and automatic PAP (APAP) have been relatively popular for treating sleep apnea in China.

36.4.2 Treatment of OSA in China

Few studies on the treatment of obstructive sleep apnea (OSA) in China have been published. Liao et al. (2018) [19] reported a survey of 4097 OSA patients (mean age 45, range between 37 and 55 years). The diagnosis and the judgment of the severity were based on the apnea-hypopnea index (AHI) on polysomnography (PSG) with the standard criteria, i.e., mild, 5–15; moderate, 16–30; and severe, >30. The treatments were composed of (1) CPAP; (2) oral appliance; (3) surgical treatment, including uvulopalatopharyngoplasty (UPPP), revised UPPP, septoplasty, radiofrequency ablation, multilevel or stepwise operations, palatal implants, and surgeries on sinus, turbinate, and tonsils; (4) behavioral therapy, including weight loss, physical exercise, changing sleep position, avoiding drinking alcohol, and/or taking sedating medications before bedtime; (5) adjunctive therapy, including pharmacotherapy, oxygen, acupuncture, massage, and bariatric surgery; and (6) integrated treatment, including the combination of surgeries with adjunctive therapy and/or behavioral therapy. Good CPAP adherence was defined as using CPAP four hours or more per night for more than 70% of the nights during the recorded period [19].

The results of multivariate regression analysis showed that the factors helping participants to use CPAP treatment were age between 45 and 59 years, female, severe OSA, and those with comorbid hypertension and/or diabetes. Of the 4097 patients, 2779 (67.8%) either did not receive any treatment or withdrew after a brief treatment. Among them, 53.4% (1485/2779) believed that their condition was not severe enough for requiring treatment, despite more than half (53.7%) of them had severe OSA. Only 32.2% (1318/4097) of patients received treatment. Mean AHI decreased from 49.3 to 26.2 in surgery treatment patients, from 52.5 to 26.9 in CPAP treatment patients, and from 54.9 to 24.0 in integrated treatment patients; statistical differences were found in all these three groups [19]. However, the AHI differences before and after treatment did not reach statistical significance in oral appliance group, behavioral treatment group, and adjunctive therapy group. The successful treatment rates were 67.1% (53/69) in the integrated treatment group, 50.0% (210/420) in CPAP group, 48.7% (304/624) in surgery group, 8.0% (2/25) in adjunctive group, 4.7% (2/43) in oral appliance group, and 3.9% (5/127) in behavioral group. Successful OSA treatment was defined as AHI decreased to below 5 or more than 50% of reduction [19].

36.4.3 Adherence to CPAP in Patients with OSA

In the abovementioned study [19] only 10.3% (420/4097) of patients used CPAP to treat their OSA. Among the 420 CPAP recipients, 58.8% (247/420) regularly used the machine. The rest (41.2%, 173/420) either received CPAP treatment initially and withdrew it later or never initiated CPAP. The reasons of withdrawing were as follows: inconvenience, 37.0% (64/173); no symptom improvement, 19.1% (33/173); intolerance, 17.3% (30/173); reported symptoms disappeared, 13.9% (24/173); partner complaining of too much noise from the machine, 9.3% (16/173); and equipment failure, 3.5% (6/173) [19].

In another study, Wang et al. (2012) [20] interviewed 193 OSA patients who received CPAP treatment. Among them, 162 were males and 31 were females. Their mean age, AHI, and CPAP pressure were 51.9 years, 60.0, and 12.1 cmH2O, respectively. While being interviewed, these patients received treatment for 59 (standard deviation: 32) months. A total of 100 (51.8%, 100/193) patients used CPAP for their treatment while they were interviewed. However, 17 of these patients did not meet the criteria of adherence. Therefore, the percentage of adherence was 43.0% (83/193) [20].

The top three reasons of poor adherence were "unable to adapt to CPAP or sleep well during titration trial," "troublesome to use CPAP every night," and "did not perceive benefit," occupying 27.3%, 18.2%, and 11.8% of those poor adherence patients, respectively. The rest of the reasons of poor adherence were "noise and discomfort of apparatus (6.4%)," "difficult to exhale and fall asleep (6.4%)," "cumbersome (5.5%)," "unable to afford the device (4.5%)," "forgot to use (2.7%)," "not satisfied with the treatment (2.7%)," "nasal dryness/sore (2.7%)," "muggy in summer (1.8%)," "sleep disruption by CPAP (1.8%)," "heart attack or transient ischemic attack (1.8%)," and "claustrophobia with mask (0.9%)" [20].

36.5 Middle East Asia

According to the data from the National Health Insurance Service in Korea, the number of patients treated for OSA (obstructive sleep apnea) surged from 29,255 in 2015 to 86,006 in 2019. This increase in the number of OSA patients is largely due to the policy that led to insurance coverage for polysomnography (level I) and CPAP therapy for OSA since July 1, 2018. Coverage requirements are one of the following based on level I polysomnography: (1) AHI 15 or higher; (2) AHI 10 or higher with insomnia, daytime sleepiness, cognitive impairment, or mood symptoms; and (3) AHI five or higher with hypertension, ischemic heart disease, history of cerebrovascular disease, or lower than 85% of O2 saturation. When patients meet the abovementioned coverage requirement, they are registered with a CPAP company according to the doctor's prescription of CPAP and receive rental service from the company. In addition, in order to maintain the reimbursement of the rental service of CPAP, at least four hours or more of use time per day for a continuous month during the first prescription of three months is required. After that, patients must visit a doctor once every three months to receive a re-prescription of the CPAP device, and the average usage time must be two hours or longer to receive continuous insurance coverage. From July 1, 2018, to December 31, 2020, 76.5% of patients passed the minimum standard of using an average of four hours or more per day during a continuous period of one month during the first three months of CPAP prescription in the Sleep Clinic of the Psychiatric Department at Seoul National University Hospital. The cost of the CPAP device rental service is 76,000 won per month, 89,000 won per month for APAP, and 126,000 won per month for BiPAP, and the patient's payment rate is 20%. I believe that this CPAP insurance system in Korea is contributing to improving the CPAP compliance of OSA patients. According to data from the Health Insurance System, 20,000 CPAP device units were leased for 6 months since July 2018, and 270,000 units in 2019, and 410,000 units as of September 2020, with a total of 700,000 units. During the last two years, the amount spent on the rental of CPAP was 12 billion won in out-of-pocket and 48.1 billion won in the national insurance system, a total of 60.1 billion won.

In Japan, medical insurance coverage is administered by the Central Government (Ministry of Health, Labor and Welfare). Full polysomnography (including EEG, EOG, EMG, EKG, Resp, and SpO2) cost is JPY 33,000 per night, of which 30% is from patient and 70% from Government. OSA screening is mandatory before full polysomnography; the cost is JPY 7200. Total CPAP therapy cost (monthly) is JPY 14,500. CPAP coverage requirements are as follows: (1) AHI 20 or higher, (2) sleepiness or headaches and difficulty in managing everyday life, and (3) sleep fragmentations or lack of deep sleep, and CPAP therapy eliminates these symptoms as confirmed by polysomnography. It means that diagnosis based on polysomnography and second night polysomnography is required for CPAP titration. The provider runs a rental contract system as the reimbursement for equipment is a fixed monthly amount of JPY 14,500. The CPAP rental contract includes delivery, service and maintenance, and all basic accessories (humidifier could be included on the contract). Under a system like this, long-term usage/adherence is important for all parties to maintain income.

A previous study in Japan showed CPAP adherence rate after a six-month period was 38% [21]. Another Japanese study reported 89.8% CPAP adherence rate at five years [22]. In a study on CPAP adherence of a Southeast Asian privately funded healthcare system, 42.2% of all patients with significant OSA rejected CPAP treatment upfront, but

adherence among those who started CPAP is comparable to other reports, which was 52.6% [23]. CPAP acceptance rate has been reported to be 39.7% in Taiwan among the elderly [24].

In summary, the CPAP compliance of patients with sleep apnea in East Asia does not seem to be very different from other regions. However, in Korea, it has not been long since insurance coverage for CPAP was introduced, so a large-scale study is needed to determine the degree of compliance in the future.

36.6   Canada

According to *Statistics Canada*, in 2016 and 2017 [3], 6.4% of Canadians reported they had been diagnosed by a healthcare professional with sleep apnea. This is an increase in comparison to the 2009 survey results, which found that the prevalence of self-reported sleep apnea was only 3% among adults 18 years and older. In a more recent article examining the global prevalence and burden of OSA, Canada was shown to have over 19 million adults ages 30–69 years old reporting having OSA with 24.5% of this population having an AHI greater or equal to five events per hour, and 4.8% having an AHI greater or equal to 15 events per hour [1]. Despite the significant demand for treatment and the increasing risk for developing OSA and its associated complications within this patient population, adherence to CPAP treatment remains problematic. CPAP adherence rates are highly individualized: how a patient perceives, experiences, and administers self-treatment differs from individual to individual [25]. Commonly cited barriers to CPAP adherence in clinical literature include, but are not limited to, air leaks, dry mouth, nasal congestion, excessive moisture in tube, tubing being disruptive when moving in bed, claustrophobia, and skin irritation. Receptiveness and support of a partner and experiencing few or mild side effects have also been correlated with higher adherence rates [25, 26].

OSA is associated with a substantial societal and economic burden within Canada, and treatment using CPAP can be quite costly depending on provincial jurisdictions. A report from the Assistive Devices Program within Ontario's Ministry of Health and Long-Term Care showed that in just 2008, approximately 72,400 new devices were being administered each year at a cost of $2000 each, totaling $145 million per year as direct expenses [25]. Currently, individual costs vary, as public coverage of OSA and access to treatment vary greatly across Canada. Table 36.2 is showcasing CPAP coverage across Canada as extracted from the Canadian Ministry of Health database [27].

Table 36.2 CPAP coverage across Canada

Province	Program name	Program description	Does the client need to demonstrate therapy compliance?	Compliance criteria	Payment of trial period
Ontario	Assistive Devices Program (OHIP)	The Ministry of Health and Long-Term Care, Assistive Devices Program (ADP) pays for CPAP devices for individuals diagnosed by a sleep physician as having OSA. CPAP machines are covered up to 75% by OHIP if purchased with a doctor prescription	No. simply renew with the ADP every 2 years to continue receiving this specific financial support	N/A	N/A
Saskatchewan	Saskatchewan Aids to Independent Living (SAIL)	Respiratory Equipment Program offers the loan of a selection of respiratory equipment. Loan of CPAP flow generator is given upon the receipt of a $275 program fee (fee includes loan of a CPAP and repairs as needed for the useful life of the machine, defined as 5 years)	No	N/A	N/A
Manitoba	Winnipeg Regional Health Authority (WRHA)	CPAP coverage includes remaining balance for the CPAP machine, mask and service fees (administration for the initial equipment purchase, 60-minute consultation fee with a vendor of choice, mask fitting, education regarding care and use, follow-up appointments for treatment issues, and auto-titration trial fee)	Yes	Use of the device for 4 hours/night for 70% of the 3–6-week trial period	WHRA funds service fees during the trial period
Alberta	Income Support (IS)	IS program provides coverage for CPAP devices for the treatment of moderate-to-severe OSA when medically essential. The IS program does not provide funding for the treatment of mild OSA or for the renting of a CPAP device. IS program may provide up to $1736.00 for fixed pressure CPAP devices, or up to $2042.00 for auto-pressure CPAP devices. Prices include a 3-year warranty, heated humidifier, hose, mask with headgear, chin strap (if needed), and 12 filters	No	N/A	N/A
	Assured Income for the Severely Handicapped (AISH)	Provides coverage for non-auto-CPAP devices to treat sleep apnea when the condition is substantiated as a life-threatening situation. AISH provides up to $1600 for CPAP supplies. Auto-pressure CPAP devices are covered up to the maximum medical equipment amount once every 3 years, while fixed pressure CPAP devices are covered up to $1736.00 once every 3 years	No	N/A	N/A
British Columbia	Employment and Assistance Regulation	The least expensive, appropriate breathing devices may be provided by the ministry under the Employment and Assistance Regulation to specific recipients that need assistance with a medically essential need	No	N/A	N/A

36.7 Conclusion

From North America to Europe and Asia, this chapter explored international perspectives concerning global CPAP adherence rates. This chapter highlights that despite the recognition of CPAP as a gold standard for OSA treatment, its adherence remains a severe problem in the global management of patients with OSA. Specifically, eco-nomic, sociocultural, adverse health effects, and cognitive barriers are cited across diverse countries as barriers to adequate CPAP initiation and usage. Given the multifactorial socioeconomic and health consequences of untreated OSA, further need for increased CPAP consumer education, patient support, and standardized, healthcare policy reform remains an imperative issue to work toward achieving.

References

1. Benjafield AV, Ayas NT, Eastwood PR, et al. Estimation of the global prevalence and burden of obstructive sleep apnoea: a literature-based analysis. Lancet Respir Med. 2019;7(8):687–98. https://doi.org/10.1016/S2213-2600(19)30198-5.

2. Rotenberg BW, Vicini C, Pang EB, Pang KP. Reconsidering first-line treatment for obstructive sleep apnea: a systematic review of the literature. J Otolaryngol Head Neck Surg. 2016;45:23. https://doi.org/10.1186/s40463-016-0136-4.

3. Statistics Canada. Sleep apnea in Canada, 2016 and 2017. 2018. https://www150.statcan.gc.ca/n1/pub/82-625-x/2018001/article/54979-eng.htm.

4. Saraei M, Najafi A, Heidarbagi E. Risk factors for obstructive sleep apnea among train drivers. Work. 2020;65(1):121–5.

5. Arshi S, Salmani M, Sadeghniiat-Haghighi K, Najafi A, Alavi S, Shamsipour M. Prevalence of obstructive sleep apnea among adults in north-west of Iran. Sleep Med. 2017;40:e18.

6. Sarokhani M, Goli M, Salarvand S, Gheshlagh RG. The prevalence of sleep apnea in Iran: a systematic review and meta-analysis. Tanaffos. 2019;18(1):1.

7. Shapiro GK, Shapiro CM. Factors that influence CPAP adherence: an overview. Sleep Breath. 2010;14(4):323–35.

8. Najafi A, Naeimabadi N, Sadeghniiat-Haghighi K, Salmani-Nodoushan M, Rahimi-Golkhandan A. Continuous positive airway pressure adherence in patients with obstructive sleep apnea syndrome. J Sleep Sci. 2017;2(3–4):67–70.

9. Nodoushan MS, Chavoshi F. Association between depression and severity of obstructive sleep apnea syndrome. J Sleep Sci. 2016;1(1):13–7.

10. Patil SP, Ayappa IA, Caples SM, Kimoff RJ, Patel SR, Harrod CG. Treatment of adult obstructive sleep apnea with positive airway pressure: an American Academy of Sleep Medicine clinical practice guideline. J Clin Sleep Med. 2019;15:335–43. https://doi.org/10.5664/jcsm.7640.

11. Wallace DM, Sawyer AM, Shafazand S. Comorbid insomnia symptoms predict lower 6-month adherence to CPAP in US veterans with obstructive sleep apnea. Sleep Breath. 2018;22:5–15. https://doi.org/10.1007/s11325-017-1605-3.

12. Borel JC, Tamisier R, Dias-Domingos S, Sapene M, Martin F, Stach B, et al. Type of mask may impact on continuous positive airway pressure adherence in apneic patients. PLoS One. 2013;8:e64382. https://doi.org/10.1371/journal.pone.0064382.

13. Suri J, Sen M, Ojha U. Acceptance and compliance issues of nasal CPAP amongst Indian patients of obstructive sleep apnea. Indian J Sleep Med. 2006;1:197–203.

14. Goyal A, Agarwal N, Pakhare A. Barriers to CPAP use in India: an exploratory study. J Clin Sleep Med. 2017;13:1385–94. https://doi.org/10.5664/jcsm.6830.

15. Ninan M, Balachandran J. CPAP compliance in patients with moderate to severe obstructive sleep apnea from three centers in South India. Int J Res Med Sci. 2017;5:4886. https://doi.org/10.18203/2320-6012.ijrms20174939.

16. Ramachandran P, Devaraj U, Sandeepa H, Kavitha V, Maheswari U, D'Souza G. Mixed method model to assess CPAP adherence among patients with moderate to severe OSA. Indian J Chest Dis Allied Sci. 2019;61:119–22.

17. Periwal P, Ali M, Talwar D. CPAP compliance in Indian OSAHS patients can be improved by correcting mask and humidifier related problems. Chest. 2014;145:590A. https://doi.org/10.1378/chest.1834845.

18. Reddy NR, Sasikala N, Karthik KVGC, Priya GK. Customized nasal prosthesis in continuous positive airway pressure treatment, current trend in treating obstructive sleep apnea for better patient compliance. J Family Med Prim Care. 2019;8:2728–31. https://doi.org/10.4103/jfmpc.jfmpc_473_19.

19. Liao WJ, Song LJ, Yi HL, Guan J, Zou JY, Xu HJ, Wang G, Ma F, Li-Bo Zhou LB, Chen YQ, Yan LB, Deng ZC, Walter T, McNicholas WT, Yin SK, Zhong NS, Zhang XW. Treatment choice by patients with obstructive sleep apnea: data from two centers in China. J Thorac Dis. 2018;10(3):1941–50.

20. Wang Y, Gao W, Sun M, Chen B. Adherence to CPAP in patients with obstructive sleep apnea in a Chinese population. Respir Care. 2012;57(2):238–43.

21. Tanahashi T, Nagano J, Yamaguchi Y, Kubo C, Sudo N. Factors that predict adherence to continuous positive airway pressure treatment in obstructive sleep apnea patients: a prospective study in Japan. Sleep Biol Rhythms. 2012;10(2):126–35.

22. Tokunaga T, Ninomiya T, Kato Y, Ito Y, Takabayashi T, Tokuriki M, et al. Long-term compliance with nasal continuous positive airway pressure therapy for sleep apnea syndrome in an otorhinolaryngological office. Eur Arch Otorhinolaryngol. 2013;270(8):2267–73.

23. Lee CHK, Leow LC, Song PR, Li H, Ong TH. Acceptance and adherence to continuous positive airway pressure therapy in patients with obstructive sleep apnea (OSA) in a Southeast Asian privately funded healthcare system. Sleep Sci. 2017;10(2):57–63.

24. Yang MC, Lin CY, Lan CC, Huang CY, Huang YC, Lim CS, et al. Factors affecting CPAP acceptance in elderly patients with obstructive sleep apnea in Taiwan. Respir Care. 2013;58(9):1504–13.

25. Kim J, Tran K, Seal K, et al. Interventions for the treatment of obstructive sleep apnea in adults: a health technology assessment. March 2017. http://search.ebscohost.com.proxy.library.nyu.edu/login.aspx?direct=true&db=mnh&AN=30601604&site=eds-live.

26. Laratta CR, Ayas NT, Povitz M, Pendharkar SR. Diagnosis and treatment of obstructive sleep apnea in adults. CMAJ. 2017;189(48):E1481. http://search.ebscohost.com.proxy.library.nyu.edu/login.aspx?direct=true&db=edb&AN=126568105&site=eds-live.

27. Tran K, Kim J, Tsoi B, et al. Interventions for the treatment of obstructive sleep apnea in adults: a health technology assessment – project protocol. Ottawa: Canadian Agency for Drugs and Technologies in Health; 2016.

The History and Future of CPAP

37

Shaista Hussain

37.1 CPAP Timeline

In the sixteenth century, an Irish poet called John V. Kelleher used a poem to describe snores, moans, and groans – an early depiction of the sleep apnea experience.

In 1836, renowned author Charles Dickens published *The Pickwick Papers*, a story that depicted an overweight character whose symptoms articulate what is now known as sleep apnea. This early clinical picture became known as "Pickwickian syndrome," throughout the nineteenth century [1].

In 1901, English Engineer Hubert Cecil Booth who was famed for designing suspension bridges and Ferris wheels, developed a machine that blew out air to raise dust from carpets into a collecting bag, and then redesigned the machine to suck air into a collecting bag. Thereafter, the machine evolved into the practical, household vacuum technology that continues to be a universal, domestic appliance [2].

In 1956, Dr. C.S. Burwell officially documented the first case of Pickwickian syndrome, in an obese man who had lost a winning hand in poker because he had fallen asleep [3].

In 1965, a team of European doctors, led by Dr. Gastaut, researched and identified three varieties of sleep apnea [4].

In 1970, from his laboratory in Toronto, Canada, Dr. Eliot Phillipson investigated airflow technology treatments in dogs who suffered from respiratory issues [5].

In 1971, Dr. George Gregory and his team applied continuous positive airway pressure to infants suffering from idiopathic respiratory distress syndrome – the then leading cause of respiratory failure in newborns – by supplying humidified positive airflow with endotracheal tubes, resulting in improved PaO2 and survival rates in all the participants (*New England Journal of Medicine* in 1971) [6].

In 1980, in Australia, Dr. Colin Sullivan treated his dog's breathing difficulties with a vacuum cleaner, then speculated that by pumping air into the respiratory tract continuously, impaired breathing could improve during sleep. He tested this theory on dogs with respiratory illnesses, and subsequently found success in human trials [7].

In 1981, Dr. Colin Sullivan and his colleagues at the University of Sydney developed the first continuous positive airway pressure (CPAP) device as the first successful, noninvasive treatment for obstructive sleep apnea (OSA). And the team went on to make CPAP a universally available, life-changing technology. Dr. Sullivan went on to continue research at the University of Toronto [7].

In 1987, Baxter International licensed and commercially developed Dr. Sullivan's CPAP patent with a mask which was released in 1988 [7].

In 1989, Dr. Peter Farrell acquired Baxter Internationals' interest in CPAP and founded the company ResCare [7, 8].

In 1995, ResCare became known as ResMed, one of the world's leading manufacturers of CPAP machines and masks [7, 8].

37.2 Now

37.2.1 Global Goals

Approximately 1 billion of the world's 7.3 billion people, aged 30 through 69 years, are estimated to have the most common type of sleep-disordered breathing, obstructive sleep apnea (OSA). A rise in global prevalence of sleep apnea is largely attributed to an increase in the prevalence of obesity, a major OSA risk factor. Males are three times more likely than females to have OSA [9]. OSA is associated with many cardiovascular and metabolic disorders and undiagnosed untreated OSA has also been shown to be associated with a reduced quality of life and an increased incidence of depression [10]. CPAP therapy aims to alleviate symptoms of fatigue and somnolence, improve activities of daily living, improve quality of life, improve cognitive function, resolve snoring, and reduce work or motor vehicle accident risks, in the short term. In the long term, CPAP aims to

S. Hussain (✉)
Medical Technology Solutions Laboratories, Riyadh, Saudi Arabia

reduce premature death, as OSA has been associated with cardiovascular and cerebrovascular disease, hypertension, impaired cognitive function (Alzheimer disease), type 2 diabetes, anxiety and depression symptoms, and impaired sexual function in both men and women [11]. The burdens of OSA, however, extend beyond the frustrated sleeper. Healthcare services and management costs increase with the increased demand for physician services [10] creating a demand for healthcare support. OSA is associated with excessive daytime sleepiness and compromised vigilance resulting in impaired work performance, reduced productivity, absenteeism, motor vehicle accidents, and significant increases in unemployment and underemployment [10]. The global sleep apnea device market size was valued at USD 3.7 billion in 2020 and is expected to expand at a compound annual growth rate of 6.2% from 2021 to 2028, and the global market size is expected to reach USD 4697.3 million by the end of 2026 [12]. The globally growing geriatric population, a product of increased life expectancy, is expected to lead to a rise in the prevalence of sleep disorders, especially OSA which affects between 13% and 32% of people above 65 years of age [13]. Furthermore, obesity rates will encourage CPAP usage as obesity is a known OSA risk factor and the estimated prevalence of obesity in the USA in 2016 was 39.8%, accounting for nearly 93.3 million adults [14].

37.2.2 Mechanisms

Prior to the invention of the CPAP machine, the most commonly prescribed therapy for severe OSA, was surgery [15]. The value of CPAP has been substantiated by research that has mapped the physiological benefits of CPAP across a multitude of diseases. CPAP remains the first-line treatment for OSA and works via pneumatic splinting of the upper airways, with airway pressure applied through oral, oronasal, and nasal devices [9]. The machines employ mechanisms which pressurize air between 4 and 20 cm H_2O (in increments of 1 or 0.5) [16]. As a result, the nighttime respiratory events and sleep fragmentation occurring in these patients disappear, and normal sleep architecture is restored with observable clinical improvement [17]. Other therapeutic mechanisms include positional therapy, weight loss regimens, behavioral modification therapies, oral appliance therapy (OAT) (e.g., mandibular advancement devices), orofacial surgery, nasal expiratory positive airway pressure (EPAP) devices, oral pressure therapy, and implantable hypoglossal nerve stimulation devices. Mandibular advancement devices reduce the apnea-hypopnea index, to various degrees, and have been shown to reduce blood pressure in patients but with no predictable pattern [18]. Some patients with OSA prefer OAT, and such devices are often recommended when CPAP is not available.

37.2.3 Designs

Modern CPAP machines have become smaller, quieter, and self-adjusting air pressure and humidification controls offer personalized comfort settings, making the patient's comfort and compliance increase [19]. Straps and masks in newer models are also more comfortable than older models, and home testing kits now offer a less intrusive, less expensive method of collecting physiological data. "Smart" CPAP machines use auto-titration to breathe with the host, based on advanced algorithms that produce optimal pressures in real time [20]. Advanced algorithms measure:
- Snoring volume
- Respiratory effort
- Sleeping position

When the machine detects a need for increased pressure, it delivers the required pressure; when the machine detects physiological relaxation, it reduces the pressure setting [15].

Most advanced CPAP and autoPAP machines contain microprocessors, which allow dense data storage, internal hardware and software self-testing to ensure optimal performance, and results are generated in parameter output reports. This type of data output enables clinicians to track patient compliance and monitor dose-response output in more detail. Current major market producers include ResMed, Philips Respironics, 3B Medical, Apex, Circadiance, Drive DeVilbiss Healthcare, Fisher & Paykel Healthcare, InnoMed Technologies, Sleepnet, and Transcend. Many manufacturers employ remote, telemedicine monitoring techniques to evaluate patient adherence to treatment [19]. New airing systems use micro-pump technology as a source of pressure from within a small nasal bud attached to a system of micro-blowers and zinc-air batteries that provide 8 hours of power [21], also enhancing the end-user experience. Advancements in medical technology are guiding the evolution of the CPAP machine.

37.2.4 Analysis of Benefits

Medical research is propagating the depth of our understanding of the physiological effects of CPAP therapy. A discussion on the benefits of CPAP in OSA, authored by the Agency for Healthcare Research and Quality (AHRQ), questioned research findings and suggested a lack of overall benefit; a subsequent response from multiple sleep boards placed some of the isolated findings that were discussed, in detailed scientific context, revealing a more optimistic outlook on the value of CPAP. In a review of 47 studies, the AHRQ criticized sleep medicine research design validation and measures of respiration, suggesting a lack of long-term morbidity and mortality benefits from CPAP use [11]. The authors suggested that evidence remains insufficient or weak, regarding the effects of CPAP on hypertension, functional status, sexual function, and days of work missed, and suggesting that future CPAP studies should include blinding elements to reduce the risk of bias. In response, the multiple sleep boards (including the American Academy of Sleep Medicine, Canadian Sleep Society, American Society of Sleep Medicine, World Sleep Society, American Academy of Dental Sleep Medicine, Sleep Research Society, American Sleep Apnea Association et al. (2021)) remarked that the draft's suggestions were not based on a totality of evidence available, thereby not adequately representing the true, measured value of CPAP. The sleep boards encouraged research revisions that acknowledge excessive sleepiness as a clinically important outcome for patients with OSA [22]. In patients with OSA, continuous positive airway pressure lowers blood pressure and rates of arrhythmia and stroke, improves left ventricular ejection fraction in patients with heart failure, and reduces fatal and nonfatal cardiovascular events. Meta-analyses on CPAP use have found that it is associated with significant reductions in blood pressure and in excessive sleepiness in compliant CPAP users [22]. The boards highlight non-randomized, comparative studies that have demonstrated striking reductions in motor vehicle accidents, in the comparison of pre- and post-CPAP usage. The authors additionally propose correlational approaches to assess a dose-response relationship between changes in apnea-hypopnea index (AHI) and clinical outcomes: i) by measuring the hours of CPAP use and specific clinical outcomes and ii) by examining the extent to which CPAP alleviates the AHI (considering the duration of CPAP use as a proportion of total sleep time, measured by the mean disease alleviation index) [22]. It is important to consider that short-term studies may yield more accurate results based on a higher likelihood of adherence to CPAP therapy, whereas long-term studies may reflect more realistic impressions of lesser compliance. The benefits of CPAP across a range of short- and long-term morbidities are statistically evident in a large base of literature, as ongoing research outcomes steer the direction that OSA therapy will take in the future.

37.3   Future

Current research and development is challenging the shadows of OSA that have haunted the nights of so many sleepers. Microprocessors, nanosize hardware, artificial intelligence recognitions, and customizable wearable medical technology are driving sleep solutions to conquer what was once known as the Pickwickian demise. Levels of healthcare service should increase to coincide with the growing compendium of information on the topic, enabling more uniformed practitioners to operate

from an evidence base. The direction of therapy in the future will be dependent on the quality of decisions made from clinical investigations, making thorough and appropriate study designs imperative for correct decision making processes. With diligent patient adherence and sound clinical research, a thorough map detailing the long-term outcomes of CPAP therapy will manifest and guide our therapeutic decisions.

The Snoring Bedmate
John V. Kelleher.
   (Sixteenth Century – Irish Poet)

You thunder at my side,
Lad of ceaseless hum;
There's not a saint would chide
My prayer that you were dumb.

The dead start from the tomb
With each blare from your nose.
I suffer, with less room,
Under these bedclothes.

With could I better bide
Since my head's already broke—
Your pipe-drone at my side,
Woodpecker's drill on oak?

Brass scraped with knicky knives
A cowbell's tinny clank,
Or the yells of tinkers' wives
Giving birth behind a bank?

A drunken, braying clown
Slapping cards down on a board
Were less easy to disown
Than the softest snore you've snored

Sweeter the grunts of swine
Than yours that win release.
Sweeter, bedmate mine,
The screech of grieving geese.

A sick calf's moan for aid,
A broken mill's mad clatter,
The snarl of flood cascade…
Christ! now what's the matter?

That was a ghastly growl!
What signified that twist?—
An old wolf's famished howl,
Wave-boom at some cliff's breast?

Storm screaming round a crag,
Bellow of raging bull,
Hoarse bell or rutting stag,
Compared with this were lull!

Ah, now a gentler fall—
Bark of a crazy hound?

Brats squabbling for a ball?
Ducks squawking on a pond?

No, rough weather's back again.
Some great ships's about to sink
And roaring bursts the main
Over the bulwark's brink!

Farewell, tonight, to sleep.
Every gust across the bed
Makes hair rise and poor flesh creep.
Would that one of us were dead!

This Irish seventeenth century poem captures some features of sleep apnea. We trust that you have enjoy this book on CPAP adherence.

References

1. EOS. A Brief History of Sleep Apnea. 2020. https://www.eossleep.com/2015/05/26/a-brief-history-of-the-causes-of-sleep-apnea/.
2. The Science Museum. The invention of the vacuum cleaner, from horse-drawn to high tech. 2020. Published: 3 April 2020 The Science Museum. https://www.sciencemuseum.org.uk/objects-and-stories/everyday-wonders/invention-vacuum-cleaner#:~:text=In%201901%2C%20if%20you%20were,of%20us%20clean%20our%20homes.&text=Hubert%20Cecil%20Booth%20(1871%E2%80%931955).
3. Ferriss JB. Obstructive sleep apnoea syndrome: the first picture? J R Soc Med. 2009;102(5):201–2. https://doi.org/10.1258/jrsm.2009.090023.
4. Bradley TD. Respiratory sleep medicine: a coming of age. Am J Respir Crit Care Med. 2008;177(4):363–4. https://doi.org/10.1164/rccm.200711-1717ED.
5. Parker JD, Brooks D, Kozar LF, Render-Teixeira CL, Horner RL, Douglas Bradley T, Phillipson EA. Acute and chronic effects of airway obstruction on canine left ventricular performance. Am J Respir Crit Care Med. 1999;160(6):1888–96. https://doi.org/10.1164/ajrccm.160.6.9807074.
6. Gregory GA, Kitterman JA, Phibbs RH, Tooley WH, Hamilton W. Treatment of the idiopathic respiratory-distress syndrome with continuous positive airway pressure. N Engl J Med. 1971;1971(284):1333–40. https://doi.org/10.1056/NEJM197106172842401.
7. Resmed. The Resmed Story. 2021. https://www.resmed.com.au/about-us/the-resmed-story.
8. Premium Author Leroy Batards A Short History and Timeline of the CPAP Machine and Sleep Apnea Health Articles. (August 23, 2011). http://www.articlesfactory.com/articles/health/a-short-history-and-timeline-of-the-cpap-machine-and-sleep-apnea.html.
9. Semelka M, Wilson J, Floyd R. Diagnosis and treatment of obstructive sleep Apnea in adults. Am Fam Physician. 2016;94(5):355–60. https://www.aafp.org/afp/2016/0901/p355.html
10. Lyons MM, Bhatt NY, Pack AI, Magalang UJ. Invited Review Series: New frontiers in sleep disordered breathing Free Access Global burden of sleep-disordered breathing and its implications. 2020. First published: 21 May 2020 https://doi.org/10.1111/resp.13838.
11. Continuous Positive Airway Pressure Treatment for Obstructive Sleep Apnea, by the Evidence-based Practice Center Program at the Agency for Healthcare Research and Quality (AHRQ).
12. GVR (Grand View Research). Sleep apnea devices market size, share & trends analysis report by product type (diagnostic devices, therapeutic devices, sleep apnea masks), by region (North America, Europe, APAC, Latin America, MEA), And Segment Forecasts, 2021–2028. 2021. (March 2021). Report ID: 978-1-68038-265-5 https://www.grandviewresearch.com/industry-analysis/sleep-apnea-devices-market.
13. Glasser M, Bailey N, McMillan A, Goff E, Morrell MJ. Sleep apnoea in older people. Breathe. 2011;7(3):248–56. https://doi.org/10.1183/20734735.021910.
14. Hales CM, Carroll MD, Fryar CD, Ogden CL. Prevalence of obesity among adults and youth: United States, 2015–2016. NCHS Data Brief No. 288, October 2017. 2017. https://www.cdc.gov/nchs/data/databriefs/db288.pdf.
15. CPAP.COM (2018).The Invention and Historical Perspective of the CPAP Machine. https://www.cpap.com/blog/cpap-invention-historical-perspective/.
16. Johnson C. CPAP Machines by Chris Johnson Posted On January 26, 2021. 2021. https://www.sleeprestfully.com/blog/best-cpap-machines-2018/.
17. Monasterio C, Vidal S, Duran J, Ferrer M, Carmona C, Barbe F, Mayos M, Gonzalez-Mangado N, Juncadella M, Navarro AM Barreira R, Capote F, Mayoralas LR, Peces-Barba G, Alonso J, Montserrat JM. Effectiveness of continuous positive airway pressure in mild sleep apnea–hypopnea syndrome. Am J Respirat Crit Care Med. 2000;164(6). https://doi.org/10.1164/ajrccm.164.6.2008010. PubMed: 11587974 Aug., 03, 2000. https://www.atsjournals.org/doi/full/10.1164/ajrccm.164.6.2008010.
18. Marklund M, Braem MJA, Verbraecken J. Update on oral appliance therapy. Eur Respir Rev. 2019;28:190083. https://doi.org/10.1183/16000617.0083-2019.
19. Sleep Review. What's New With CPAP Technology? Posted by Sleep Review Staff | Jul 2, 2002 | Heart, Obstructive Sleep Apnea, Oral Appliances, Skin, Snoring, Weight. https://www.sleepreviewmag.com/sleep-treatments/therapy-devices/oral-appliances/whats-new-with-cpap-technology-2/.
20. Ma Z, Hyde P, Drinnan M, Munguia J. Development of a smart-fit system for CPAP interface selection. Proc Inst Mech Eng H. 2021;235(1):44–53. https://doi.org/10.1177/0954411920959879.
21. Sistema Blog. New CPAP Developments and Alternatives New CPAP Developments and Alternatives. 2019. Apr 20, 2019 https://sistemmacpap.com/blog/new-cpap-developments-and-alternatives/.
22. Patil S, Gay P, Johnson K, Kimoff RJ, Pack A. AHRQ Response from Multiple Sleep Boards. CPAP – Sleep Apnea Report. 2021. Sent via email to: epc@ahrq.hhs.gov.

Index

A

Acceptable apnea-hypopnea index, 284
Active listening, 39
Adaptive servo ventilation (ASV), 4, 183, 284, 285
Adenoid facies, 240
Adenoid hypertrophy, 240
Adherence, 136
  arbitrary thresholds, 63
  baseline factors, 64–66
  behavioural interventions, 65, 66
  cardiometabolic outcomes, 63
  clinical and practical relevance, 32
  clinical setting, 33
  combined focus interventions, 33
  cost-effectiveness research, 33, 64
  CPAP usage pattern, 67
  daytime sleepiness, 64, 141
  diagnostic groupings, 33
  education, 65
  effectiveness, 141
  follow-up period duration, 31, 67
  health and functional benefits, 32
  health professional-related factors, 142, 145
  implications, 33, 34
  interface, 66, 67
  measures and outcomes, 32
  metrics, 63
  network theory, 35
  objective sleepiness, 63, 64
  OSA, 14
  overview, 14
  patient-directed interventions
    education, 30
    myofunctional therapy, 31
    patient behavior and affective state, 31
    upper airway, 31
  patient-related factors, 142–144
  patients' failure, 14
  peer buddy interventions, 33
  phenotypes
    age-related phenotypes, 146
    clinical manifestations, 145
    congenital abnormalities, 147
    craniofacial abnormalities, 147
    definition, 145
    EDS, 145, 146
    ethnic population, 146
    gender-related phenotypes, 146
    insomnia, 147, 148
    pathophysiological causes, 145
    REM-related OSA, 147

    risk factors, 145
    sedative use, 147
    strategies, 145
    supine position-related OSA, 147
  QALY, 64
  randomized trial, 142
  recommendations, 13, 14
  reimbursement, 64
  search procedure and inclusion criteria
    data extraction, 16
    data synthesis, 16
    diagnosis, 30
    intervention strategies, 16, 30
    publications, 16
    risk of bias, 16, 30
    search strategy, 16–29
    study characteristics, 30
    study design, 30
    study origin and setting, 30
    study size, 30
  sleep related quality of life, 63, 64
  socio-economic differences (*see* Socio-economic differences)
  subjective sleepiness, 63, 64
  support and troubleshooting, 68, 69
  technology-targeted interventions
    auto-adjusting pressure, 31
    humidity, 31
    masks types, 31
    pressure relief machines, 31
  telemonitoring, 67, 68
  therapy- and medication-related factors, 142, 144
  therapy discontinuation, 141, 142
  treatment benefits, 141
  upper airway, 141
Adherence barriers to CPAP questionnaire [ABCQ], 293
Adjusting positive airway pressure device (APAP), 66
Agency for Healthcare Research and Quality (AHRQ), 384
AHRQ criticized sleep medicine research design, 384
Air pressure treatments, 347
Airflow generator. *See* Continuous positive airway pressure (CPAP) device
Alzheimer's disease (AD), 158, 159, 168
Anxiety, 51, 76–79, 157
Apnea hypopnea index (AHI), 4, 30, 50, 141, 214, 231, 280, 317, 359
Arousal index, 257
Atrial fibrillation (AF), 6, 91, 179
Attention deficit hyperactivity disorder (ADHD), 155, 156
Attitudes to CPAP treatment inventory (ACTI), 295, 296
Autism spectrum disorder (ASD), 157
Auto-adjusting BPAP, 4
Auto-titrating PAP (APAP), 229, 248

B

Bariatric surgery
   auto titrating PAP, 229
   CPAP adherence, 228, 229
Best evidence synthesis approach, 16
Big data analysis, 97
Bi-level positive airway pressure (BPAP), 4, 160, 257, 337
Biopsychosocial (BPS) model, 51
   clinical facility, 45
   elements, 45
   motivational interviewing, 45–47
   resources, 45
   style of interaction
      adherence, 40, 41
      aphorism, 42
      appointment, 44
      beneficial behavior, 40
      comorbid conditions, 41
      components, 40
      CPAP device feedback, 44
      diagnostic information, 44
      disability, 43
      doctor–patient communication, 39
      education, 42, 43
      EGBDF, 41
      end-stage renal disease, 40
      family support, 44
      fast acquisition, 44
      genetics, 43
      issues, 44, 45
      NICE review, 40
      patient centric, 42
      patient's view referrals, 44
      psychological and sociological factors, 40
      recognition, 39
      referring physician/agency, 39, 40
      socioeconomic status, 39
      symptom and sign, 39
      usage and apnea rate, 41
Biot's respiration, 159
Bradyarrhythmias, 6
Brief behavioral therapy, 190
Bruxism, 163

C

Calgary sleep apnea QoL index (SAQLI), 5
Cardiac arrhythmia, 179, 180
Cardiovascular (CV) system, 55, 177
Cardiovascular disease (CVD)
   atrial fibrillation, 6
   bradyarrhythmias, 6
   CAD, 5
   CHF, 6
   endothelial dysfunction, 5
   hypertension, 6
   prevalence, 5
   stroke, 6
   type 2 diabetes, 7
Center for Epidemiological Studies Depression (CES-D)
      Scale, 205
Centers for Medicare and Medicaid Services (CMS), 97
Central respiratory drive, 232
Central serous chorioretinopathy (CSC), 221
Central sleep apnea
   emergence of, 7
   respiratory instability, 7

   treatment success
      adherence, 9, 10
      daytime sleepiness assessment, 8, 9
      quality of life instruments, 8
      self-report, 8
Centre for Medicare and Medicaid Services (CMS) funding, 49
Cheyne-Stokes respiration (CSA-CSR), 159, 340
Children with medical complexity (CMC)
   characteristics, 255
Children with special health care needs (CSHCN)
   definition, 255
   functional abilities, 255
   positive airway pressure
      acclimatization phase, 268–270
      behavioral interventions, 263
      definition, 259
      device, 259
      disease and mode of therapy, 262, 263
      expiration, 258
      family and social factors, 262
      functional interfaces, 270
      hypnosis techniques, 263
      indication and functionality, 258
      individual factors, 262
      initial phase, 268, 269
      initiation phase, 268
      inspiration, 258
      interfaces, 259, 261
      maintenance phase, 268, 270
      modes of ventilation, 258
      parent and patient engagement programmes, 263
      socioeconomic factors, 270
      specific PAP adherence factors, 264–267
   prevalence, 255
   sleep disordered breathing
      craniofacial features, 255, 256
      impact of untreated OSA, 257
      muscle weakness, 256
      obesity, 256, 257
      PAP therapy, 257
      prevalence, 255, 256
      therapeutic interventions, 257
   social health determinants, 255
   typical development, 255
Chronic headaches, 7
Chronic illness, 114
Chronic kidney disease (CKD), 7
Chronic sinus, 162, 163
Claustrophobia, 143
Clinician-administered PTSD scale (CAPS) score, 215
Coexistent sleep disorders, 87
Cognitive behavioural therapy (CBT), 65, 71, 213
Cognitive-behavioral therapy for insomnia (CBTi), 76
   administration, 189
   bed allocation, 191
   comorbidity, 192
   compensatory behaviors, 192
   efficacy of, 189
   first-line treatment, 189
   initial sleep window, 191
   intervention with behavioral strategies, 190
   multicomponent intervention, 190
   PAP initiation, 190
   perpetuating factors, 190
   precipitating factors, 190
   predisposing factors, 190
   protocol, 190

sleep efficiency, 191
sleep restriction strategies, 191
Spielman 3-P model, 190
stimulus control and sleep restriction, 191
stimulus control strategies, 190
symptoms, 189
Comorbid obstructive sleep apnea and insomnia (COMISA)
antidepressants, 198, 199
eszopiclone, 199
first-line treatment, 195
hypnotic medications, 197
identification, 195
new dual orexin receptor antagonists, 197
non-benzodiazepines, 197, 199
sedative/hypnotic agents
benzodiazepines, 196
effects, 195
non-benzodiazepines, 196
non-benzodiazepines, with CPAP, 197
non-benzodiazepines, without CPAP, 196
zolpidem, 199
Co-morbid OSA and insomnia (COMISA), 88
Compliance, 13, 136
Compliance vs. adherence vs. concordance (CAC), 299
by bridging bias in therapeutic options, 301, 302
effective therapy, 304, 305
evolution, 306, 307
impact of, 300
OAT, 302–304, 307–309
approaches, 312
vs. PAP therapy, 309–311
participation, 299
personalization, 299
prediction, 299
prevention, 299
by reducing barriers to care, 301
by reducing bias in restrictive definition of OAT, 305, 306
SRBD therapies, 311, 312
Congestive heart failure, 340, 341
Congestive heart failure (CHF), 6
Continuous positive airway pressure (CPAP) device, 257
adherence, 341, 342
analysis of benefits, 384, 385
care and equipment cleaning and maintenance, 352
clinical conditions, 340
congestive heart failure, 340
obesity hypoventilation syndrome, 340
stable hypercapnic COPD, 340
contraindications, 341
in COVID-19 environment, 344
designs, 384
education and follow-up, 364, 365
future aspects, 385
global goals, 384
historical background, 337
history, 383
initiation, 338, 339
machine, 347, 348
mask technology, 338, 349–351
mechanisms, 384
motivational enhancement therapy, 367
obesity hypoventilation syndrome, 340
congestive heart failure, 341
remote monitoring, 343, 344
side effects, 342
technological advances, 337, 338
Continuous positive airway pressure (CPAP) therapy, 195

Continuous positive airway pressure (CPAP) trial
hospital admission, 90
lack of effectiveness, 86
failure to control OSA, 86
mild OSA, 86
non-classical OSA symptoms, 86, 87
persistent sleepiness, 87, 88
mixed obstructive and central sleep apnea, 89, 90
obstructive sleep apnea
atrial fibrillation, 91
fibromyalgia, 91
insomnia, 92
periodic leg movements, 91
residual daytime sleepiness, 92
patterns of, 89
perception questionnaire, 294, 295
poor adherence, 84, 85
psychosocial aspects, 365, 366
reasons for failure, 85, 86
sanitizers, 353
side effects, 368
spousal support, 366, 367
suboptimal compliance vs. lack of effectiveness, 84
technical factors, 85
threshold for, 83, 84
treatment coordinator's role
medical suppliers and equipment manufacturers, 357, 358
ongoing therapy compliance monitoring, 359–361
stages of grief, 355, 356
therapy expectation and troubleshooting, 358, 359
treatment options and accessibility, 356, 357
Continuous positive airway pressure therapy (CPAP), 178
Coronary artery disease (CAD), 5, 180–182
Cost-effectiveness analysis, 136
COVID-19 pandemic, 68, 85, 333
CPAP-associated retrograde air escape via the nasolacrimal system (CRANS), 222
Craniosynostosis, 246
C-reactive protein (CRP), 178

D
Daytime sleepiness, 281
Demyelinating disease, 163, 164
Dental/oral appliances (OA), 285
Depression, 51, 64
Diabetic retinopathy (DR), 220, 221
Dialectical behavioral therapy (DBT), 119
Doctor–patient communication, 39
Dry eye syndrome, 222
Durable medical equipment (DME), 53, 96

E
Education and behavioral strategies, 65, 267
eHealth, 65
Endothelial function index (EFI), 232
Epilepsy, 155–157
Epworth sleepiness scale (ESS), 50, 289, 290, 292, 319, 320
Excessive daytime sleepiness (EDS), 4, 126, 158, 159, 204
adverse effects, 317
motor vehicle crash risk, 317
prevalence, 317
risk factors, 318
self-report questionnaires, 319, 320
subjective symptoms, 318
unmet need and objective, 318

Excessive sleepiness (EDS), 145, 146
Expiratory positive airway pressure (EPAP), 258

F
Familial aggregation, 168
Fatigue severity scale [FSS], 290–292
Fibromyalgia, 91
Floppy eyelid syndrome (FES), 223
Full face masks, 350, 351
Function residual capacity (FRC), 231
Functional outcomes of sleep questionnaire (FOSQ), 8

G
Gastroesophageal reflux disease (GERD), 7, 55
Glaucoma, 222

H
Headache, 162, 163
Health belief model (HBM), 51
Healthcare professionals (HCPs), 363, 364, 367, 368
Health literacy screening (HLS) questionnaire, 294
Heart failure (HF), 182, 183
Hospital anxiety and depression scale (HADS), 205
Hypertension (HTN), 6, 178, 179, 280
Hypnosis techniques, 263
Hypoglossal nerve stimulators, 285

I
Idiopathic intracranial hypertension (IIH), 220
IF SLEEPY questionnaire, 289
Imagery rehearsal therapy (IRT), 80
Immature defense mechanisms, 119
Index for non-adherence to positive airway pressure (I-NAP),
    53, 294
Information motivation strategy model, 40
Insomnia, 51, 75, 76
Inspiratory positive airway pressure (IPAP), 258, 337
Intraocular pressure (IOP), 222

K
Kaplan-Meir plot, 66
Karolinska sleepiness scale (KSS), 320

M
Maintenance of wakefulness test (MWT), 43, 321, 322
Major depressive disorder, 205
MATRx auto-titrating OA, 304
MatrX sleep study, 357
Maxillary hypoplasia, 240
Mental health problems, 79, 80
Mentalization-based therapy (MBT), 120
Mild cognitive impairment (MCI), 158
Mild neurocognitive disorder, 55
Motivation to use CPAP scale (MUC-S), 295, 296
Motivational enhancement therapy (MET), 65, 75, 367
Motivational interviewing, 45–47, 51, 55, 72, 73
Motor vehicle accidents (MVAs), 125, 127
Multiple sclerosis (MS), 163, 164
Multiple sleep latency test (MSLT), 44, 289, 321, 322
Myofunctional therapy, 242

N
Nasal masks, 259, 350
Nasal obstruction, 240
Nasal pillows, 259
Nasal resistance, 143
National adaptive trial for PTSD-related insomnia (NAP), 215
National institutes of health stroke scale (NIHSS) scores, 184
Neighborhood SES, 104
Neurocognitive function (NCF)
    alerting agents, 172
    cognitive changes, 172, 173
    comorbidity, 171, 172
    electroencephalogram(EEG)-epochs, 170, 171
    neuroimaging findings, 170
    nocturnal hypoxia, 172
    obstructive sleep apnea
        CPAP therapy, 169, 170
        daytime sleepiness, 167
        objective NCF, 168
        severity spectrum, 168, 169
        subjective cognitive complaints, 167, 168
    optimization, 173
    oropharyngeal exercises, 172
    pulmonary rehabilitation, 172
    sleep fragmentation, 172
Neurodegenerative disorder
    EDS, 158, 159
    Parkinson's disease, 158
    RBD, 158
Neurodevelopmental disorders (NDD), 157, 158
Neurologic deficits, 163
Neuromuscular disease (NMD)
    abnormalities, 159
    attended in-lab polysomnography, 159, 160
    BPAP therapy, 160
    Duchenne muscular dystrophy, 159
    mechanisms, 159
    sleep disordered breathing, 160–162
Nocturnal ventricular premature beats (VPBs), 180
Nonadherence, 14
Non-alcoholic fatty liver disease, 7
Non-arteritic anterior ischemic optic neuropathy (NAION), 219, 220
Nonrestorative sleep, 189

O
Obesity, 50, 331
    OSA, prevalence of, 227
Obesity hypoventilation syndrome, 340
    congestive heart failure, 341
Objective/subjective sleepiness, 50
Obstructive apnea hypopnea index (OAHI), 257
Obstructive sleep apnea (OSA), 14
    adherence, 332
    Canada, 379, 380
    and cardiovascular complications
        cardiac arrhythmia, 179, 180
        continuous positive airway pressure therapy, 178
        coronary artery disease, 180–182
        heart failure, 182, 183
        hypertension, 178, 179
        mechanism of, 177
        stroke, 183, 184
    China, 377, 378
    chronic headaches, 7
    CKD, 7
    clinical application, 209

clinical features of, 204
cognitive and psychological features, 203
cognitive issues, 5
CPAP, 227, 332
CPAP adherence
    depression, 208
    therapy, 207, 208
CPAP therapy, 207
C-reactive protein (CRP), 178
CVD
    atrial fibrillation, 6
    bradyarrhythmias, 6
    CAD, 5
    CHF, 6
    endothelial dysfunction, 5
    hypertension, 6
    prevalence, 5
    stroke, 6
    type 2 diabetes, 7
daytime sleepiness, 167
definition of, 203, 281
depression, 204, 205
direct and indirect economic impacts, 204
excessive daytime sleepiness, 4, 204
general depression questionnaires, 205
GERD, 7
India, 376, 377
inflammation, 5, 178
Iran
    future perspectives, 375
    government issues, 375
    health care system, 375
    PAP device-related factors, 375
    patients-related factors, 374, 375
    physician-related factors, 375
    prevalence, 374
major depressive disorder, 205
Middle East Asia, 378, 379
mood, 5
multiple interrelated mechanisms, 203
new-onset atrial fibrillation, 178
non-alcoholic fatty liver disease, 7
obesity, 227
objective NCF, 168
ophthalmic disease
    central serous chorioretinopathy, 221
    diabetic retinopathy, 220, 221
    dry eye syndrome, 222
    floppy eyelid syndrome, 223
    glaucoma, 222
    idiopathic intracranial hypertension, 220
    intraocular pressure, 222
    non-arteritic anterior ischemic optic neuropathy, 219, 220
    papilledema, 220
    postoperative considerations, 223
    retinal vein occlusion, 221
partners and family members, 109, 110
pathogenesis, 331
potential mechanisms, 206, 207
prevalence of, 203
PTSD
    positive pressure therapy, 214, 215
    prevalence, 214
pulmonary hypertension, 7
quality of life, 5
sequelae of, 203
Serbia, 377

severity of, 4, 7
severity spectrum, 168, 169
signs and symptoms, 347
sleep quality, 4
snoring/apnea, 4
subjective cognitive complaints, 167, 168
symptoms and consequences, 204, 331
treatment, 331, 332
    decision, 7
    options, 207
Obstructive sleep apnea syndrome (OSAS), 136
    pathophysiology
        arousal response, 241
        loss of volume of oropharynx, 240, 241
        nasal obstruction, 240
        reduced tone of oropharynx, 241
    positive airway pressure
        with craniofacial anomalies, 246
        with down syndrome, 247
        in infancy, 247
        obesity, 246
        residual, 245, 246
    treatment options, 241, 242
Obstructive sleep apnoea (OSA)
    benefits, 127, 128
    cost-effectiveness
        mild OSA, 132
        OAT, 132, 133
        socioeconomic impact, 129–132
        surgery, 132, 133
    definition, 136
    diagnosis, 128, 129
    direct costs, 135
    end-to-end assessment, 135
    indirect costs, 135
    non-adherence
        clinical costs, 134
        clinical factors, 133, 134
        prevalence, 133
        socioeconomic costs, 135
        socioeconomic factors, 134
    prevalence, 125
    socioeconomic burden
        geographic factors, 126, 127
        MVA, 127
        patient factors, 126
        work productivity, 127
        workplace accidents, 127
    treatment, 128, 129
    untreated OSA
        clinical burden, 125
        societal and economic burden, 126
    work-related barriers, 136
Open and blocked airways, 348
Ophthalmic disease
    with obstructive sleep apnea
        central serous chorioretinopathy, 221
        diabetic retinopathy, 220, 221
        dry eye syndrome, 222
        floppy eyelid syndrome, 223
        glaucoma, 222
        idiopathic intracranial hypertension, 220
        intraocular pressure, 222
        non-arteritic anterior ischemic optic neuropathy, 219, 220
        papilledema, 220
        postoperative considerations, 223
        retinal vein occlusion, 221

Oral appliance therapy (OAT), 132, 133, 302–304, 307–309
    approaches, 312
    vs. PAP therapy, 309–311
Oro-nasal mask, 259
Oxford sleep resistance (OSLER) test, 322
Oxygen desaturation index, 281
Oxygen nadir, 257
Oxygen saturation, 50

P
Papilledema, 220
Parent and patient engagement programmes (PEP), 263
Parkinson's disease (PD), 158
Patient health questionnaire (PHQ-9), 205
Patient monitoring
    acceptable adherence level, 284
    acceptable apnea-hypopnea index, 284
    adaptive servo ventilation, 284, 285
    anatomical challenges, 282
    automatic mode, 282
    bariatric surgery, 286
    chief complaint, 281
    co-morbid conditions, 282
    CPAP *vs.* bilevel PAP, 284
    dental or oral appliances, 285
    education, 283
    environmental factors, 283
    gender differences, 283
    obstructive sleep apnea, 281
    patient acceptance, 283
    psychological acceptance, 283
    SAVE trial, 281
    socioeconomic status, 283
    special population, 282
    STAR trial, 286
    surgical referal, 285, 286
    symptomatology, 282
Periodic leg movements (PLMs), 88
Persistence of fatigue/EDS, 163, 164
Personality disorders
    adherence, 120–123
    diagnosis, 118–120
    follow-up appointment, 117
    obstructive sleep apnea therapies, 120–122
    patterns of, 117
    prevalence, 117
Philips Respironics device, 344
Pickwickian syndrome, 203
Pierre-Robin sequence, 246
Positive airway pressure (PAP) therapy, 3, 4, 279, 280, 376
    adherence
        definition, 248
        factors, 249, 250
        interventions, 251, 252
        quantifying, 248, 249
    child management, 246
    in chidren
        acclimatization phase, 268–270
        behavioral interventions, 263
        definition, 259
        device, 259
        disease and mode of therapy, 262, 263
        expiration, 258
        family and social factors, 262
        functional interfaces, 270

        hypnosis techniques, 263
        indication and functionality, 258
        individual factors, 262
        initial phase, 268, 269
        initiation phase, 268
        inspiration, 258
        interfaces, 259, 261
        maintenance phase, 268, 270
        modes of ventilation, 258
        parent and patient engagement programmes, 263
        socioeconomic factors, 270
        specific PAP adherence factors, 264–267
    clinical practice, 95
    compliance
        auto-titrating technologies, 97
        claustrophobia, 97, 98
        CMS definition, 97
        cognitive therapy, 98
        ear, nose, and throat (ENT) specialists, 98
        matching patient and treatment, 96
        medical equipment provider, 96
        non-compliance, 97
        optimal interface, 95, 96
        patient education, 96
        patient feedback, 98, 99
        sedative-hypnotic use, 98
        smartphone-based technologies, 98
        social support, 98
        telephone follow-up, 96
    forms of, 247, 248
    mechanisms, 247
    OSAS
        with craniofacial anomalies, 246
        with down syndrome, 247
        in infancy, 247
        obesity, 246
        residual, 245, 246
    partners and family members
        daytime functioning, 110
        family involvement, 111, 114
        partner involvement, 112–114
        partners' sleep, 110
        spouse/living with partner, 110, 111
        untreated OSA, 109, 110
Positive airway pressure devices, 279
Positive pressure therapy, PTSD
    national adaptive trial for PTSD-related insomnia, 215
    prospective study, 214, 215
    retrospective chart reviews, 214
Post-traumatic stress disorder (PTSD), 51
    obstructive sleep apnea
        positive pressure therapy, 214, 215
        prevalence, 214
    prevalence of, 213
    sleep disturbances, 213
    treatment choices, 213
Potable PAP devices, 353
Pregnancy
    chemical/hormonal changes, 232
        chest and volume changes, 231, 232
        upper airway changes, 232
    CPAP interventions, 233
    outcomes
        endothelium insult, 232
        metabolic/inflammatory mechanism, 233
    sleep disorders, 231

Proangiogenic placental growth factor (PlGF), 232
Procedural memory, 43
Pseudocentrals, 159
Psychologist-behavioural sleep specialist
    behavioural sleep specialist, 71
    client-clinician communication
        annual medical visit, 72
        anxiety, 76–79
        collaborative relationship, 74
        insomnia, 75, 76
        ME therapy, 75
        mental health problems, 79, 80
        motivational interviewing, 72, 73
    cognitive behavioural therapy, 71
    evidence-based methods, 71
    interventions, 71
    motivational enhancement, 71
Psychomotor vigilance task (PVT), 322
Pulmonary hypertension, 7

Q

Quality adjusted life year (QALY), 64
Quality of life (QoL), 5, 8
Quality-adjusted life years (QALYs), 136

R

Relaxation strategies, 190
REM behavior disorder (RBD), 158
Remote health information technologies (RHIT), 56, 57
ResMed device, 343
Respiratory disturbance index (RDI), 232, 257
Retinal vein occlusion (RVO), 221
Rhinitis, 232

S

Schema focused therapy (SFT), 120
Self-determination theory (SDT), 52
Self-efficacy measure for sleep apnea (SEMSA), 293
Self-report questionnaires, 319, 320
Sensory processing disorders, 157
Sleep apnea, 39, 43
Sleep apnea cardiovascular endpoints trial (SAVE), 181
Sleep apnea quality of life instrument (SAQLI), 8
Sleep apnea severity index (SASI), 50
Sleep-disordered breathing (SDB), 183
    adherence, 95
    children with special health care needs
        craniofacial features, 255, 256
        impact of untreated OSA, 257
        muscle weakness, 256
        obesity, 256, 257
        PAP therapy, 257
        prevalence, 255, 256
        therapeutic interventions, 257
    clinical practice, 95
    compliance
        auto-titrating PAP technologies, 97
        claustrophobia, 97, 98
        cognitive therapy, 98
        ear, nose, and throat (ENT) specialists, 98
        matching patient and treatment, 96
        medical equipment provider, 96

        non-compliance, 97
        optimal interface, 95, 96
        PAP adherence, 97
        patient education, 96
        patient feedback, 98, 99
        sedative-hypnotic use, 98
        smartphone-based technologies, 98
        social support, 98
        telephone follow-up, 96
    guidelines, 95
    pregnancy, 231
Sleep efficiency, 191
Sleep health disparities, 103, 104
Sleep medicine fellowship training program, 375
Sleep medicine global distribution, 373–374
Sleep quality, 4
Sleep regulation, 190
Sleep restriction strategies, 191
Sleepiness, 55
Snoring solution, 352
Social-cognitive theory (SCT), 51
Social cognitive theory questionnaire, 294
Social learning theory (SLT), 51
Socio-economic differences
    evidence, 104
    factors, 104, 105
Socio-economic status (SES), 39, 49, 51, 65
    evidence, 104
    factors, 104, 105
Socioeconomic system (SES), 53
SoClean vs. Lumin, 352
Soft/non-mechanical methods
    adherence and acceptance, 49, 50
    adherence measurement, 53
    in children and adolescents, 55, 56
    delivery of service, 54
    demographic variables, 49, 50
    educational, supportive, and behavioral interventions,
        54–56
    hypnotic use, 54
    inconsistent self-reported pretreatment bedtime, 51
    insomnia, 51
    lack of awareness/training, 53
    major mental illness, 50, 51
    non-supine sleep, 51
    OSA disease factors, 50
    patient-related factors, 49
    personalized medicine approach, 57
    physical side effects, 49
    psychological variables, 51–54
    RHIT, 56, 57
    self-report questionnaires, 53
    short sleep duration, 51
    sleep latency, 51
    sleeping locations, 51
    spousal and partner support, 52, 53
Spielman 3-P model, 190
Spontaneous timed (ST) mode, 4
Stanford sleepiness scale (SSS), 319, 320
Stimulation therapy for apnea reduction (STAR) trial, 286
Stimulus control strategies, 190
STOP BANG questionnaire, 289
Stressful life event, 143
Stroke, 6, 162–164, 183, 184
Sundowning, 159

T

Telehealth, 57
  COVID-19 pandemic, 333
  CPAP compliance, 333
  definition, 333
  programs, 334
Telemonitoring, 65, 67, 68
Toronto hospital alertness test (THAT), 292–293
Tracheostomy, 242
Transference-focused psychotherapy (TFP), 119
Transtheoretical model (TTM), 51
Transtheoretical model of change, 40
Type 2 diabetes, 7
Typical development (TD), 255

U

Upper airway resistance syndrome (UARS), 241

V

Vacuum-cleaner blower motor based device, 279

W

Wake promoting drugs, CPAP therapy

evaluation
  differential diagnosis, 321
  EEG-based objective assessments, 323
  objective assessments, 319, 321–323
  optimization, 320
  self-report assessment, 322
  subjective symptoms, 322
excessive daytime sleepiness
  adverse effects, 317
  motor vehicle crash risk, 317
  prevalence, 317
  risk factors, 318
  self-report questionnaires, 319, 320
  subjective symptoms, 318
  unmet need and objective, 318
risk factors, 318
treatment, 323–324
  agent's efficacy and safety profile, cost, and patient
    characteristics, 326
  armodafinil, 325, 326
  follow-up, 326
  modafinil, 325, 326
  pitolisant, 325–327
  sleep specialist, referral to, 327
  solriamfetol, 325, 326
  stimulants, 326